Disease and Democracy

Disease and Democracy

The Industrialized World Faces AIDS

PETER BALDWIN

University of California Press

BERKELEY   LOS ANGELES   LONDON

Milbank Memorial Fund

NEW YORK

The Milbank Memorial Fund is an endowed operating foundation that engages in nonpartisan analysis, study, research, and communication on significant issues in health policy. In the Fund's own publications, in reports or books it publishes with other organizations, and in articles it commissions for publication by other organizations, the Fund endeavors to maintain the highest standards for accuracy and fairness. Statements by individual authors, however, do not necessarily reflect opinions or factual determinations of the Fund.

University of California Press
Berkeley and Los Angeles, California

University of California Press, Ltd.
London, England

Library of Congress Cataloging-in-Publication Data

Baldwin, Peter.
    Disease and democracy : the industrialized world faces AIDS / Peter Baldwin.
        p.   cm. —   (California/Milbank books on health and the public ; 13)
    Includes bibliographical references and index.
    ISBN 0–520–24350–1 (cloth : alk. paper)
    1. AIDS (Disease)—Developed countries.
    [DNLM: 1. Acquired Immunodeficiency Syndrome—prevention & control.   2. Public Health Practice.   3. Democracy.   4. Developed Countries.   5. Disease Outbreaks—history.   WC 503.6 B182d 2005]
I. Title.   II. Series.

RA643.8B35 2004   2005
362.196'9792'0091722—dc22   2004008793

Manufactured in the United States of America
13   12   11   10   09   08   07   06   05
10   9   8   7   6   5   4   3   2   1

The paper used in this publication meets the minimum requirements of ANSI/NISO Z39.48–1992 (R 1997) (Permanence of Paper).

For
John W. Baldwin
and
Jenny Jochens,
parents and colleagues

Contents

Foreword

The Milbank Memorial Fund is an endowed operating foundation that engages in nonpartisan analysis, study, research, and communication on significant issues in health policy. Since 1905 the Fund has worked to improve and maintain health by encouraging persons who make and implement health policy to use the best available evidence. The Fund makes available the results of its work in meetings with decision makers and publishes reports, books, and the *Milbank Quarterly*, a multidisciplinary journal of population health and health policy.

This is the thirteenth of the California/Milbank Books on Health and the Public. The publishing partnership between the Fund and the press seeks to encourage the synthesis and communication of findings from research that could contribute to more effective health policy.

Peter Baldwin is an internationally admired historian of health and social policy who has a great deal to contribute to policy making for the global epidemic of AIDS/HIV. In this book Baldwin emphasizes differences in how the industrialized countries of Europe and North America responded to the epidemic. He traces these differences to the policies for prevention and treatment that countries adopted to address epidemics of contagious disease in the nineteenth century.

Baldwin's analysis and conclusions are relevant for policy makers, and the people they serve, in every country. He offers considerable evidence that a comparative approach enhances understanding of why countries choose particular policies, but he also recognizes that the AIDS/HIV epidemic and the recent outbreaks of SARS offer compelling evidence that what he calls "mutual dependence" and "self-protection" have become global as well as national issues.

Daniel M. Fox, President

Samuel L. Milbank, Chairman

Acknowledgments

As always, comparative studies leave the scholar in a state of pleasantly genteel bankruptcy, hopelessly indebted to others who have helped along the way.

Grants from the National Institutes of Health and the Robert Wood Johnson Foundation allowed leave time to pursue research and writing, as did other funding from the National Science Foundation; the Deutscher Akademischer Austausch Dienst; and, at the University of California, Los Angeles, the Academic Senate, the Center for American Politics and Public Policy and what was then the International Study and Overseas Program.

The Parliamentary Library in Copenhagen once again allowed me the run of their well-organized holdings of European parliamentary papers. Research assistants who have dug up obscure references and otherwise smoothed my path include Sumithra Rajashekara, Sung Choi, Amy Sueyoshi, Chelsea Neel, Howard Padwa, and Harald Braun. Anne Hoy gave the manuscript a thorough and much-needed working over.

My colleagues in the History Department at UCLA have given me a wonderfully lively and encouraging intellectual home. I thank especially six successive Chairs for being patient, understanding, and flexible far beyond the call of duty: Peter Reill, Scott Waugh, Ronald Mellor, Richard von Glahn, Brenda Stevenson, and Teofilo Ruiz.

My wife, Lisbet Rausing, took time to bring to the manuscript both scholarly and editorial talents—besides being my utter joy.

The dedication of this book to my parents reflects a debt, accumulated over a lifetime, that can never fully be repaid.

Abbreviations

ADA	Americans with Disabilities Act
BT	Bundestag
CARE Act	Ryan White Comprehensive AIDS Resources Emergency Act
CDC	Centers for Disease Control and Prevention
IDHL	*International Digest of Health Legislation*
JAMA	*Journal of the American Medical Association*
MSM	men who have sex with men
RD Prot	*Riksdagens Protokoll*
SARS	sudden acute respiratory syndrome
SFS	*Svensk Författnings-Samling*
STD	sexually transmitted disease
VD	venereal disease
WHO	World Health Organization
WSW	women who have sex with women

Introduction

Slaves to the Past

This is a book about the influence of the past on the present. Its central arguments are three. First, faced with the acquired immunodeficiency syndrome (AIDS) epidemic, the developed nations adopted surprisingly different approaches to a public health problem that confronted them all with similar challenges. Second, some of these industrialized liberal democracies were markedly more interventionist than others, favoring the commonweal over the rights of infected and at-risk citizens. Which nations subordinated individual liberties to the collective good, and which instead employed voluntary and consensual tactics, was sometimes surprising. Restrictive polities were often otherwise concerned with civil liberties: the United States, for example, and Sweden. Others, including nations usually willing to allow the state to impose on its citizens, like France and Germany, adopted a much more laissez-faire attitude. The general political ideologies of developed nations certainly influenced their public health policies. But it was not obvious what the connection would be. Often, it was the reverse of what one might expect.

Third, the industrialized nations of Europe and North America took divergent approaches that broadly corresponded to the preventive tactics they had adopted during the nineteenth century when dealing with earlier epidemics of contagious disease: plague, cholera, yellow fever, smallpox, and syphilis. In each country, policy makers were convinced that they were now responding in ways dictated by the nature of the threat they faced. In fact, their actions bespoke the influence of past decisions. As this book shows, such divergences among the industrialized nations are due to precedence—a kind of deep historical public health memory.

The variety of preventive approaches was remarkable, too, when held up against most observers' implicit presumptions that these nations employed

1

broadly similar public health tactics. This common approach in democratic polities—so the argument goes—to a disease that was initially transmitted through often illicit and always intensely private behavior was not to impose harsh and therefore dysfunctional measures on groups that were frequently social outcasts even before becoming infected. Instead the emphasis was on education, counseling, behavioral change, and voluntary treatment. Though the welcome arrival of new and effective treatments during the 1990s meant a comeback for certain traditional public health techniques, especially reporting and contact tracing, the voluntarist, consensual strategy, this widely accepted narrative continued, had become common dogma. Unlike other contagious diseases, for which harsh public health interventions remained applicable, AIDS was supposedly treated in an exceptional manner.

Cholera victims used to be quarantined. Lepers were compulsorily institutionalized well into the twentieth century. Syphilitic prostitutes were once, and sometimes continue to be, locked up and forcibly treated. In many countries they were registered with the police and had to show up for periodic inspections. In sum, it was common to violate the civil rights of the ill to spare the still healthy. By this standard, an exception was made for AIDS. Public health authorities believed that, in the late twentieth century, you could no longer order the ill to act in certain ways or restrict their liberties. Instead, educational campaigns sought to convince citizens to change their behavior voluntarily to make them less vulnerable to infection.

This book shows that, on the contrary, Western nations took widely different approaches to the common problem of the AIDS epidemic. Some countries sought a cure, hoping to avoid the tricky politics of imposing behavioral strictures on powerful high-risk groups or to sidestep drastic statutory impositions that were incompatible with other political traditions. In other countries the state was allowed a nearly free hand in limiting individuals' rights on behalf of overall epidemiological security. Some saw the threat as coming from without, and imposed controls at the borders. Others recognized frontier patrols as fruitless and staked their hopes on domestic interventions. Some shied away from making uniform recommendations about nontransmissive behavior to a multicultural population of variegated customs, habits, and morals. Others were confident that implicit national norms of conduct could be relied on to guide behavior. Even more interesting, which nations took which approach was rarely intuitively obvious. Countries commonly considered to be laissez-faire (the United States) and concerned with civil rights (Sweden) took the most old-fashioned and restrictive approach. Others with traditions of statutory initiative that were longer (France) and sometimes drastic (Germany) were markedly hands-off.

This book analyzes why nations took such different approaches to a largely common problem and why the strategies adopted were so surprisingly and counterintuitively different. It thus goes beyond AIDS as a public health issue to examine the basic political problem created by contagious disease and its prevention. Attempts to curtail epidemics raise—in the guise of public health—the most enduring political dilemma: how to reconcile the individual's claim to autonomy and liberty with the community's concern with safety. How does the polity treat the patient who is both citizen and disease carrier? How are individual rights and the public good pursued simultaneously? Public health thus allows a deeper plumbing of political instincts and attitudes than the surface foam of officially expressed ideology. Nations that claimed to be hands-off in fact intervened drastically. Others, from whom one might have expected firm interventions, shied away. What was a given polity willing to do to spare the still-healthy majority from the dangers threatened by an infected minority? How important was the relative balance of rights between those spared and those infected? Did political cultures focus on the lives saved by traditional public health interventions or on the liberties violated? What was most important, the rights of patients or of the uninfected?

This book accounts for the many different factors that explain these divergent choices in the industrialized world during the first phase of the epidemic, from the early 1980s to the turn of the millennium: the balance of political forces; the importance attached to privacy; the different approaches to sexuality; the commitment to personal liberty; the value placed on voluntarism; and the role of historical and political traditions, governmental and administrative structures, and interactions with existing legislation. Yet despite the undeniable influence of such factors, each nation tailored its AIDS strategy largely to its long domestic traditions of public health, as the book shows. Basic decisions on how to deal with contagious disease were taken during the nineteenth century, above all in response to the cholera epidemics that ravaged western Europe from 1832 on. Tactics adopted 150 years earlier created a template for the responses to AIDS. This book thus continues some of the arguments advanced in my work *Contagion and the State in Europe, 1830–1930* (Cambridge University Press, 1999) while bringing them into the current era and expanding them to include the United States as well as Europe.

For a historian to argue that the past matters is not surprising. That the past determines the present is not a claim, however, whose acceptance can be taken for granted. Economists, sociologists, and political scientists often do not believe that the past matters in such ways. For example, if humans are rational interest maximizers—as many neoclassical economists and some sociologists think—then past decisions have little influence on current choices.[1] Choice, and ultimately the ordering of society, is the outcome of a rational weighing of present costs and benefits.

Increasingly, however, even the harder social sciences have begun to allow the past a causal role in the present, by means of the concept of path dependence.[2] Path dependence theory argues that first (and therefore past) decisions are more important than later ones, in that they initiate a primary movement in a certain direction, narrowing future possible choices and increasing costs of subsequent changes. Because initial choices are crucial, subsequent decisions may respond not to later circumstances but to those at the very outset. It follows, too, that causes which, at the outset, may have been rational, with time become more arbitrary—though nonetheless remaining important for all that.

The classic example of path dependence is the QWERTY layout of most English-language typewriter keyboards.[3] Although the superiority of alternatives has been questioned, the claim is that QWERTY (which was worked out by trial and error to avoid type bar clashes on early machines) is not the best possible layout. Its eventual dominance reflected precedence—the snowball effect of first investments in a particular technology—rather than a reasoned choice or the ideal solution. Another example of path dependence, but here of policy rather than technology, is pay-as-you-go pension systems. Once started, they become almost impossible to change, since current contributors then must pay both for current retirees and for their own future, funded benefits.[4] Reformers seeking to change policies on a supposed tabula rasa, whether Germany after 1945 or eastern Europe after 1990, know only too well the continuing influence of dismantled institutions and long-lingering mentalities.[5]

This book shows how path dependence has structured public health even today. Decisions taken in the early nineteenth century to control cholera and syphilis continue to influence the response to AIDS. Public health officials and politicians commonly believed that AIDS must be treated differently than cholera or even syphilis. Yet in nations like Sweden and the United States, old mentalities and old ways of doing things remained markedly consistent. Next to path dependence, broad geoepidemiological factors that pushed nineteenth-century policy makers to adopt one set of tactics over another continue to influence us even today. This book thus focuses on the deepest and most perduring causal factors at work in what otherwise appear as the fleeting incidentalities of the present: it offers a neo-Braudellian emphasis on historical bedrock, as it were.

This is a book about public health. But it uses public health as a means of getting at broader questions of how political cultures and states differ across the industrialized world. It goes beyond official political ideology and its bromides, investigating instead what is actually done in a broad array of developed nations, and why. It argues that traditional political analysis of the response to the epidemic is inadequate. Left and right, conservative and liberal, are not labels that help explain why administrations and nations adopted their approaches to the epidemic. Such decisions were taken in accord with deeper, prepolitical policy structures already set in place during the previous century.

Much has been written on AIDS, but much of it is journalistic and of the first generation. Little of it is broadly synthetic, most is restricted to evidence from one nation or in one language, and almost none applies a longer historical perspective. Now that the epidemic has come under some semblance of control in the developed world, it is time to begin to understand it in its historical context. This is a work of comparative public policy history. Although it is contemporary history, it is still a historical book. It is thus not about how the epidemic will develop or how it is developing now. It deals with the recent past, from the first phases of the epidemic during the early 1980s to the end of the century. Because it is a work of history and thus based on dense empirical detail, it covers a select group of nations (the United States, Britain, France, Germany, and Sweden) most closely. On this basis—for historical work a very broad one—it seeks to draw wider conclusions about the response of the developed world in general.

This is a book about the developed, democratic world and not the Third World epidemic. It does not discuss this newer, and most horrifying, phase of AIDS as it unfolds among developing nations. And yet the conclusions drawn here are not without interest for the Third and Second Worlds. These nations are likely to address similar policy questions of how to deal with the epidemic. Many of the basic political dilemmas that the First World confronted when choosing its preventive strategies will reoccur elsewhere, especially among those nations that are democratizing as the epidemic ravages them. How to balance the interests of the healthy and the infected, how to treat minorities whose habits and practices differ from the mainstream, where and how to change behavior, even when contrary to instinct, proclivity, or custom: such issues affect all peoples and nations of the world.

It remains only to add that writing about the AIDS epidemic is an impossible task. As one of the most horrific events of the twentieth century—

an era with more than its share—and a foreshadowing of worse to come in the new millennium, it poses once again the oft-noted inadequacy of language, much less scholarly investigation, to do justice to the sufferings of its victims. The abstraction and distancing that are part of any attempt to contextualize and historicize an event, the tension between understanding and empathizing, are all but unavoidable. It goes without saying that the horror of being torn out of the cautiously optimistic and pacific last decades of the century by an unexpected microbiological attack, and even more the relentless suffering now added to those who do not yet enjoy the advantages of global prosperity, is more important than anything that can be written here. Yet it must be said.

1. Bodily Fluids and Citizenship

Whatever else you may think of him, General Jack D. Ripper, Doctor Strangelove's nemesis, had a point: democracy requires uncorrupted bodily fluids, whether precious or merely quotidian. Blood, sweat, and tears were, in Churchill's rhetoric, what stood between democracy and totalitarianism. Whether fluoride in the drinking water will help us flash our brightest or a nefarious conspiracy of health communists has set out to administer chemicals unbeknownst to the citizenry, ruining the branch water for our bourbon in the process, is a matter on which even those of goodwill can disagree. But bodily fluids are the sap of the body politic.

Our early modern ancestors learned to keep their fingers out of the soup bowl and their snot away from their neighbors. Our great-great-grandparents started covering their mouths when they coughed or sneezed. Their children were weaned off the habit of public expectoration and taught to breathe through their noses at about the same time that the practice of kissing children and acquaintances was discouraged, becoming instead an act reserved for erotic intimacy.[1] We, in turn, have come to fear intimate contact without the interposition of latex. In the absence of a human version of pasteurization, which renders bovine bodily fluids harmless and allows us to be gustatorially promiscuous with our four-legged compatriots, civilization rests on our ability to keep our bodily fluids apart. In the AIDS era, the discovery that nations dependent on plasma products collected in the United States were also at the mercy of America's epidemiology led to expressions of blood-based nationalism, calls for serological self-sufficiency, and a revival of explicit considerations of whose blood is the purest—subjects one might otherwise have thought no longer discussable.[2]

Bodily fluids are our individual essence. Bacteriology has replaced crude clinical symptoms—patient and physician collaborating in a diagnosis as

7

witness and interpreter—with impartial tests as the determination of our epidemiological status. Once genetic testing becomes commonplace, it will confront us starkly with the issue, revealing our genetic foibles and weaknesses even when we are in the rudest of health. Testing unveils our dirtiest secrets: that we are too drunk to drive, too infected to reproduce, too under the influence to work, too damaged to be actuarially underwritable. Our essences now belong to the public domain. As drivers or workers, we can be obliged to surrender them for screening.[3] Although Strangelove's cold war is over, we are still obsessed with bodily fluids and their purity. The mania for drug testing at work has led to a black market in drug-free urine and micturation under observation.[4] *Gattaca* is the movie for the AIDS era, as *Strangelove* was that for the cold war. Arlo Guthrie's cloyingly faux-innocent request for supplemental urine at his army induction in *Alice's Restaurant* now seems quaintly naive. The quality, not quantity, of your fluids is what counts today.

Bodily fluids are politically important, indicating our status as viable members of the community. Inebriated, infected, or influenced, we are less than fully capable and responsible citizens. In the case that concerns us here—public health—citizens stricken by contagious disease pose a threat, and the community must decide how to protect itself. Illness, in the best of circumstances a private misfortune, becomes public and political. How is the infectious patient to be treated? Much depends, of course, on the disease in question: whether transmissible via mere proximity, as with tuberculosis and smallpox, or whether limited to deliberate, usually voluntary and purposive contacts, like syphilis or AIDS. Requiring isolation and possibly treatment makes sense in the former case yet seems less persuasive in the latter. But how to deal with contagious disease is more than a technocratic public health matter. Basic political decisions are involved. How much deference does the community's interest deserve? How much protection the rights of the afflicted citizen? Where should the line run between the imperatives of the group and the liberty of the patient? It seems intuitively plausible that different political systems, varying ideologies and cultures, do not answer such questions uniformly. What is the same biological problem in each polity—infection with a particular microorganism—might be dealt with in quite different ways.

The AIDS epidemic in the developed world presented much the same challenge in each nation. True, the epidemic manifested itself differently in various countries, especially afflicting gays in some, drug injectors elsewhere, hemophiliacs in yet others, or heterosexuals across the board, as in the Third World. It was spread via blood donations in China, drug injections in the Mediterranean, homosexual sex in America, and heterosexual intercourse in Africa. Moreover, there were various strains of human immunodeficiency virus (HIV) whose differences had epidemiological repercussions. Some were more infectious and readily transmissible through heterosexual intercourse. Others were passed more via needle sharing, unprotected anal sex, and other forms of potential blood contact. Nonetheless, in broad terms, the problem was much the same for each polity of the industrialized world. When Cubans joked that their form of AIDS was invincible while the American variety was merely incurable, they highlighted the similarity of the threat.[5] And yet not every nation responded to this common challenge in the same way. Some pursued education and voluntary behavioral change as the best means of prevention. Others were willing to impose drastic limitations on the infected. Even more puzzling are the identities of the lenient and strict nations. The United States and Sweden, normally considered polities considerate of civil rights, have been among the most drastic public health interveners. France and Germany, countries with long statist traditions, have taken a markedly more laissez-faire approach. Why a common public health threat has been dealt with in such unpredictably various ways is the subject of this book. But before we return to that theme, some context is required.

DISEASE AS METAPHOR

Henry Sigerist, the distinguished historian of medicine, argued in 1928 that each society and era gets the epidemic that best fits its social circumstances—that, in a word, it deserves. The Middle Ages suffered the plague, a communal disease that struck indiscriminately. The individualistic Renaissance was tormented by syphilis, transmitted in discrete acts of will.[6] The idea is apparently irresistible that illness has moral intent and implication, whether in societies as a whole or in individuals. Just as VD strikes sinners in the member with which they err, consumption is the occupational hazard of genius, gout the result of gluttony, rabies the product of domesticated canines' sexual frustration, and cancer the outcome of bourgeois society's strictures on emotional release, so AIDS is seen as the outward manifestation of inner imbalance and disruption.[7] The temptation to interpret diseases and especially epidemics metaphorically and morally, as bearers of significance beyond the death, dismemberment, and disfigurement they wreak, was famously lamented by Susan Sontag. Sometimes a disease is just a disease.[8]

The battles fought in the nineteenth century over syphilis and prostitution were not just about public health. They were part of larger debates over
relations between the sexes and the changing role of women, over the de-
mise of traditional values and the hollowing out of patriarchal power.
Syphilis was seen as retribution—perhaps divine, perhaps natural—for the
collapse of sexual and social boundaries, which resulted from women's new
freedoms, the first stirrings of the gay movement, and other challenges to
the inherited order. Conservatives seized on syphilis as exemplifying the
ravages likely to befall the society that abandoned chastity and monogamy.
Radicals saw it as the outcome of bourgeois decadence and a product of
treating women as property.[9]

Similar fears lay behind disputes over AIDS. Did promiscuity (whether
hetero- or homosexual) undermine the family and society? How did drug
use and sexual unorthodoxy interrelate? The socially transgressive connections among blood, sex, premature death, gayness, and drugs occasioned
much facile metaphorizing of AIDS. The disease combined the metaphorical
punches of tuberculosis and cancer, being transmissible and laying bare a
fundamental internal rot. Like tuberculosis, it was romanticized, associated
with heightened artistic awareness and tragically early death. Society's reactions to the disease mirrored those to drugs, homosexuality, death, racial
minorities, and foreigners—most generally to that ubiquitous foil of contemporary thought, the "Other." Its rendering the immune system incapable of warding off otherwise harmless attacks portended larger social
problems, a disorientation of values, and a general inability to stave off dangers.[10] AIDS was emblematic of the mutual dissolution of everything: this
might be a summary, if indeed anything could be, of the position taken on it
by that sporadically brilliant mystifier Jean Baudrillard.[11]

Sex, blood, and death were not the whole of it. For AIDS conjured up
even more fundamental transgressions. It violated the species line, invoking
biblical admonitions against abomination of the most basic sort. The epidemiological connection between ape and human evoked the same horror at
cross-species pollination that smallpox vaccination had earlier. Edward Jenner's use of cowpox to combat smallpox had provoked violent reactions during the nineteenth century to this literal brutalization. In 1915, Hideyo
Noguchi's derivation of animal lymph from rabbit testicles to inject into babies for immunization sparked revulsion and resistance.[12] Syphilis too was
thought to arise from encounters between different orders of beings (sometimes the eating of iguanas or monkeys). Now, similar themes were evoked
again.[13] Africans, or Haitians, sodomizing, or at least eating, apes became an
image, both bestial and utterly racist.[14]

So cumbersome was its metaphorical baggage that AIDS was sometimes regarded less as a disease in a biological or epidemiological sense than as a social and symbolic phenomenon with medical consequences—or so argued those who themselves were still healthy.[15] AIDS was pronounced an epidemiological Rorschach test whose handling revealed the essence of our culture. In selecting preventive strategies against the epidemic, society was also revealing its core values. Individual rights, liberty, and democracy, on the one hand, or compulsion, exclusion, and force, on the other: thus ran the Manichaean choice offered by many observers.[16] The epidemic allowed the fronts of an ongoing Kulturkampf to define themselves anew in mutual opposition. Cultural conservatives, aghast at relaxed sexual mores and patterns of reproductive sociability other than the conventional family, lashed out at those who sought to fight the disease alone and not its supposed concomitants of promiscuity and decadence.[17] Conversely, those gays who were willing to combine self-pity with conspiracy theory gave AIDS, and especially the public responses to it, equally wild metaphorical readings: as an excuse to impose a totalitarian, biomedicalized, dystopian set of nuclear family values on the sexual polymorphosity of erotic reality, or a new form of sexual apartheid whose ultimate purpose, according to the cultural critic Simon Watney, was "to purge the entire planet of the regrettable existence of black Africans, injecting drug users, workers in the sex industry, the 'promiscuous,' and, above all gay men."[18]

SOIL, SEED, AND HOST:
BIOMEDICINE AND PUBLIC HEALTH

Over the long course of medical thought, three fundamental factors of disease etiology have coexisted in parallel, determining in different combinations how illness is understood: contagion, surroundings, and personal predisposition—or agent, environment, and host. Perhaps it would be more accurate to say two and a half factors. Since antiquity, medical thinkers have distinguished between the seed and the soil in which disease flourishes, the contagion and the environmental circumstances that hinder or encourage its dissemination. Personal predisposition and behavior have in turn tipped the scales in either direction, helping explain why not all those exposed to the cause of illness (microbe or environment) in fact succumb. In rough, but not lockstep, correlation, there have also been three basic approaches to prevention: quarantinism, sanitationism, and support for individual health.

Focusing on contagion meant seeing transmissible disease as arising

from an outside source, propagated among humans directly or through in-
termediaries. From this vantage, combating epidemics meant interrupting
chains of transmission, whether by isolating victims or by breaking the
cycle of disease through disinfection, barriers to trade and travel, vaccination, food inspection, and other means of arresting contagion's peregrination. Regarding disease as arising from unhealthy surroundings, in turn,
meant that humans' contact with each other was not the primary concern.
Instead, the noxious environment needed correction. This was to be
achieved through public works and collective actions, whether burning
pyres to scorch miasma out of the atmosphere during the Middle Ages or
laying in sewers during the nineteenth century; assuring minimum standards of space, ventilation, and light; separating residences from sources of
noxious production; and other means of sanitizing the urban environment.
Finally, the question of personal predisposition has been dealt with by encouraging healthy habits and unobjectionable conduct, enabling individuals
to resist both poisonous environments and predatory microbes.

The ideological and ethical valences of each of these positions have not
been historically fixed or stable. Contagionism once meant that those feared
as infectious, such as lepers or plague victims, were shunned and excluded.
But once the bacteriological revolution illuminated the mechanisms of
transmission, it also morally neutralized disease. It became clear that illness
often struck with Olympian impartiality, carrying away the virtuous and
virginal and sparing gluttons and drunkards. An ill-fated encounter with
malevolent microorganisms had little, if any, moral import. An environmental understanding of disease, in turn, was often socially reformist, concerned to provide all urban dwellers with the basic infrastructure of hygienic life and to improve their living conditions. But sanitationism also had
a technocratic, top-down aspect. At its most messianic, it demanded fundamental social change as a precondition for a healthy environment. Poverty
and health were mutually incompatible. If focused on filth rather than social
inequity, however, sanitationism could serve functionalist efforts to preserve the status quo. Then it provided workers with the minimum needed
for effective productivity, while shunning more fundamental change.[19] And,
of course, it assumed that urbanites had to live by the precepts of modern
hygiene. After the middle of the nineteenth century, for example, the poor
could no longer share their dwellings with pigs. If that is social control, then
socially controlled they were.

A focus on predisposing factors, in turn, could be socially reformist and
concerned with alleviating factors beyond the individual's control: the unhealthy diets and living conditions, say, of the poorest. Or, it could be hec-

toring and moralizing, blaming disease on victims for behaviors under their control: the gluttony of the gout sufferer, the overindulgence once thought to be a source of cholera, the sexual irregularity associated with gonorrhea and its spread, the emotional repression alleged to be the root of cancer. Even more ambiguous was what the individual was considered capable of controlling, or not. Social determinists argued that, ultimately, there is no purely personal and undetermined factor, that the personal is political and social: the stress and sleeplessness of the unemployed, the temptation to smoke and drink encouraged by advertising, the sexual and drug risk-taking of the ghetto dweller with few prospects for the future and no motive to delay gratification.

Though views of disease causation and how best to prevent or curtail epidemics have varied and different ones often been held at once simultaneously and inconsistently, some general patterns of historical development may be traced. During the Middle Ages, the plague was attacked primarily with the methods of quarantinism. Attempts to improve environmental circumstances were tried (burning pyres, enforcing market regulations on food, and the like), but nothing more ambitious. Cutting chains of transmission by means of quarantines and sequestrations, in contrast, was the most common approach. As part of the Enlightenment's attempt to better the condition of humanity, the idea was developed by medical men, like the Scots William Cullen and William Pulteney Alison, that poverty, poor diet, inadequate clothing and shelter, overwork, and putrid surroundings were among the causes of fevers. Misery caused illness.[20] The key to better public health was a better body politic. During the mid–nineteenth century, burgeoning democratic movements in Europe rallied to the idea that health and liberty were mutually dependent. Louis-René Villermé in France, Rudolf Virchow in Germany, Edwin Chadwick and Southwood Smith in Britain: all saw democracy and public health as connected and believed that, until life was improved for the poor, disease could not be prevented.[21] Such hopes of improving the urban environment were given practical expression especially in Britain during the mid-1800s, the heroic age of sanitary engineering. "Think of what our nation stands for," John Betjeman, the poet laureate, exhorted in verse, "Democracy and proper drains."

Toward the end of the nineteenth century, this socially reforming approach to public health faded in all nations. It was partly a victim of its own success. With the construction of the necessary infrastructure, both legislative and concrete—plumbing, sewers, zoning and building codes—the ambitions of the movement's heroic phase were gradually realized. But equally important, science undercut the sanitationist approach. The bacteriological revolution, starting in the 1880s with the work of Louis Pasteur and Robert Koch, changed both the understanding of disease and how it was prevented. Biomedicine's new leading idea of "one disease, one cause, one cure" implied that the best method of prevention was to avoid contact with the pertinent microorganism. If disease was not caused by unfortunate environmental circumstances, but by microorganisms and their dissemination, then the point was no longer to remove filth or improve the physical circumstances of all citizens but, at best, to ameliorate the immediate surroundings of those who were ill or, at the least, to ensure that the contagious spread no germs.

Rather than taking aim at every distasteful metropolitan odor, or crudely equating dirt and disease, the new, bacteriologically informed public health official could now target those who were carriers, isolating a few people rather than cleaning up entire environments.[22] Why improve the living conditions of one hundred million Americans, argued enthusiastic proponents of the new bacteriologically inspired public health in the United States, when all you had to do was to confine the infective discharges of two hundred thousand active tuberculosis cases?[23] Germ theory and bacteriology narrowed the scope of public health, substituting general environmental sanitation, or improvements in living conditions, with a focus on the transmission of microorganisms.[24] During the yellow fever epidemic in Memphis in 1878, when this was still primarily considered a disease caused by filth, the city had been cleansed and a model sewer system constructed. Ten years later, the epidemic hit Jacksonville. With the disease now increasingly viewed as transmissible and caused by some as yet unidentified germ, the response was a massive disinfection campaign aimed at neutralizing the germ, not at filth in general. The impetus for urban sanitary reform had weakened.[25]

In a larger sense, the habits required by the new knowledge of microorganisms meant that individual hygiene of a scientifically informed sort now played an important role. The onus of precaution shifted to the newly well-to-do and educated citizens of emerging democracies. Appropriate habits became part of the conduct of good burghers. Citizens could take responsibility for their actions; indeed, the democratic ethos required them to do so.[26] Controls shifted from the outward impositions of a predemocratic state to the internal restrictions each put on his or her own behavior.[27]

As part of this new approach, citizens were encouraged to adopt habits to ensure their health. The lessons of the laboratory, the ability of unseeable microorganisms to spread disease, were translated into strict codes of personal hygiene and conduct that meant minimizing physical contact, avoiding common objects, ending the indiscriminate discharge of bodily fluids, trimming men's beards, shortening women's hemlines, and making untold other behavioral changes that we now regard as second nature. Bacteriology thus partly individualized public health. The older miasmatic or environmentalist approach to disease had of necessity required a collective response. When the plague struck during the Middle Ages, it was seen not as an attack on the individual but as a collective affront, hitting the city or the region.[28] Bacteriology helped shift matters away from such public concerns, but only because it could assume a vast, existing infrastructure of communal benefit: salubrious housing, potable water, efficient waste removal, and the like, all accomplishments of the sanitationist phase of public hygiene during the nineteenth century. With such benefits in place, private behavior at the margins now made the difference between catching disease or not. On the basis of a vast collective effort, in other words, public health shifted in an individualized and privatized direction. Though infant mortality was highest in slum neighborhoods, public health authorities now focused their attention not on widespread social reform but on the personal—on health education, promotion of breast-feeding, higher standards of domestic hygiene, and the like.[29]

Mass persuasion and education became the preferred techniques of public health, replacing the coercion that lay implicit as a last resort in old-fashioned measures. As subjects became citizens, they were expected to take their own affairs in hand, no longer at the behest of the authorities. Hygienic behavior belonged to the self-control that was assumed of members of the democratic body politic. Public health concentrated increasingly on the personal behavior and habits that transmitted disease: spitting, coughing, having sex with the wrong people, and generally engaging in what the archbacteriologist Charles Chapin charmingly called the "universal trade in human saliva."[30] Sneezing and suffrage were linked. The person who failed to cover his mouth when coughing, who expectorated in public, could not distinguish the functions of his water closet from his sink, or exposed his smallpox-stricken children in public was unlikely to be entrusted with the right to govern himself.

The French Revolution had made it a requirement of membership in the polity that citizens conduct themselves so as to remain healthy. While the state was now recognized as having a duty to foster the well-being of its members, they in turn had obligations in not acting to destroy the common property that was their weal.[31] Begun in the spirit of the Enlightenment, such trends continued during the interwar years as liberal democracy declined. All industrialized nations fell prey to the collectivist engineering of eugenics. Right-wing and fascist regimes of the period were not alone in pursuing such goals. Sweden and the United States practiced sterilization widely, and the left turned to eugenics with much the same enthusiasm as the right.[32] In the hyperpopulism of the totalitarian regimes, such matters were carried to their extreme, exemplified by the Nazi slogan "Your health does not belong to you."[33]

As the victories of the sanitary revolution were registered, an epidemiological shift in the nature of the most significant diseases followed. The growing prevalence of chronic disease in the mid– to late twentieth century added weight to the new emphasis on personal responsibility. Many of the problems that now caused the highest mortality—obesity, cardiovascular disease, some cancers—were in part the outcome of poor diet, smoking, and lack of exercise, and public health turned to changing such unsalutary conduct.[34] Individual behavior became paramount to health, and lifestyle issues gained prominence. With chronic disease, promotion of health rather than prevention of illness became the focal point.[35] Individual behavior was the concern: overeating, overworking, overdrinking, underexercising, overcopulating. The law was invoked to discourage risky behavior: mandating seat belts and motorcycle helmets, requiring (primarily of prostitutes) condom use, outlawing certain drugs and testing to ensure compliance, clamping down on smoking, and raising the legal age of drinking. Democracies could not, however, mandate their citizens' behavior except at the margin. Healthy lifestyles, insofar as they involved abstinence from pleasurable behaviors, could not be legislated. For citizens to live lives of moderation and good health, they would have to be convinced of their innate virtue and pursue them voluntarily. The lifestyles of contemporary democracies had to be shaped via persuasion and consent—through promoting the merits of diets low in fat, of little alcohol and less nicotine, sufficient exercise, the liberal use of sunscreen, sexual parsimony, and so forth.

Modern, democratic public health rested on the belief that individuals should be responsible for their own well-being. And yet, though control had been internalized, voluntarily adopted by citizens rather than imposed on subjects, it remained as strong as ever. Indeed, the behavioral precepts of modern life were arguably stricter than before.[36] The new individualized approach, with its emphasis on wholesome habits, has been caricatured as the reign of the monogamous jogger or, most extremely, dismissed as "health fascism."[37] Such an individualized strategy, it is argued, ignores how any given choice springs from broader social forces: the adolescent is encouraged by glamorous advertising to smoke, the wife hesitates to ask her husband to use a condom in fear of his wrath at the implication of unfaithfulness, those at the bottom of the social totem pole may not postpone or avoid the immediate gratifications available—fatty food, smoking, drugs, or sex.[38] Few, alas, have been willing to come straight out and say that bad habits are mostly fun and that it should be one of medicine's tasks to allow us as many years of indulgence as possible. Few have mentioned that, actuarially, some bad habits are in fact cost-effective. The drunk dies younger than the teetotaler, saving the pension and health insurance systems the price of octogenarians.[39]

The field of public health declined from its heyday during the mid–nineteenth century, when its ambition was to reorder society as a whole. Bacteriology narrowed its focus, and the triumphs of biomedicine during the mid–twentieth century meant that other medical specialties grew dominant. Public health, a victim of its own success, was increasingly relegated to the suburbs of professional prestige.[40] The study of the social and behavioral context of disease was shunted aside. Of the three factors classically the focus of epidemiology—agent, host, and environment—the emphasis now shifted to the first and away from the latter two. And yet, though battered, the old environmentalist approach was far from defeated.

Its roots lay in the nineteenth century. The French workers' movement claimed that Koch's bacillus was irrelevant as a cause of tuberculosis in comparison to the misery of working-class life under capitalism. Starting with the First World War, health disparities between blacks and whites in the United States became increasingly recognized—both prompting an environmentalist approach and perpetuating racial categorizations.[41] Investigations of beriberi and pellagra offered classic vindications of environmentalism early on.[42] While the medical world, dazzled by the explanatory power of bacteriology, searched for the responsible microorganism, simple nutritional deficiencies proved to be the cause.[43] During the interwar years, the idea of what we can call (broadly speaking, to avoid fruitless terminological wrangles) "social medicine" continued the environmentalist tradition. In most European countries, including the Soviet Union in its first flush of revolution, social medicine advanced the idea that health could be understood and promoted only in its societal context.

Later in the twentieth century, social medicine focused on environmental pollutants, psychosocial factors such as the stress of unemployment, the risks inherent in modern technology and urban environments, climate change, health differentials among classes, and other broadly contextual aspects of morbidity.[44] Next to the detrimental results of poverty and squalid

social circumstance, the psychosocial effects of hierarchy and class stratification became an issue—factors, in other words, that were built into the very
framework of market societies.[45] Clinical ecology, or environmental medicine, expanded this approach. Starting with the nutritional causes of allergies, its purview broadened after the Second World War to include radiation,
agricultural chemicals, and the potential ill effects of industrial civilization
generally.[46] Modern social medicine grew preoccupied with the avoidance of
dangers imposed on unwitting citizens by technology—nuclear power, genetic engineering, climate alteration, and the like. Why worry about trivial
individual risks when threatened by major and potentially catastrophic
ones?[47] Don't bother adding roughage to your diet, so the logic went, when
you share a postal code with Chernobyl. Modern social medicine believed,
often as eschatologically as its predecessors, that illness could not be conquered without fundamental social change. It discounted mere technical
fixes—biomedical tinkering, cures, vaccinations—so long as the unhealthy
social circumstances that allegedly caused, or at least promoted, illness remained in place.[48]

Social reform appeared to be the key to health. As though to compensate
for their lowered prestige in the biomedical era, public health professionals
often sought to expand their bailiwick from health to wholesale social reform. Public health, one textbook earnestly insisted, "must really be regarded as an ethical enterprise, an agent of social change, not just for the
sake of change, but to make possible the achievement of the improved lot of
mankind."[49] In 1946, the preamble to the constitution of the World Health
Organization defined health as "a state of complete physical, mental and social well-being, and not merely the absence of disease or infirmity." Health
was utopia. As the Ottawa Charter for Health Promotion put it forty years
later, "The fundamental conditions and resources for health are peace, shelter, education, food, income, a stable eco-system, sustainable resources, social justice and equity."[50] To achieve this state of perfection, mere public
health work was insufficient; political action would achieve plenitude, empowerment, autonomy, and sociability. The aim was not just a subjective
sense of well-being (biomedicine's ambition) since, inducible by drugs, this
could be delusionary, but also a broader concept of an objective standard of
the good life.[51]

Modern social medicine and its adherents argued that quarantinist disease prevention was outmoded in the era of chronic, noninfectious diseases,
and that illness could not be understood except in its social context. Biomedicine, in turn, pointed both to its obvious triumphs and to the continued
vigor of classic ailments (cholera in developing nations and tuberculosis in

the inner cities of the First World) that still required traditional quarantinist attempts to break chains of transmission.

This clash of worldviews can be summed up in two examples. Multiple chemical sensitivity, the alleged hyperallergy to even minute traces of chemicals in the environment, is scarcely recognized as an illness by orthodox biomedicine. Yet its victim advocates regard it as the outcome of a generalized toxicity of our surroundings caused by modern technology. As part of an updated miasmatic theory, it is seen as treatable not through biomedical tinkering but by radical environmental cleanup and social reforms.[52] Conversely, peptic ulcers have provided the biomedical camp with the poster illness that pellagra was for the social medicine faithful. Once (and in the popular mind still) thought to be the result of stress and the dysfunctional aspects of modern, overcaffeinated life, ulcers are now known to result from a particular microorganism, treatable by antibiotics. In the choice between specific biomedical intervention and broad social reform, such diseases emblematize the opposing morals of this medical Kulturkampf.

POLITICS BY OTHER MEANS

Public health, we may agree, mangling Clausewitz, is a continuation of politics by other means. What tactics to fight transmissible disease were acceptable? Which incursions were overly draconian? These have been political issues. Politics determined whether one should combat cholera by breaking chains of transmission, quarantining the infected, disinfecting goods, and shutting down trade and travel, or whether one should seek to improve the filthy urban environment that at least encouraged, if it did not actually cause, disease. Should all citizens be inoculated and, later, vaccinated against smallpox? Should syphilis be prevented by regulating and inspecting prostitutes, providing in the process an epidemiologically unobjectionable class of public women? Or should one impose similar strictures on all citizens, male or female, who indulged in irregular sex? Should one seek to combat sin by targeting the error itself, advocating abstinence and monogamy, and punishing fornication? Or should the state abstain from controlling its citizens' sexual transactions—seeing them as perhaps misjudged but ultimately private and voluntary? All these choices were fraught with political valuations and judgments.

It has been plausibly argued that drastic curtailments of individual rights were more likely to be pursued by autocratic or at least conservative regimes.[53] The most extreme political definition of public health came from the Nazis. They assimilated bacteriology to anti-Semitism, portraying Jews as like microorganisms, to be exterminated for the public good. They walled off the Warsaw ghetto under the pretext of typhus quarantine and took this fiction to its grotesque extreme in the fake delousing showers of the death camps.[54] From the other end of the totalitarian spectrum, Lenin worried about the petty bourgeois bacillus.[55] Conversely, sanitationists, who hoped to maintain public health by improving the living conditions of the poor without requiring punitive impositions, have been seen as typically liberal or left of center.

Nonetheless, the left has also subordinated individual rights to the community's interests. Requiring smallpox vaccination, for example, was an incursion into the body politic required of individuals for the benefit of all. Liberals and conservatives alike supported or rejected this. The alternative—barring a fatalistic acceptance of pustulous epidemics—threatened to violate rights even more: isolating all who had been exposed. It is, consequently, hard to identify consistent political correlations with preventive stances on this issue. Similar ambiguities also held true for syphilis in the late nineteenth century. The incipient women's movement and its allies on the left rejected the regulationist system for singling out women who sold sex and leaving their male clients largely untroubled. Conservatives saw such precautions as necessary to spare society the ravages of disease. While the political inflections of this divide were clear, those of the alternatives were not. The left in Britain sought to repeal regulationism. On the Continent, in contrast, the same camp concluded that the problem was too urgent to be ignored. Equity demanded not the abolition of regulation but its de facto extension to the entire sexually active population, male or female, prostitute or paterfamilias.[56] Though preventive tactics have had obvious political implications, it is not always possible to predict precisely which.

Into this broad and unstable field of political and prophylactic tension, AIDS erupted. The epidemic was fraught by the enduring dilemma of public health, whether to see transmissible disease primarily as the result of a contagion, whose pathways were to be obstructed, or as that of noxious environments, which should be improved. From the vantage of biomedicine, once the retrovirus eventually named HIV was discovered, the cause had been established. The goal then was to cure AIDS and to ensure that it did not spread. From the vantage of social medicine, however, things were not so simple. It approached the disease in its social and environmental context.[57]

Most extremely, some observers denied that HIV was, in fact, the root of the disease. One of the epidemic's most peculiar aspects was how strongly biomedicine's authority was challenged—not just by quacks (both well intentioned and predatory) and by those desperate for hope but also from within its own, and sometimes highest, ranks. Partly, this was due to biomedicine's inability to find an effective cure, however rapid the growth of its understanding of the disease. Partly, it was the result of the unparalleled mobilization of victims—the health care populism of the AIDS era—which spawned heterodox opinion.

The idea that AIDS was not caused by a single microorganism and that a purely biomedical approach was insufficient remained remarkably persistent, spawning a school of so-called AIDS dissidents, or denialists.[58] Rejected by the biomedical establishment, they received a hearing far beyond unorthodox opinion on other ailments, enlisting the full spectrum of cultural producers, from Nobel Prize–winners (Kary Mullis) to rock bands (Foo Fighters).[59] In March 2000, the South African president, Thabo Mbeki, an economist with a degree from the University of Sussex, a penchant for micromanagement, and a habit of trawling the Web for information on his own, sought advice from such dissenters. He appointed Peter Duesberg, a Berkeley cell biologist who denied that HIV causes AIDS, to the same government panel as Luc Montagnier, codiscoverer of HIV, at the same time that his government decided to stop providing AZT (zidovudine, one of the first effective anti-HIV drugs) to expectant mothers in public hospitals.[60] In July of that year, at the thirteenth annual AIDS conference in Durban, more than five thousand scientists felt called on to publish a declaration affirming HIV as the cause of AIDS, an issue that most people had assumed was settled.[61]

AIDS denialists argued either that HIV was not the cause of AIDS or—more moderately—that, though perhaps it was implicated, other factors were equally required to explain why clinical cases arose. They continued an environmentalist approach to disease, questioning or minimizing the role of HIV as the (single) cause of AIDS and focusing instead on the effects of poor nutrition, bad sanitation, "environmental insults," compromised immune systems, poor access to medical care, and other alleged cofactors. In sum, they applied a social analysis to what virologists insisted was purely, or at least largely, a microbiological problem.[62] In attempting to counter this unusually persistent argument, biomedical orthodoxy, as formulated in the Durban Declaration, acknowledged that, while poverty, malnourishment, age, other diseases, and similar cofactors might leave some more susceptible than others, ultimately, "HIV is the enemy."[63] Many of the AIDS dissidents, in contrast, saw the epidemic as "an aspect of worldwide ecological crisis and as part of a complex of immune-related illnesses caused by malnutrition, man-made toxins and pollutants, abuse of psychoactive and medicinal drugs, multiple sexually transmitted diseases, and other by-products of urban civilization." The antidotes were "sound nutrition and various alternative therapies."[64] These dissidents suggested replacing the "infection model" of AIDS with a "pollution model" that saw it as a multiplicity of diseases generated by the stresses of modern life, social conditions, and medical practices.[65]

At their most vehement, AIDS dissidents followed Peter Duesberg. He claimed that AIDS, far from being the outcome of HIV, was the result, in the industrialized world, of drug use, including AZT, and, in Africa, of poor environmental conditions, malnutrition, and parasitic infections. The conceptual dominance of germ theory had misled science to believe that HIV was both the necessary and sufficient cause of AIDS.[66] Others, including the Nobel laureate Kary Mullis, and the Group for the Scientific Reappraisal of the HIV/AIDS Hypothesis, were unwilling to follow him this far, remaining content with an emphasis on the cofactors that were allegedly also necessary to explain the disease.[67] This approach received a much needed infusion of scientific prestige when Montagnier concluded that his virus perhaps required a cofactor, a mycoplasma, to become virulent.[68] But the position was weakened as protease and entry inhibitors, along with other treatments, enjoyed their successes starting in the mid-1990s. The continued vitality of an environmentalist approach had little to do with its scientific validity. Rather, it stemmed from deeper currents of thought and feeling, a rejection of science and orthodox medicine that sprang from a long-standing belief in disease as a sign of imbalance between humans and nature, a cosmic and moral indication that things were out of joint.

At their more moderate, such dissidents insisted on an insight that would be disputed by few: that HIV was a necessary, but perhaps not invariably a sufficient, cause of the AIDS epidemic. A social analysis of the epidemic was essential.[69] Peculiar etiological ecologies arising from new moral, sexual, demographic, and medical circumstances in the late twentieth century allowed it to spread. Ecological pressures on untouched areas brought human and animal carrier into contact. The new mobility of peoples enabled microorganisms to hitchhike globally at astonishing speed. Medical technology using large quantities of blood products, trans-species transplants, and drug use by injection—all made human bloodstreams promiscuous. The customs of certain social groups, whether First World gays and drug users or African men of the social elite, favored the rapid spread of sexually transmitted disease—as did changes in sexual mores, both the private promiscuity of relations and the flourishing sex trade. The *disease*, in other words, would obviously not have existed without the necessary cause of HIV, but the *epidemic* was made possible by social factors.[70]

The battle between social medicine and biomedicine was joined once again. Even those perfectly willing to accept HIV as the necessary cause of AIDS pointed to the epidemic's social inflections, arguing that a fixation on the retrovirus alone and the hope of preventing its transmission were insufficient. A disease for which there was, as yet, no biomedical solution left prevention by default as the truest arrow in medicine's quiver.[71] Having long stood in second place behind biomedicine, as cure and treatment took precedence over prevention, public health found itself back at center stage.[72] The environment of the afflicted and the societal determinants of their conduct came back into view. The heroic tradition of public health gained a new lease on life. A sick society could not rid itself of disease. Regarding prevention as something more than a narrowly medical exercise in avoidance and treatment, a revived social medicine understood the *salus populi* in terms of broad social reform.

Discrimination, marginalization, stigmatization: all heightened vulnerability to HIV, it was now argued. The best-demonstrated cofactors were social inequalities.[73] Without basic social change, so it was implied, the epidemic would rage on. One account earnestly claimed that, to prevent sexual transmission of HIV, universal peace had to be attained to end machismo and its attendant rape; global wealth had to be redistributed to make condoms available and obviate the need for prostitution; and religious leaders needed to support nonpenetrative and therefore nonprocreative sex.[74] With a logic that would have warmed the heart of Villermé or Virchow, President Mbeki asked why the South African government should administer powerful and expensive drugs like AZT while ignoring "the underlying poverty." At his opening address to the Durban AIDS conference, he again presented poverty as Africa's main problem, implicitly de-emphasizing HIV as the primary concern.[75]

Even more messianically, Jonathan Mann, the former head of the World Health Organization's AIDS program, called in 1994 for a wholly new approach to the epidemic. Social discrimination, that factor most strongly correlated with infection, must be fought. Tackling AIDS, he had written a few years earlier, required a new conception of social solidarity that redefined the boundaries between self and other and refused to separate the fate of the few from the many.[76] Poverty, in the eyes of well-meaning observers, including the World Health Organization, was the root cause of HIV and therefore had to be eradicated to end the epidemic.[77] Long-term change in society's structure and power relations was one modest prescription for combating the epidemic.[78] Work, decent housing, and cultural projects for the victims composed a slightly more realizable recipe for an end to the epidemic.[79] To prevent HIV among addicts, more was required than the merely individualistic approach of needle exchanges and counseling: racism, gender inequality, and poverty would have to be cured before harm reduction strategies could succeed.[80] At its most heroic, the fight against AIDS was seen as inseparable from a major reform of the status quo. In a world without AIDS, all people would be taught about sexuality, drugs, and health; all drug addicts would be treated; everyone would have access to basic health care; no one would maltreat gays or ethnic minorities; and there would be no homeless.[81]

UNPRECEDENTED YET FAMILIAR

Analytical distance from a subject should be a function of methodology, not mere time elapsed. The AIDS epidemic is still very much upon us. Seen globally, the worst is yet to come. Yet that should not prevent us from approaching AIDS historically, understanding and analyzing it in terms of its context and precedence. Though the contrary is often claimed, the AIDS epidemic is far from unprecedented. It is not the first major epidemic of contagious disease to strike in the era when such illnesses were thought a thing of the past. Hepatitis B and herpes had already raised similar issues, though they had not sparked as much fear because they are not fatal.[82] Nor was AIDS the first disease regarded as a global problem and treated as such.[83] From the mid–nineteenth century up through the 1930s, the International Sanitary Conferences had united many nations in intense negotiation on how to counter plague, cholera, and yellow fever.[84]

Nor was AIDS the first disease to be ambiguously classified as both sexually transmitted and less salaciously conveyed.[85] In the narrow sense, no disease is a sexually transmitted disease (STD) only. Transmission is channeled through sexual intercourse first when our habits of personal hygiene have become so abstemious that the only permeable membranes in sufficiently prolonged contact are those of the genitalia. Syphilis was once transmitted by quotidian interactions in rustic circumstances of indiscriminate physical contact and bad hygiene. Venereal diseases were created as a separate and especially stigmatized class of illness not only by a puritan sense of the sinfulness of sex but equally by the triumph of personal hygiene that eventually left sexual contact as their predominant mode of transmission.[86]

AIDS was also not the first disease to add stigma to affliction, turning its patients into pariahs. Leprosy and syphilis had done so for centuries. It was certainly not the first disease to force a confrontation between individual rights and community prerogatives. All contagious illnesses raise this classic dilemma of political theory in its most pressing and unavoidable form. The AIDS debates paled in comparison to the battles fought over smallpox vaccination—one of the most vigorous, though now forgotten, struggles of the nineteenth-century Kulturkämpfe.[87] The "book cholera" of writings on that disease, diagnosed during the nineteenth century, was as striking as the output today on AIDS.[88] AIDS has perhaps provoked more attention, discussion, and reflection than previous illnesses, but only in the trivial sense that today we jabber on more topics in every conceivable medium.[89] Logorrhea about the unspeakable no longer seems a paradox.[90]

What remains true is that AIDS caught the industrialized West unaware. It laid bare its epidemiological complacency, undermined its assumptions of controlling, or at least of keeping at arm's length, the world of malevolent microorganisms, and unmasked its pretensions to tolerance and sympathy. For a culture that celebrates the clinical antisepticism of Richard Meier's architecture as appropriately convivial domestic surroundings, pestilence and putrefaction rudely remind us that the microscopic is still with us—indeed that we humans are but ambulatory appetizers for the masters of an unseen world. AIDS helped undermine a trust in biomedical science that, whatever its discontents, swallows an ever increasing portion of the gross national product in testimony to its ability to spare us the worst slings and arrows of mortality. It revealed that habits many considered unsavory were in fact widespread. It hauled topics from the back of the closet and plastered them across the front page.[91] The eighties became the AIDIES, and positive was negative. While its spread in the industrialized world has been such as to make "plague" and "Black Death" merely overused journalistic analogies, the terms are, alas, highly applicable to sub-Saharan Africa and, increasingly, Asia. There, the sociodemographic effects of AIDS will likely prove to match the worst historical epidemics. By 2000, it caused 21 percent of all deaths in sub-Saharan Africa, leaving malaria as a distant second at about 9 percent. Average life expectancies declined tragically from near age seventy to levels not seen for a century: twenty-nine in Botswana, thirty in Swaziland, and thirty-three in Namibia and Zimbabwe.[92] However much the epidemic seems under control in the First World, its effect in underdeveloped nations threatens global security.[93] As one French minister of health put it, hunger is not transmissible, AIDS is.[94] What happened in the Third World could not be ignored by the First.

AIDS took the industrialized West on an epidemiological voyage back to the future. Its prevention evoked institutional precedence, historical resonance, and public-health deja vu. In an era that fancied acute contagious disease a thing of the past, that had trained its prophylactic cannons on chronic ailments, AIDS rudely reminded us that transmissible illness was still current.[95] The Spanish flu pandemic of 1918 had been but a brief, though horrific, return to the earlier pattern of urban epidemics striking victims indiscriminately. But it was thought to have marked the end of the era of contagious disease.[96] In 1979, when one of the great historic killers, smallpox, was officially declared eradicated, it was an unprecedented triumph of medical technology and public health organization. Ironically, it was also a victory perched on the cusp of the AIDS era.

The venerable epidemics of the past had seemingly been conquered by better living conditions, more circumspect personal hygiene, and targeted biomedical interventions. Life spans in the developed world were now limited only by industrial successes—sedentary, overfed, and exposed to the by-products of material prosperity as we are. The circumstances for which evolution had prepared the human body and those in which average Westerners found themselves differed ever more: from hunt and gather to hunt and peck, from scarcity to supersized caloric surfeit.[97] Our chronic diseases were ones in which personal habits and environmental factors played a large role. Their prevention required changes in lifestyle and surroundings.

Though surgeons general sometimes, like their military colleagues, prepare for the previous war, public health slowly turned in response to this epidemiological sea change. It gradually abandoned the old techniques of breaking chains of transmission to focus instead on convincing people to change their bad habits. AIDS in this context came like an unannounced visitor from the past, a reminder that even half a century of triumphant medical progress could not promise immunity from transmissible disease. AIDS does not stand alone in this respect. Ebola, Marburg, hantavirus, and other hot-button and highly infectious illnesses—so virulent that they burned themselves out in a horrifying swath of destruction ventilated in tabloid headlines—not to mention the use of anthrax as a terrorist weapon and the sudden acute respiratory syndrome (SARS) epidemic of 2003, added emphasis to reawakened concerns about transmissible illness.[98] Illness like salmonella food poisoning and Legionnaires' disease have exposed the public health machinery as complacent in its belief that such problems were of the past. Old killers, like cholera and tuberculosis, came out of retirement to rattle epidemiological cages. Many diseases formerly thought of as degenerative or related to lifestyle and environment are also now understood to be infectious, through the discovery of new microbiological agents—prions (responsible for mad cow disease) or retroviruses.[99]

A PRISM OF PERSPECTIVES

Faced, as all developed nations were, with this epidemic return of the past, history was initially thought to offer guidance.[100] Because the vast bureaucratic machine of public health could turn only slowly, historical factors continued to have influence long after their time. Much of the early approach to AIDS was framed in terms of whether traditional measures should be applied in this case too, or whether they had been outmoded.[101] Outmoded meant that, despite its similarities to past epidemics, AIDS would be better treated in a new style of public health—one that sought less to require than persuade potential victims to change risky behavior. Whether to see AIDS as a reoccurrence of past diseases and thus best dealt with through inherited procedures, or as one for which voluntary behavioral change was the appropriate technique depended, in turn, on how the epidemic was conceptualized. And that varied remarkably.

The taxonomy of the first hour, as the disease was first identified during the early 1980s, saw it as an affliction associated with homosexual men and therefore a gay cancer or a gay-related immune deficiency (GRID)—a disease of the diseased, as those who drew negative implications from this coincidence put it.[102] Before the nature of HIV was understood, the connection between gayness and the illness remained mysterious. Once revealed, it became clear that certain practices were the problem—above all anal sex, allowing transmission in the first place and then promiscuity to spread it widely. From this original connection between the new ailment and the erotic practices that identified gay men as a social group, AIDS was defined as a sexually transmitted disease, even though, as with all so-called STDs, sex was only one means of transmission.[103]

Around 1983, it became clear that others beyond homosexuals also fell ill, above all the infamous "H group" of AIDS victims: Haitians, heroin addicts, hemophiliacs, and hookers. Despite the denialists' insistence that something other than HIV caused AIDS, no denominator beyond a joint microbiological assault was common to these five disparate groups. AIDS was therefore soon recognized as a disease transmitted through blood contact. When the microorganism that would eventually be called HIV was identified and isolated in 1983–84, most observers agreed that the cause of AIDS had been found. Cofactors and questions of lifestyle and environment accordingly became less important.

Conceptualizing AIDS as transmissible, and not the result of environmental or lifestyle factors, allowed it to be perceived during the mid-1980s as a return of problems once considered vanquished: acute epidemic transmissible disease—a return, as the much exercised analogy had it, of the plague. As experience with the illness accumulated, however, such historical analogies began to fade. Partly because of its nature, with an often long-drawn-out development, and partly because new treatments managed to stave off, sometimes for years, its inevitable course, AIDS came to be viewed during the late 1980s as a chronic disease. The increasing use of aerosolized pentamidine against pneumocystis carinii pneumonia and of AZT, the herring and salmon sperm derivative that became one of the first effective therapies, served to shift the analogies. The illness was managed rather than cured; life was prolonged rather than health restored. AIDS was seen through the conceptual prism of cancer rather than cholera.[104]

Viewing AIDS as an infectious disease, whether acute or chronic, shifted the emphasis from its social background—the soil—to the seed itself. In part, this was an obvious result of biomedicine's prowess in identifying its immediate cause. But such displacement also sprang from demands by victims—gays, drug addicts, prostitutes—who objected to the lifestyle approach, which explained their vulnerability by their social identity. In April 1990, fifty thousand Haitians demonstrated in New York, claiming that AIDS was spread by individuals, not groups.[105] Sexual unorthodoxy and addiction had initially been adduced as causes of disease, rather than the accidental mechanisms by which the microorganism gained access to parts of the general population. Such prejudice added insult to the injury of an already heightened mortality for stigmatized groups. A purely biomedical focus on HIV promised to shift attention away from the social identity of marginalized groups and to the particular behavior that set them—but not them alone—at risk. Risk behavior, not risk groups, was now to be the concern, and that was not something on which the H group had a monopoly. The Republican businessman who slept with a prostitute, paying extra for condomless pleasure, and then had anal sex with his wife was a greater epidemiological risk than a monogamous gay couple or an addict who did not share needles.

Such attention to risk behavior rather than risk groups was part of a general insistence on the potential danger threatening the entire population. This "degaying" of the epidemic also shifted the focus away from other risk groups of the first hour. From having been seen as an "undemocratic" epidemic, mainly afflicting minorities, AIDS came to be understood as especially democratic, potentially concerning all who were carnally active.[106] In 1986, the French minister of health declared AIDS a "grande cause nationale" of concern to all citizens, not just the marginal.[107] Gay prostitutes had sex with married men, drug users with the nonaddicted. The distinctions between normal and liminal were obscure and fading.[108] Everyone was a minority now. Degaying the epidemic diffused questions of responsibility. All were potentially at risk, no particular groups were the epidemic's source, and no limited categories should bear the onus of prevention alone.

But the flip side of generalizing the epidemic was to fuel more potent fears whipped up by advocates of drastic interventions. With all at risk, the stakes were higher than if just marginal groups had been exposed. A groundswell of anxiety might encourage draconian precautions.[109] The National Front in France played on such fears, arguing that HIV transmission via saliva or mosquitoes had never been irrefutably disproven, that the disease might have multifactoral etiologies and cofactors, broadening the threat of epidemic spread, and that more precautions were therefore needed, including reporting seropositives, isolating the ill, and imposing border restrictions. AIDS victims, claimed the National Front's leader, Jean-Marie Le Pen, were contagious through their sweat, tears, and saliva; they were modern lepers.[110] American conservatives, like Pat Buchanan, argued a similar line.[111]

As the feared spread of disease out of high-risk groups into the population at large failed to materialize in the developed world, yet another sea change in conceptions took place. With the advantage of precocity, the recognition that the epidemic was only slowly crossing over into the general population took hold in 1987–88 in the United States, just as the European nations were preparing for precisely this eventuality.[112] The venerable venereologists William Masters and Virginia Johnson made a last, miscalculated entrance on the sexological stage with a book arguing that the epidemic would soon be abroad in the heterosexual population. But their arguments were poorly received, and they were accused of irresponsibly encouraging panic. In contrast, the science writer Michael Fumento's controversial work, begun in 1987, argued that a heterosexual AIDS epidemic was a myth, or at least an exaggeration.[113] As it grew apparent that the epidemic did not especially threaten average First World citizens, the disease grew more "normal" in the sense that, like many others, it was becoming an affliction of the marginal and poor, of ethnic minorities and drug users. While heterosexual transmission became more common in developed nations, it was also primarily limited to impoverished minority and marginal groups, for whom cofactors such as drug use, infection with other STDs, and unequal access to health care played a role.[114]

The AIDS epidemic in the First World thus passed through various conceptual phases: from being a gay disease, to one of high-risk groups, to a threat for the entire population, and back to an ailment afflicting disadvantaged minorities. Biologically speaking, AIDS was largely the same disease everywhere in the West (though globally, there were different strains of HIV with various effects and epidemiological implications). But in terms of its social incidence, it presented differing faces in different places. Five American states had more than two-thirds of all cases in the United States. At one point New York City harbored almost one-half of the country's AIDS cases, and thirteen states contained 93 percent of all those related to intravenous drugs. Most of San Francisco's early patients were white and gay; in New York City, a larger fraction were black, Hispanic, and/or drug addicts.[115] In Europe, the incidence varied dramatically. It was three times higher in France than in the United Kingdom. Within France, Paris and the south were hard hit, Brittany and the Limousin spared. Rates per capita were five times higher in Denmark than in Sweden.[116] Once the numbers of drug-related cases took off during the 1990s, the Mediterranean countries had an incidence at least three times that of northern Europe. Half of all European pediatric cases were found in Romania alone.[117]

The identity of the most afflicted social groups also varied at first. In Australia, the epidemic remained largely one of sexual transmission among gay and bisexual men, little affecting drug users or the heterosexual population.[118] Early on in Scandinavia and the Netherlands, it was a disease first and foremost of gay men. In Germany, France, and the United Kingdom, with the notable exception of Scotland, where it was heavily intravenous-drug related, most cases were gay men, but there were other groups as well.[119] In the late 1980s, 60 percent of Italian cases were among drug users, only 20 percent among gays, as was typical for the Mediterranean world. In Japan, hemophiliacs were the hardest hit, infected by imported blood products. In Africa, it was spread primarily by sexual contact among heterosexuals, but in certain First World places this was also the case—in Greenland and Bulgaria.[120]

For the obvious reason of ethnic homogeneity, European nations initially experienced the epidemic as one of sexual, more than racial or ethnic, minorities. In the United Kingdom, of some five hundred AIDS victims by the mid-1980s, only seventeen were nonwhites.[121] Belgium was an exception, with the epidemic concentrated among Africans from former colonies.

Other nations with colonial ties to Africa—France and Britain—later discovered that ethnic minorities were especially afflicted.[122] In the United States, the epidemic was initially perceived as attacking gay men. Only later did its particular ravages among ethnic minorities become evident. In retrospect, it was clear that these groups had borne a disproportional burden from the start. Blacks and Hispanics were overrepresented among AIDS cases, and among those attributed only to intravenous drug use, the vast majority (89 percent) were ethnic minorities. In contrast, most white victims were gay males (78 percent).[123] The number of hemophiliacs infected varied among nations, in large measure in relation to the dependence on American plasma.[124] The clinical picture of the epidemic also varied. Pneumocystis carinii pneumonia, cytomegalovirus infections, and Kaposi's sarcoma were more frequent, and patients survived longer, in northern Europe. In the south, toxoplasmosis and extrapulmonary tuberculosis were characteristic and survival rates were lower. AIDS had different clinical manifestations in the United States than in Haiti, different ones in Africa than the West.[125]

THE EVOLVING RESPONSE

Just as the perception of the epidemic changed as it developed, so too the response evolved. The unprecedentedly rapid growth of medical knowledge naturally affected the measures implemented to counteract the spread of AIDS. At the onset, with the disease believed to afflict especially the outcast and marginal, the precautions broached included traditional sanctions that would probably have been disapproved if mainstream groups had been the primary victims.[126] When the disease was later thought to threaten the population at large, and as the risk groups of the first hour mobilized against becoming epidemiological scapegoats, tactics changed to a more voluntary and consensual approach. Since HIV was usually transmitted through sex and drug use—purposive and conscious acts—the rules needed to halt illnesses like tuberculosis, where a sneeze could be an epidemiological offense, were unnecessary. Second, traditional public health measures were likely to drive already ostracized high-risk groups underground, out of treatment's reach. Rather than seeking to compel behavioral change to reduce transmission, public health officials increasingly emphasized education on risks and a voluntary change of conduct. Compared to previous epidemics, AIDS was treated in what was seen as an exceptionalist manner. The techniques of voluntary behavioral change developed for chronic diseases were applied.[127]

Still later, the wheel came full circle as a new approach, taken because of the growing promise of treatment, partly rehabilitated traditional precautions. AZT in 1989, protease inhibitors in 1995, and entry inhibitors in 2000: these new treatments, Highly Active Antiretroviral Therapy (HAART), and especially their use early in the course of illness, created good reason to identify, report, and care for the infected. Traditional control measures that, back when no treatment was in sight, had been dismissed as pointless, were appreciated anew.[128] Even gay groups, once against testing, came to support it. Physicians were eager to presume consent for HIV screening along with other normal blood work. Contact tracing was valued again to identify those who had been unknowingly exposed.[129] Changing its policy in 1995, the Los Angeles AIDS Healthcare Foundation now supported the routine offering of HIV screening for hospital patients and newborns. Because undetected seropositivity threatened to obscure the results of tuberculosis tests, mandatory HIV screening of those tested for tuberculosis was advocated.[130]

Coupled to epidemiological and medical reasons for a revised approach came a sociological and political change: the wider spread of the disease among powerless minorities. Unlike gays, they were less able to demand respect for their civil rights. Nor, perhaps, did they have the same concern for privacy. Resistance to measures that subordinated individuals to the group weakened accordingly.[131] Early in the epidemic, prevention had been dominated by concerns with civil rights and privacy. With the broadening of transmissive routes beyond sexual relations to include drug use, perinatal contact, and blood transfusions, such a primarily negative approach made less sense. The political initiative shifted away from the coalition of public health officials, civil libertarians, and gay activists that had dominated the early phase, as decision making was taken over by a broader range of institutions and actors, some less reluctant to apply traditional tactics. The Hobson's choice between public health and civil liberties that had apparently been sidestepped during the consensus phase now reemerged, and AIDS was no longer treated as an exceptional disease.[132] Duties and not just rights became increasingly important.

A CURE?

Strategies against the epidemic thus varied over its course. Simultaneously, there was a remarkable spectrum of preventive policies among nations. Seen globally, countries differed dramatically in how they countered AIDS. Most simply, the efforts marshaled to achieve a preventive vaccine or cure varied widely. Curing or biomedically preventing the disease would, of course, have been the most painless approach. Once salvarsan and then penicillin were available against syphilis, old-fashioned, moralizing attempts to regulate or change sexual behavior were left largely superfluous. The sexual insouciance of the late twentieth century was made possible by antibiotics, along with effective contraception. Victims were treated, nipping transmission in the bud, without having to alter their behavior.[133] AIDS prevention, in contrast, remained at the presalvarsan stage of syphilis control, seeking to alter behavior rather than merely to mop up its unfortunate results.

A biomedical cure—or the eradication through vaccination—of a disease so fraught with stigma and sin, so closely related to lifestyles regarded by many as immoral, will eventually solve the problem in the most radical way. Curing will sidestep traditional prevention, which violates individual rights.[134] But a cure will also allow us to snap our fingers at practices that transmit the disease. Technologically enchanting, a cure is an amoral solution in its disregard of objections to the habits and conduct associated with transmission. It will reduce the externalities of desire to practically nil and free allegedly noxious habits of their consequences. To cure or prevent AIDS means it is back to business as usual at the bathhouse or the shooting gallery.[135] Already in 1772, such a technical fix had plunged the physician Guilbert de Préval into trouble. He was expelled from the University of Paris medical faculty for claiming to have discovered how to prevent syphilis and thus, in the eyes of his detractors, for giving libertinage free rein.[136] The promise of a cure has sent moralists into frenzies of self-righteousness ever since. Early in the twentieth century, they foresaw a "moral syphilization" of society, an infection that threatened, as the German reformer Katarina Scheven claimed, to be even more pernicious than the merely corporeal version.[137]

Such ideas now resurfaced.[138] The Conservative Family Campaign in Britain argued that modern society's permissiveness was to blame for the epidemic.[139] Norman Podhoretz, the neoconservative journalist, phrased it analogously: seeking a biomedical solution to a moral problem would spread "a kind of AIDS in the moral and spiritual realm." Like a Westside Jehovah of the New Right, he thundered that a crash program for a vaccine meant that researchers gave "social sanction to what can only be described as brutish degradation," allowing gays "to resume buggering each other by the hundreds with complete medical impunity."[140] Even the humble condom was suspect as a technical fix that allowed indulgence without consequences.[141] As one of Newt Gingrich's constituents put it, "I do not want to see condom ads on TV, that give the impression that one can have it all—a sexually promiscuous lifestyle and protection from sexually transmitted disease."[142] Real behavioral change emphasizing sexual fidelity was the solution proposed by Edmund Stoiber, then Bavarian interior minister, not just "promiscuity wearing a condom."[143]

Such concerns with the lifestyle of infection were not, however, monopolized by the socially conservative right. Those who fancied themselves progressive—alert to the needs of the epidemic's victims and concerned with social reform—including gays troubled by aspects of homosexual behavior, also argued that curing AIDS, vaccinating against it, and even adopting the technical fix of condoms all failed to address the fundamental problem raised by the conduct that spread the epidemic. Rather than advocate such narrow means of avoiding disease, they demanded broad social and sexual reform: changes in behavior to eliminate intravenous drug use, promiscuity, and the anonymous anal sex at the root of the problem.[144] Curing the disease also threatened radicals of the left, who were convinced that AIDS had social causes or at least cofactors. Without changing society as a whole, they insisted, the epidemic could not be vanquished: "Without institutional change, the virus wins." A cure would solve the problem "while allowing the distribution of power and health to remain the same."[145]

Two nations in particular sought a biomedical solution to the problem, a technological shortcut to eliminate endless public health strategizing: the United States and, at a vast remove, France. The French, as one observer put it, were good at research and treatment, poor at prevention.[146] The Americans, in turn, poured far greater resources into a biomedical solution than all other nations put together. Though administratively decentralized in other respects, the United States had national funding of scientific research. In the postwar period, its biomedical research establishment had become without equal in the world.[147] The bulk of federal spending on AIDS went to basic biomedical research, vaccine development, clinical trials, and epidemiological surveillance, rather than to public health education and prevention programs.[148] Most European nations, in contrast, spent their monies on care of the ill.[149] As with national defense, they freeloaded on the public goods provided by American research efforts. In the 1980s, American research spending was one hundredfold that of the British, ten times per inhabitant the Swedes'.[150] In 1993, French spending (in a nation one-fifth the size of the United States) was only 3 percent of the American expenditure (and it dropped to 2 percent in 1997), but even this modest sum was a third more than the British, its nearest competitor, and three times that of Germany. The United States provided some 90 percent of global governmental AIDS research funding.[151] The equivalent French budget, one critic calculated, would have paid for constructing four kilometers of mountainous highway.[152] Insofar as Europeans studied the disease, Americans often provided the money. During the mid-1980s, the American government provided Swedish researchers with more resources than Sweden's own authorities did.[153] Other than France, only Germany and Britain were making a comparable effort, though the decentralized nature of German research was arguably not giving value for money and even modest levels of funding were threatened with cuts.[154] The British worried that the trans-Atlantic brain drain would worsen if gross disparities in research opportunities on this topic continued. When in 1998 Montagnier went to Queens College in New York, supplementing the cream of French science with the promise of $20 million in research funds, even the French were concerned.[155]

PUBLIC HEALTH FACES THE EPIDEMIC

In the absence of a cure, vaccination, or effective treatment, prevention was the only means of controlling the epidemic. And here we again take up the theme of national variation in response to AIDS that was broached at the outset. For despite the fact that, in biological terms, the problem faced by each polity was much the same, nations adopted remarkably divergent strategies for dealing with the epidemic. At one extreme, a bevy of poor and peripheral countries (which this book will not assess) imposed drastic measures of traditional contagious disease control on the sick and infected. China, Iraq, and Syria demanded testing of aliens entering for long stays and nationals returning from abroad. In China, anyone with reason to believe that another citizen suffered from AIDS was required to report that person for isolation and treatment. Seropositives and their contacts were detained for examination, restricted in their activities and movements, and obliged to carry registration cards.[156] In the Indian state of Goa, no one could refuse HIV testing if disease was suspected, and seropositives were isolated. In India generally, AIDS patients could travel by rail only with permission of the stationmaster and only if willing to pay for the entire compartment.[157] Cuba imposed screening on broadly defined groups (travelers abroad, hospital and STD patients, pregnant women, and the sexual contacts of seropositives) and, ultimately, on the entire population through its inevitable contacts with the national health system. Seropositives were isolated in sanatoriums where, though they were quarantined, their salaries were paid. They were allowed to pursue their educations, permitted home visits, and otherwise treated (by most accounts) in a humane fashion.[158] In

Mongolia, HIV screening was compulsory for all citizens, enforced if necessary by direct police action. AIDS patients who did not follow medical prescription could be isolated and treated by force, and pregnancies among seropositive or sick women were to be terminated.[159]

At the other extreme, there was the voluntaristic tactic of seeking to convince the healthy to shun risky behavior and seropositives to avoid transmissive conduct, aiming to educate citizens on potential pitfalls and providing what treatment was possible but otherwise enforcing few injunctions on the ill. This was the consensual strategy that was adopted most clearly in nations such as the Netherlands, Britain, and Germany. The details of this approach will occupy us throughout most of this book.

Seen globally, there was a wide spectrum of approaches. But what if we turn to the narrower realm of the industrialized West? Was there a similarly broad palette of responses?

Some observers have argued that Western industrialized democracies eventually adopted largely comparable strategies based on education, voluntary testing, and behavioral change. While some nations may at first have implemented traditional measures, all eventually recognized their dysfunctional effects and abandoned them. Only Sweden, Bavaria, sometimes Austria, and in certain respects the United States were recognized as partial exceptions to the consensus that was achieved around a voluntary strategy.[160] In the most optimistic accounts, this consensual strategy finally resolved the perennial public health dilemma between the rights of the individual, even when infectious, to autonomy, bodily inviolability, freedom of movement and occupation, and other activities of potential threat to others, and the claims of the community to protect itself against contagion. If a consensual approach to AIDS alone provided effective prevention, so the argument went, there was no contradiction between individual rights and the public weal.[161] AIDS was thus treated in an exceptionalist manner.

In fact, however, such epidemiological optimism does not hold. Even in the heyday of traditional prophylaxis for contagious disease, during the late nineteenth century, Western nations varied starkly in their choice between coercive and voluntary measures.[162] During the AIDS epidemic, they diverged equally—in large measure in tandem with the approach taken already a century or more ago. The tactics for dealing with this epidemic were therefore not determined only by the nature of the new disease itself, or by etiological and epidemiological insights won during the AIDS era. They were also influenced by historical factors that, over a long period of development, had helped cement approaches to contagious disease, indeed to public health in general. Despite commonalities in many other respects, in this most recent epidemic Western nations continued to differ markedly in their preventive tactics and in their ideologies of statutory intervention.[163]

The timing of the response varied, for example. It was more rapid in northern Europe, especially Scandinavia and the Netherlands, than in the United States and in the Mediterranean.[164] Some nations introduced many new laws to deal with the epidemic: Sweden, for example, and America.[165] Other countries, like Germany and Britain, passed almost nothing novel, relying instead on the existing armamentarium of precautions, however reinterpreted.[166] In more specific matters, the differences were also drastic. All American states required the reporting of AIDS, and about half of them the reporting of seropositives. The Germans and the Dutch did not have nominative notification of even full-blown cases. The Americans screened and excluded foreigners on the basis of serostatus, as did nations to which they generally did not compare themselves: Indonesia, China, South Africa, and Japan, for example, not to mention the then-socialist nations of the East Bloc.[167] In contrast, with a few exceptions, their European allies did not. The Swedes, otherwise among the most drastic interveners, were laissez-faire at the borders. The Americans required screening of certain civil servants, as did, to some extent, the Germans. The French and British shied away from any such measure. The military was screened in the United States, but, with a few exceptions like French soldiers on duty in Africa, not in Europe. HIV screening was strictly anonymous in Germany; but in Sweden anonymity was ruled out on principle. Testing, though voluntary, was considered much more important to preventive efforts in France and Sweden than in Britain. In Austria, Sweden, Bavaria, and some American states, prostitutes were screened and forbidden to work; they were left alone in most other nations.

Contact tracing was required in Sweden and some American states, but few other countries. Medical confidentiality was still considered an absolute in France, so strictly upheld that sometimes patients themselves were not told. In other nations, especially the Anglo-Saxon, the concern to warn endangered third parties limited patients' privacy. All nations were laggards in terms of funding basic research compared to the United States. But many produced far more frank and effective public education campaigns. Blinded seroprevalence studies were accepted without alarm in America but hotly resisted in Britain, the Netherlands, and Germany. Transmissive behavior was criminalized and prosecuted in the United States and Germany, while largely ignored in Britain. Gay bathhouses were closed in some American cities and in Sweden and Bavaria, yet left largely untouched in other American cities and in France and the Netherlands.

To put the contrasts in a pointed form: American soldiers were subject to one of the most draconian regimes of HIV surveillance anywhere. They were screened, obliged to follow rules of conduct to prevent transmission, required to inform their sexual partners and medical caregivers of their serostatus, and had to practice safe sex. The soldiers' spouses could be informed of their condition, their contacts traced; their sex partners could be identified, counseled, and tested without consent. They were, in other words, treated only slightly more harshly than all Swedish citizens. Conversely, the seropositive Dutch, non-Bavarian Germans, and French, other than being potentially excluded from private life insurance coverage and possibly sued for damages if they knowingly transmitted the disease, had few curtailments of their activities and rights.

STRATEGIES OF CONSENSUS AND CONTROL

Within this panoply of variations in public health tactics, there were, broadly speaking, two choices. The names varied, but the essence of the positions remained stable. The first involved traditional transmissible-disease control: identifying and reporting the infected and tracing their contacts, isolating and quarantining them, treating potentially dangerous carriers, and taking steps to destroy the contagion through disinfection, cleansing, or other antimicrobial means. Proponents of the second approach claimed that such techniques were antiquated, ineffective, and counterproductive. Instead of seeking to control the infected, health officials should encourage voluntary compliance with procedures of identification, testing, and treatment and reward behavioral change that lessened transmission. To this binary choice might be added a third approach, that of heroically reformist social medicine, which would rest content only with the eradication of social evil. Since supporters of this strategy were better at stating than realizing their ambitions, the first two were what mattered in terms of implemented policies.

A taxonomist is not a Manichaean, any more than an oenophile divides wines merely into red and white. But in fact the preventive tactics were largely binary. Almost uniformly, the two public health strategies available to Western health authorities were described as some variant of a division into a compulsive, reactionary line and a voluntary, progressive approach, a contain-and-control strategy and one based on cooperation and inclusion.[168]

The political valences attached to these respective strategies are evident in the vocabulary itself. Conservative opinion often favored measures, early in the epidemic especially, to identify, isolate, and render the infected harmless. This had worked in the past for other diseases; there was no reason not to apply such techniques again. Progressive opinion, in contrast, tended to understand AIDS in its broad environmental context, to worry lest its victims be ostracized, to argue that coercion would drive victims underground, and to insist that, in the absence of a cure, behavioral change to minimize transmissive conduct was the hope—which meant education and not compulsion. Words were not minced on this Manichaean dichotomy. In the battles between these two strategies, old-fashioned public health control was routinely labeled by its opponents as fascist, authoritarian, totalitarian, or, among the Finns, communist.[169] In Germany, associations were common between the traditional precautions implemented in Bavaria, discussed in chapter 3, and measures imposed by the Nazis on Jews, making for pungent polemics.[170]

Conversely, believers in traditional public health precautions applied also to AIDS naturally took umbrage at being portrayed as violators of individual liberty.[171] Whose liberty, was one obvious issue: that of the unfortunates who were stricken or the vast majority who were, as yet, only threatened by disease? The extreme argument was that, faced with a lethal epidemic, sacrificing the civil rights of a minority was a small price to pay for sparing many pain and death. Ronald Bolton, a prominent British physician, put this most starkly. Screening all individuals and quarantining seropositives would halt the epidemic. Had such precautions been rigorously imposed at the onset, millions would have been saved. Isolating, say, fifty thousand seropositives would have been worth it, had it meant sparing the lives of many more.[172] Hoping to avoid any painful weighing of the contradictory claims of sick and healthy, supporters of a traditional approach invoked the long historical continuity of such strategies. The rightist National Front in France argued that left-wingers had supported making tuberculosis notifiable in the early postwar years, and similar restrictions on syphilis victims had found backing across the political spectrum. That the collective interest should take precedence over individual rights in such cases was not a controversial position. Similar arguments were advanced for the measures imposed in Bavaria. In California in 1986, Lyndon LaRouche's Proposition 64 claimed disingenuously to impose on AIDS only the venerable measures applied to other communicable diseases.[173]

Voluntary measures, the right argued, were insufficient. A virulent threat required drastic restrictions. AIDS should be dealt with using the customary instruments of disease control. Exemption was an unjustified privilege.[174] If applicants for civil service jobs were rejected for having diabetes or multiple sclerosis, why should HIV not entail similar consequences? Pilots were grounded if they were diabetic or syphilitic; why not if afflicted with AIDS? Cancer victims could not buy life insurance; why should those with AIDS? Foreign victims of lymphogranuloma venereum were forbidden to enter the United States without permission. Why should seropositives be treated any differently?[175] Curable VD was reportable in Germany and America. Why not incurable AIDS? Victims of malaria, syphilis, or whooping cough could be reported and isolated. Why not AIDS?[176] Children who were not immunized or who suffered from other contagious diseases were barred from school. Why not seropositive pupils? Prostitutes were inspected for syphilis; why not gays for AIDS? Heterosexual brothels were illegal. Why not gay bathhouses? Liberals who resisted interfering with gay sexual habits often wanted to ban smoking in public places. Why not abstinence for both bad habits?[177] And so forth. Continuity was conservatism in the clearest sense.

Indeed the dialectic was double-edged; special treatment could be good or bad. If AIDS victims were not to be stigmatized but treated like any other patient, should they be subject to the restrictions imposed on sufferers of other ailments? Should insurance companies screen for HIV as part of routine underwriting, as for other diseases, so as to normalize AIDS? Was applying the penal code to potentially transmissive behavior, as was the case for other illnesses, not a way to regularize treatment of the disease and its victims?[178] Or was the exceptionalism of the approach to AIDS now to set the standard? Was it the onset of a trend that would end such restrictions altogether? Much like the logic of race-blind policies in the face of affirmative action, such reasoning allowed proponents of traditional tactics to portray their position as the democratic and fair one. The same rules applied for all illnesses; there were to be no exemptions for anyone.[179]

The vast literature on the epidemic is saturated with the often implicit assumption that politics and preventive strategies ran in tandem.[180] Broadly speaking, the contain-and-control strategy is seen as having been advocated by the right, the cooperation-and-inclusion approach by the left. Yet as we shall see, such simple correlations did not hold. Indeed, when examined comparatively across a broad range of nations, politics and prevention bore remarkably little resemblance to each other. The question then arises, how do we best explain why industrialized nations faced with much the same epidemiological problem responded so variously?

2.   What Came First

At the dawn of the AIDS era, in the early 1980s, public health's traditional, quarantinist approach to contagious disease was widely thought to have outlived its time. Growing irrelevant in the era of chronic disease, it remained on the books only as a reminder of a bygone age. But then came AIDS and a resurgence of the classic enemies, such as cholera, tuberculosis, and even the plague, as well as new outbreaks of horrifyingly transmissible emergent diseases. The inherited laws and regulations on contagious disease had not been modified for many decades. In principle, therefore, the classic techniques of testing, reporting, contact tracing, isolation, quarantine, and compulsory treatment generally still applied to the diseases for which they had originally been formulated.

All nations confronting AIDS were equipped with a series of legal instruments fashioned to deal with contagious and venereal diseases. In most cases, these had been developed and implemented during the late 1800s and early 1900s. Even in those cases where the laws were more recent (West Germany in 1961, Switzerland in 1970, East Germany in 1982, Czechoslovakia in 1984, Finland in 1986), the ideas codified were of venerable pre- and interwar stock. Their goal was to break chains of transmission. To this end, they imposed restrictions on the movements and activities permitted the victims of transmissible illness, sometimes also mandating treatment and care. With the general decrease of communicable disease, most of these laws had lain fallow during the middle decades of the century. Heart disease required no quarantine. And antibiotics and vaccination had replaced the lazaretto as the most effective weapon against infection. Epidemiological developments thus obscured the potential clash between traditional public health procedures and individual liberties.

The AIDS epidemic now forced a question whose resolution had been conveniently sidestepped for over half a century. Did it make sense, epidemiologically and politically, to invoke old instruments against the new epidemic? Should seropositives be exempt from the rules of reporting, isolation, tracing, and treatment that applied to the victims of other ailments? If a German physician, for example, diagnosed a sexually transmitted disease other than AIDS, he could be fined if he failed to report the patient. But if he diagnosed AIDS, he was equally obligated to respect professional confidentiality.[1] Was this fair, sensible, or desirable?

The inherited regulations were based on premises formulated during the heyday of bacteriology. Their basic assumption was that transmissible disease was caused by particular microorganisms. To prevent epidemics thus meant to hinder their transmission by identifying, reporting, and quarantining carriers and disinfecting the persons, effects, and dwellings of the afflicted. Largely absent was any concern with the broader environment—the squalor, misery, and filth that helped spread illness. These laws ignored an earlier, prebacteriological approach to disease that had found a voice in the tradition of social medicine. The laws also, however, sought to sidestep the moral context of illness, especially the venereal sort. The contagious disease and VD laws passed during the first third of the twentieth century in most developed nations focused on microorganisms rather than morals. They aimed to treat diseases as purely biological phenomena with few ethical overtones. In many respects, they dealt with STDs in the same, nonstigmatizing fashion as other transmissible ailments. The West German Contagious Disease Law of 1961 exemplified this heavy but impartial hand, treating all transmissible ailments alike and regarding even syphilis as an illness with no particular implications for public order, morality, or anything else that might smack of the old system of vice squads and regulated prostitution.[2] Yet, while perhaps no longer moralizing, laws intended to prevent the spread of STDs imposed draconian controls on individual behavior.

In nations that, like Sweden, had adopted a form of sanitary statism for VD—imposing rules on all adults rather than regulating prostitutes—the new view of sexually transmitted disease was strict and uncompromising.[3] All citizens were considered potentially infected, were required to report themselves and, if ill, submit to treatment. VD was no longer regarded as the sporting result of pleasure's pursuit, as in the seventeenth and eighteenth centuries, nor as a largely moral blemish, as in the Victorians' picture of bourgeois domesticity and romantic marital love. With the growing awareness in the late nineteenth century of its widespread ravages, VD shifted from being seen as an individual misfortune to a devastating social scourge. Increasingly the cannons of law were trained on the problem. Legal liability for transmission, especially between spouses, was enforced, helping to undermine the strict confidentiality of relations between physician and patient. Infection became regarded as a crime, and the penalties for being ill, yet not following the procedures of treatment and prevention, were now defined by the penal code.[4] STD legislation in the United States, for example, often criminalized the intentional transmission of VD but not other communicable diseases.[5]

During both world wars, many nations imposed more drastic measures to curb VD among the armed forces and the civilians with whom they fraternized. Wartime controls often included case reporting, testing, treatment at public expense, and the promotion of prophylaxis, both chemicals and condoms. The mass roundups of thousands of prostitutes in the United States during the First World War have entered the annals of both injustice and ineffectiveness.[6] But citizens who were not prostitutes were also subject to strict controls. A Denver ordinance allowed those arrested for sex-related offenses to be detained for examination and treatment. During the 1940s in New Jersey, migrant laborers were required to undergo VD exams ninety days prior to entering the state. In New York State, VD patients could be reported by name and compulsorily examined, and their contacts could be traced. As late as the 1960s, New Jersey, Pennsylvania, and Ohio allowed health officers to quarantine recalcitrants suspected of syphilis until they had been examined and treated. Persons convicted of vagrancy could be compelled to undergo testing. Mass screenings for VD were conducted on occasion, with 31 percent of Chicago's population taking Wassermann tests during the late 1930s. In California, New York, and Texas, it was punishable to expose others to VD infection. In Texas, it was a felony knowingly to conceal one's status as a disease carrier, and the infected were forbidden to attend public places or gatherings.[7]

For other transmissible diseases, strict control of the infected was also the rule before the AIDS era. In America, states could impose significant restrictions on the movements and liberties of contagious disease patients. Laws dating from the nineteenth century continued to grant authorities broad powers of epidemiological investigation, inspection, and identification, including the removal and isolation of the contagiously ill.[8] Until late in the twentieth century, tuberculosis patients who refused to follow infection control instructions might be isolated at home or in an institution.[9] Occupational restrictions could be imposed, forbidding persons with salmonellosis, for example, to work in food handling or childcare. Milk sellers in New York were tested for typhoid and excluded if infected; syphilitics were barred from food-related jobs in Texas. Lepers could be quarantined, as could those who had come into contact with smallpox carriers, however fleetingly. Pupils with transmissible diseases were routinely excluded from school. Prisoners incarcerated longer than seven days were examined for VD in New Jersey.[10]

In contrast to the United States, many European countries had national—not just regional—laws to control transmissible disease. In Germany, the Imperial Contagious Disease Law of 1900 and the VD law of 1927 set the tone for subsequent measures well into the AIDS era. The latter required those suspected of infection to be examined, the ill to be treated and their contacts traced, and the infected to refrain from sex. The Nazi regime, whatever its effects in other respects, did not fundamentally alter the German approach to disease prevention. Prostitutes were regulated for the army's use, and VD victims were denounced as parasites.[11] But in other ways, the Nazis left unchanged the basic principles of epidemic disease prevention inherited from the earlier laws. The VD law was given a few minor embellishments.[12] During the 1930s, the 1900 Contagious Disease Law was expanded to encompass psittacosis, afflicting parakeets and parrots, and it could be extended to other diseases.[13] As part of its attack on Jews and other supposed racial enemies, the Nazi regime invoked the tenets of bacteriology to justify its oppression and eventual genocide, presenting Slavs and especially Jews as the social equivalent of microbes that had to be eradicated to preserve the health of the body politic.[14] Yet domestically, the minor fine-tuning of public health legislation indicated that the regime did not consider transmissible disease a priority. After the war, when they criticized harsh public health measures, Germans turned not to the experience of totalitarianism, nor to the laws of the imperial and Weimar periods, but rather to the emergency legislation imposed by the occupying Allies.[15] These measures sought, for example, to deal with the flood of refugees into war-ravaged territories by extending obligatory reporting by name and by enforcing mandatory treatment.[16]

When the West Germans themselves took up such matters, the continuity with prewar and pre-Nazi practices was striking. In 1953, the old VD law was modernized but not fundamentally changed.[17] Hoping to cut through the confusion of wartime and postwar emergency statutes, some of which had caused elderly matrons to be trucked off together with prostitutes for VD treatment, the Germans sprang back over the totalitarian interlude to what now seemed to be the liberalism of the 1927 law.[18] Those who suspected they had VD were—on pain of compulsory hospitalization—to be examined and treated and to follow prescriptions on nontransmissive behavior. The occupations permitted the ill were restricted, and prostitutes and the promiscuous were to be reported and tested for syphilis. VD patients in the infectious stage were forbidden to have sex. The formerly syphilitic were examined before marriage and, if still infectious, were allowed to wed only if they informed their spouses-to-be. Syphilitics were not allowed to donate blood or breast milk, nor to nurse other women's children. VD victims were reported by name if they refused treatment, posed a threat of transmission, or withheld information on their contacts. Attending physicians were to trace contacts, who in turn could be reported if the doctors feared interruption of treatment or transmissive behavior. In the absence of other options, all measures could be carried out with direct force, though potentially harmful medical interventions required the patient's consent.

In 1961 West Germany passed a new Contagious Disease Law. It too continued the earlier tradition for all contagious diseases other than STDs.[19] Like its predecessor of 1900, it classified the objects of its interventions in five subtle, complicated, and exhaustive categories: the ill, those suspected of illness, those suspected of infectiousness, carriers, and finally those suspected of being carriers. The law mandated reporting the victims of various illnesses by name. Unlike the VD law, it did not require the ill to be treated, but it did obligate symptomless carriers to register changes of address and work and to warn of their condition if hospitalized. It restricted the employment of the diseased. During epidemics, it allowed the authorities to limit individual freedom of movement and bodily autonomy and to ignore the inviolability of the home. It permitted authorities to enter property and inspect it; required those with information on the presence of illness to report it; and obliged the infected to submit to the necessary examinations, x rays, and tests, although it pursued more extensive medical interventions (removing stomach contents, spinal taps, etc.) only with consent. It allowed the authorities to prescribe behavior to prevent transmission and, in the worst cases, permitted the isolation of victims (though carriers were constrained only when they did not follow prescriptions or endangered others). This included having their mail opened and other measures to prevent their escape from isolation wards. It also threatened with jail those who transmitted certain diseases.

In Sweden, the Epidemic Disease Law of 1919 had instituted traditional quarantinist public health measures against contagious illness. The Lex Veneris of 1918 applied to VD in particular, treating it largely like other contagious diseases. Its point was to end the regulation of prostitution and the focus on commercial sex, shifting attention instead to all carriers of VD, whether call girl or family man. In turn, the Contagious Disease Law of 1968 broke new ground by subjecting all transmissible diseases, venereal or

otherwise, to the same measures, thus lessening the particular, peculiar position of STDs.[20] Passing this modernized version of inherited public health
measures, the Swedes consciously rejected the voluntary approach to VD
that had been followed in Britain and the Netherlands—which were exceptions among industrialized nations. The Swedes prided themselves on the
extent to which their approach to STDs had been emulated abroad, and decided that the traditional approach had proven its worth.[21] Victims of transmissible diseases were classified, much on the German precedent, into four
groups: the ill, asymptomatic carriers, those suspected of being ill, and suspected carriers. Those suffering from notifiable diseases were examined and
tested, and they could be limited in their freedom of movement, even isolated in a hospital. During epidemics, disinfection of dwellings and destruction of clothing and bedding were authorized. The populations of hard-hit
areas could be isolated; prohibiting the use of certain property or destroying
it was possible. In times of war or national emergency, entire areas could be
cut off to prevent the spread of disease.

Though included in the same law as other transmissible diseases, STDs
were still treated differently in Sweden. Individual liberties were more restricted than for other ailments, largely because prostitutes were most likely
to be afflicted and they were considered unwilling to undergo treatment or
to conduct themselves in a nontransmissive manner.[22] Those who suspected
that they had VD were obliged to be examined and treated and to follow
measures prescribed by the attending physician. Recalcitrants were subject
to compulsory examination, isolation, and treatment. Attending physicians
were to trace contacts, and contacts were subject to examination and treatment, at police behest if necessary. As the quid for the quo of such strict obligations, medical examination and treatment for VD were provided free of
charge. The ill, including those who only suspected they were afflicted,
could be punished for having sex with others.[23]

In Britain, the pertinent text was the 1936 Public Health Act, a vast portmanteau measure that covered notifiable contagious diseases other than
VD, forbade transmission, prohibited the sick from various occupations and
activities, and allowed hospitalization of the ill who could not be treated at
home.[24] Later legislation altered only details of this traditional approach.
The 1961 Public Health Act permitted compulsory examination of suspected sufferers of a notifiable disease. The 1968 Health Services and Public
Health Act required reporting the names of victims of cholera, plague, re-
lapsing fever, smallpox, and typhus and the testing of carriers. The Public
Health (Control of Disease) Act of 1984 continued this approach into the
AIDS era, though it did not include the new disease. In quaintly anachro-

nistic language often copied verbatim from nineteenth-century precedents, the act obliged physicians to report the names and addresses of patients with notifiable diseases and threatened to fine those who exposed others to infection, including by lending or selling bedding and rags or taking undisinfected laundry to public washhouses. It removed the infected from certain occupations, though with compensation, and banished afflicted children from school and other public places. It forbade the infected from borrowing books at public libraries and allowed the destruction of those in their possession, insisted on disclosure of disease in rooms being let and disinfection before renting, prohibited the use of public transport by the infected, mandated examinations of the diseased and carriers, and required the ill who could not be cared for at home to be removed to hospitals.

Unlike Sweden and Germany, however, the United Kingdom did not have a specific statute covering VD. The Contagious Disease Acts of the mid–nineteenth century had been hotly contested and were abolished in 1886, thus ending a form of regulated prostitution that had applied to certain women in garrison towns. Thereafter, the authorities had adhered to a fastidiously voluntary approach to STDs. In 1913, a royal commission on VD recommended making free medical treatment in clinics widely available. This reliance on voluntary rather than coercive tactics then remained the strategy of choice.

In France, perennially retarded in matters of public health, the legislation in question was of more recent vintage. The 1902 law on public hygiene finally brought France up to par with other European nations.[25] Basic contagious disease procedures were introduced: notification of certain ailments, disinfection and cleansing of infected goods and property, and isolation of the ill. On VD, however, the French changed prophylactic horses only after the Second World War. Although the late nineteenth century had seen desultory attempts to reform or abolish the system of regulated prostitution—perfected and institutionalized, if not invented, during the reign of the first Napoleon—little had come of such efforts before 1945.[26] Not until the 1960s was the preventive focus on prostitutes abandoned. The new reforms emulated the Scandinavian approach, although there were also domestic precedents, both from the Popular Front era of the late 1930s and the Vichy regime.

In all nations, such inherited laws meant that fin de siècle measures were still in effect a century later, when the HIV epidemic began. For contagious diseases other than AIDS, traditional precautions remained on the books and were enforced on those increasingly seldom occasions when required. For STDs, strictures were still regularly imposed on prostitutes, but for other diseases the intervals between applications lengthened. A rare example of measures that had once been common occurred in Bavaria in 1965. When three cases of smallpox came to light, eighty-four neighbors were quarantined, including a man whose only offense was to have read the water meter.[27] The question now, as AIDS hit, was whether this new disease was to be treated in the same way as classic epidemics. Or had the rules changed in the meantime?

ON THE BOOKS, OUT OF USE?

Like the proverbial generals fighting the previous war, the first instinct of policy makers in most nations was to wheel out the prophylactic artillery available to them. Just as cholera, when it struck Europe in the early 1830s, had initially been fought with weapons developed for the plague, so too AIDS was at first seen through the crosshairs of existing legislation on contagious disease. In this, public health officials were supported, and often egged on, by a public that—faced with a new disease of unknown provenance, unpleasant associations, inscrutable routes of transmission, and merciless lethality—assumed the worst, called for strict measures, and hoped to be pleasantly surprised rather than sorry in retrospect. And yet, as we will see, things quickly changed. Once the nature of the disease was better understood, once powerful groups of its initial victims organized in defense of their rights, and once the public health sector considered its options, the old-fashioned approach was often resisted.

The most common arguments about why traditional techniques of transmissible disease control should now be bypassed were technical. HIV was not easily communicable, requiring some form of direct blood contact. Hence the measures, used for more directly transmissible diseases like smallpox or tuberculosis, which involved isolating the stricken, were ill suited in this case. Because of AIDS's lengthy estimated latency period (which kept expanding as seropositives appeared who had remained asymptomatic for years and sometimes decades), contact tracing and reporting were rendered almost useless. Because the number of seropositives worldwide quickly expanded into six and then seven figures, isolation of the potentially infectious was logistically impractical. Because travel was no longer an upper-class privilege but a mass pleasure, quarantine in harbors and, now, airports seemed all but impossible to organize. Because HIV was transmitted not in a blunderbuss manner widely among the population but selectively to close contacts of infected persons, targeted measures—rather than universal ones—had logic on their side.[28]

Yet such technical considerations alone cannot explain why traditional public health techniques were not used uniformly against AIDS. True, measures untuned to the nature of the disease and blind to the social context of their implementation were unlikely to be successful. In polities that were not dictatorships, public health could not be compulsory in any rigorous way. "Public health agencies," as one observer put it, "possess the authority, but not really the power, to coerce."[29] And yet, granting limits to what could have been imposed, the spectrum of possible responses—not to mention the smorgasbord of tactics actually applied in the nations studied here—indicates that there was little about AIDS in a technical, biological, or even epidemiological sense that directly stipulated how it could be fought. There was nothing inherent in AIDS that excluded traditional techniques.

Since there was as yet no cure, prevention was the only way of limiting the epidemic. But prevention did not necessarily mean just education and voluntary behavioral change. Prevention could, in theory, just as well have included testing the entire population at regular intervals and isolating or imposing behavioral prescriptions on seropositives. Precisely because a cure was not forthcoming, a German liberal argued, precautions like making AIDS reportable were necessary.[30] It was not for scientific or epidemiological reasons that a traditional course was resisted in certain countries, but for political ones. The lifestyles of the infected and those at risk determined whether the epidemic spread or not. From this it might follow that voluntary behavioral change was necessary and the best prophylactic hope. But it could just as well suggest, as the Swedish government concluded from the same evidence, that compulsory hospitalization was necessary and justifiable when behavioral change was not forthcoming.[31]

There was nothing in the character of AIDS that led necessarily to one form of prevention or another. Those who argued against restrictive measures often sought to portray their position as flowing naturally from the very nature of the disease.[32] Sex and drug use were private behaviors largely beyond the state's ken. Hence hopes of influencing such conduct would have to rely not on statutory strong-arming but on cooperation with the victims, education, and behavior modification. But in fact there was nothing inherent in such behavior that put it beyond the state's grasp. Where statutory interventions end and where personal privacy begins is, of course, a political, not an epidemiological, decision. Sexual conduct has never been free of state interference. Sodomy remains technically illegal in many American states. Over the nineteenth century, the legal age of sexual majority rose, even as the biological age of sexual maturity fell. In the late twentieth century, marital rape, a form of (mis)conduct hardly recognized in law earlier, was forbidden by statute.[33] What a few years before would have been dismissed as harmless flirting now merited legal sanction as sexual harassment. If it was not the nature of the disease itself that dictated the response, then what did? But before tackling that question, we need to determine what, exactly, the response was.

3. Fighting the Previous War

Traditional Public Health Strategies and AIDS

The first question was whether to treat AIDS as just another contagious disease and its victims as subject to traditional precautions. The second, broader question was whether the venerable quarantinist strategies of prevention could and should be applied. Should screening (possibly of the entire population, perhaps only of certain high-risk groups) to identify seropositives be undertaken? When identified, should the ill or even the infected have their sexual and intravenous drug contacts traced, and could these be warned? Should the infected, in turn, be required to undergo what treatment was available? Should they be obliged to follow behavioral prescriptions to minimize transmission, with criminal and civil liabilities in default? Could they be isolated if, despite warnings, they persisted in risky behavior that endangered third parties? The answers varied dramatically from country to country.

Because of existing contagious-disease legislation, those who favored interventionist measures against AIDS did not have to pass new legislation, but had only to include HIV disease among those already covered. Bavaria's draconian precautions were simply the application of what, in principle, was already allowed in the German Contagious Disease Law. When America sought to keep out seropositives among immigrants, it did so by having the Public Health Service add HIV infection to the list of excludable diseases in the existing federal regulations. Colorado adopted a restrictive approach, fully conscious of continuing traditional public health tactics in the new epidemic.[1] Conservative politicians in the United States sought to portray restrictive precautions for AIDS as reasonable by stressing their continuity with measures already in place for other diseases.[2]

One of the first questions was to decide what sort of disease AIDS in fact was: generally transmissible, including via sexual contact; sexually transmissible in a specific sense, analogous to syphilis and gonorrhea; or perhaps fitting into neither of these categories? Speaking purely biologically, if that is possible, there is no such thing as an STD. Most diseases transmitted via genital contact can also be communicated through other membranes or directly via blood. What creates an STD are the habits of sociability that—evolving as societies industrialize and urbanize—restrict potentially transmissive contacts to acts of sexual, and not also social, intercourse. Earlier conduct and customs facilitated transmission through everyday as well as sexual interactions. As personal hygiene and habits of contact avoidance began to define civilized behavior, transmissive intercourse became that permitted only our most intimate acquaintances. Well into the nineteenth century, syphilis was considered not a sexually transmitted disease in any exclusive sense, but one spread also through quotidian interactions. When travelers bunked with their hosts en route, when families slept in one bed, and when mothers sucked the penises of infant boys to calm them, licked sties from their children's eyes, and chewed their food for them before spitting it in their mouths, then clearly syphilis had avenues of transmission other than merely the genitals.[3] Personal hygiene—and the general rule that immediate physical contact is avoided with all but children and lovers—created STDs as a particular category of diseases.

Such issues were raised anew by AIDS. Of all its routes of transmission, only one, however predominant in some nations, involved sex. The hysteria surrounding seropositive children attending school posed the question of transmission via casual contact. Quacks peddled devices and cleansers promising to render harmless everyday contacts, testifying to the fear that AIDS might not be an STD in the narrow sense.[4] Observers in Haiti traded on similar fears when they claimed that women mixed menstrual blood in food to keep their men faithful.[5]

Whether to classify AIDS as a communicable or sexually transmitted disease was thus as much a political as a biological or epidemiological decision. In some nations, much hung on the distinction. Communicable diseases were often treated differently from STDs. Contact tracing was mandated for VD, for example, while detention of the ill was possible for certain transmissible illnesses. Conscious transmission of VD, but not other ailments, was criminally liable. Medical confidentiality was enforced more strictly for VD than for other diseases.[6] In Sweden, the decision to treat seropositivity and AIDS as STDs meant that sequestered seropositives were denied certain benefits that would otherwise have been theirs.[7] Some nations resisted classifying AIDS as an STD precisely to avoid the preventive consequences. Despite the urging of right-wing parties, the Danes chose not to include AIDS under their Contagious Disease Law, which allowed mandatory testing, internment, and the like. And when they decided that the similar VD law also did not suit the requirements of this new epidemic, they abolished it altogether.[8] The Dutch decided to include AIDS neither under legislation on contagious diseases nor VD, thus exempting its victims from rigorous strictures.[9] Most American states, with some exceptions like Florida, Illinois, and Kentucky, did not classify HIV as an STD. In New York, had not the state commissioner of health, David Axelrod, refused in 1990 to classify AIDS as a venereal disease, victims would have been reported and screened, had their contacts traced, and possibly been isolated.[10]

In France, AIDS was at first classified as a contagious disease in 1986. This entailed consequences such as the requirement that the deceased be immediately enclosed in a coffin and hermetically sealed in case of transport. The following year, however, AIDS was reclassified. It was given its own section in the Health Code to avoid the strict penalties attached to transgression, including the possibility of prison for the ill who did not undergo treatment. This also kept the issue out of the hands of local politicians, especially the right-wing National Front in southern departments. Policy prerogatives were thus reserved for the Parisian authorities, who resisted an old-fashioned approach.[11] In contrast, the Italians and Swiss included AIDS on their list of contagious diseases, which implied various restrictions for victims.[12] Different Australian states classified HIV infection as either a transmissible or a venereal disease. Consequences varied, from reporting the afflicted, to prohibiting them from having sex without informing their partners, to making it an offense (in West Australia) for a seropositive to board a public bus without notifying the driver.[13]

THE TRADITIONALIST ODD COUPLE: SWEDEN AND BAVARIA

Perhaps Sweden's and Germany's different approaches best illustrate the choices facing public health authorities. In Sweden, one of the first official acts, in September 1985, was to classify AIDS as a venereal disease within the scope of the Contagious Disease Law of 1968.[14] The continuity with traditional ways of preventing epidemics was marked here.[15] In 1985 and then again in 1988, laws were passed that revised the 1968 Contagious Disease Law to cover not just full-blown AIDS but also seropositivity alone, thereby amalgamating the two at a very early stage in the epidemic.[16] The full arsenal of precautions that applied to other transmissible illnesses was thus mobilized here. On pain of possible isolation, all who suspected that they were infected had to seek medical care and follow the attending physician's behavioral prescriptions. Testing could be required. Their contacts had to be traced and made to submit to the same procedures.

Physicians advised seropositives on safe sex techniques that were to be followed: they could have sex only with a single constant partner, who had been informed of their serostatus. They could, in any case, have only safe sex (mutual masturbation was allowed, but oral sex was considered highly risky, and condoms had to be worn throughout intercourse). They could not use drugs and certainly not share needles. They had to inform attending medical personnel of their condition. If they ignored such prescriptions, they could be reported and isolated in a hospital. Isolation could, at first, be indefinite, but this was later changed to a duration of up to three months, extendable in half-year segments thereafter.[17] Those who had had sex or shared needles with someone they knew to be infected were to regard themselves as infected. They too had to be examined and had to follow the physician's prescriptions. Seropositives who failed to inform their partners before sex or to follow the prescribed medical regimen could be jailed. Swedish law did not require evidence that disease had been deliberately transmitted. A mere suspicion that the infected would not follow the rules was enough. If an infected drug abuser, for example, said he would have unprotected sex, a court could incarcerate him initially for three months.[18]

The law also recognized, however, that the heavy hand of statutory intervention might hamper the goal of curbing the epidemic by scaring the infected away from treatment. Thus, it ended the punishment of those who had sex while infected, since the penal code could, in any case, be used in cases of transmission. Physicians were required to report even suspicions of such behavior. Like other STDs, HIV and AIDS were to be reported anonymously, using a system of coding derived from the personal identification number of the infected citizen. Contacts were to be reported by name, unless the physician believed they would voluntarily go for testing.[19] Though the National Board of Health and Welfare specifically ruled out taking the lifestyle of high-risk groups as reason to suspect disease and thus to compel examination, it did agree that high-risk circumstances should prompt a suspicion of infection.[20] Apparently, while the fact of being gay, a drug addict, or a prostitute itself was not sufficient to mandate examinations, any act of anal or commercial sex or drug injection was. At issue was not the lifestyle, in other words, just the act of living. Isolation was used a number of times. In 1986, an addict was isolated (with two guards present and the lights always on). In April 1987, it was the turn of a seropositive prostitute who refused to use condoms. By the mid-1990s, the 1988 Contagious Disease Law had been invoked over sixty times. Its victims were isolated on average for a year, but in one case at least for several.[21]

In Germany, one of the major battles of the epidemic was fought over whether to include HIV and AIDS under the precepts of the 1961 Contagious Disease Law. Among the nations under analysis here, Germany perhaps could bring the heaviest legislative firepower to bear. The Contagious Disease Law allowed the authorities broad and, indeed, drastic powers of intervention.[22] Precisely the blankness of the check thus issued, however, made it politically difficult, and ultimately unfeasible, to cash.

That AIDS was a transmissible disease in the legal sense was not disputed.[23] If applied to this epidemic, the 1961 law would have allowed screening and examination of those suspected of infection, their periodic appearance before the health authorities, and the testing of prostitutes and their clients, by force if necessary, at regular intervals. It could have required the infected to report changes of address and employment and permitted them to be banned from certain jobs or even isolated. Medical surveillance of the ill and infected was allowed, as was the closing of public institutions and meeting places that facilitated transmission. It gave the authorities access to private property, including the dwellings of the infected and suspected, and permitted them to forbid prostitutes and physicians to practice if infected. It would have authorized health officials to prescribe behavior to prevent transmission, including using condoms, informing spouses and partners, not donating blood, organs, or sperm, and not nursing infants. The law did not, however, permit compulsory medical treatment, as it did for other diseases. Nor would it have required the reporting by name of the infected and ill.[24] Nor was it likely that the application of the law to AIDS would allow isolation of the infected, since the possibility of casual transmission was slight, excepting perhaps those who refused to act nontransmissively. Whether the law would have prohibited the infected from pursuing certain professions, except perhaps prostitution, was also unclear, since, again, transmissibility was low.[25]

The most drastic of the 1961 law's potential implications rested on its almost limitless definition of the infected. This had been inherited from the law's predecessor of 1900. Five groups of potential targets were identified. Formulated in terms of AIDS, they were the ill (seropositive, with symptoms), those suspected of being ill (symptoms but no positive HIV test result), carriers (a positive HIV test, but symptomless), those suspected of being carriers (suspected of being infected, but with neither symptoms nor a positive test result), and those suspected of being infectious (suspected of having received HIV, but not ill, suspected of being ill, or carriers). The authorities' ability to intervene rested on how a person was classified. The categories, in turn, were so elastic and expandable that almost anyone would have fit—perhaps excluding Howard Hughes, perambulating in his Kleenex-box shoes in the throes of acute germophobia. One could be suspected of being a carrier or of infectiousness without any medically measurable indication of disease or contact with it. Some observers held that all those who had previously lived "at risk" should be suspected of infectiousness, with prostitutes and their clients, and gays who patronized saunas or bathhouses, falling under this heading. The Bavarian authorities automatically suspected prostitutes and intravenous drug addicts of being infectious.[26] Others asserted that if every risky behavior counted equally, then all sexually active citizens would be liable to strictures. Anyone, after all, could have had extramarital sex or other possibly dangerous contacts.[27] Potentially, the law would have allowed the authorities to suspect, say, any male found in a public toilet in a major city of being infectious or a carrier and, thereby, subject to massive limitations of his personal freedom.[28]

Equipped with such formidable powers, the German government did not consistently seek to apply the inherited techniques of epidemic control. Invoking the Contagious Disease and VD Laws and their wide reach, the authorities argued against the need for new statutes.[29] With such legislative sabers to rattle, they could both keep demands for more drastic interventions at bay and threaten recalcitrants who refused to change risky behavior, while in the main not actually wielding force.[30] AIDS was assumed to fall within the scope of the Contagious Disease Law, but few, if any, of its provisions were actually marshaled against it.[31]

More explicit application of the Contagious Disease and VD Laws remained politically unfeasible, however. In 1984, most federal states rejected a draft law that promised to apply many such measures to AIDS, and the following year the health ministers of the states unanimously rejected making AIDS notifiable. This helped focus the Bonn authorities' attentions on a more consensual and voluntary approach.[32] By around 1986 or 1987, Germany had developed a lumbering consensus behind a voluntary approach. In an important historical shift, the country turned away from older responses to epidemics. The ruling Christian Democrats and Free Democrats, supported by the Social Democrats, agreed that education and voluntary behavioral change should be the basis for prevention. Though they still kept in reserve the possibility of extending the Contagious Disease Law, they concurred that AIDS would not be reportable. Nor would there be routine or compulsory screening of risk groups.[33] The AIDS Enquête Commission, established in 1987, broadly supported this approach.[34] Its final report urged education and information as the main strategies, with harsher interventions reserved for recalcitrants only.[35]

This consensus unraveled, however, on a regional basis. Insisting on applying inherited disease-prevention techniques to this epidemic, Bavaria struck out along its own preventive *Sonderweg* in 1986. In part, electoral tactics were at play; the Christian Socialists hoped to distinguish themselves from their coalition allies during the spring 1987 elections.[36] Ministries in Hesse and North Rhine–Westphalia also broke ranks with other federal states in not rejecting out of hand the idea of making AIDS reportable.[37] But the Bavarians were most assiduous in continuing traditional measures. They also vainly sought in the Bundesrat to convince the other states to adopt their approach. Controversy followed within the federal government coalition. The Christian Socialists pushed the Bavarian position; a more liberal approach was represented by the Christian Democrat Rita Süssmuth and her portmanteau Ministry of Youth, Family, Women, and Health.[38] The federal government papered over such disagreements, unable and unwilling to rein in local divergence from national policy.[39]

In Germany's federal system, disease control falls to local prerogative. Thus, the Bavarians could in large measure follow their own proclivities. Because they were simply extending existing legislation to this epidemic, they did not have to seek new legal instruments (with all the debate that this threatened). They attacked the problem through administrative regulation instead.[40] Once having added AIDS to notifiable diseases, the Bavarians required screening of a broad variety of groups. Most other federal states argued that membership in a high-risk group should not per se subject someone to testing, without evidence of potentially transmissive behavior. Bavaria, in contrast, screened prostitutes and addicts by virtue of their membership alone.[41]

The Bavarian measures issued in 1987 focused on prostitutes and intravenous drug addicts. Nonetheless, in theory anyone suspected of infection could be screened (by force if necessary).[42] A judicial decision in 1988 specifically allowed health authorities to act even on only moderate suspicion.[43] In addition, Bavaria screened civil service applicants, non-EU foreigners seeking residence permits, and prisoners. Infected aliens could be denied residence. Resident aliens who might transmit disease could be deported. And alien addicts and prostitutes could be deported even if not infected. The measures also forbade the infected from donating blood, sperm, or organs, infected women from nursing infants. Seropositives were required to warn their sex partners and health care providers. Prostitutes, male and female, were obliged to be screened, to use condoms in their work, and forbidden to ply their trade if infected. Razzias and closings of gay bathhouses and brothels were possible. Bars, discos, saunas, and other public establishments could be closely regulated.[44] The infected were warned that transmission of disease was punishable, and those who refused to curb potentially transmissive behavior could be isolated.

Sweden and Bavaria were thus united in their decisions to apply inherited contagious disease controls to this new epidemic. While the odd couple of a Scandinavian Protestant and a south German Catholic polity was most decisive in setting off down their well-trodden prophylactic path, other nations also adopted venerable precedents, sometimes piecemeal.

QUARANTINE AND ISOLATION

Nations took a variety of approaches to quarantine, the quintessential feature of the classic public health strategy on contagious disease. Cuba was the only nation to impose systematic quarantine of the infected.[45] At the other end of the spectrum, the Netherlands and Denmark refused to incarcerate even those whose actions threatened transmission. In other developed nations, however, besides what was possible in Sweden and Bavaria, isolation was also used on occasion. Icelandic seropositives who persisted in unprotected sexual relations could be put under house arrest, and the Swiss authorities had similar powers.[46] The Anglo-Saxon nations had legal instruments to isolate the infected who refused to minimize the risk of transmission. Every American state had powers to isolate the communicably ill; a dozen acted specifically to include seropositives whose behavior posed a risk.[47] Such statutes were used sparingly, primarily to warn rather than to incarcerate victims, and were hedged about with restrictions to prevent abuse.[48] In various Canadian provinces, including New Brunswick and British Columbia, AIDS victims, and sometimes also their contacts, could be quarantined.[49]

In the United Kingdom, the broad provisions of the 1984 Public Health (Control of Disease) Act were extended the following year to include AIDS. AIDS was not made a notifiable disease, but victims (although not seropositives) who might knowingly spread it could be isolated. Medical examination could be ordered of seropositives, and certain precautions with respect to corpses required.[50] The measure was merely a means of last resort, having been intended to quiet backbench objections to the government's refusal to make AIDS notifiable.[51] Its powers were invoked only once. In September 1985, a Manchester man, manifestly incapable of caring for himself, was isolated for some ten days. Thanks to the ensuing protests, the statute was never used again.[52]

Some nations also imposed various regulations to ensure that victims' remains could not spread disease. Though not among those countries that quarantined the quick, the French took drastic precautions against the dead: like the victims of highly contagious diseases, they were immediately placed in hermetically sealed caskets with air purifiers.[53] In Britain, the 1988 Public Health (Infectious Diseases) Regulations prohibited wakes and open coffins for AIDS victims.

SCREENING

As of mid-1985, AIDS screening was technically possible, and debate raged over its use. Knowledge of their negativity was thought to be important for uninfected members of risk groups, motivating them to take precautions. For the infected, screening permitted measures to prevent transmission. Identifying seropositives allowed a targeting of information and care. It facilitated knowledge of the spread of the epidemic and helped trace and limit sources of the disease. It was also part of a broader strategy of safer sex that promised to limit the need for condoms: after testing, seronegative couples could have unprotected intercourse with each other, sheathing up only for encounters outside their protected circle. Screening's most ardent proponents supported it so long as isolation of seropositives was also possible.[54] Others argued, in contrast, that, since little could as yet be done to help the infected, why screen them? If anything, the consequences, discrimination and stigma, were negative. The infected were unlikely to act differently just on the basis of knowing their serostatus, and behavioral change should, in any case, be encouraged among all sexually active citizens, not just seropositives.[55] The lengthy period during which infection was possible without testable antibodies, as well as the problem of false negatives, meant that, until the eventual advent of accurate tests measuring the direct presence of HIV, screening remained a wide-meshed sieve.

Most nations forbade testing against the patient's wishes, or at least limited it to exceptional cases. Physicians were left open to damages and prosecution for battery (or negligence in the United Kingdom) if they failed to inform patients that blood taken for other purposes was tested.[56] Some American states required specific written consent for HIV testing, rather than just assuming implicit agreement in the course of treatment and other blood work.[57] In Germany, testing without consent violated the right to informational self-determination, as well as being an act of bodily injury. Some observers argued, however, that physicians not only had the right to test patients without explicit consent but also would have neglected their duties if they did not screen when it was medically indicated.[58] In Sweden, the situation was ambiguous. Whether the Contagious Disease Law of 1968 allowed testing without consent was unclear, but official opinion considered permissible the tests required for a diagnosis, even against the patient's will.[59] In Britain, the dispute was over whether a patient's agreement to diagnosis and treatment implied consent to testing. The government and the main physicians' organizations argued for a specific consent to HIV screening because of the lack of any cure and the drastic consequences of a positive result. At the same time, some medical organizations insisted on a surgeon's right to test patients, if necessary without consent.[60] In Iceland, testing of prisoners, alcoholics, and drug abusers was in principle voluntary, but the test had to be actively refused, rather than consented to.[61] Italy allowed testing without special permission when in the medical interests of the affected.[62]

General screening of the population threatened to be unfeasible, requiring a vast and expensive apparatus, made costlier by the need for regular repetition. Occasionally, mass testing was advocated.[63] But most often, it was rejected on the basis of cost, inefficiency, and the potential sacrifice of civil rights.[64] Screening only high-risk groups threatened to be discriminatory and raised the problem of how to identify targets. Testing high-risk groups in toto discriminated against those who did not practice the behavior associated with their communal identity. Among those at greatest risk, only hemophiliacs could be easily identified without their own cooperation. Unless bisexuals, gays, drug users, and promiscuous heterosexuals came forth voluntarily, how could they be selected for screening?[65] During the early phases of the epidemic, high-risk groups often opposed testing, not only mandatory but also voluntary. Ignorance might not be bliss, but given AIDS's deadliness and the absence of any useful treatment, it did not seem to be much of a disadvantage.[66]

Yet not all high-risk groups could exempt themselves. Many nations had provisions for compulsorily testing those arrested for crimes, usually sexual, that threatened transmission. Accused prisoners could not be tested against their will in Austria or Switzerland, but in Germany the code of criminal procedure foresaw testing to establish the facts of a case (though not if it threatened the accused's health).[67] In Sweden, the parties of the center and right proposed screening for certain crimes.[68] With support in the main AIDS advisory body, the government revised the Contagious Disease Law in 1988 to allow mandatory testing of criminals who might have transmitted disease and to curtail medical confidentiality for them.[69] In Finland, accused criminals facing lengthier punishments could be medically examined, including HIV screening.[70] In over forty American states, compulsory testing was possible on those arrested for rape or other sexual offenses, sometimes including prostitutes' clients. In 1996, the Violence against Women Act allowed victims of sex crimes to be told the perpetrator's HIV status.[71] In contrast, Germany and France offered no such possibilities of compulsorily testing criminals.[72]

Police, medics, and others exposed to infection during their duties naturally had an interest in being allowed to screen perpetrators. In many nations, those who, when arrested, might have transmitted disease to medical or law enforcement personnel could also be screened. In Sweden, police wounded by a criminal could require the aggressor to be tested.[73] Authorities in Florida could insist on testing those who injured law or medical personnel. The 1990 Ryan White Comprehensive AIDS Resources Emergency Act (CARE Act) made federal funds contingent on the state prison systems allowing their personnel to know whether they had been exposed to disease by a prisoner.[74]

People about to marry were also occasionally screened. Some nations required premarital testing for syphilis. During the 1930s, various American states had pioneered this, and about half retained such tests into the new epidemic. Sweden had restricted the marriage of infectious syphilitics in 1918 and, two years later, required prenuptial testing. France introduced similar measures in 1942. The Germans required disclosure of disease to the prospective spouse, while the British had nothing of this sort. But generally speaking, such testing had been gradually abandoned, partly as an inefficient and costly means of finding cases, and partly in recognition that sexual activity was less and less contingent on marriage.[75] To these precedents, such as they were, HIV screening was occasionally attached. Some American states, like Louisiana, Illinois, and Texas, demanded premarital screening. California required the offer of testing. Though the ban was quickly overturned, Utah forbade seropositives from marrying.[76] Once authorities discovered the practical difficulties of implementing such measures, however, they abandoned them. Illinois and Louisiana rescinded their laws when the unfavorable cost-benefit ratios became clear. During the first six months of premarital screening in Illinois, eight of seventy thousand applicants proved seropositive. The cost (charged to the applicants) was approximately $2.5 million.[77] In any case, couples wishing to wed without benefit of screening were voting with their feet for the registry offices of neighboring states. In Germany, calls for marital testing were heard, but with no effect. In France, screening was offered but not required during prenuptial examinations.[78]

In contrast, a consensus around screening of blood donors quickly emerged across developed nations, although globally less than half of all countries had such procedures on the books. As of 1985, all Western nations had instituted these precautions, though the French tarried for a few crucial months, foolishly impelled by national *amour-propre* to give a local test competitive advantage over the already developed American version.[79] Sperm banks, in contrast, were less thoroughly covered. Despite the recommendations of the Centers for Disease Control and the Federal Drug Administration that donors be tested both initially and again after six months, and that sperm be quarantined for half a year, most American states had no formal rules. Up to a third of banks did not test donors. Screening was, however, demanded of organ donors.[80] British sperm donors were required to be tested twice during a three-month period. Their Swedish counterparts had to be tested too, and high-risk groups were excluded. French sperm donations had to be tested, as of August 1985.[81] More fraught with ethical difficulties was the question of testing pregnant women and newborns. The interests of mother and child had to be weighed against each other. On the one hand, knowledge of serostatus allowed women to make informed decisions on terminating pregnancy, taking AZT, giving birth via Caesarian, or other means of minimizing risk. On the other, testing infants meant testing their mothers by proxy.

Despite such general trends, screening played very different roles among polities. In eastern Europe, both before and after the fall of Communism, screening was crucial to preventive strategies. Besides testing foreigners, the Soviet Union screened transfusion recipients, drug addicts, gays, prostitutes, and those in contact with the infected. Bulgaria sought to test all adults, and Hungary victims of STDs and sexual partners of AIDS victims, prostitutes, prisoners, criminals, and drug users. The Czechs tested all with a record of venereal disease.[82] Swedish preventive strategies rested on widespread voluntary screening undergirded by contact tracing and other compulsory testing. Parties from the center and right advocated even broader policies, seeking, ideally, to test all adults.[83] Even as it stood, however, the system achieved near-saturation levels. Some 70 percent of Swedish women between the ages of twenty-five and thirty-four were tested. By 1992, about a quarter of all men and one-third of all women had been screened. This was one of the highest per capita rates in the world, though still below the almost 100 percent level achieved in Cuba by the early 1990s.[84] In some parts of Sweden, 80 percent of drug addicts had been screened on a voluntary basis.[85] (In comparison, by 1990 between 13 and 20 percent of citizens from age sixteen to thirty-five in Denmark, and 22 percent of Germans over sixteen had been screened.)[86]

Compulsory screening in Sweden was possible for drug abusers and alcoholics. As noted earlier, all patients suspected by a physician of infection were required to submit to screening, as were the sexual and needle-sharing contacts of the infected.[87] It was, moreover, impossible to be tested anonymously in Sweden. Anyone could choose to be tested, but if the results proved positive the patient's identity was required. Such information was restricted: results were coded and there were general rules of medical confidentiality. But within these limits, seropositives could not remain anonymous.[88] Despite repeated attempts in Parliament by Communists, Liberals, and some renegade Social Democrats, as well as by parliamentary committees and physicians, the government and its Social Democratic support adamantly rejected anonymity for seropositives.[89] Anonymity was allowed only where testing proved negative. This was, of course, a largely pointless concession, reminiscent of the agreement between the old peasant couple—that on matters where they agreed, the husband was allowed to decide, but on those where they did not, it was the wife's turn. Physicians protested and took out newspaper ads illegally promising anonymity even for seropositives—at least until they showed symptoms, at which point their names too would be reported.[90] The government, however, saw anonymity as incompatible with the Swedish tradition of drastic restrictions on those whose conduct threatened transmission. How could one ensure strict interventions if the infected were allowed to remain anonymous?[91] It was not logical, as a Social Democratic defender of the government's position put it, to exempt one group of the infected from the consequences of the law by promising them anonymity.[92] Anonymous testing was also impossible in Iceland.[93]

Other than for organ and blood donors, the French had no mandatory screening. Instead, they encouraged widespread voluntary testing, with the exception of obligatory screening for soldiers having served in Africa.[94] After the National Front's calls in 1987 for broad compulsory screening (followed by similar proposals from the minister of health in the new Socialist government in July 1988), the government decided to offer—but not require—screening of certain groups, such as hospital patients, pregnant women, and couples about to marry.[95] Nonetheless, the issue erupted again several times during the 1990s. Draft bills requiring screening during prenatal and prenuptial examinations, and of the tubercular and prisoners, were supported in the Senate by parties of the center and right and, on some points, by medical organizations, but opposed by the government and defeated in the National Assembly.[96] In the United States, the position was ambiguous. On the one hand, there developed an early consensus that mass mandatory testing made little sense. At the same time, several required screening programs were put in place: for some civil servants, for the military, for prisoners, and for certain categories of foreigners. As the possibilities of treating victims increased, however, especially after AZT use began in mid-1989, matters changed. As in all other nations, the logic behind screening strengthened as it made increasing sense to identify and bring the infected into the ambit of medical care and counseling.[97]

Excepting Bavaria, the Germans did not emphasize screening. The government rejected routine or compulsory testing of risk groups in 1986. The AIDS Enquête Commission could not bring itself to advocate even voluntary testing, since the results would psychically disturb without helping the victims. It split over compulsory screening. The majority favored it only when a positive result would allow further public health precautions. A dissident minority wanted screening in each instance of possible transmission.[98] Civil service applicants in some federal states and various categories of foreign scholarship students were, however, tested as groups. The United Kingdom, in turn, refused compulsory screening lest this discourage voluntary testing among high-risk groups.[99] The government rejected calls for widespread or compulsory screening as pointless so long as no treatment was on offer for the infected. The authorities resisted promoting even voluntary tests among the general public.[100] The Netherlands and Switzerland went further, making few attempts to encourage even risk groups to test voluntarily (except, in Switzerland, those at risk who wished to have children).[101]

Thus, the approach to even an arguably obvious tactic like testing varied widely across the Western world during the first phase of the epidemic. In Sweden and the United States, compulsory testing was implemented for certain groups. Some nations, like Sweden and France, also emphasized voluntary testing, believing that it encouraged the infected to practice safe behavior. Others, like Britain, the Netherlands, and Germany, discounted voluntary screening. They held that, in the absence of treatment, little was gained; indeed, it might discourage high-risk groups from care and counseling.[102] As a result, the rate of voluntary testing even among high-risk groups varied dramatically among nations. Over half of Dutch gays decided, after counseling, not to be tested.[103] In 1991, 65 percent of all gays in the Netherlands and 53 percent in Britain had never been tested. In France and Denmark, where testing was encouraged, the corresponding figures were 21 and 24 percent.[104]

Even anonymous screening—blinded seroprevalence studies—an issue of apparently soothing uncontroversiality, raised hackles and provoked varying responses. The aim was largely statistical and epidemiological: accurately mapping the spread and incidence of the epidemic. By testing blood samples taken for other reasons (after stripping them of all identifying markers), authorities hoped to achieve this more accurately than through testing at blood banks, STD clinics, and other venues where incidence rates might be skewed. Because such screening was anonymous, informed consent was impossible, and so of course were notification and counseling of the infected. The arguments against blinded seroprevalence studies were partly practical (they did not provide much information about incidence rates in specific populations) but mostly ethical (they did not allow the authorities to help, or even notify, the infected). The German Green Party argued that epidemiological knowledge already sufficed without resort to such measures; the interests of medical confidentiality outweighed those of research. Humans should not be degraded, as they put it, into objects of science. The right of individuals to determine what was known about them took priority over a mere increase in knowledge.[105] Similar arguments were decisive in Britain. Ian Kennedy, professor of medical law and ethics at Kings College, London, managed to convince the pertinent parliamentary committee that ignorance was better than immorality, and that screening should confer at least some benefit on the patient. If the results promised by seroprevalence studies could be had only by such devious means, then better not to partake of this epidemiological apple.[106]

The United States practiced blinded testing from 1985 with few, if any, objections raised.[107] In contrast, the United Kingdom at first shied away. In 1990, however, the British introduced a limited scheme for testing at genitourinary, prenatal, and drug dependence clinics and other venues, though with broad patients' rights of refusal. The following year, the scheme was expanded to include National Health Service patients generally.[108] In the Netherlands, blinded testing, like testing in general, was not pursued.[109] In Denmark, delayed by objections, such programs started only in 1990. In Norway and Iceland, where anonymous testing was not possible, blinded testing was also ruled out.[110] But the Swedes, who also rejected anonymous testing, did have various programs of blinded screening.[111] In Germany, the legal situation was ambiguous.[112] The Laboratory Reporting Ordinance of 1987, discussed below, required laboratories to anonymously report infected blood samples for statistical purposes. It was, like so many laws in postwar West Germany, a tortuous ethical compromise, where an innocent and well-intentioned technique was resisted against a background of implicit fears of totalitarianism. The use of the population census of 1939 to identify Jews for deportation had sensitized Germans to the potential misuses of otherwise apparently innocuous official information gathering.[113] Such worries continued in disputes over the census planned during the mid-1980s as well as in fears that the 1987 AIDS Enquête Commission, established by the government to make recommendations on the epidemic, might seek more information than its mandate allowed.[114] There were some initial studies of representative sentinel populations, including a Bavarian one in 1991. But not until 1993 did the government decide to conduct a test program of anonymously screening newborns.[115] Unsurprisingly, therefore, in the early stages of the epidemic, the standards of statistical knowledge of HIV incidence varied greatly among countries. It was better, for example, in the United States, spotty in Germany.[116]

REPORTING, NOTIFICATION, AND CONTACT TRACING

Reporting and notifying victims' identities to the authorities and tracing the infected's sexual contacts—other ways to control contagious disease—were used only contingently when it came to AIDS.[117] Most observers agreed that reporting was ill suited to curb the epidemic, because of the limited means by which the disease was transmitted and its long incubation period. It might also discourage voluntary testing and counseling.[118] Every nation classified certain diseases as of public consequence and reportable to the authorities. Whether to include AIDS and HIV was the question. At a minimum, most countries required reporting full-blown AIDS cases, nonnominatively (without the patient's name), in order to develop a statistical picture of the epidemic. In some countries, seropositivity was also notifiable. More contentious was whether the identities of individual patients should be made known to the authorities. But even anonymous reporting was an issue in some nations.

In the United States, as of 1983, all states required nominative reporting of AIDS by physicians, hospitals, laboratories, and indeed by "any other person knowing of or attending a case" to confidential public health registries, adding it to the already established lists of notifiable diseases. In contrast, named HIV reporting raised objections from gay and civil liberties interests and had become policy in only half the states by the mid-1990s.[119] In California, the Health and Safety Code was amended in 1985 to ensure that there would be no compulsion to identify anyone who had been HIV tested. In 1989, after major political skirmishing in New York City, a compromise was eventually achieved that excluded named reporting.[120] As the benefits of early treatment became clearer, however, and as more seropositives lived longer without passing to a clinically identifiable AIDS stage, the tide changed. The Presidential Commission on the Human Immunodeficiency Virus Epidemic supported making seropositivity reportable in 1988, and in 1990 the CDC urged states to undertake named notification as part of its increasing emphasis on contact tracing and early intervention. The 1990 CARE Act required states to have partner notification in place to receive federal monies.[121] As of 1998, reporting of seropositives by name or other identifying markers, with confidentiality, was American federal policy, and the CDC provided funds on the basis of states' ability to meet such criteria. By 2002, thirty-five states or territories required named reporting of seropositives.[122]

In March 1983, Sweden became the first European nation to legislate on AIDS when it was made a notifiable disease. Similar requirements followed in 1985 for seropositivity.[123] Denmark, Norway, and Finland required nominative reporting of AIDS; Iceland and Sweden used a code to ensure confidentiality. For seropositives, the Danes, Icelanders, and Norwegians collected only anonymous statistical data, the Finns used social security numbers, and the Swedes an abbreviated code.[124] As of 1986 those tested and found positive in Sweden had to be reported.[125] Negative tests were without consequence, but for those who proved infected, there was no such thing as anonymous screening—unsurprisingly, the system was described as "rat trap anonymity."[126] Attending physicians were to report victims, coding their identities with the first two and last four digits of the national registration number. Since this did not guarantee anonymity in a small country that routinely uses the personal identification number for nearly every official and commercial transaction, down to credit card purchases, some physicians broke the law, performing testing anonymously.[127] More important still were the consequences of reporting. So long as patients followed instructions, in theory they remained hidden behind the abbreviated code. If, however, they violated the attending physician's instructions (by leaving the hospital, say, or continuing to have unprotected sex), their identity could be reported to the health authorities.[128]

In Finland, patients with clinical AIDS symptoms had to reveal their identities; the asymptomatic did not. The Swiss had a similar system, reporting by name all AIDS patients and the seropositives who did not act responsibly.[129] In Italy, AIDS patients were reportable by name; in Austria, only by their initials.[130] In 1986, the French made AIDS cases compulsorily but anonymously notifiable (with initials). Seropositivity alone was not. In order to reimburse their medical costs fully, however, they were reported by name, but with strict confidentiality protection, to the social security authorities.[131] French Polynesia, on the other hand, took a Swedish approach, reporting seropositives who refused to attend regular medical consultations.[132] The British, in contrast, had no specific measures on reporting AIDS or HIV infection. The Public Health (Control of Disease) Act of 1984 in theory allowed compulsory medical examination of seropositives and hospitalization of AIDS patients. But, for fear of driving the infected underground, the law was not used to make the disease notifiable.[133] Otherwise, there was only a voluntary system of reporting cases of AIDS and seropositivity to the Communicable Disease Surveillance Centre. The government, committed to the voluntary system adopted at the turn of the century for syphilis and other STDs, had no ambitions to introduce compulsion.[134]

Among major nations, it was the Germans, however—with the exception as always of the Bavarians—who were the odd nation out. Along with the Dutch, they were the only developed country that did not, with one minor exception, have even an anonymous reporting requirement for AIDS, much less for seropositivity.[135] The federal authorities and the health ministers of the states other than Bavaria agreed not to extend notification requirements to AIDS, fearing that otherwise victims would shun voluntary measures.[136] The issue was discussed at length in Parliament, with Social Democrats joined by Christian Democrats and Free Democrats in their support of anonymous screening.[137] The AIDS Enquête Commission, however, split on the issue, with dissident Christian Democrats holding up the American example as proof that sooner or later nominative reporting would be required.[138] Though there was some discussion about whether tests and reporting should be required of prostitutes, all parties and the government agreed that screening should remain strictly anonymous and that AIDS should not be nominatively reportable.[139]

The one exception, which reveals the allergic German reaction to such matters, was the Laboratory Reporting Ordinance. This modest and attenuated piece of legislation made it to the books in part as the result of the Bavarians' prodding. They wished for something along Swedish lines, of generally anonymous notification, but with nominative reporting for recalcitrants.[140] In 1987, negotiations between the Christian and Free Democrats over formation of the new coalition government led to the reporting ordinance. Aiming for a statistical overview of the epidemic, it required an anonymous report of infected blood samples, including only age, sex, and the first two numbers of the victim's postal code. This eliminated any reliable coding. Anonymity was complete, but statistical accuracy had been undermined, with no means of excluding multiple reporting of the same case.[141] Since only positive results were registered, there was no way of knowing whether an increase reflected a proportional worsening of the epidemic or merely more tests undertaken. Other than this, and a limited Bavarian pilot study during the early 1990s, reporting was not required. The German authorities were therefore hampered in developing a reliable picture of the epidemic's progress.[142] The state health ministers were reduced to making hapless appeals to hospitals that they report AIDS cases to the Federal Health Office.[143]

Contact tracing, or partner notification, was another venerable technique of contagious disease control. In Sweden, it brought contacts under restrictions similar to those imposed on individuals already known to be infected. In most other countries, it meant merely notifying contacts that they had been exposed to risk. In practical terms, short of applying extreme methods, contact tracing required the patient's cooperation. Yet, the infected could be put under varying degrees of pressure to identify contacts. In Colorado, for example, cease and desist orders prohibited the infected from having sex without warning partners of their serostatus.[144] Contact tracing and its inevitable breach of confidentiality set two classic medical principles at odds: the duty of physicians to treat information gained professionally in confidence and their obligation not to harm others. Shifting the burden to the infected themselves—transforming contact tracing into partner notification—preserved medical confidentiality through an ethical legerdemain on the part of doctors, but only by roping in the patient for these purposes.[145] Generally speaking, having the physician trace contacts (provider referral) was more effective than asking patients to do so (patient referral).[146] Contact tracing thus stood in opposition to strict medical confidentiality. Those favoring ironclad confidentiality argued that, despite the obvious benefits of warning unsuspecting third parties, disrupting the physician-patient relationship meant that the ill would withdraw from treatment, continuing to infect others who could no longer be warned.[147] Those supporting partner notification were unimpressed by this exclusive concern for the patient.

They argued that, since AIDS often spread through specific and knowing actions, each patient posed a potential threat to his or her intimates. Therefore, privacy could not be an absolute.

Tracing made most sense where disease density did not surpass saturation levels. In the gay ghettos of New York or San Francisco, it would have been largely useless, leading from one infected person to practically the entire community by only a degree of sexual separation or two. In areas where gays were less thickly populated, however, a given person might not be aware that he had been exposed, and tracing promised greater payoffs.[148] Contact tracing in shooting galleries also threatened to be a waste of effort.[149] But for women without other risk factors whose partners endangered them, contact tracing held out potentially greater benefits.[150] Indeed, in Denmark, the logical conclusion was drawn in the argument that contact tracing was most appropriate for heterosexuals with fewer sexual contacts.[151] Conversely, the prudent Norwegians pondered the question of whether contact tracing made sense for them. Nordic gays were, so they claimed, less promiscuous than their American brothers.[152] This was also a general problem: people worldwide were more promiscuous now than a century earlier, when contact tracing had first been developed as a preventive technique. Like other drastic interventions, compulsory tracing also threatened to discourage voluntary testing. But as early identification increased in usefulness with the emergence of life-preserving treatments, tracing, like other traditional measures, became appreciated anew.[153]

In American law, physicians had a well-established duty to protect potential victims of dangerous patients. Doctors could be liable in tort for failure to warn family members or others close to contagious patients.[154] In 1987, California enacted a partner notification law allowing physicians to notify spouses of a patient's positive HIV test. A year later, this was limited to patients who refused to do so themselves, but the category of notifiable persons was broadened to include sexual and needle-sharing partners.[155] At the same time, both the American Medical Association and the Presidential Commission on the HIV Epidemic came out in favor of warning AIDS patients' sex partners and other endangered third parties.[156] By the end of the 1980s, approximately fifteen states had some form of partner notification program that went beyond the purely voluntary; by the mid-1990s, more than half of all states did.[157] In February 1988, the CDC made partner notification a condition for states receiving funds from its HIV prevention program; two years later, the CARE Act refused monies to states without such programs.[158]

Similarly, there was a duty of care imposed on the infected that required them to warn others before engaging in potentially transmissive contacts. First broached for syphilis early in the century, and extended to herpes simplex during the 1980s, this obligation now included AIDS.[159] American juries on occasion awarded significant sums for what they considered to be the egregious conduct of not disclosing infection to sex partners. The case of the movie star Rock Hudson is among the best remembered. Many states introduced criminal penalties for failing to inform a sex partner of infection. By using criminal liability in civil cases as evidence that an obligation had been breached, this created, in effect, a duty for the HIV infected to warn or to risk liability to their sex partners.[160] In Florida, the infected were expected to tell partners of their status before sex. In 1992, a seropositive woman in North Carolina was ordered to inform her partners and use condoms. When she nonetheless became pregnant, she was jailed.[161]

The Scandinavians, whose systems of syphilis control had long required contact tracing, were happy to continue such techniques into the current crisis. In Sweden, Finland, and Iceland—but not Norway and Denmark—physicians were required to trace contacts and offer them testing.[162] The Germans inevitably divided along a north-south axis. The Bavarians explicitly required the infected to notify sexual partners and medical personnel. Elsewhere, things were spelled out less clearly. But several high-profile court cases, discussed in chapter 4, holding liable the infected who had sex without informing, made it clear that partner notification was expected.

France, in contrast, had no requirements that seropositives notify partners, and tracing was not mandated.[163] Swiss doctors could not inform third parties without their patient's consent, and seropositives were under no obligation to tell partners, though they might be held liable if they did not use condoms.[164] Nor did the Dutch instigate partner notification or contact tracing.[165] In Britain, the National Health Service (Venereal Disease) Regulations of 1974 required confidentiality in cases of STDs, though they opened a loophole when informing the authorities was necessary to ensure treatment or prevent the spread of disease. In cases where the disease might be transmitted sexually, this allowed telling the spouse of an AIDS patient.[166] In the absence of clear legal guidance, judges determined cases individually as they juggled the conflicting demands of public health and confidentiality. Except on a local basis, contact tracing was not generally pursued, although in the early 1990s, partly in response to a dramatic case of transmission and no tracing, more formalized procedures were instituted. VD clinics kept information on the identity of their patients confidentially, using it for tracing only when others were deemed at serious risk.[167]

CONFIDENTIALITY

During the nineteenth century, the ethical dilemmas of contact tracing and reporting syphilitics had been endlessly discussed. The absurd results of an overly punctilious understanding of medical confidentiality were investigated at length, dramatized to pungent effect in plays like Henrik Ibsen's *Ghosts* (1881) and Eugène Brieux's *Damaged Goods* (1902). Confidentiality had been a cornerstone of an old-fashioned, preinsurance view of the doctor as a private practitioner and a liberal professional with a privileged relationship to his patients. Physicians everywhere had resisted the demands of public health authorities that they help gather information and report patients with dangerous diseases.[168] The medical profession's concern to protect traditional prerogatives also motivated its ambition not to dilute confidentiality during the AIDS epidemic. Then, as now, physicians hoped to avoid becoming informational conduits for public health authorities. They feared alienating patients with the threat of passing information along.[169]

Yet, things had also changed during the intervening century. With the spread of insurance, whether private or social, third-party payers had now muscled in on the once exclusive relationship between physician and patient. Demanding to know what it was they were being asked to underwrite, they undermined the very possibility of confidentiality. With the rise of managed care, insurance bureaucrats were not only granted access to medical decisions. They became part of the therapeutic process itself. As holders of the purse strings, they were the ultimate arbiters of treatment. The political valences of professional secrecy also shifted. In the nineteenth century, it had been unknowing married women, and sometimes wet nurses and other caregivers to syphilitic infants, who were endangered by sexually errant husbands. Confidentiality had then been attacked by progressive opinion as a bulwark of male prerogative and philandering husbands—the medical profession conniving with male dalliance against female fidelity and innocence. In the AIDS era, when the culprit was often the infected gay lover who saw no reason to limit his enjoyment, progressive opinion regarded professional secrecy as protective of privacy and civil liberties, a bulwark against an overly inquisitorial state.

Like nature, appreciated only in the moment of its loss, confidentiality seemed more attractive as it became less possible or even justifiable. It was increasingly seen as a right of patients not to have their health status revealed, as part of their claim to privacy. From having been the aggressor, the infected patient became the victim. The self-proclaimed voice of progress in Germany, the Green Party, and the AIDS Enquête Commission, for example, wanted to expand the already long list of professions granted immunity from testifying in court to include employees of AIDS counseling centers. Drug addicts and others who might otherwise fear being reported would thus be encouraged to use such facilities. Expanding professional secrecy meant protecting individual rights.[170] Conversely, it was often conservatives who argued that confidentiality should be tempered to weigh the interests of the community over those of the individual.[171] The temptation to allow breaches of medical confidentiality was also heightened when the issue was posed, as was now often the case, as a balancing between the interests of a drug-addicted criminal and the police or medical personnel he had wounded. As one Swedish conservative asked, was it reasonable to insist on strict secrecy so that the police officer might not know whether he had been harmed?[172]

A cynic might be tempted to argue that confidentiality had been defended in the nineteenth century, when men's interests were pitted against women's, but that support softened when the opposition was not so clearly defined along gender lines, and when men could be found as both infectors and infectees. Less jaded observers might note that more stigma attached to AIDS, with the high likelihood that the infected were homosexuals or injecting drug addicts, than to syphilis in its era, when infection had revealed mainly that the patient was a functioning heterosexual. There was more at stake in confidentiality now than earlier. Most modern statutes that permitted a breach of confidentiality also shifted the focus from the nineteenth century's obsession with the marital union, to include a broader range of epidemiologically relevant contacts. They allowed a weighing of the interests of patients and, on the other hand, those who might have had contact with them, including fellow addicts, sexual partners other than spouses (including the victims of sexual assault), medical and law enforcement personnel, embalmers, and so forth.

As during the nineteenth century, the importance of medical confidentiality varied among nations, strictly upheld in some, laxer in others. The World Medical Assembly, meeting in Madrid in 1987, adopted a resolution allowing physicians to abandon confidentiality and alert the authorities if a patient appeared to endanger others.[173] Yet not all countries followed this advice. Some nations interpreted confidentiality absolutely. In Denmark, a seropositive husband's unwillingness to inform his pregnant wife did not seem reason enough to make an exception to secrecy, though such attitudes changed in the early 1990s. In the Netherlands, confidentiality remained an inviolable principle even when infected patients continued having sex with unsuspecting partners. In France, informing the sexual partner of a seropositive was denounced as treachery. Conversely, the Swiss civil code had anchored a duty of spouses to disclose upon important issues. A seropositive was obliged to reveal his status to his spouse, though whether it would require testing after risky behavior was debated.[174]

In the United States, confidentiality was, comparatively speaking, weakly interpreted and enforced. Partly this was a characteristic shared with the British legal tradition. Partly it may have reflected the powerful influence of lawyers. The legal and medical professions were continually engaged in an antagonistic pas de deux stretching back at least to the first wave of medical malpractice suits in the 1840s.[175] Confidentiality was rooted in the common law principle that physicians had a duty not to disclose information and in the constitutional right to privacy. *Whalen v. Roe* (1977) was interpreted by federal circuit courts to give a constitutionally protected right to privacy of medical records. Not every state, however, had laws on medical confidentiality, and those on the books were a mélange of differing rules. Thirty-three states had legislation specifically prohibiting disclosure of HIV-related information about patients without their consent.[176] There was, in contrast, no federal confidentiality law protecting HIV test results, though the Americans with Disabilities Act did provide some protection for medical records relating to employment. The Medical Records Confidentiality Bill, introduced to Congress in 1995, sought to strengthen such protection but failed to become law.[177]

Confidentiality was thus far from absolute. Early in the nineteenth century, American courts and legislatures had adopted legal norms that imposed on physicians a duty to inform, though with the decline of infectious diseases by midcentury such requirements had lost much of their urgency. Already in 1796, New York State required doctors to report the names of infectious patients, though the measure does not appear to have been enforced.[178] Two centuries later, the Tarasoff case of 1976 nailed fast the principle that physicians' duties to avoid potential harm to third parties outweighed the confidential nature of their relationship to patients.[179] "The protective privilege ends," as the California Supreme Court put it in a weighing of the classic public health dilemma between individual and community, "where the public peril begins."[180] Some states did adopt the Tarasoff doctrine, and confidentiality statutes were often relaxed to allow physicians to warn. And yet, the doctrine of physicians' mandatory disclosure to threatened parties was not widely enacted during the AIDS era, largely in fear that its effects would be counterproductive. Of the twenty-one states that passed legislation on the matter during the late 1980s, only two allowed for mandatory notification. The California Health and Safety Code, which formulated a strict definition of confidentiality and foresaw criminal penalties for disclosure of HIV status to third parties, was amended in 1987, but only to allow disclosure to a patient's spouse. A year later, it was broadened to include all sexual partners. New York State's confidentiality law of 1988 carefully limited the circumstances under which physicians could warn endangered third parties.[181] On the other hand, spouses who had not been informed of their partner's infection could sue for damages.[182]

The British had little explicit legislation on medical confidentiality.[183] Disclosure to third parties was considered a matter for the responsible physician and was normally contingent on the patient's consent.[184] On the other hand, British physicians could not, as in France, refuse to testify in court. Medical secrecy was considered subordinate to the public interest, and prosecution of crime was generally deemed the higher good. As in the United States, the right to confidentiality was not absolute. Exceptions came in the form of court orders, other legal duties, and limited instances required by the public interest (as in the investigation of serious crime or a health risk to others). The General Medical Council, the organization that registered physicians, thought that confidential information could be disclosed when dangers to specific persons were posed. In 1985, the British Medical Association ruled that physicians could tell a spouse or lover of their partner's AIDS diagnosis even without consent.[185] The National Health Service (Venereal Diseases) Regulations of 1974 specifically allowed sharing health data when necessary to prevent the spread of infection. Government policy on the confidentiality of HIV tests also allowed disclosure to prevent the spread of infection, with such circumstances to be judged by the attending physician.[186]

Added to problems of medical confidentiality was the broader question of privacy. During the mid-1980s, the concept of privacy began to be recognized as a right in common law, and at the beginning of the new millennium the European Human Rights Convention expanded its protection in Britain.[187] The 1988 Access to Medical Records Act was an ad hoc piece of legislation. Originating in the absence of government initiatives as a private member's bill, it sought to address some of the privacy problems caused by the epidemic—in particular the reports from patients' personal physicians requested by insurance company underwriters.[188] Nonetheless, in the absence of any law of privacy, information that elsewhere was considered confidential was still distributed on the open market in Britain. As late as 1992, insurance companies asked applicants whether they had received blood products from abroad or had sexual relationships with foreign residents. Gays were asked whether they were in a stable relationship and how many partners they had had over the past two years.[189]

In Sweden, the issue was regulated in the Secrecy Act of 1980. This foresaw exceptions to medical confidentiality as part of fulfilling official duties, where other statutes required release of information and for certain crimes and emergency situations. The epidemic now prompted changes. The old, stricter, approach to professional secrecy impeded the fight against HIV, the government argued, and a "breakthrough in confidentiality" was required. Drug-addicted prostitutes who continued to ply their trade though infected were especially worrisome. Disease transmission by such individuals would not be tolerated, the minister of social affairs warned. Their confidentiality protections were to be valued lower than the threat they posed to others. In 1986, matters were loosened up specifically for HIV as authorities were granted new powers of collecting and sharing information on seropositives who did not follow behavioral prescriptions. The aim was to allow a pooling of data to ensure enforcement of public health regulations, especially among drug addicts, whose unpredictable lifestyle hindered compliance.[190]

In Germany, the right to privacy, or informational self-determination, was anchored in the Basic Law. Confidentiality was an issue colored by its coincidence with a major political battle during the mid-1980s over the national census.[191] In certain respects, confidentiality was strictly protected. Physicians were on the long list of occupations with a right to refuse to testify in court. Since AIDS was not a notifiable illness, physicians were not required to report it either to the authorities or third parties. The penal code forbade physicians from revealing medical information without authorization. What determined authorization, however, depended on the circumstances. Emergencies justified disclosure, and it was commonly accepted that protecting a seropositive's healthy partner could outweigh a patient's right to confidentiality. Physicians had the right (and, some argued, the duty) to warn endangered third parties, especially if they had first sought to convince their patient to act nontransmissively.[192]

As in the nineteenth century, France remained among the nations most concerned to uphold medical confidentiality.[193] This inherited emphasis on physicians' prerogatives, the inviolability of the private relationship between professional and client, was now continued, surprisingly unchanged, into the twentieth century. Indeed, so absolutely was confidentiality interpreted that patients were among those not to be told of their condition, unless a third party would thereby be put at risk. In 1984, when the philosopher Michel Foucault died, it was still common for French doctors not to inform their patients of what they suffered.[194] This mentality, which existed independently for other diseases like cancer, was extended also to AIDS in part because, in the mid-1980s, many physicians still believed that not all seropositives developed the full-blown disease. Why worry them, so the paternalist logic went, when only some would actually become ill? Daniel Defert, Foucault's partner, was motivated to found AIDES, the main French AIDS organization, in part to end this state of affairs, giving patients the chance to dispose of what time remained to them.[195]

With respect to others as well, confidentiality was interpreted strictly. With a few exceptions, like child abuse and other sexual violence, it remained absolute.[196] Contact tracing, with its inevitable breach of confidentiality, was rejected as a dead end by the onetime head of the French agency devoted to fighting AIDS. When the American Medical Association decided to allow partner notification, its French colleagues worried lest this mean betraying the profession's most sacred tenets.[197] AIDES supported the right not to have patients' secrets revealed even for seropositives who took no precautions to prevent transmission. Sexual contacts could not be informed by anyone other than the infected themselves. Just as in the nineteenth century, physicians were enjoined from informing patients' spouses, even at the request of the patient.[198] In 1994, the Academy of Medicine recommended reforms, but only allowing the patient to release his physician from confidentiality. It added a few other changes, such as telling the father of a seropositive newborn, even though this meant revealing the mother's affliction. It also gingerly suggested that perhaps physicians should be permitted to warn third parties on their own initiative. This would have brought France only to the starting point of most other nations. But even that was considered too far. The National AIDS Council rejected such changes with the usual arguments about driving the infected underground. Not even the AIDS epidemic justified changing the rules of confidentiality: so ran the conclusion of a report delivered to the minister of health; she agreed, and nothing changed.[199]

DEFENDING THE RAMPARTS

Among the most venerable measures of contagious disease prevention were screenings of outsiders and quarantining of the suspected. Much as the first germ panics were associated—especially in the United States—with the turn-of-the-century wave of immigration from southern and eastern Europe, so current concerns coincided with a new era of mass migration.[200]

Quarantines could be imposed internally, by cutting off infected places. But usually they restricted the movement of travelers. Screening foreigners and limiting the access of the infected made sense only from the parochial vantage of any given country hoping to remain off the map of microbial peregrination. As a public health strategy, such measures deliberately ignored the broader, transnational aspects of epidemics. International health organizations, above all the World Health Organization, therefore—and almost by definition—rejected testing travelers or certifying visitors.[201] Nonetheless, and despite their obvious limitations, quarantine and the exclusion of foreigners (or natives returning from abroad) were widely adopted, especially early in the epidemic. Several, if admittedly less developed, nations—Cuba, Iran, Iraq, Libya, Saudi Arabia, Syria, China, the Soviet Union, and post-Communist Russia, among others—sought to hold the disease at bay by restricting the access of foreigners other than tourists, screening long-term alien residents, and testing returning nationals.[202]

This was not a wholly irrational response, even as applied to a disease like AIDS, with its long latency and lifelong presence, and despite the disfunctionalities of quarantine in the modern world, with its Brownian motion of countless carriers across frontiers. Nations that, early on, were still free of the disease had reason to limit access. But only some were in a geoepidemiological position to do so. Cuba sought to hinder entry of infected outsiders and to isolate its own citizens who returned diseased from abroad—especially military advisors to Africa. Given the discount of individual liberty in its official ideology, this was both rational and politically feasible. Cuba, after all, had relatively few drug problems and open homosexuality was rare. The most common risk factor was sexual relations with a foreigner, either directly or at one remove.[203] Similarly, it was arguably rational for the Soviet Union (as for the other East Bloc nations that followed suit) to require HIV tests of long-term visitors, since a majority of early cases were found among such individuals. Bulgaria, for example, reported that 42 percent of its AIDS cases were among international seafarers.[204] More debatable was the accuracy of the claim, made in 1994 by a Russian deputy, that sexual contact with a foreigner was now a hundred times more dangerous than with a native.[205]

Much like the Austrian plague wall against the Ottoman Empire during the seventeenth and eighteenth centuries, the Iron Curtain played an incidental role for a while as a cordon sanitaire for the East Bloc. The Berlin Wall was described by one wag as the world's largest condom.[206] The absence of a drug and gay scene in East Germany during the mid-1980s, at least in the form of transmissive hot spots like bathhouses and sex tourism, meant that the epidemic spread more slowly than in the West. The lack of convertible currency blessedly spared hemophiliacs from tainted imported blood products.[207] Swedes and Danes too regarded themselves as threatened from the outside, with over half of heterosexual transmission cases having been infected abroad. Finland—remote, isolated, and with a highly restrictive immigration policy—thought itself able to control the epidemic by such tactics.[208] There were even American proponents of excluding seropositive foreigners from the nation that was, in fact, the major developed exporter of HIV. Their peculiar logic was bolstered by the argument that keeping out the infected might prevent ingress of the HIV-2 strain, prevalent in certain parts of Africa, apparently more easily spread via heterosexual intercourse and thus more dangerous.[209]

In all, at least forty-eight countries imposed HIV testing for certain entrants, sometimes contingent on the length of the intended stay, other times on their occupation or other allegedly relevant personal characteristics. In Cyprus, cabaret artists were tested; Egypt, in contrast, screened defense contractors. In South Korea, foreigners intending to stay long-term were tested, while artists and sports figures accompanied by their spouses were exempted.[210] The French, much like the Cubans, tested soldiers returning from specific African countries and from French Guiana. The South Africans, in restricting the entry of seropositives in 1987, aimed mainly at migrant mine workers from neighboring states.[211] In Norway, 244 Africans were found to be seropositive in the mid-1990s; almost a hundred were deported or had residence permits denied.[212] Testing foreign students was motivated by similar hopes of preventing the epidemic but also, for those on scholarships, by a chilling Benthamite calculation: to keep scarce resources for those most likely to make productive use of them. The screening of applicants to the Job Corps, an employment program for poor youths in the United States, was analogous in its purpose. In Syria and Poland all foreign students were tested, in Belgium only students from central Africa on scholarships, and in Spain and India all African students.[213] In Germany, mainly African students holding certain scholarships underwent screening and in some cases were tested without their knowledge as part of general health examinations. Some were deported.[214]

Many nations required those seeking permanent abode to be free of HIV infection—Chile and Costa Rica, for example. Australia allowed immigration officials broad discretion to keep out foreigners seeking to stay longer than twelve months. After reforms in 1989 this was largely eliminated for seropositives. On the other hand, all applicants for residence permits were now required to undergo HIV testing. There was no official policy on tourist visas, and on occasion they were refused to seropositives. The Finns required screening of anyone intending to stay more than three months, and of foreign workers and students, with provision for the expulsion of seropositive aliens. Canadian law required medical examination of immigrants and, apparently, held the possibility of excluding the infected and ill.[215]

In Germany two levels of legislation complicated matters. National legislation regulated the presence of foreigners who threatened the public health, while the individual states established criteria for residence. On the federal level, foreigners who represented a risk could be turned back. Prostitutes and drug addicts, for example, could be refused entry on this basis, without the need to demonstrate their infection. In 1987, controversy erupted when the border police were issued instructions reminding them that they were authorized to deny entry to foreigners suspected of HIV infection. A supplement, emphasizing that one could not tell by visual inspection alone whether a traveler was ill or infected, was intended to limit arbitrary decisions by the police. But it was not forwarded to those actually manning the frontiers. The government had clearly blundered in seeking to control HIV at the frontiers. It was rewarded for its misstep by quick and intemperate reactions from the parties of the center and left. At the same time, its examples of how the law might be used indicated that the authorities had no intention of allowing in just any seropositive. An African businessman who was known from the newspapers to have infected several people in Belgium, should not, it was argued, be allowed entry. In 1987, eight AIDS or HIV-infected foreigners were identified at the frontier, usually because of what they themselves said or from evidence in their possession. Four of them (one Senegalese, one Austrian, and two Swiss citizens) were turned back.[216]

At the second level of legislation, individual German states required health examinations before allowing foreigners to stay longer than three months. But what these tests included varied. The Bavarians required a HIV test and could deny permission if it were positive. Other states had similar powers.[217] Both levels of restriction were, however, also governed by supranational law. European Union (EU) citizens could not be denied residence because of HIV infection, although they could be for certain other diseases (active tuberculosis, syphilis) or if their conduct threatened transmission. Nor could asylum seekers claiming political persecution, although they could for acting in ways judged to be irresponsible and dangerous—for example, by having unprotected sex if infected.[218] In vain, the Bavarians sought authorization to deny seropositive EU citizens residence, since a distinction between EU and other foreigners made little epidemiological sense. Foreigners were on occasion expelled from Germany for HIV infection, mainly students from Africa on scholarships. In 1986, immigration authorities seeking to deport a Philippino woman, infected by her German husband and now widowed, lost on appeal.[219]

In a bizarre revival of medieval municipal corporatism, the Austrian city of Klagenfurt required foreigners to certify their seronegativity for residence permits.[220] *Stadtluft macht gesund.* In France, foreigners from outside the EU could be refused residence if they suffered from certain contagious diseases, or if they were drug abusers or severely mentally retarded. In 1987, it was decided, however, that they could not be required to undergo HIV testing unless they presented clinical AIDS symptoms, and that seropositivity alone was not cause for denial of residence, though full-blown AIDS could be.[221] In Sweden, despite demands that access be denied to foreigners unable to prove they were uninfected, nothing was done. Voluntary tests were made available on behalf of parents of adoptive children from abroad. Asylum seekers were also offered testing, though the seropositive were not repatriated. No doubt there was an element of informal pressure, since they were hardly in a position to be uncooperative.[222] Having instituted rigorous controls domestically, Sweden evidently believed that defenses at the border did not have to bristle quite so menacingly.

In Britain, an absence of formal regulations on HIV combined with administrative discretion at the frontier. Though students were mentioned as a special concern, nothing targeting them in particular seems to have been instituted. Port medical inspectors had wide latitude on admitting foreigners. When arriving long-term aliens mentioned health or medical reasons as the cause of their visit, or appeared to be in ill health, the authorities looked more closely. They could refuse admission to victims of dangerous communicable disease, determine whether their ailments precluded maintaining themselves, and estimate their ability to cover medical expenses. As part of this medical examination, foreigners could be screened for HIV antibodies and refused entry.[223] Though there were early instances of the infected being sent back, the government's position was that HIV infection was not reason alone to refuse entry. The requirement that foreigners cover their own medical costs was used only sparingly to block access.[224] This combination of official laissez-faire with the ability to deny entry meant that widely divergent interpretations of British policy were possible, from self-congratulation for avoiding the restrictive American approach, to the conviction that they had imposed drastic restrictions.[225]

Though there were variations—from the hands-off approach of the French and Swedes to the controls kept in reserve by the British and Germans—most European nations were relatively liberal in allowing infected foreigners access. The United States, in contrast, levied the most drastic controls in the Western industrialized world. Given that the country admitted more immigrants than all other developed nations combined, and that the epidemic coincided with a new wave of immigration unprecedented since the late nineteenth century, the issue was posed in particularly acute terms here. Some observers were surprised that the United States, allegedly liberal in its prophylactic instincts, adopted policies similar to those imposed in autocracies, dictatorships, and various Third World nations. Americans themselves were often aghast at how widely their country's policies differed from those of nations usually regarded as its peers.[226] Indeed, testing foreigners occasioned spectacular conflicts among industrialized nations, leading to the threatened and partly fulfilled boycott of the 1990 Sixth International AIDS Conference in San Francisco. Large-scale defection was avoided only by the Bush administration's last-minute tactical tergiversations. Following successful protests against American immigration and travel restrictions for seropositives, the 1992 conference was then shifted from Cambridge to Amsterdam.[227] While others may be surprised to hear the French congratulate themselves for persuading the Americans to moderate their policies, clearly international outrage was not without effect, though it was ultimately unable to offset countervailing domestic factors.[228] Among these was the way such screening of immigrants, far from being a peculiar tactic adopted in this particular case, in fact continued long-standing American traditions.

Diseases that already precluded immigration to the United States included five STDs, infectious leprosy, and active tuberculosis. In 1987, AIDS was included on this list.[229] The addition of AIDS (and later infection with HIV) was brokered in a political horse trade. The Public Health Service and the CDC supported it, while Jesse Helms, the conservative senator from North Carolina, made his support for providing AZT to needy patients contingent on expanding the list of excludable diseases. The Senate backed the change unanimously, partly because it had the blessing of the Public Health Service and partly because it believed that only immigration, not all travel, was affected. In 1989, the implications of the new policy became glaringly apparent when a Dutch seropositive en route to a conference was denied entrance, sparking international and domestic outrage.[230] When the issue flared up again during preparations for the 1990 AIDS conference in San Francisco, the Bush administration sought to parry criticism with various fine tunings: preserving the confidentiality of foreigners' medical information, avoiding permanent markings in seropositives' passports, and the like. In fact, such adjustments did not touch the heart of the matter: that foreigners, even those simply seeking tourist visas, could be tested and barred if infected.

In 1990, after the presidential commission had recommended rethinking the policy, the Immigration Act redefined the medical exclusion so as to bar persons only if they had a "communicable disease of public health significance," and not one considered to be a "dangerous contagious disease." In February of that year, the CDC recommended that AIDS and diseases other than infectious tuberculosis be removed from the list that barred entry. In January of 1991, Louis Sullivan, secretary of the Department of Health and Human Services, agreed. This emerging consensus was torpedoed, however, by protests led by Republican Congressmen William Dannemeyer and Dana Rohrabacher and TV evangelists, in the form of forty thousand letters. The Department of Justice, with jurisdiction over the Immigration and Naturalization Service (INS), objected to eliminating AIDS from the list, too, because it had not been sufficiently consulted. Though even President George H. W. Bush favored removing AIDS, in the end policy remained unchanged. Seropositives continued to be barred from permanent residence and could visit temporarily only with special permission. The INS began conducting the largest required HIV-testing program in the world. Annually, close to half a million immigrants, nonimmigrants, and refugees were tested. In addition, some 2.5 million aliens already present were required to undergo screening to qualify for legal residence.[231]

In practice, however, the policy was to maintain testing for immigrants while dropping it, except in special cases, for temporary visitors. Visitors, including even long-term students, were not routinely screened, though they were asked to indicate their HIV status on visa applications. But immigration officers could require a test if there was reason to suspect infection.[232] Approximately three hundred to six hundred seropositive aliens were denied admittance to the United States annually. Though this meant fewer potential sources of infection, it made little practical difference in a nation with one million seropositive residents already.[233] Besides the controversies already mentioned occasioned by this American *Sonderweg*, such policies put the United States in the continually embarrassing position of having to make exceptions to the ban on infected foreigners. In 1994, participants in the Gay Games in New York were given blanket waivers, only to have them retracted after protest from conservatives. It also sparked exclusionary reprisals—as when Indonesia refused to allow Magic Johnson to play in an exhibition basketball game.[234]

The policy spectrum regarding access of foreigners was thus as wide as for other tactics used against the AIDS epidemic, ranging from the laissez-faire approach of France and Sweden to the mass screenings imposed in America. The range of responses can be understood only by placing the specific issue of admitting infected travelers in the broader context of the rules and regulations governing access to nations. One problem was tourism, by some measures the world's third largest industry. Did border controls threaten it? Europe especially, host to over two-thirds of international tourists, and a region that increasingly preserved in aspic its past glories for outside consumption, had to heed such concerns. Would tourism suffer from restrictions at the frontiers? In cities like Amsterdam, the gay-tourist guilder was nearly as important a source of income as the usual specimen of discretionary currency and helped temper overly drastic restrictions.[235] The colonial past of different countries was another issue. The Belgians were especially worried about transmission from Africa, not just because their former colonies encompassed the most afflicted sub-Saharan regions (Burundi, Rwanda, and Zaire), but also because they maintained dense social and sexual connections with the ex-colonies.[236]

More important still was the issue of access in general. The United States imposed public health restrictions, as it had since the nineteenth century, precisely because immigration was large and increasing. The European nations, in contrast, had choked off immigration much more thoroughly. "Fortress Europe," the idea that all access had been shut down, was an exaggeration. The market for both cheap, unskilled labor and computer expertise still sucked in workers from abroad. And yet the numbers were lower than across the Atlantic. Immigration in the American sense of the word had been shut down starting with the oil crisis of the 1970s, leaving only the avenue of asylum-seeking, which was increasingly force-fed by the new waves of transmigration during the 1980s.[237] The result was, to put it baldly, that what remained an issue for the public health authorities in America was effectively transferred to the immigration police in Europe. With sharp restrictions imposed on ingress for reasons extraneous to public health, the need for screening and other forms of access limitation was lessened in Europe, and, in any case, it was sufficiently covered by the measures applied to the few immigrants allowed in.

Also, most foreign entrants among the European nations were EU nationals. Whatever the wishes of local zealots like the Bavarians, EU citizens could not be excluded under supranational law. It is therefore not the case that the Americans imposed restrictions on the entry of foreigners while the Europeans did not. More accurately, they each did so, though in different ways. Both allowed seropositives in as visitors, and neither as immigrants. What the Europeans were protesting in American strictures, the cynic might argue, was not that limitations were imposed on foreigners as such, but that they were imposed on them.

4. Patients into Prisoners

Responsibility, Crime, and Health

AIDS is a disease that was spread, at first in the developed world, mainly by conscious, though rarely intentional, behavior. Questions of individual responsibility and liability, both moral and legal, were vital. The infected often transmitted disease by actions they could have avoided. How could they be discouraged before the fact? How could they be punished afterward? Criminal and civil law, not just public health, were seen as part of the solution in all developed nations. The penal and civil codes were used to control transmissive behaviors and to hold transgressors liable. Indeed, in certain respects, the criminal law helped the accused by including more procedural protections of individual rights (such as clear determination in court whether crimes had been committed, and sentences of specified duration) than public health law, where, in extreme cases, quarantine or hospitalization could be indefinite.[1]

Whether use of criminal and civil law made sense for HIV transmission was, nonetheless, hotly debated. During the eighteenth and nineteenth centuries, criminal law commonly had been deployed to regulate behavior deemed unsociable, obnoxious, or immoral, and not just illegal.[2] During the twentieth century, in contrast, citizens were socialized into appropriate epidemiological conduct. In effect, behavioral restrictions were imposed "voluntarily" by individuals on themselves, thereby reducing the role of official prescriptions codified in law and enforced by uniformed authority.[3] And yet formal external control had in no sense been wholly abandoned. Though the distinction between law and morality had widened during the twentieth century, the two still overlapped, whether in legislation that regulated inebriants, restricted smoking, prohibited gambling, or outlawed certain sexual acts. In some senses, lawlike regulation was used increasingly, counteracting the trend toward informal control: in reintroducing sartorial codes, say, that banned gang insignia in California schools and Muslim head coverings in Parisian ones; in codifying sexual conduct in the workplace or relations between adults and minors ever more minutely; in hemming in free speech with codes of verbal etiquette.[4] Indeed, as public health aimed at chronic diseases caused by modern lifestyles and thereby focused on behavioral change, the logic of discouraging certain conduct strengthened, not only through public education campaigns, but also in the fine-tuned paragraphs of the penal code.

Occasionally, the penal code had been used effectively to modify dangerous behavior: seat-belt and motorcycle helmet laws, for instance. Here compliance could be easily monitored and the results measured for effectiveness. In other respects, the penal code was largely symbolic, especially where common opinion held morality to be the governing code. Laws punishing adultery were useless, though they remained on the books with surprising longevity—up until 1942 in Sweden, for example. Even more absurdly, fornication remained an offense in forty American states in 1965, fifteen in 1987, nine today. Prohibitions of sodomy, both anal and oral, also remained on the books in America and abroad.[5]

Whether legal intervention could reduce potentially transmissive behavior, however, remained an open question. For diseases such as tuberculosis, cholera, plague, or smallpox, where exhalation, expectoration, or excretion transmitted the illness, it was hard to hold individuals liable. Yet there was a logic to punishing the infected who exposed others. Everyday actions that cost the ill little, and the public potentially a great deal more, could in this way be discouraged. Did the same hold for diseases spread by purposive and voluntary acts in situations of intimacy beyond the state's ken? The question had been hotly debated for syphilis during the nineteenth century, especially whether to prosecute actual transmission alone or mere endangerment as well.[6] Criminalizing exposure of others to other contagious diseases was common. In Britain, smallpox victims could not appear in public, use public transportation, or check out library books. Herpes had provided a more recent dress rehearsal for such issues. In the United States during the 1980s, the knowing transmission of herpes was found actionable, and a legal duty to abstain from sex or warn potential partners was imposed on the infected.[7]

Ignoring for the moment rape and perinatal transmission, such illnesses were spread largely through voluntary and conscious behavior. Should the authorities seek to discourage transmissive conduct or rely on voluntary self-protection? Was it the state's duty to guarantee that your sex partner was uninfected or your shooting needle clean? Was it likely, especially with a fatal disease like AIDS, that people would act more circumspectly if threatened with legal sanctions?[8] More technically, the window period between transmission and the formation of antibodies was so long that, barring the development of tests to detect the virus itself, assigning responsibility for transmission was difficult. Infected with a lethal disease, perpetrators were unlikely to serve their sentences or, in civil cases, to offer much restitution. AIDS's long latency period meant that the statute of limitations would often have expired in the interim. The principle of adequacy required that it should be possible for the action prosecuted to accomplish the effect imputed to it. This shed doubt on whether biting or spitting were criminally liable actions, since the likelihood of transmission was small.[9] Murder or bodily harm were crimes hard to prove, as they required evidence that the perpetrator had had sex, or shared needles, with the intent of killing the victim—years later. Indeed, the entire issue of intent was nebulous in HIV transmission. As one observer put it, having sex is a highly indirect modus operandi for a murderer.[10] Reckless, negligent, or attempted homicide or harm were crimes more likely to result in conviction.[11] And yet some observers still argued that criminalizing sodomy promised to reduce HIV transmission.[12]

Exposing others to the risk of HIV transmission was rarely prosecuted. By the nature of the act, unless infection resulted, the victim would often not even be aware that a crime had been committed. If infection did follow, it was still difficult to prove that the perpetrator had been infected at the time and knew it. The most general argument against criminalizing transmission or endangerment was that—ignoring rape, which existing statutes already punished—no one had to engage in risky behavior. Prophylaxis should therefore center on personal protection rather than on enforcing specific behavior through the legal code.[13] On the other hand, because potentially transmissive actions were purposive and deliberate—to the extent not caused by instincts beyond control, whether sex or addiction—the actors could be held responsible. As widespread educational and media campaigns were mobilized against the epidemic, transmissive behavior could no longer be excused as the result of ignorance and might justly be targeted for prosecution. Though criminalization might not have much of a practical effect, society thereby drew a line in the sand. The legal code served to reinforce ethical values. At a minimum, it offered leverage against reckless perpetrators who knowingly and callously exposed others to danger. In turn, civil law held out, at least for those victims who survived long enough, a promise of financial compensation and not just the pleasure of seeing justice done.[14]

Measures like criminalizing transmission or endangerment were an intermediate step between the extremes of compulsion and laissez-faire. Isolating the infectious would have been a more direct and effective means of preventing them from transmitting. Criminalization tackled the same problem only indirectly. It assumed implicitly that most citizens could be expected to behave so as to minimize transmission, that there would be only a few recalcitrants to worry about.[15] Use of the criminal code also presupposed other tactics that in some nations were ruled out. As long as medical confidentiality restricted the authorities' ability to identify the infected, and if nominative reporting was not common practice, the criminal code was hobbled. In the most general sense, if AIDS prevention rested on cooperating with the infected, then the repression implicit in the criminal law threatened to counteract such tactics, driving victims away from efforts to reach them voluntarily.[16] The potentially dysfunctional effect on voluntary testing of possible prosecution was the classic case.

To convict for transmissive behavior, it had to be shown that perpetrators knew of their serostatus. This put a legal premium on not knowing whether one was infected, and it was thus a disincentive to voluntary testing. Such were the concerns when Senator Helms sought to punish seropositive medical personnel who failed to disclose their status before operating.[17] Such was the result when the main German AIDS organization, the Deutsche AIDS-Hilfe, reacted to the 1988 German Supreme Court decision—to allow punishing seropositives who had unprotected sex with uninformed partners—by recommending against voluntary HIV testing altogether.[18] Similarly, in Norway, voluntary testing declined after the justice minister announced that the penal code might be used against seropositives.[19] American courts hoped to avoid this problem by not requiring actual knowledge of infection to find potentially transmissive conduct liable. If an individual ought to have known of possible risks because of past activities, ignorance was inadmissible as a defense. Thus, the courts could impose a duty to test on those at risk so as to determine whether they were, in fact, infected.[20] This, of course, solved the problem only—if at all—by an even more drastic invasion of individual liberties, and required a legal determination of which risky behaviors obliged voluntary testing: all anal sex between males, or only that with strangers, for example? Another instance of potential dysfunctions concerned abortion. If the transmission of HIV perinatally were also criminalized, the likelihood of seropositive mothers aborting might well increase.[21]

Nonetheless, whatever the difficulties of controlling transmissive behavior by law, there remained instances of conduct that everyone agreed should be punished. Some of these were AIDS variants of urban myths. In the 1980s, modernized stories of revenge infections reemerged, tales recounted by Boccaccio in the *Decameron*'s account of the plague in fourteenth-century Florence, and later by Daniel Defoe for sixteenth-century London. Chief among these contemporary myths was the persistent story—told both in gay and straight versions—of a nocturnal pickup, of anonymous sex sufficiently vigorous to raise the audience's moralistic hackles, and then the morning-after message (in lipstick on the mirror or some other suitably theatrical medium): "Welcome to the AIDS club."[22] And yet, whatever the exaggerations of such stories, consider the cases that most would agree deserved censure: the epidemic's Typhoid Marvin, Gaetan Dugas, the spectacularly promiscuous and conscienceless airline steward who disseminated HIV transcontinentally; the man who injected his son with seropositive blood to avoid paying child support; the physician who infected his former girlfriend when she ended their relationship; the seropositive who injected his girlfriend with his blood for having drunk the last sip of his cola; or the infected man who knowingly had unprotected sex with up to three hundred women, some as young as thirteen.[23]

Different nations took various approaches to such monsters of the epidemic. Theorists working in code-based legal traditions performed feats of definitional hairsplitting, hoping to clear up the concepts before many cases presented themselves. How much responsibility could the victim of infection resulting from consensual sex be expected to bear? Should an act of transmission be considered bodily harm, or (since the disease was eventually fatal) attempted manslaughter? If HIV caused damage, was it harm to body or to health? How to determine whether a transmitter had intended actually to kill, to convey an illness, or merely to enjoy someone carnally with no forethought? Could seropositivity be an illness in terms of health insurance (thus permitting treatment) but not in terms of labor law (thus not allowing termination of employment)?[24] In Germany entire legal schools did battle over such issues as whether transmission, or even just (what only a lawyer could describe as) the intercorporeal emission of seropositive ejaculate, could be seen as a purposive attempt to bring about death through sex, and more generally whether the penal code had a role to play in combating the epidemic.[25] In 1988–89 a lower court—later overruled—exonerated a seropositive of bodily harm for repeated consensual sex with a woman. It reasoned that, even had she been infected, seropositivity did not damage her health because she would have felt fine in the immediate aftermath, and because, as a willing partner, she bore part of the responsibility. In France, the penal code's strictures on bodily harm resulting in incapacity to work were considered inapplicable to HIV transmission because the newly infected would be capable of employment. During the late 1980s, American courts debated whether asymptomatic seropositives suffered measurable impairment and whether they could be considered handicapped.[26] Perhaps the adjective *dismal* has been applied to the wrong science.

Despite their markedly different legal traditions, Germany and the United States used criminal law most heavily, providing sanctions against transmissive behavior.[27] Yet all nations put their penal codes to use. All had provisions for bodily injury, sometimes specifically focused on actions like poisoning, that could in theory be used against the knowing transmission of contagious disease.[28] In Denmark in 1994, the penal code specifically targeted those who endangered others with life-threatening and incurable disease. Though in 1985 Sweden abolished the provision in the Contagious Disease Law punishing sex while knowingly infected, prosecutions for bodily harm were possible under the penal code. During the early 1990s, lower courts sentenced seropositives to significant jail terms for having sex without informing their partners. Because Swedish law required that seropositives be issued behavioral prescriptions to reduce the risk of transmission, convicting violators was easier than in nations where ignorance provided a more plausible defense.[29] In France, however, transmission of and endangerment with VD were not outlawed until 1960, and then only indirectly, in that the infected who shunned treatment could be punished, the crime being the refusal. Though it was argued that the penal code's strictures on bodily harm and homicide might be applied to HIV transmission, attempts to enshrine this in law failed. On occasion, however, the infected were prosecuted. In Metz in 1993, a seropositive woman who had not informed her companion was charged with involuntary homicide; in Mulhouse in 1992 a seropositive who had bitten a policeman was convicted.[30]

In Britain, the 1861 Act Relating to Offenses against the Person concerned wounding or harming, but not directly via disease transmission. In *R. v. Clarence* (1897), a man who had knowingly infected his wife with gonorrhea was found not guilty under the statute because their sex had been consensual, and thus not assaultive, though with her ignorance of his sickness. Despite hopes that the act's section on poisoning might be used against transmission, little resulted.[31] Not until the summer of 1992, with the case of an infected hemophiliac who may have sought deliberately to infect his sex partners, was there much concern for possible criminal charges. Then, in *R. v. Brown and Ors* (1992), men who had engaged in consensual sadomasochistic acts resulting in minor injuries were convicted under the act, and the possibility opened that seropositives having had consensual sex might be subject to prosecution.[32] In 1992, the Law Commission, seeking to codify the criminal law, aimed to include transmission in the criminal code's concept of "causing injury," thus avoiding the problem inherited from the Clarence case that infection did not constitute assault.[33] In Victoria, Australia, a new offense—punishable by up to a quarter century in jail—was defined in 1993 as intentionally infecting a person with a serious disease.[34]

Many nations also enacted legislation specific to HIV. Often they sought to avoid the problems of prosecuting under traditional criminal statutes by sidestepping the need for a proof of harm (endangerment rather than actual transmission) or state of mind (intent to harm).[35] In the United States, using the penal code in hopes of changing behavior became evermore accepted in the late 1980s, encouraged by the recommendations of the presidential commission. The CARE Act of 1990 made federal monies to states dependent on their criminalizing the knowing donation of infected bodily fluids, and sex or needle sharing by seropositives except with informed partners. As of 1994, some twenty-seven states had criminal penalties for knowingly transmitting or exposing others to HIV. These statutes did not require that perpetrators intended to harm their victim, only that they knew they were infected and nonetheless engaged in dangerous behavior. Most of the statutes either mandated disclosure of serostatus, proscribed certain actions, or enhanced penalties for actions already illegal, like prostitution.[36] Various Australian states also introduced measures mandating disclosure of serostatus to sex partners.[37]

In Germany, Bavarian measures required seropositives to inform sex partners, needle-sharing partners, and medical personnel of their status.[38] German courts gradually created the duty of seropositives to inform their partners and to practice safe sex. A 1987 Nuremberg court jail sentence for an American army cook who had partly protected sex while infected was one of the first.[39] Infected prostitutes who did not warn clients could be charged with poisoning, bodily harm, or even murder.[40] In France, attempts to create a statute specific to the transmission of HIV failed, leaving only the usual measures against bodily harm and their requirement that intent be proven.[41] Most nations had cases, too, of seropositives punished because they sought to bite or otherwise infect arresting policemen or attending medical personnel: the United States, France, Germany, Belgium, the Netherlands.[42]

In some nations, only actual HIV transmission was actionable. This raised the issue of proving that a particular act of sex or needle sharing had in fact caused a specific infection, a difficult task at best given the long latency period. Courts therefore often sought to convict for the attempt, rather than for the actual offense. The problem here was that this presupposed an intent to achieve the result envisaged, not mere negligent action. In hopes of addressing this problem, German and Swiss law relied on a complex legal notion of "rashness": the perpetrator foreseeing the possible consequences of his actions and accepting them. But in cases where the perpetrator was aware of the potential results of his conduct, but did not intend them, it was hard to convict even under such assumptions. While courts in central Europe recognized the concept of rashness, the French did not.[43]

In other nations, mere endangerment or exposure, whether infection resulted or not, was a crime. This avoided the need to prove that X was the cause of Y's infection. On the other hand, it raised problems of its own concerning the amount of risk that the infectee had assumed in having unprotected sex in the first place.[44] The concept of putting oneself in harm's way—contributory negligence or assumption of risk—and the extent to which it mitigated the guilt of anyone having sex, or sharing needles, while infected was debated at great length, especially in Germany.[45] In a case widely commented on in 1989, eventually overturned, a lower court exonerated a seropositive because his partner had initiated the relations despite knowing of his infection. In contrast, in Hamburg the same year, the principle of *Selbstgefährdung* was rejected in a case where a man had deceived his girlfriend as to the nature of his ailment.[46] The Soviets, Czechs, Estonians, and Ukrainians, too, punished endangerment.[47] In America, certain states (Louisiana, Idaho, and Florida) forbade endangerment.[48] Nonetheless, consent to sex with a seropositive undercut the plaintiff's ability to recover for damages from transmission.[49] In Britain as well, consent was legally considered to imply acceptance of the consequences. Barring rape, it was therefore hard to prosecute for transmission.[50] By contrast, in Sweden and Norway, even knowingly consenting to an act of sex with an infected person did not eliminate the perpetrator's legal liability. Nor did the use of condoms or other protection mitigate responsibility for the transmission of VD.[51]

MOTHER'S MILK AND PERINATAL TRANSMISSION

Preventing the spread of HIV also meant dealing with mother's milk. This was a venerable public health issue. During the eighteenth and nineteenth centuries, wet nurses both infected and were infected with syphilis by the infants they suckled.[52] In the AIDS era, faint echoes of earlier disputes could still be heard. Rare cases of nursing women being infected by seropositive infants were reported from the USSR.[53] But generally speaking, with HIV, mothers infected children. While not preventing infected mothers from nursing, the French prohibited donations of unpasteurized human milk in 1987. The Bavarians forbade seropositive mothers from nursing or donating their milk, while the Germans in general only advised them against breast-feeding.[54] The Norwegians screened all donations to milk banks; the Danes counseled seropositive mothers not to breast-feed. The Swedes did not consider pasteurization by itself sufficiently safe. The authorities instructed seropositive women not to breast-feed and rejected the use of breast milk from high-risk groups, requiring screenings of donors and heat treatment of their milk.[55] In the United States, the presidential commission recommended that seropositive mothers not breast-feed. But except in Idaho, where they were forbidden to nurse, the matter was regulated only theoretically: a woman who thus infected an infant might be liable to criminal penalties.[56]

In the Third World, one of the epidemic's many tragic ironies was that international health organizations' efforts to encourage breast-feeding, offsetting reliance on costly imported milk substitutes, were undermined when mother's milk proved dangerous. Women in developing countries now had to balance the risks of transmission with those attendant on not breast-feeding. Biostatisticians calculated with gloomy precision that, on balance, in areas where infectious disease was the predominant cause of infant mortality, even seropositive women should breast-feed.[57] For women facing this terrible, negative Hobson's choice, the testimony of aggregate numbers must have provided only the coldest comfort.

Perinatal transmission, in turn, raised particular ethical and political issues of its own.[58] The conflict was between the child's interest in being born healthy and its mother's in avoiding unwanted statutory incursions and investigations. Requiring testing and drug treatments of pregnant women obviously discriminated against them, but equally obviously it protected unborn and defenseless future citizens. AZT, given during pregnancy and to the infant just after birth, reduced the risk of infection. If mothers also gave birth via Caesarian and avoided breast-feeding, the chances of partum and postpartum infection could be halved. Beyond this, identifying an infected expectant mother made sense only if aborting the fetus was an option.[59] But one could hardly then claim to be vouchsafing the future child's interests, except by invoking the wood sprite Silenus's Nietzschean admonition: Better not to have been born at all, but if born, better to die as quickly as possible.[60] Even more drastically, identifying them made purely epidemiological sense if seropositive women were denied the right to bear children. The consensual tactics so widely adopted against AIDS had little purchase in such considerations. For all other means of transmission, the potential victim could avoid infection. But here, the risk consisted of being conceived and born, matters on which we are all notoriously underconsulted, and which, from the mother's point of view, were fundamental human rights.

Perinatal transmission was thus a politically ticklish issue. Screening pregnant women for syphilis had been accepted by the mid-1920s in the United States as standard procedure.[61] Screening for HIV, advocated by many obstetricians and pediatricians, promised to identify those who might transmit to their infants, but—as for any generally low-risk group—only at the cost of many false positives. Universal screening, as practiced for hepatitis B, syphilis, and various congenital conditions, had the virtue of not singling out any particular women as inherently high risk. In nations like the United States, where ethnic minorities predominated among the infected, attempts to target screening invoked specters of discrimination or even racially based eugenics.[62] If testing expectant women was problematic, screening infants, by introducing an involuntary backdoor investigation of their progenitor's serological status, raised the issue of the mother's consent.

Identifying those at risk of transmitting to the unborn was one thing. Holding them liable for any such infection was quite another. During the AIDS era, many countries began to make mothers accountable for other sorts of damage potentially wrought on their fetuses. Perinatal transmission might allow an action by a child against its mother for injuries. Or authorities, using statutes outlawing knowing transmission or endangerment, might charge an infected woman for becoming pregnant or giving birth.[63] Most American courts had long refused to allow actions between a minor child and parent for personal torts. But since the early 1960s, more than half of states had abrogated parent-child immunity. During the late 1980s and early 1990s, some went as far as to hold parents liable for negligent or intentional prenatal injury, especially in cases where the mother took illegal drugs. In South Carolina, women were charged with child abuse if their newborns had traces of illegal drugs in their blood. HIV transmission might, it was thought, be seen on this analogy.[64] The 1990 federal CARE Act did not make perinatal HIV infection actionable, but among the states, only Texas and Oklahoma specifically excluded it from the scope of their laws criminalizing HIV transmission.[65] On the other hand, few American jurisdictions recognized so-called wrongful life actions: claims that, where infection and damage were unavoidable, conception or birth should have been avoided.

Because wrongful life actions might prompt abortions, some states even outlawed them.[66]

In Germany, a pregnant seropositive woman whose child died of HIV-related causes in utero might be charged with illegal abortion, but not if the child was born seropositive and then died. Had she become infected during her pregnancy, she might be charged with bodily harm if the child seroconverted after birth. In civil law, a child infected by its parents might have a case against them if it had already been conceived when the parent was infected (in which case it had been damaged by negligence), but not if it was conceived by already seropositive parents, who would have had the same right as the uninfected to reproduce.[67]

The possibility of abortion raised ideological and moral dust storms. An infant's chances of being infected in utero or during birth by a seropositive mother was about 30 percent if no precautions were taken. It was half, and often much less, of that if due medical care was given. Were such risks sufficient reason (if anything was) to terminate a pregnancy? In Cuba, fetuses of seropositive mothers were routinely aborted. In the developed world, however, most pregnant women, informed of their seropositivity, carried their children to term.[68] In the United States, an unholy alliance of women's rights advocates, concerned to protect the pregnant from medical paternalism, and antiabortion activists, eager to avoid more terminations, opposed mandatory testing for expectant mothers. Much medical opinion here wished to have pregnant seropositives counseled to abort and bridled at the Reagan government's opposition. But even this conservative administration was internally divided on the issue.[69] In most European nations—in Britain, Sweden, and France, for example—seropositivity was generally regarded as sufficient reason to abort. In Denmark, seropositive women were counseled to abort, even after the twelfth week. In Germany, the Federal Chamber of Physicians recommended advising infected expectant mothers not to give birth, and the Federal Health Office criticized as irresponsible and immoral the support by AIDS groups for seropositive mothers' right to carry pregnancies to term.[70]

The issue was especially clouded in the United States not just thanks to the abortion dilemma but also because most women at risk—drug users or the sexual partners of addicts—were black or Hispanic and, therefore, members of those groups which had suffered most under earlier sterilization and eugenic policies. In response, civil libertarians and feminists had helped carve out and protect a realm of reproductive freedom, leaving final decisions to mothers regardless of the likely health of the baby. Public health officials therefore had a hard time recommending voluntary testing for high-risk women, much less counseling them to terminate pregnancies if infected: charges of racism and genocide were too easily leveled.[71] On the other hand, the increasing possibility of treatment and care during the mid- and late-1990s encouraged screening of pregnant women and newborns. In 1996 the AMA changed its position to support mandatory screening of expectant women. That year, with reauthorization of the Ryan White CARE Act, the loss of federal funds was threatened if states chose not to test newborns and infant AIDS case levels did not decline.[72] Some states permitted the testing of newborns or pregnant women, and in 1997 New York required HIV screening of all infants.[73] In Sweden, HIV tests were available to all pregnant women. For those found infected, contact tracing was instituted; sexual partners and previous children were tested. In France, though there were proposals to include HIV screening in routine antenatal medical examinations, in fact only voluntary testing was offered pregnant women. In Britain, all who were admitted to prenatal clinics were screened, with consent presumed unless they objected.[74]

Civil law also offered a means of modifying behavior through the legal system, or at least a way to sanction the socially unacceptable. Few nations employed civil law to impose liability for transmission as eagerly as the United States. Nor did liability law in general play such a major role elsewhere. Tort law of negligence allowed individual compensation where someone had been wronged by another person with a duty of care. Though the exact legal standing of sexual partners, especially if not married, was unclear, litigation in America affirmed such a duty. It thus allowed civil actions for transmission, or threatened infection, via sex. One of the first and most celebrated cases was that of Marc Christian, the film star Rock Hudson's former lover, who was awarded damages even though not infected.[75] Other nations had their share of civil law cases too. In Germany, infection with contagious disease was actionable in civil law. Instances of civil actions in France included traffic accidents requiring blood transfusion, employers who posted news of an employee's seropositivity in public, and diagnostic errors. In Sweden, civil law was used less frequently to compensate for damages than in the United States. Though most such injuries were dealt with through private and social insurance, some were tried in civil court. In 1990 a police officer received compensation for her anxieties after she was bitten while arresting a person who claimed to be infected.[76]

The most tragic cases involved infection via blood products, a subject that deserves—and has been granted—entire books to itself. In many nations, both civil and criminal charges were brought against public officials, the staff of blood transfusion services, and personnel from pharmaceutical companies. Most dramatic of these were the trials in France during the 1990s against high-ranking public health officials, including a former prime minister and several other ministers. Similar charges were also brought against the director of the Swiss Red Cross Central Laboratory and leading personnel of a German company found to have sold infected blood products. In Japan, at least two high-ranking figures in the medical world were charged with murder.[77]

5. Discrimination and Its Discontents

Protecting the Victims

Throughout the industrialized world, the law was used to discourage and punish risky behavior. Typically, it both outlawed potentially transmissive conduct and increased sentences for acts aggravated by the threat of infection: rape, child abuse, and assault, especially on police or medical personnel. But in other cases, the interaction of the law and HIV meant attempts at mercy and moderation. Compassionate release of prisoners was one example. Should an incurable and lethal ailment be considered when sentencing or paroling inmates or setting them free? In Poland, prisoners deliberately infected themselves in hopes of having their terms reduced. Courts, in turn, were prompted to stop releasing infected inmates early.[1] But the law could also work more positively, by protecting the infected against prejudice and discrimination.

That AIDS was a disease fraught with stigma is clear, though it was surely an excess of good intentions that led one German parliamentarian to claim that discrimination was sometimes worse than the virus itself.[2] With syphilis, a pointed distinction had been drawn in the nineteenth century between its morally culpable victims and the innocent, afflicted by *Syphilis insontium:* unsuspecting wives, clueless babies, and honest craftsmen, such as glassblowers, in trades where the oral sphincter served as a professional tool. For AIDS, such distinctions were drawn even more strongly. It was not just sex associated with its transmission, it was anal sodomy and injected drugs. The links between disease and deviancy were impressively forged. "People get AIDS by doing things most people do not do and of which most people do not approve," asserted C. Everett Koop, the surgeon general appointed by President Ronald Reagan. Koop nonetheless contradicted his conservative views on other subjects to take up the cudgel for a nondiscriminatory approach to the epidemic.[3] But could such fears and prejudices—of a disease transmitted by sex, borne by blood, and invariably fatal—be countered by legal remedies? Working against discrimination was not just socially tolerant, it was also a tactically necessary move. Discrimination threatened to drive the afflicted underground, where they avoided public health precautions. As one observer put it, protecting the rights of seropositives was not a luxury, but a necessity. Otherwise hopes of encouraging voluntary compliance would founder. The safety of the majority depended on protecting the rights of the infected.[4]

The first and most obvious act of discrimination came with initial efforts to distinguish high-risk groups on the basis of the still poorly understood epidemiology of AIDS.[5] Before serological testing was possible, precautions such as prohibiting certain people from donating blood could be based only on risk-group membership. In March 1983 in the United States, the following groups could not donate blood: Haitians who had entered the country since 1977, men who had slept with men since that time, intravenous drug users past or present, prostitutes and their clients, hemophiliacs, sexual partners of AIDS victims, and the sexual contacts of all these categories. Blood collection agencies questioned donors to elicit information about high-risk behavior.[6] In various Australian states, male donors had to sign a statement that they had not had sex with men or injected unprescribed drugs during the previous five years, had no symptoms, had no symptomatic or drug-injecting sex partner, and had not recently received acupuncture, tattoos, or body piercings.[7]

Similar categorizations of high-risk groups who were prohibited from donating blood held in other countries as well. In Britain, men who had had even a single homosexual encounter since 1977 were included, as were sexual partners of Africans.[8] The Swedish list encompassed, in addition to the usual suspects, the sex partners and parents of hemophiliacs, as well as anyone with enlarged lymph nodes. French military posted abroad were forbidden to donate blood for half a year after their return.[9] The Czech Republic included long-term residents of America and western Europe and their sex partners, not just Africans, among those prohibited from donating. Italy excluded those who had had sex with persons unknown, and Costa Rica all promiscuous men.[10] As in many other nations, French and Danish gays protested such distinctions as discriminatory.[11] By way of contrast, the Swedish gay organization itself recommended that its members not donate blood.[12] Informal discrimination took place among gays themselves in an understandable attempt to avoid risk: European homosexuals warned against sex with Americans, Oxford gays cautioned against relations with Londoners, and Japanese gay saunas barred foreigners.[13] As of mid-1985, with the coming of HIV antibody tests, however, the need for such lifestyle discrimination diminished. Nonetheless, the Food and Drug Administration continued banning Haitians from donating blood as late as 1990, before massive demonstrations in Miami and New York prompted a reversal. In 1996, Ethiopian Jews (recently airlifted to Israel and widely infected) rioted, protesting that their blood donations had been secretly dumped.[14] Even after the onset of serological testing, high-risk groups were still discouraged from donation because of false negatives and the long period before antibodies formed.

Western nations differed significantly in how they countered discrimination against the infected. The United States implemented more legislation to protect AIDS victims from discrimination than most of Europe, especially at the state and sometimes municipal level. Ultimately, it classified seropositives as handicapped, with all the privileges and rights that followed. Moreover, to the extent that specific HIV-related protections were not implemented, it was largely because the existing panoply of antidiscrimination laws could simply be extended to HIV without further effort.[15] For reasons that go far beyond the scope of this study, the United States had more elaborate legal protections in favor of the handicapped than most European nations. Thus, seropositives found an already existing regulatory niche. Gay rights ordinances were also passed at the state, local, and municipal levels, though sometimes they were rescinded or defeated. More than in Europe, the courts played an important role in protecting the infected against discrimination.[16] With the partial exception of France, European countries shied away from special treatment of AIDS victims. But at the same time the ill benefited from legislation, above all employment termination laws, that left their position stronger than that of their American peers, wholly independently of AIDS.[17] Protection against discrimination on the basis of sexual orientation was also more widespread in northern Europe than America.

Attitudes toward AIDS victims varied in tandem with the legal protection offered the handicapped, women, and ethnic and other minorities in the legal systems considered here. In Europe, positive discrimination on behalf of the disadvantaged was regarded more skeptically than across the Atlantic. In Germany, antidiscrimination measures were the concern primarily of the Green Party, which at the start of the epidemic still dwelt in the suburbs of political respectability.[18] A substantial, long-oppressed, and impoverished ethnic minority was not the same factor in Europe—ignoring Roma and Sinti—as across the Atlantic. With the increase of ethnically distinct immigration in the 1960s, however, similar problems arrived also in Europe. The women's movement of continental Europe had a long-held ideology of sep-

arate spheres. It attached less value to equality of job opportunity for females, making legislation guaranteeing such rights less pressing.[19] Age discrimination, an important and classic equal-opportunities issue in America,
was actively practiced in Europe, as sclerotic labor markets sought to shed
older workers. When the question arose of classifying seropositives as needing special protection, Europeans held up allegedly bad experiences with
similar provisions for women as reason to shun this path. More generally, it
was argued that, in nations without traditions of singling out certain groups
for favorable treatment, a focus on AIDS victims could actually be to their
disadvantage.[20]

In the United States, antidiscrimination legislation based on ethnicity
stretched back to the 1930s on the state level. On the national stage, it began
in earnest during the Second World War with attempts to halt discrimination against blacks in war industries. During the postwar period, Title VII of
the 1964 Civil Rights Act and the 1972 Equal Employment Opportunity Act
outlawed discrimination on the basis of ethnicity, religion, nationality, or
sex.[21] Attempts to prohibit discrimination by sexual orientation were less
successful. *Bowers v. Hardwick* (1986) failed to extend privacy protections
to gay sodomy (though the ruling was overturned in 2003), and the Civil
Rights Act did not cover sexual orientation. Yet local and state measures did
protect sexual orientation—for example, in California, New Jersey, New
York, Massachusetts, the District of Columbia, and over one hundred municipalities.[22]

In Europe, penal codes or constitutions, and sometimes specific statutes,
outlawed discrimination (most often and clearly in employment) on the
basis of sex, ethnicity, union membership, nationality, sometimes religion,
and occasionally sexual orientation. Handicap, however, including disease
infection, was, as a rule, not similarly protected.[23] The Norwegians outlawed
discrimination on the basis of sexual orientation in 1981, the French four
years later, and the Danes in 1987. The German state of Brandenburg included such protection in its constitution in 1992, the same year that the
Dutch took similar steps. By contrast, the European Community implemented little coverage against discrimination by sexual preference.[24] In
Britain, however, discrimination on the basis of sexual orientation remained
legal.[25]

What protection existed for the handicapped was generally provided by
existing labor legislation determining the conditions of termination and the
like, supplemented with provisions on privacy.[26] After fitful attempts, the
British passed the Disability Discrimination Act in 1995, intended to emulate the Americans with Disabilities Act. It protected AIDS patients but did

not apply to the 95 percent of British firms employing twenty or fewer workers. Nor did it include protection against discrimination based on serostatus alone.[27] In Germany the Law on the Severely Handicapped of 1986 gave some protection against termination, and extra benefits, to the disabled. Asymptomatic seropositives were not regarded as handicapped, but individuals in later stages of the disease qualified on a sliding scale.[28] In France, a law of 12 July 1990 forbade discrimination on the basis of handicap and various illnesses.[29]

In some instances, legal protections against gender or ethnic discrimination were used against actions taken because of handicap. British legislation had already outlawed employment discrimination on the basis of sex and race. Since most initial AIDS victims were men and some were African, claims for protection on this basis were possible.[30] In 1987, using the 1975 Sex Discrimination Act, Dan Air was forced to rescind its policy—which sought to avoid the HIV problem—of hiring only women as flight personnel. In an American case the same year, the court found an employer's exclusion of AIDS-related treatments discriminatory because 90 percent of those with the disease at the time were men.[31]

Workplace discrimination against infected and potentially seropositive applicants and employees was a major problem across the industrialized world. Many employers sought to screen applicants or even current employees: Dan Air, British Air, and Texaco in the United Kingdom; Philips in the Netherlands; the airline SAS in Sweden; Lufthansa, Daimler, and AEG in Germany; the Eastern Nebraska Community Office of Retardation in the United States; the Union Bank of Finland; and the Paris municipality and the SNCF in France.[32] Even the most high-minded institutions found that their interests as employers contradicted their noble aspirations. The World Health Organization and the International Labor Office recommended against employment-related HIV screening. In January 1988, the European Union nonetheless announced HIV screening for its applicants. Six months later, when this proved too controversial, it reversed itself to make the tests voluntary. Job candidates who refused were instead often subjected to a battery of other examinations to determine their serostatus indirectly. Similarly, the UN, otherwise so Olympian in issuing moral advice, screened personnel in at least some of its agencies.[33]

Employment protection varied across nations. Generally speaking, European legislation did not allow routine HIV testing as a precondition of employment and required that candidates' exams relate specifically to necessary job qualifications. It thus broadly banned queries about serostatus, and allowed candidates to lie about or omit such information. But it did not prohibit questions about full-blown AIDS, which might in fact affect the terms of employment.[34] Across Europe, those who fell sick with AIDS and failed to perform their duties could be dismissed for that reason, if not for the disease itself. From the patient's point of view, this was, of course, an exercise in exculpatory hairsplitting.[35] Most nations also restricted the occupations that the infected could pursue, ruling out food services and medicine, for example, where the risk of transmission was real, but sometimes also occupations involving any skin penetration.[36]

British employers, however, could ask job applicants about their serostatus, and even their membership in risk groups. They could also ask for HIV testing either before or during employment, though they could not fire an employee for refusing. So long as they did not discriminate on the basis of race or sex, employers could also refuse to hire seropositives.[37] In Denmark, applicants who did not inform prospective employers of an AIDS diagnosis—though not seropositivity—risked forfeiting the right to sick pay and certain protections against termination. Swedish employers had the right to refuse employment to seropositives and to screen during the course of the job.[38] In Germany, employers had similarly extensive freedom to screen. Inquiries had to relate directly to job qualifications but could touch on HIV as it affected applicants' ability to perform their duties or the dangers they posed to fellow employees or clients. Employers could ask candidates whether they were suffering from AIDS or related symptoms and could require medical examination or certification. Applicants denied a job because of their serostatus had no claims against employers. Though German employers could not routinely require a preemployment medical examination, applicants who refused one could be turned down without any recourse.[39] French employers were also equipped with unusual powers. Though systematic HIV screening was not allowed during the term of employment, employees who presented suspicious symptoms could be examined by the company physician to determine fitness for continued work.[40]

Dismissal of infected or ill employees also presented a varied picture. In both Germany and Britain, though HIV infection alone was not a reason for termination, other factors might permit it: when there were risks to others, as with medical personnel, or when coworkers or customers demanded firing the infected person.[41] Swedish employees enjoyed strong protection against dismissal for seropositivity or an AIDS diagnosis. Employers, in turn, had broad latitude in redeploying them on tasks compatible with their illness. In Norway, in contrast, termination was possible for seropositivity alone, and rental contracts of limited duration could also be ended for this reason. If an employer could show that he would be hurt by retaining a seropositive (for example, if other employees balked at working with that person or customers mutinied, and if he could not find alternative duties for the seropositive), then firing was allowed.[42] In France, the law of 12 July 1990 forbade dismissal for health reasons, including seropositivity, unless unfitness to work was medically certified. If an employee was found to be infected during the annual medical exams that were a unique feature of French labor practice, and hence incapable of performing his duties, the employer could reassign him to other functions, even at a lower salary, or fire him.[43]

In the United States, the issue of discrimination against the victims of HIV was incorporated as part of broader protections for the handicapped. Already in November 1986, a federal district judge ruled AIDS to be a handicap under the Rehabilitation Act of 1973, which protected participants in federally funded programs. An infected kindergartner, expelled for biting a fellow pupil, was ordered readmitted, and the school district was required to accommodate the child's disability. In 1987, with the Arline case, contagious disease was accepted by the Supreme Court as a handicap. Gene Arline was a tubercular teacher dismissed in fear that she might transmit disease. Not only was she to be considered handicapped, the Court ruled, but to be so because her employer feared she was contagious, even though she in fact posed no danger. Following the Rehabilitation Act, the Court thus defined impairment to include those who, though not necessarily physically ill, were thought so.[44] During the following three years, the jurisprudence evolved that allowed seropositives to be considered handicapped in the eyes of the law.[45]

In 1988 Congress passed the Civil Rights Restoration Act of 1987, which extended to seropositives the coverage of the 1973 Rehabilitation Act and so protected them unless they constituted a direct threat to the health or safety of others. The Rehabilitation Act applied only to programs receiving federal monies. But the federal Fair Housing Amendments Act of 1989 extended protection for the disabled under Title VIII of the Civil Rights Act to private landlords and owners, forbidding discrimination against the handicapped, and thus seropositives, in the sale or rental of dwellings.[46] The Americans with Disabilities Act (ADA) of 1990 (which took effect two years later) took the next step. It extended protection against discrimination to those employed in the private sector, as well as to individuals using public accommodation, transportation, and services. An exception was made in the case of insurance underwriting. The ADA adopted the Rehabilitation Act's broad definition of disability, but also its exclusion of those who posed a direct threat to the health or safety of others.[47] Since HIV was not easily transmitted by casual contact, this meant that seropositives could not be excluded from most forms of work, even though—to take an obvious example—they might not be allowed to perform invasive medical procedures. The law also allowed preemployment medical examinations and tests only if they were job related.[48] Congress deliberately excluded homosexuality and current drug use from the list of disabilities. But since disability was defined to include also those who were *regarded* as being handicapped, a gay denied employment might be protected if he could show that he had been disadvantaged not because of his homosexuality but out of a belief that he was likely to be HIV infected.[49] A modest protection against discrimination because of sexual orientation was thus introduced, almost accidentally, thanks to the epidemiological link between gays and HIV.

Legislation at the state level generally preceded federal measures, complementing and adding to them. All states had laws protecting the handicapped against discrimination, and half extended these to include HIV. In 1983, just two years after the disease had first been identified, New York State's disability statute was interpreted to protect many of those affected by HIV against discrimination. Several other states also passed measures forbidding employment discrimination on the basis of HIV status or HIV screening used for employment purposes.[50]

CIVIL SERVANTS AND THE MILITARY

Civil servants enjoyed special perks in employment. Accordingly, they were sometimes held to particular requirements. In return for salaries often uncompetitive with the private sector, the state took greater responsibility for its employees, providing them with generous health insurance, disability payments, and old age pensions. The state, and ultimately the voter and taxpayer, thus had a vested interest in remaining free of employees who might skew its actuarial burdens. Hence, civil service applicants were often asked to demonstrate a continued ability to fulfill their duties. With increasingly generous employment conditions came stricter controls at the point of access. The armed forces were in a similar position, since recruits and personnel had duties that might be undermined by HIV.

Medical examinations for civil service positions were common but often did not include HIV, as in Italy and Sweden. Norwegian applicants could be tested, but denied a position only if they were already too ill to perform their functions or if there was a risk of transmission.[51] In France, after inconsistent practices, the government ruled out systematic HIV screening and agreed to hire seropositives, but retained the ability to reject AIDS patients too sick to carry out their duties.[52] The British civil service was not screened, and ministers disavowed any intention of introducing such measures.[53]

In Germany, the home of Europe's perhaps most venerable civil service, the issue was particularly fraught. Applicants who might suffer prolonged illness and disability before normal retirement were not to be appointed. While full-blown AIDS was generally admitted as cause to reject a candidate, whether screening was allowed and whether the same consequences attended seropositivity was debated.[54] In 1986, German foreign service applicants were HIV tested, some without their knowledge, in examinations for duty in the tropics. As of the following year, however, such screening was performed only voluntarily, and refusal to submit had no career consequences. No other branch of federal government made use of screening.[55]

In Bavaria, however, tests were required as of 1987. Applicants were asked about their sexual habits and whether they were gays, prostitutes, or drug addicts. In a technical sense, confidentiality was preserved in that test results, if positive, would be communicated to state authorities only with the candidate's permission. Otherwise, their refusal was noted and the employer could draw his conclusions. Were a seropositive candidate hired nonetheless, he was required to accept the possibility of early retirement because of long-term unfitness for service.[56] No other federal states followed the Bavarian example, however. Even within Bavaria, Nuremberg (in the Protestant and Social Democratic enclave of Franconia) rejected such screening. In 1988, the federal government explicitly rejected the Bavarian example and permitted the employment of asymptomatic seropositives as civil servants. The move partly reflected a fear that, if the state discriminated against the infected, then private employers would follow suit.[57]

Curiously, the United States, with a civil service apparatus perhaps least imbued with Continental-style corporatism, actively screened certain segments of its bureaucracy. In 1988, civil service guidelines took a moderate approach, allowing the infected to continue to work as long as possible and threatening uncooperative coworkers with disciplinary action.[58] From 1986 on, however, the foreign service screened its members and their families biannually, and seropositive applicants were not hired. The already hired infected were either deployed only domestically or, if asymptomatic, were assigned to one of the nineteen nations where medical services were considered up to snuff. Allowed to continue their functions so long as they were able and harmless to others, they could, at their request, be retired on an invalidity pension. The reasoning was that foreign service officers were often assigned to posts abroad where medical provisioning was insufficient, and the necessary vaccinations and potential local infections might challenge their weakened immune systems. Since such conditions were pertinent only to members of the foreign service, other civil servants were not screened. In the German case, the main concern was the reciprocal obligations of the corporatist relationship between civil servant and state. The logic in the United States was that testing served the best interests of the employees themselves.[59]

A similar logic applied to the armed services and Justice Department employees working in penal institutions, who were tested if exposed in the course of their duties. Employees of local administrations were sometimes screened, too: firefighters, paramedics, and police. Schoolteachers were often required to certify good health, and half the states required proof of freedom from various contagious diseases. As of 1987, schoolteachers in Georgia could be asked for evidence of seronegativity if they appeared to suffer symptoms of AIDS. But they could not be fired so long as they performed their duties.[60]

The armed forces were treated much like civil servants. Among the strictest nations was the United States. For a while, until sometime in the 1990s, when others followed suit, only the American military tested all applicants, screening active soldiers and reservists at regular intervals, as well as when they were symptomatic, donating blood, or being admitted to the hospital. Infected applicants were not accepted; ROTC and military academy students were disenrolled. The infected who were already enlisted were deployed only within America. They could be reassigned and, though adverse personnel actions against seropositives were prohibited, in certain senses they might be demoted (denial of security clearances and suspension of access to confidential information). They were obliged to follow rules of conduct to prevent transmission: informing their sexual partners and medical caregivers, not donating blood, and practicing safe sex, which meant not exchanging blood or bodily fluids, including saliva, during intercourse. Soldiers also had their contacts traced, with the names of civilians released to the health authorities unless prohibited by local law, and military sex partners identified, counseled, and tested without consent. Military physicians could also contact the spouses of infected reservists.[61]

In Europe, the tendency was not to screen recruits or soldiers. The Italians at first screened but then made this voluntary. The Spaniards informally excluded seropositives from armed service by using the tests required of blood donors. The Belgians screened certain categories of personnel (pilots in training, those returning from high-risk countries). So did the

French, who also tested soldiers seeking to be posted abroad, but otherwise they screened only on a voluntary basis during enlistment.[62] In Germany, the government intended initially to screen recruits from risk groups. Tests were possible, too, when the inspecting physician suspected AIDS. In 1987–88, however, it was decided that the law requiring recruits to be medically examined did not apply to symptomless seropositives. About half of all recruits agreed to testing, but it remained voluntary, except for those wishing to train in the United States.[63] Even the Swedes, always ready to test civilians, postponed screening the armed forces because it was too costly. Nor did the British screen the military, though—like the Americans—they refused to accept gays, until 2000.[64]

Differences in the nature of the respective armies, above all the distinction between conscript and professional forces, help explain such variations. American troops were tested because long-serving professional soldiers presented a needless and avoidable burden if infected. The conscript Continental armies had short service periods, and national health insurance systems took responsibility for ailing former draftees. That does not, of course, explain why Britain, also with a voluntary, professional force, did not screen. Since private sector employers were forbidden to screen for HIV, it was argued there, neither should the army.[65] During the late nineteenth and early twentieth centuries, British military authorities had feared that drastic inspections, of the sort common among the Continental conscript armies, would discourage recruitment for their voluntary forces.[66] A similar logic appears to have applied to HIV screening. The American army recruited heavily from minorities and may therefore have had more cause to screen and exclude than did conscript armies, which enlisted from all ranks of society.[67] Finally, as the only military force in the Western world intended for serious use during this period (excepting the British and arguably the French), the American army had an incentive to exclude seropositive troops in order to keep its worldwide deployable strength at a maximum in times of low manpower levels.[68]

PROSTITUTION

The strictures imposed by certain nations on prostitution were an occupationally targeted form of prophylaxis, on par with those on other potentially risky professions. Though often suspected of transmitting disease, female prostitutes in fact had dramatically varying infection rates. Sometimes, as in Nevada or Germany, incidence was very low. A seropositive prostitute posed an epidemiological danger no different, of course, from any girl with a full dance card—or a deb's delight. As one commentator noted, charging money for sex does not, in itself, transmit disease.[69] Vaginal sex was among the least efficient transmissive routes, especially female to male. Most commercial transactions involved oral sex, which was even less dangerous. Prostitutes' infection rates were largely proportional to their use of intravenous drugs, and the problem they posed was thus part of the larger issue of drug abuse, not directly one of sexual habits.[70]

In contrast, male prostitutes posed a greater danger, since anal intercourse was an effective means of transmission. In addition, they were a potential gateway to the heterosexual population through the wives of their bisexual clients. How, in any case, was prostitution to be defined? One researcher found that up to a quarter of gay men at some time had accepted money for sex. Include sex tourism and the poverty of Third World "companions," and distinctions between mercenary and affectionate relations faded even more. (In Africa, similar issues arose where "transactional sex" exchanges, or barter of favors for value, made hash of education campaigns that relied on Western distinctions between sex and commerce.)[71]

National strictures on prostitution reflected the varied role that it played, both legally and in fact, in each country. Nations that banned prostitution could not suddenly recognize it in law by imposing special precautions on commercial copulation.[72] In other countries, sex workers, like workers in any other regulated profession, were put out of business if they threatened public health. Why, one observer demanded to know, should a butcher, a chef, or a waiter be prevented from spreading salmonella, but a prostitute be exempt from similar controls? Subjecting sex workers to screening and reporting if infected gave consumers a clear choice, proponents argued: the government-certified flesh of the Eros Center or a risky street corner encounter with a clandestine hooker.[73] On the other hand, consumers might understand screening and certification as a statutory imprimatur of a disease-free status, a status that was impossible to guarantee, leading to more rather than less risky behavior. The Germans—falling for that irresistible combination of pleasures, locomotion, and copulation—called this screening an AIDS-TÜV (car inspection). Indeed, in Bavaria, prostitutes were required to submit to screening, yet forbidden to advertise their status with certificates of seronegativity.[74] For male homosexual prostitution, the problems were compounded. Though of venerable pedigree, such work had flourished especially in the era after regulation's decline. For this and other reasons, many European laws dealing with prostitution simply turned a blind eye to the male variant. In some nations, as in Austria in 1989, male prostitution was legalized precisely so that it could be dealt with in terms of the law.[75]

Nations that regulated prostitution could most easily forbid the sale of sex by the infected. On the other hand, those localities—like Hamburg—whose red-light districts were major employers also faced a Hobson's choice. How great a loss of tax revenues were they willing to accept when restricting potentially infectious sex?[76] In other places, a more circuitous route was taken by criminalizing participation in sex while infected. This applied to all citizens, whether the bespectacled family father or the street-walker, though obviously as a matter of practice the merchants of venery were most often affected. In some instances, the endless debates of the late nineteenth century over the regulation of prostitution and especially the virtues of official brothels were replayed in shorthand. Inspecting prostitutes promised to take some infected ones out of circulation. On the other hand, only a fraction of the sex traded on the venereal market would be affected. HIV's long period of antibody-free infection also threatened to undercut the usefulness of testing. Infected prostitutes would have to be forbidden to ply their trade for life. Barring generous disability or superannuation payments, many would disappear underground, thus defeating the intent.[77] In France during the late 1980s and early nineties, proposals were made, including one supported by the discoverer of HIV, Luc Montagnier, to reopen official brothels, abolished since the 1960s. They were now to be glorified with the peculiar name *espaces de liberté*. The new climate of women's rights, however, forbade such ventures and relegated them to the shelves of outmoded prophylactic practices.[78]

Calls were also heard to prosecute prostitutes' clients, to suppress pornography, and forbid mail-order brides. Various unholy alliances sprang from such attempts—in Sweden, for example, of conservatives, ready to pounce on any extramarital sex, and leftist feminists, happy to restrict yet another expression of male sexual prerogative.[79] The Swedes in fact recriminalized prostitution in 1999 and threatened with fines those soliciting sex for money.[80] The right-wing National Front sought to close military brothels in French Africa. In Germany and the Netherlands, in contrast, the trend was to regularize the sex trade, preventing police suppression of prostitutes who cooperated with public health measures and making prostitution a legally recognized (and socially insured) profession.[81]

Austria was among the first to impose HIV-related restrictions on prostitutes. In 1986, it required quarterly HIV screenings and forbade the infected from working.[82] The Bavarians did the same, and required clients to use condoms.[83] In Britain, regulation had been repealed amid great controversy in 1886, and the policy on prostitution had been largely hands-off thereafter. The government had no intention of traveling such prophylactic paths again (though the possibility of legalized brothels was briefly broached). Nor did it attempt to screen prostitutes for HIV.[84] The Swedes forbade infected prostitutes from plying their trade, while the Greeks only strongly recommended that they cease work.[85] Most East Bloc nations screened prostitutes.[86] Prostitutes in Nevada were tested monthly and inspected weekly, and the infected were prohibited from working.[87] Other American states sought to increase, for the infected, the penalties already imposed on commercial copulation. In Newark, New Jersey, anyone arrested for a prostitution-related offense, including clients, could be tested.[88]

Gay sex tourism in Haiti, the Dominican Republic, and other Caribbean venues had played a crucial role in disseminating HIV early on.[89] Even male prostitution with female clients, which was otherwise uncommon—excepting the Hollywood fantasies of *American Gigolo*—became part of sex tourism, especially in Kenya, Haiti, Bali, and the Gambia.[90] During the AIDS era, sex work grew increasingly global, with prostitutes from the Second and Third Worlds a ubiquitous feature of European and North American cities. Moreover, Mohammed now also traveled to the mountain. Sex tourism, especially among Japanese and northern European men, became an ever more common form of vacationing. The brothels of Thailand, the Philippines, and other Asian countries served an international market, as well as indulged Western males whose tastes had been outlawed at home—such as the rape of children. The attempt to deal legally with such issues, by criminalizing, for example, the sexual abuse of minors by Western nationals even when committed abroad, is a chapter that is only slowly being written.[91]

PRISONERS

Being incarcerated may not be an occupation in the usual sense. Yet given the incidence of male-to-male sex in prison, incarceration and AIDS were closely linked. Jail for even a misdemeanor often came with the added punishment of a potential death sentence via infection. Such dissemination also posed dangers to the rest of society as prisoners who might otherwise have remained healthy were freed to become vectors of disease.[92]

As of the early 1990s, at least seventeen state correctional systems in America had programs of mass prisoner screening. But the trend was declining, despite the eagerness with which such measures had been embraced during the previous decade. Some states tested all prisoners, and some only those who had been convicted of certain crimes, such as rape. The Federal Bureau of Prisons had started in 1987 by screening all incoming inmates, and all continuing inmates half-yearly and at release. Later, it shifted to a more selective testing of certain inmates. In 1990 the CARE Act made federal monies contingent on states testing prisoners on entry and release, and on providing the results to personnel who might have been exposed, spouses paying conjugal visits, and the victims of those sentenced for sexual crimes.[93]

In contrast, in most western European countries, testing in prison was voluntary, with the exception of Portugal (mandatory for all prisoners) and Spain (for all high-risk groups), though informal pressure could be well-nigh irresistible.[94] In Germany, compulsory testing of prisoners was practiced only in Bavaria, Hesse, Schleswig-Holstein, and, for a time, North Rhine–Westphalia. Even there it was carried out on a nominally voluntary basis, encouraged by the explicit threat of compulsory screening for at least high-risk groups. Screening ratios were correspondingly high: 97 percent in Munich, a tad less in Nuremberg. Similarly impressive results were achieved also in other states: 90 percent in Hesse, 80 percent in North Rhine–Westphalia, and 99 percent in Hamburg, though figures were much lower in Berlin and Bremen. Prisoners accepted "voluntary" screening, since otherwise they were treated as though infected and were isolated and kept from certain desirable jobs.[95] Iceland achieved similar results by requiring inmates actively to refuse testing, and the Swedes, too, had high rates of acceptance for voluntary testing.[96]

The Dutch did not screen. In Britain, routine and compulsory testing of prisoners was rejected as being out of line with procedures for the general community.[97] But informal pressure was also exerted. In the infamous Wandsworth Prison, a wing in the basement, formerly the dungeon, reportedly housed inmates until they agreed to submit. The Irish, in contrast, allowed compulsory testing of high-risk prisoners and routinely isolated seropositives.[98] The French outlawed systematic testing of prisoners in 1985, though various localities, like Marseilles, continued the practice.[99] The Italians permitted compulsory testing. They also distinguished themselves with a 1993 law that exempted AIDS patients from prison. The result was a well-publicized case two years later of a bank-robbing spree in Turin prompted by the criminals' assurance that they could not be jailed.[100]

In most nations, medical confidentiality for prisoners was not as strictly enforced as for the general population. Authorities were often informed of test results, and infected inmates were identified during transports.[101] In some German states and parts of Spain, release was contingent on screening and informing the prisoner's partner of his status. In the United States, seropositive prisoners were often denied conjugal visits. Some correctional systems required seropositive prisoners to disclose their status to family members, former sex partners, and potential employers.[102] In terms of housing prisoners, the interests of the infected in not being isolated and stigmatized had to be weighed against the other inmates' concerns to avoid exposure. The American trend favored mainstreaming infected prisoners, and by the early 1990s, only twenty correctional systems segregated AIDS victims, and even fewer seropositives. In France and Belgium, seropositives were not isolated, but AIDS patients were confined to prison hospitals or sent to special centers.[103] Some German states, like Hesse, isolated seropositives at night to prevent sexual contact.[104] In Britain, procedures were irregular. Many seropositives were housed in single cells, others together in communal arrangements. Segregation was reported especially at Leeds and Wandsworth prisons, but not at Bristol.[105] Russia opened a special prison for seropositives at Tver in 1999. Some Australian states also isolated seropositives.[106]

Allowing prisoners to protect themselves, by giving them condoms and clean needles or the means of sterilizing them, raised dilemmas because it implied toleration of illicit activities, whether homosexual sex or drug use. Even the Council of Europe, otherwise heartily liberal in proposing condoms and syringe disinfectants, stopped short of needle exchanges.[107] In the United States, only a handful of correctional systems gave inmates condoms, and none allowed prisoners sterile needles or bleach.[108] The British did not allow access to condoms, except eventually to confirmed homosexuals, or syringes.[109] The Swedes and eventually the French distributed condoms.[110] The Danes, who otherwise made syringes available, forbade them in prisons.[111] Germany banned clean needles at first, though disinfectants were accessible in Bavaria and Berlin. Then, from 1992, disposable syringes for addicts were legalized and distributed in prisons.[112]

MEDICAL PERSONNEL

Medical personnel, in turn, with their threat of reciprocal dangers, were a special case. Patients might infect caregivers, and they, in turn, could transmit to precisely those whom the Hippocratic oath enjoined them not to harm. The two parties danced a delicate pas de deux of rights and obligations.

To start with physicians' duties and responsibilities, courts tended to enforce the obligation to treat seropositives despite the risk. But gray areas emerged for elective or cosmetic procedures. Conversely, medical personnel occasionally asserted their rights as employees under occupational safety and health rules not to undertake dangerous tasks. More generally, while a requirement to treat may have obliged the profession as a whole, individual practitioners—excepting perhaps public hospital and emergency room personnel—were largely within their rights when they shunned risks.[113] Though many physicians (a quarter in some surveys) considered it ethical to refuse treatment to AIDS victims, the American Medical Association (AMA), and equivalent bodies elsewhere, rejected such triage. Given their obligation and its attendant dangers, physicians understandably sought to secure information on patients' status. In certain circumstances, they insisted on their prerogative to test them, especially if undergoing surgery, though many professional organizations disagreed.[114]

In some countries, AIDS patients were treated with the same precautions as for acutely transmissible diseases: they were isolated in single rooms and confronted with medical personnel in full protective regalia. The Swedes extended this policy even to eye examinations. Dentists here, too, were allowed to demand a HIV test and to treat those who refused as though infected. Recalcitrant patients who changed dentists could expect their file to indicate that they posed a risk. Indeed, seropositives were required to inform medical caregivers of their status. General screening of hospital admissions, however, was rejected in 1988. Instead, personnel were asked to keep an eye out for suspicious symptoms or risky behavior. Norway, however, required screening of hospital admissions. Some institutions also tested pregnant women, treating those who refused as infected.[115]

In Germany, other than Bavaria, whether infected patients had to inform caregivers of their serostatus was unclear. The Contagious Disease Law of 1961 required carriers to tell medical personnel of their condition. However, a technicality of wording limited this to *Ausscheidungen* (excrement), which arguably did not include bodily fluids (with the possible exception of menstrual blood).[116] In Britain, the Royal College of Surgeons accepted testing of unconscious patients who appeared to belong to risk groups. Screening without consent could be performed if surgical staff were wounded during an operation on a high-risk patient.[117] The French, in contrast, forbade systematic screening of hospital patients and testing without consent in 1987, though actually there were frequent violations.[118] In the United States, the CDC and other government agencies recommended against routine testing of patients. Instead, they advocated universal precautions—treating all patients as though infected.[119] In theory, hospitals could require screening for admission, so long as the results were not used to discriminate against seropositives. In reality, few did. Illinois and Arkansas allowed HIV testing on the basis of a general consent to medical treatment when deemed necessary. Texas and Wisconsin permitted nonconsensual testing if a procedure exposed physicians to infection.[120] The CARE Act allowed emergency response personnel to determine whether they had been exposed. Otherwise only army personnel entering military hospitals could be tested.[121]

On the other side of the equation, the public wanted to be protected against iatrogenic infection. Statistically, transmission was far more likely from patient to caregiver than vice versa. Yet the fears generated by the Kimberly Bergalis case during the early 1990s in the United States, where a patient apparently was infected by her dentist, led to demands for screening of all medical personnel and exclusion of the infected from active practice. The inherent vulnerability of patients in the hands of physicians may have been enhanced by semiconscious fears among heterosexuals of coming into unwitting bodily contact with gays.[122] Jesse Helms, always one to shoot from the hip, sponsored an amendment in 1991 that passed by a landslide majority in the Senate. It threatened to jail infected physicians performing invasive procedures who failed to disclose their serostatus. It was never, however, enacted into law, largely thanks to the resistance of the medical profession—which was dismayed to see actions formerly a matter of professional conduct suddenly become the province of the penal code.[123] Among homosexuals, the sad joke was that, since so many of their doctors were themselves infected, "the urban gay male worries less about transmission from his physician than whether or not he will survive him."[124]

Physicians fought demands that their serostatus be revealed to patients. Since caregivers were not rigorously tested for other ailments, and patients were not warned of the relative success rates of procedures at different hospitals, why should HIV be treated differently?[125] Such arguments, that sought to privilege one particular ailment, were attempts without much hope to buck the swelling tide of knowledge placed—in large measure by the Web—in patients' hands. For the first time in history, consumers of medical care could take informed decisions. The insistence on patients' rights to know their caregivers' status was but part of a broader movement to make relations between physician and patient ever more transparent.

Whether concerned with breast cancer or schizophrenia, later activists used tactics pioneered during the AIDS epidemic. These, in turn, followed the autonomous patient mobilization initiated by Alcoholics Anonymous.[126] Against demands for disclosure stood the rights of infected medical personnel not to be discriminated against. Physicians had already successfully fought being tested for hepatitis B.[127] In the United States, once HIV infection became recognized as a handicap in law, employers could restrict the duties of personnel—whether teachers, chefs, or brain surgeons—only if significant risks of transmission were posed. Conversely, infected medical personnel shared the same interests as everyone else in increasingly routine testing as the treatments for the disease improved.

In America, the CDC reversed itself during the late 1980s, moving from earlier recommendations that infected health care workers be allowed to work freely so long as barrier protection was employed, to more cautious policies of restricting activities with the risk of transmission. In June 1991, during the Bergalis affair, the AMA concluded that physicians should know their own serostatus and cease invasive procedures if infected, or at least inform their patients. Some states, like Florida and Louisiana, required testing of seropositive health care workers and informed consent from patients.[128] In Germany in 1991, medical and government representatives agreed to ask personnel involved in possibly transmissive procedures for voluntary testing, with seropositives not to perform them. In Britain, the General Medical Council accepted that health care workers who knew of infected colleagues should seek to persuade them to abstain from invasive procedures and report them if they refused. In 1993, Department of Health guidelines agreed that patients had a right to know when treated by infected staff and that such personnel should abstain from invasive procedures.[129] The Finns required screening of all employed in health care. In some German states and in Sweden, hygienic precautions were required of professions involving epidermal puncturing (hair dressing, beauty treatment, chiropody, acupuncture, tattooing, and ear piercing). In New South Wales, seropositives were not allowed to practice these professions at all.[130]

The consensus was thus that, since the risk of transmission was minimal—even in health care settings—seropositive medical personnel should be allowed to perform duties other than invasive procedures. The general solution was to use universal barrier precautions of the sort applicable to other infectious diseases.[131]

INSURANCE COVERAGE

Insurance coverage broached many discriminatory possibilities, but the issues depended on the kind of coverage and the broader national context. A risk like HIV, which could in part both be consciously assumed and hidden, posed the moral hazard of a selection against the fund. Should HIV be treated differently from other risks that insurance carriers were allowed to detect and exclude? Insurance, particularly health insurance, was more than just a business, especially in nations like the United States where coverage was largely assured through private companies, and it also involved ticklish political calculations. Were large and vocal groups of victims to be excluded from coverage? Were the costs of their care to be shifted to public providers of last resort, and thus ultimately to the taxpayer?

Least vexed by other considerations was life insurance. The salience of the issue varied among nations. In Britain and France, mortgages were often contingent on life insurance policies. Over 60 percent of first mortgages advanced by building societies in the United Kingdom in 1993 were endowment mortgages (involving a life insurance policy that matured to pay off the mortgage). Many of the remaining mortgages required life insurance coverage as well.[132] Indeed, so important was this connection that the interests of the banking and mortgage industries put them at cross-purposes with the insurance companies. In Switzerland, business loans to professionals were often contingent on an insurance policy.[133] In Germany and the United States, in contrast, loans were commonly secured by a lien on the property itself, and in Germany home ownership was in any case low by industrialized standards. But life insurance played an important role in the underdeveloped social policy landscape of America, assuring support of surviving dependents in a way that was less pressing in Europe. Varying tax structures also played a role. Americans used life insurance to sidestep high personal inheritance rates, while in Europe, taxes on inherited wealth were lower.[134]

For health insurance, matters became more complicated. Since illness and not death was the liability in question, problems were raised by the long latency period and the peculiar nature of a syndrome that permitted opportunistic infections free rein while it was not a clinically definable disease in the traditional sense. When did the illness begin? What were preexisting conditions? What counted as treatment? Were insurers obliged to pay the costs of assuaging symptoms in the absence of any effective treatment? Should they pay for experimental and, as yet, unproven therapies?[135] Nations with either national health systems or compulsory health insurance differed markedly from the United States, with its patchwork of national insurance for the poor, the old, and the formerly armed, on the one hand, and voluntary private provision for most—but far from all—people.

In the former systems, private health insurance, if it existed at all, either covered those few who were not required to enroll in the general coverage or provided supplemental benefits. Where private insurance remained supplemental, as in Britain, such policies often excluded AIDS, the burdens of which fell to the national system. In the European national health insurance systems, AIDS was included as a covered disease from the very beginning. Few, if any, distinctions were drawn between it and other ailments, and only minor haggles were undertaken over costs (whether, for example, to cover HIV tests motivated without reason to suspect infection). Some systems, however, included an element of personal responsibility. Where victims had some control over their liability, they could find their benefits reduced. In Switzerland in 1987, for example, an infected female drug addict found her hospital benefits cut by a third because of gross negligence.[136]

In contrast, the American discussion was bedeviled by the problem of risk skimming. Private insurance companies sought to cut costs by excluding on the basis of lifestyle or by requiring negative tests. Not only did the victims of such exclusion have cause to protest, so did the authorities—local, state, and federal—who administered the statutory systems of last resort, for they were already overtaxed by the usual problems of illness, drug abuse, and poverty. Fearing that public programs would be saddled with burdens that were deemed unprofitable by the private sector, some states sought to restrict HIV screening by insurance companies. In fact, the percentage of AIDS health costs paid for by private insurance was low and decreasing during the mid-1980s.[137] Adding a note of absurdity, poverty was the price of admission to Medicaid. Middle-class gays, perfectly capable of paying private insurance premiums, had to spend down their assets in order to become poor, adding to the burdens of a system already struggling to care for the needy. Since HIV was only one of many points of failure in Medicaid, should disproportional resources be devoted to it, when more systemic issues were neglected?[138] The geographic concentration of the epidemic also conspired with the state and local funding of Medicaid and public hospitals to accumulate burdens in areas already hard pressed by other social problems.

Some voluntary and private health insurance carriers, as in Germany, could select clients with advantageous risk profiles. But in general the risk pools of the European systems were larger, and skimming was not as troublesome. Nonetheless, even there, similar problems arose with the most marginal and least-covered groups. In France, those who were not members of national health insurance, including many drug addicts, had to be covered by social assistance, which was based on family means tests and complicated eligibility requirements. Illegal aliens, who did not belong to the system, were also a problem.[139]

The American system distributed access to medical services primarily through the workplace.[140] Since health insurance was typically a perquisite of employment, how should one cover those who changed or lost jobs? To maintain proper coverage, federal and state authorities cobbled together continuation and conversion requirements, including the bizarrely acronymed COBRA (Consolidated Omnibus Budget Reconciliation Act) program.[141] Also, since coverage was heavily workplace-dependent and linked to families of workers, gays—barred from marriage—were excluded from benefits open to heterosexuals. Some employers provided coverage to spousal equivalents, regardless of sex, but this only papered over cracks in the system. Battles over discrimination and actuarial skimming were thus fought in Europe over life insurance, and in the United States over both health and life insurance.

The French law of 12 July 1990, which otherwise outlawed discrimination based on health and handicap, excepted insurance carriers. The following year, after public protest and objections in the National AIDS Council, however, an agreement was worked out whereby the carriers would cease asking about sexual behavior, though not necessarily about medically pertinent details such as serostatus or opportunistic infections. If an applicant refused a proposed HIV test, the carriers could draw whatever conclusion they wished. The asymptomatic infected were no longer excluded from life insurance and thus mortgages. They could take out policies for up to one million francs, maturing over a decade, paying a premium of 4 to 6 percent above normal rates, though in fact very few made use of this alleged privilege. Because of this extra charge, those privy to someone's financial details—a bank issuing a mortgage, for example—had little trouble guessing its cause.[142]

Holland and Italy similarly decided that insurance policies above a certain limit were not basic necessities. They allowed screening in such cases and, in the Italian case, also for lesser amounts if risk was suspected.[143] In Denmark, though nothing prevented carriers from screening applicants, public criticism encouraged them to desist. Norwegian insurance carriers were allowed to test applicants and could postpone decisions for up to five years on the asymptomatic infected. In Sweden, carriers could test high-risk groups and reject seropositives.[144] Australian insurers might test, and some carriers asked questions meant to determine the sexual orientation of applicants. Swiss insurers followed similar policies. The Germans, too, allowed policies to be dependent on screening, though questions about lifestyle and sexual preference were thought to violate privacy protections.[145]

In Britain, insurers could ask questions about lifestyle and risky habits. Starting in 1986, most carriers queried applicants about previous HIV tests, regardless of outcome, and AIDS counseling. The insurance carriers' initial reaction to the epidemic was to increase premiums up to 150 percent for single males, to question applicants as to membership in high-risk groups, and to deny policies to those infected or at risk. In 1992, some companies began asking applicants about sexual relationships with foreigners and gays, how stable their partnerships were, and how often they changed lovers—questions without compare in other nations. In 1993, the Terence Higgins Trust, the main AIDS activist organization, sponsored a private member's bill to restrict questions about previous negative tests. To sweeten the pot, the government actuary concluded that, thanks to a decline in the projected number of AIDS cases, the insurance companies could reduce the reserves set aside to cover potential claims. When the bill drew wide support, the industry agreed in 1994 to withdraw questions about previous negative tests.[146]

In the United States, insurance companies eventually won the right to consider HIV for life and health insurance policies. During the early stages of the epidemic, they sought to exclude applicants on the basis of characteristics believed to reveal homosexuality: residence in certain zip codes, marital status, occupations of particular sorts. After pressure from gay and civil rights groups, the industry voluntarily ceased taking alleged sexual preference into account. But it continued to exclude on the basis of more tangible evidence of infection and sickness.[147] Various localities sought to prevent carriers from using screening or seropositivity in underwriting. At one point, Washington, D.C., and eight states had restricted such use of testing.[148] The tide turned quickly, however, as insurance companies drew attention to the higher costs for all policyholders in the absence of selection and threatened to pull out of restrictive local markets. In the nation's capital, Senator Helms joined forces with black ministers to make political hay out of the favoritism allegedly shown to AIDS victims and the dire consequences as insurance companies closed down operations.[149] Eventually, restrictions on insurers' ability to underwrite as they saw fit were ended in most states. California long held out in prohibiting the consideration of HIV in selling health insurance, though it abandoned such strictures on life insurance. Excepting Wisconsin, all states allowed HIV screening for life insurance, though in practice it was generally required only for policies over a certain amount. Questions that aimed indirectly at the same knowledge—about lifestyle, drug use, and sexual preference—were largely ruled out by antidiscrimination legislation. Also, although they were in principle able to consider HIV, American companies generally refrained for the group policies under which most Americans found health coverage. Some states that allowed such discrimination for individual policies forbade it for group ones.[150]

The nations that allowed most discrimination in insurance were European: Sweden, Norway, and Britain. With the caveat that health insurance raised problems that, in Europe, were largely sidestepped, the United States fell into the camp where such practices were resisted and not broadly practiced. The European peers here include France and Germany. The respective topographies of the insurance landscape help explain such differences. Nations like Sweden, where private insurance played a role of little importance because of its well-developed welfare state, could afford to treat it as a luxury, subject to actuarial calculations that did not need modification on behalf of HIV for political or humanitarian reasons. In the United States, in contrast, life and especially health insurance coverage on the open market were necessities in a system predicated on more individual responsibility and self-maintenance. Allowing private insurance to exclude bad risks threatened the stability of the systems of last resort, which were intended mainly for the underclass and not for all AIDS victims. Moreover, it also violated the implicit social compact by which the middle classes were expected to assure their own security in return for being spared the taxes otherwise required to pay for national or broadly compulsory systems.

MARRIAGE

Tying the knot presented another bottleneck at which restrictions might slow the spread of disease. In certain nations, marriage by the infected was obstructed; in some it was forbidden outright, as in Vietnam and Syria. The Poles barred those with venereal disease from marrying, but in practice health certificates were rarely demanded. In Germany, prenuptial examinations were not required, but the betrothed had to inform each other of venereal afflictions, though not including HIV. France approached the issue gingerly—which was not surprising for a nation with long natalist traditions. Though prenuptial medical examinations were required, HIV screening was only recommended. Many feared that severe restrictions might discourage marriages.[151] Sweden had no legislation regarding HIV and marriage, largely because its existing strictures on venereal disease were already broadly encompassing. Seropositivity was neither an impediment to marriage nor a reason for its dissolution, but a person's infection could be told to the spouse and seropositives were obliged to inform sexual partners. Utah forbade seropositives from marrying, but this was invalidated in 1993 for being incompatible with the Americans with Disabilities Act. During the mid-1980s, Illinois and Louisiana required HIV tests for marriage licenses. The marriage rate in Illinois plummeted to the lowest in the nation the year the measure took effect, and it was repealed shortly thereafter, in Louisiana in 1988.[152]

In terms of ending marriages, practices also differed. In Austria divorce might be granted if one partner suffered from a contagious or particularly repugnant disease. In the United Kingdom, concealment of a venereal disease from a future spouse could be grounds for annulment, although it was unclear whether HIV counted in this respect.[153] Contagious or incurable diseases that threatened the offspring were grounds for dissolution of a marriage in Germany. If seropositivity was hidden, marriage could be ended on the basis of willful deceit. Engagements could be broken if one party proved to be infected, and claims to compensation for damages depended on how the disease had been contracted.[154] In France, a spouse who discovered the partner's seropositivity after marriage might be granted an annulment. Seropositivity did not serve as cause for divorce as such, but it might belong to the larger category of reasons for such action, as proof of adultery, for example. It could also justify a demand for divorce *pour faute* if one party could show that it had been infected by the other.[155] In the United States, the situation was ambiguous. Marriages could be annulled if one party had been induced into the bond by fraud. The failure to inform of infection might possibly constitute such. In terms of divorce, infection could serve as evidence of adultery subsequent to the marriage and thus as a basis for ending it. Statutes often allowed divorce if one spouse had infected the other with venereal disease. Concealment of infection was also considered grounds for divorce and possible liability for damages.[156]

How protected the victims of AIDS were thus varied substantially among nations. Europeans enjoyed the advantages of extensive social insurance and employment coverage. Yet the very generosity of the benefits to which they were entitled also allowed employers wide latitude to investigate their epidemiological circumstances. Americans, in turn, had instituted an extensive apparatus of legislation to protect the handicapped against discrimination. When victims of the epidemic were included in this category, a major victory had been won.

6. Every Man His Own Quarantine Officer

The Voluntary Approach

At first, many observers assumed that inherited public health policies could be used without friction against AIDS. Events proved otherwise. AIDS threw a fistful of wrenches into the works of traditional contagious disease control. Caused by a new, scarcely understood, and extremely protean class of infectious agents—retroviruses—it was a disease whose nature resisted treatment and cure. There was little hope of a technical fix, and none for a quick one. On the other hand, the extraordinarily rapid development of knowledge about the disease allowed interventions more precisely targeted at risk behaviors and risk groups than had been possible with previous epidemics. Half a century ago, quarantine may have been the least restrictive means of controlling epidemic disease. With AIDS, once it was clear to public health officials that it was not spreading indiscriminately into the general population, such restrictions made little scientific sense.[1]

In any case, the universal mobility of modern life rendered unrealistic any hope of preventing movement by the infected. In the first half of 1987, for example, 223 million travelers crossed the borders into West Germany. Seventy-six million were foreigners, and of those over two-thirds were European Union citizens, whose movements could not be restricted. With such figures, traditional public health instruments barely functioned. Quarantine threatened to involve logistical nightmares. It might have worked in certain nations able to restrict access, and in others early in the epidemic, when there were few identifiable infected. But once the disease had spread, such efforts were useless.[2]

The scale of potential infection also made old-fashioned precautions very costly. Illinois's prenuptial screening requirement identified eight seropositives out of seventy thousand tests performed during six months, at a cost of $2.5 million. Had prenuptial screenings been extended throughout the country, $100 million spent annually for four million tests might have spotted some thirteen hundred not otherwise identified seropositives. Screening the German population would have meant testing forty million sexually active adults twice annually—a total of eighty million tests costing some two hundred marks each—and would have required four hundred health authorities to run two tests per minute during each working day.[3] Testing low-risk groups (pregnant women, couples marrying, visiting foreigners, and so forth) threatened to be vastly expensive. The problem of false negatives and positives was large, too. Since HIV mutated rapidly, tests for one strain might not detect others.[4]

If testing the entire population at regular intervals was prohibitive, screening high-risk groups presented ethical and political problems of discrimination: why all gays, say, when monogamous homosexual couples posed less risk than promiscuous heterosexuals? If aimed at all who engaged in high-risk activity, the basis for action would be presumptions about future behavior based on the past, with all the ticklish issues of how to justify extrapolating from one to the other.[5]

Since AIDS was spread by blood contact, not through air like tuberculosis or African hemorrhagic fever, possible precautions were limited. For the latter diseases, where a simple cough might be an epidemiological offense, it made sense to identify and isolate the ill. For diseases like typhoid, notification could be justified as a way of tracing infected food and water sources. But since HIV was only rarely transmitted via casual contact, isolation or quarantine was unnecessary.[6] Because the illness was incurable, even if isolation made sense it would have to be for life, adding immeasurably to the problems of implementation. The German VD law's prohibition on the ill having sex was intended for curable diseases. Extended to AIDS, it implied a lifelong end to carnal relations—not necessarily an illogical measure, but certainly one with an entirely different human and political import than if applied to syphilitics.[7] The restrictions imposed for other STDs sought to bring into treatment those who might otherwise avoid it. Compulsion for recalcitrants made sense because of the chance of cure, less so in its absence. But once therapeutic possibilities for AIDS, however limited, appeared in the 1990s, the situation changed. Even vehement critics of testing grudgingly admitted the logic of identifying victims if they could be helped.[8]

During the epidemic's early phases, however, the absence of therapeutic possibilities undercut the logic of testing. Knowledge of serostatus had no curative implications and therefore little value for the individual. If anything, the worth of knowing was negative: discrimination, stigma, possible legal consequences. Testing made sense only if those who now knew changed their behavior. Yet knowledge of serostatus appeared to have an ambiguous effect. Devil-may-care conduct was not unheard of. Gaetan Dugas, the French Canadian airplane steward immortalized by Randy Shilts as Patient Zero in *And the Band Played On,* refused to change his globally transmissive behavior or to warn his partners. In Cyril Collard's movie *Les Nuits Fauves,* a woman proved her love by having unprotected intercourse with her infected lover. Seronegative gays, haunted by survivor guilt, often indulged in psychologically compensatory bouts of unsafe sex, as dramatized in Tony Kushner's *Angels in America.*[9]

Moreover, the window of time between infection and the formation of antibodies meant that even those screened might unknowingly be infectious. With the numbers involved in mass screening, even highly accurate procedures threatened to leave behind many false positives and negatives. Given the long incubation period of AIDS, notification made little sense. Contact tracing was also hindered because of the virus's saturation density in the most afflicted communities.[10] In the sexually sociable gay neighborhoods of New York City or San Francisco, contact tracing would have led investigators to virtually every other denizen, and thus nowhere. Because the activities associated with HIV's spread were both stigmatized and often illegal, contact tracing meant implicating others in questionable acts.[11]

To proponents of consensual tactics, traditional compulsory methods and a voluntary approach seemed incompatible at heart, and the choice between them was either/or. AIDS was incurable and stigmatized; it afflicted marginalized groups with justified fears of statutory interventions; and it was transmitted largely in private circumstances far removed from the state's purview. In their view, it therefore required, as the main means of prophylaxis, voluntary behavioral change. Preventive strategies should avoid coercion and threats to privacy lest the epidemic be driven even further underground.[12] As critics of traditional techniques in Germany pointed out, targeting aliens, for example, would primarily affect groups such as foreign prostitutes who would go into hiding, far from the reach of counseling and treatment.[13] Hopes of encouraging high-risk groups to be tested, and to practice safe sex, abstain if infected, seek care and counseling, and so forth would be dashed if punitive sanctions otherwise threatened. The stick spoiled the carrot's allure. Criminalizing transmission or weakening medical confidentiality to allow for contact tracing or notification would discourage voluntary testing. If insurance carriers took the very act of having had a HIV test as evidence of possible risk, as in Britain, then who would voluntarily screen? Using the possession of condoms as evidence of commercial sex when arresting suspected prostitutes, as the police in many American states and in the United Kingdom did, undercut hopes of encouraging prostitutes to suit up clients in latex. If needles were evidence of drug abuse, then addicts would be more likely to share works in shooting galleries.[14]

INDIVIDUAL RESPONSIBILITY

By the AIDS era, many observers thought that public health had moved on from both its quarantinist and its sanitationist roots. Basic sanitary infrastructure was standard in all developed urban areas. The conquest of classic epidemic diseases, and the displacement of mortality to chronic ailments, shifted the focus to individual factors. Public health became increasingly individualized, with an emphasis on lifestyle, habit, and custom. Individuals were held responsible for their own well-being. Insurance companies too were concerned with individual guilt and responsibility. Activities that earlier had prompted no reprobation now had a price. Those who smoked, avoided exercise, or indulged in extreme sports paid higher premiums than the risk averse.[15] The actuarially self-indulgent found themselves excluded from limited medical resources; liver transplants were refused to alcoholics and hearts to heavy smokers. One American company, though later forced to back down after adverse publicity, refused to insure "personal lifestyle decisions" in its health plan, meaning problems arising from AIDS, alcohol or drug abuse, or self-inflicted wounds.[16] Swiss drug addicts found their hospital benefits reduced as the damage was considered self-inflicted. A Swedish store owner interpreted the law's strictures against selling tobacco to minors to apply also to the unborn and thus their mothers.[17] Pregnant women were routinely refused service in bars in America.

Seen from the old public health tradition, such a focus on individual responsibility ignored the social factors that collectively influenced each citizen. The inheritors of medicine's socially reformist tradition, updated now as "social medicine" and "social environmentalism," rejected a focus on individual habits as blaming victims for behaviors over which they had little control. Seen positively, however, this shift toward individual responsibility empowered the citizen and lessened the community's demands. Control shifted from externally imposed requirements to internally accepted restrictions. Self-control, voluntary compliance, and individual responsibility rather than coercion, compulsion, and collective action were the watchwords. Democratic public health was based on an implicit assumption that individuals would curb harmful behavior and develop healthy habits.

The individualized approach to AIDS prevention exemplified this democratic style of public health. Since HIV was spread—with exceptions like perinatal transmission—in discrete and voluntary acts, all could and should protect themselves: such was the argument advanced for dealing with AIDS. During the mid–nineteenth century, when it was gradually accepted that cholera spread via water, and not miasmatically or indiscriminately, it followed that it could be avoided by shunning infected water. John Snow, who is famous for having identified the waterborne transmission of cholera in the Broad Street pump episode of the London epidemic of 1853, put it thus: "Every man may be his own quarantine officer and go about during an epidemic among the sick almost as if no epidemic were present."[18] So, too, in the early phases of the AIDS epidemic, it was widely thought that everyone could be his or her own quarantine officer, taking the precautions required to avoid transmission. Public health was an individual good, for which each citizen could assume responsibility. Collective strictures intended to enforce acceptable behavior were largely superfluous (beyond the universally accepted prohibition on HIV-contaminated blood donation). Practically speaking, there was no need to identify and isolate the ill, deport infected foreigners, trace contacts, criminalize sex while infected, or punish transmission. After all, individuals could ensure their own safety by insisting on a condom or by not sharing needles. Bathhouses need not be closed, because customers were responsible for their own behavior and its consequences. Anyone wishing to stay out of harm's way could opt for more anodyne pleasures.[19] Liberty, it turned out, rested on moderation, hygiene, and latex.

The condomization of society became seen as the basis of its freedom, both sexual and political. Individual precautions allowed citizens to avoid infection while permitting democratic society to sidestep drastic statutory interventions. The same preventive rules applied to all, infected or not: all must act as though at risk.[20] Gay organizations and their allies frequently argued that condoms obviated the need for screening, and that it was unnecessary to advise sex partners of serostatus since you were protecting them by using latex. Promiscuity was fine so long as each encounter was rubberized.[21] The German Green Party rejected any requirement of notifying partners of serostatus. Each should assume infection in the other, excepting only cases of special trust, as between long-term partners. An American court condemned a drug addiction clinic's decision to reveal a client's serostatus to his partners as unnecessary, since all clients were counseled to avoid risky behavior. Either partner, whether in needle sharing or sex, could protect himself; whether infected or not, the positions of both were epidemiologically symmetrical. Behavior counted, not serostatus.[22]

To individualize self-protection, rather than to trust society to protect you by punishing negligent partners, avoided the paternalism of asking the state to shield its citizens from the consequences of their free actions.[23] Liberty and equality could best be ensured by holding each accountable for his or her own protection. After years of public education on the risks of unprotected sex, there were no delinquents or victims any longer. All knew the dangers and could avoid them. When couples tested themselves in starting a relationship, or as atonement for infidelity, it was considered the modern version of marriage, the sign of a cemented partnership—though now based on a lack of commitment and trust.[24] "Vertrauen," as Lenin says in a quotation that rings truest in its German translation, "ist gut, Kontrolle ist besser." The updated version was: "Trust is good, condoms are better."[25] Latex was the technical fix that obviated the need for honesty, trust, or solidarity.

Against such widespread arguments for individualizing protection stood the claim that, however responsible citizens should be for their own wellbeing, the infected must not be relieved of all consequences of transmissive behavior. The penal code still had a role to play in indicating that not every behavior was morally acceptable. Special obligations rested on the infected because of their particular knowledge. In this view, insisting that each individual, regardless of serostatus, alone bore the onus of protection was egotistical and irresponsible. Even the complete condomization of society would not have answered all questions of responsibility and liability. Condoms were not infallible, and the risk that remained for the potential recipient of infected fluids even in coitus condomatus was not an allowable one.[26]

The basic assumption of a voluntaristic public health approach to AIDS was that citizens of democratic polities could be expected to conduct themselves such that old-fashioned forms of mass, collective behavioral control were no longer necessary. Citizens were presumed to possess the competence for self-control.[27] But self-control was a two-edged sword. Since AIDS was often a self-inflicted illness, avoidable through prudence, restraint, and self-control, were its victims not responsible for their fates? If so, did this temper society's obligations to help them? Fault, guilt, and responsibility—questions that had long been part of understanding disease before the antibiotical age—were thus reintroduced to medicine.[28]

Those who defended the epidemic's victims argued that the behavior that led to infection had not been autonomously determined and was therefore not morally reprehensible. Most generally, sex was an instinct, only partly controllable. "Avoiding HIV by the 'correct procedure,'" as one observer described safe sex, "is thus similar to avoiding a cold by keeping one's mouth closed all the time. They are both theoretically possible, but not safe in practice."[29] Victims' advocates also argued that risky behavior, especially promiscuity, was socially determined, and thus involuntary and morally neutral. The gay rejection of inherited sexual mores for polymorphous pleasures was often presented as a social pathology. Once homosexuals were accepted as "normal," they would be free to settle into the bourgeois propriety and monogamous coupledom, or at least emotional intimacy, characteristic of straight society. Anonymous multiple sex was, in this view (which must have led many gays to ponder the fine line between friends and enemies), a desperate and inauthentic search to counter the myth of homosexual effemininity.[30] "The . . . discrimination of gay people," as Jo Richardson, member of Parliament for Barking, plaintively put it, "sometimes brings pressures which result in their having a high number of sexual partners."[31] The apogee of such sexual paternalism—as always motivated by the best of intentions—was reached in the Swedish government's defense of its decision to close gay bathhouses and all other establishments that might facilitate anonymous sex, whether homo- or heterosexual. Such institutions, it argued, were reprehensible because they assumed that sexuality was separate from other human relations. The government hoped to encourage instead the development of meeting places for homosexuals where they could watch movies, join study groups, listen to lectures, dance, and pursue other similarly anodyne activities.[32] As though knitting circles could purge Dionysus from the loins!

While a focus on the involuntary, socially determined nature of behavior may here have reached implausible extremes, the argument carried more conviction when applied to pathologies of drug addiction. Advising addicts not to share needles made little sense when injection equipment was not available for sale and when, indeed, possession was criminalized. In the absence of sufficient drug rehabilitation programs, appeals to addicts' self-reliance also seemed unrealistic.[33]

THE VOLUNTARY APPROACH

As the main problem posed to public health in the industrialized world shifted from acute contagious diseases to chronic lifestyle ailments, the nature of prevention changed. Rather than imposing strictures to break chains of transmission or drawing legal lines to shape behavior, the state now sought to change its citizens' conduct by educating and counseling them to undertake less risky behavior. The connection between information and behavioral change, however, was far from straightforward and direct.

A large literature—some of it of dunderheaded complexity, some of it common horse sense—arose to explore the intricacies of the connection.[34] If citizens were rational self-interest maximizers, presenting evidence of the self-destructive quality of certain habits would lead automatically to their discontinuance. But of course they were not. Bad habits were also, alas, often pleasurable or at least part of a broad and multidetermined web of behaviors not easily changed. Risky behavior was not the result of ignorance alone. Cultural and subcultural influences were strong, the determinants bred in the bone or quaffed with mother's milk, all fomenting resistance to otherwise rational behaviors. What seemed irrational in one context (unsafe sex) may have been reasonable in another (pursuit of pleasure). Perhaps rationality could be judged only within its situational context.[35] Why should one accept the assumption of safer sex campaigns, that it was rational to give up sex in order to live?[36] Consider the Polish prisoners who deliberately sought infection to shorten their jail terms, the Scottish heroin junkies who did so to be included in methadone programs, the Cubans who injected themselves with infected blood to pass the few years before a cure was certain in the relative comfort of the camps for seropositives, or the Botswanans who, faced with the statistical probability of an early death, discounted future prospects in favor of present pleasures and ignored condoms: they were being feckless, perhaps, but not irrational.[37]

Risk, like everything else, was socially constructed. Different social groups approached it quite differently.[38] Individuals' willingness to entertain risks depended on their social context, their cultural baggage, and their negotiational circumstances (a prostitute haggling over the price of foregoing a condom, as might the young lover of a wealthy, older gay man). How far to postpone gratification depended on life prospects as much as rational calculation.[39] Knowledge did not determine or change behavior in any simple sense. Education campaigns, as their critics charged, presumed that individuals rationally chose their actions. In fact, however, social contexts and determinations rendered largely illusory the deliberateness of such decisions.[40] None of this, naturally, was specific to epidemiologically risky actions. It pertained as much to the pleasures of nicotine, alcohol, and fatty foods or the rush of the main line. Yet, given the instinctual overdetermination of our reproductive behavior, the power of pleasure-seeking over reason may have been especially strong for the sexual conduct at the root of most HIV transmission.[41]

How correct was the implicit assumption that there were objectively healthy ways of living and correspondingly impartial choices to be made? What is overweight? How many lovers make one promiscuous? When, if at all, can sexual attraction be considered an addiction? Which chemicals may we use for recreational pleasures? And who wields the power to determine the content of the educational message broadcast? Early in the epidemic, for example, Dutch health authorities (as well as the British Terence Higgins Trust and the Scottish AIDS Monitor) preferred discouraging anal sex among gays to promoting condoms. All other nations, in contrast, sought widespread use of condoms.[42] The implications of such differences for gay sex were stark: business as usual behind the latex barrier or a new chastity and a refocusing of the libido from one orifice to another.

The various good intentions of information campaigns also sometimes ran at cross purposes. Should drug users be accepted as potentially rational interest maximizers, susceptible to influence by educational campaigns, or were they treated more compassionately by emphasizing the oppressive social circumstances that undercut hopes of reaching them via reason and persuasion?[43] If individual rights and autonomy were the basis of prevention, then how to reconcile the right not to know (embodied, for example, in Dutch, Swiss, and Belgian law and discussed in Germany)—that is, the right not to take a HIV test or the right to remain in ignorance of its results—with a strategy founded on knowledge, information, and behavioral change?[44] Once education campaigns were in place and the average citizen was aware of HIV's dangers, the penal sanctions that remained for recalcitrants could justifiably be more strictly enforced. Ignorance no longer served as an excuse. Liminal minorities should perhaps not be driven underground by ham-fisted tactics. But, short of intrusive information-gathering by public health authorities, how could one measure whether a voluntary approach in fact worked among the marginal?[45]

Inherent tensions also freighted the dissemination of information on practices commonly regarded as reprehensible: teaching adolescents about safe sex and distributing condoms in conservative communities, instructing gays on similar techniques where homosexual acts remained criminal offenses, and showing addicts how to bleach needles when the purpose they were put to violated the law. Some groups were simply inaccessible to information and education—not just the hard core of addicts but also otherwise respectable patrons of prostitutes who were unlikely to welcome being addressed in their capacity as johns. Contradictions plagued relations between generalized campaigns aimed at the average citizen and ones targeted at high-risk groups. Too sharp a focus and the average Joe turned away, dismissing the issue as a problem for deviants. Too wide, and resources were squandered on the worried well and those least at risk.[46] The initial British educational campaign addressed the general population. It deliberately sought to avoid stigmatizing gays by targeting risk behaviors rather than groups. It thereby also spent its energies on those with least cause to alter their conduct. Critics argued that its generalized focus rested on a "nationalistic fantasy" of a broad public undifferentiated by religion, class, or gender and yet united in opposition to all those outside the institution of marriage. Similar in their focus on the general public were the Swedish, Dutch, French, and Australian informational efforts. Though gays were the most immediate victims, they were ignored as such by these campaigns.[47]

Education and information could have unintended effects, encouraging risky behavior if, say, someone learned that an act of unprotected intercourse was in fact less dangerous than feared. Or preventive information could prompt precautions of little use that encouraged a false sense of security—as when the British Football Association counseled its members not to kiss and cuddle when celebrating goals, not to drink victory champagne from common bottles, not to exchange shirts at the end of a game, and not to take communal baths. Educational campaigns could also be seen as fig leaves, salving the authorities' bad conscience for refusing to take more effective measures. On the one hand, they could be used tactically to defuse pressure from conservatives for more drastic strictures. On the other, they justified avoiding politically explosive, but effective, techniques, like needle exchanges or condom dispensing in jails.[48]

Despite the problems of an information-based strategy, many thought that it was the only means of curbing AIDS. Shaped by a confluence of gays, civil rights activists, and public health officials, this strategy came, despite the persistence in some nations of a more old-fashioned approach, to dominate the first decade of the epidemic.

EDUCATION CAMPAIGNS

At the core of the voluntary, information-based approach lay the educational campaigns sponsored in each nation. The United States put in a decidedly mixed performance. It was late in underwriting a national education campaign (with a pamphlet in 1988 that made up the largest single act of direct mail ever—the postage alone cost ten million dollars), though it shared this dubious distinction with France and Austria, which had done equally little as of the early 1990s.[49] Initial attempts at effective efforts were hobbled by strictures imposed by conservatives. Senator Helms sponsored an amendment eliminating federal monies for activities allegedly promoting homosexuality and promiscuity, and condoms could not be dispensed to minors without parental consent. Despite broad public support for more liberal educational efforts (60 percent of Americans favored condom advertisements on TV), and despite the ability in some states to distribute reasonably explicit literature, vocal minorities of religious leaders and social conservatives still managed to block any quick movement in this direction.[50] The media resisted explicit language and pulled their punches in describing risky sexual practices. On the whole, early educational programs in America were deemed to have failed their objective by overly emphasizing the unattainable goal of abstinence while neglecting the practicalities of safe sex. Not until the late 1980s, and especially during the Clinton administration, were more aggressive campaigns for condoms possible.[51]

It became apparent, too, that no single national campaign could address the issues in a common idiom. Faced with a culturally polymorphous society, the American programs had to target messages at different ethnic, religious, and national subcultures. The Public Health Service quickly concluded that community-specific campaigns were the tactic of choice. The presidential commission recognized the need for local control over education campaigns, allowing the message on such ticklish matters to be adjusted to grassroots customs and mores. It was not for the federal government, it concluded, to dictate values to local communities, and representatives of minority and other groups were increasingly included in the process of formulating such campaigns.[52]

In Britain, the national AIDS information campaign, started in 1986, was among the first and most encompassing. It was widely praised for being frank, daring, and effective, though the British themselves admired the Dutch efforts even more. The British campaign's focus was the general public, not just risk groups, though drug users received special attention. Gays were left to be enlightened by the Terence Higgins Trust.[53] Much like the Helms amendment in the United States, the Local Government Act of 1988 forbade the promotion of homosexuality. Along with various local restrictions, this dampened educational efforts. Producers of allegedly salacious materials were occasionally prosecuted, and gay publications from abroad confiscated. The Terence Higgins Trust's safe sex materials for gay men were financed from private charitable funds to avoid accusations that the government was subsidizing pornography.[54]

The Swedish education campaign was also notable for its attention to the public at large. It was criticized for whipping up unnecessary anxieties, as well as for demonizing groups that in contexts outside Sweden would not seem particularly insidious—the allegedly loose-living Danes, for example (citizens who in inter-Nordic rivalries are dismissed as Italians pretending to be Germans).[55] The Italian, Dutch, and French campaigns also primarily addressed the general public. Seeking to prevent stigmatization, they focused on risk behaviors and not groups.[56] In France, the ideology of republican universalism, which regarded group-defined identities as illegitimate, hampered any targeting of a message that was seen as pertaining to all. After 1990, however, efforts were targeted more specifically at risk groups.[57] The Germans, in turn, divided their educational efforts, with federal authorities taking the average citizen in their sights, while the quasi-private Deutsche AIDS-Hilfe concentrated on gays and other high-risk groups.[58]

Cultural differences also colored the respective education campaigns. In the United States, conservatives prevented discussion of subjects that were commonplace elsewhere—condoms, for example. The general sexual timidity of public advertising was reflected also in the preventive effort.[59] In France, Italy, Austria, and other Catholic nations, initial campaigns were equally vapid and inexplicit, with the Church encouraging a less revealing approach than in the north.[60] In Germany and Scandinavia, which had long traditions of frankness about the human body, campaigns were more unflinching. Even where municipal government was Christian Democratic, condom use was encouraged in ways that would be unthinkable in America. Yet even here, the squeamishness that afflicts public discussions of sex was present. A brochure with photographs of condom use was forbidden in the German army, though considered tame enough for the navy's sailors: as in most nations, the latter were long the object of antivenereal campaigns and still considered salty dogs who knew which end was up.[61]

Parents' abilities to exempt their children from sex education, or at least that part concerned with AIDS, also varied nationally. In the United States, with its federalized school system, the issue was decided locally, parents sometimes being allowed to withdraw pupils, sometimes not. In New York City, parents could ask to have children exempted only from those parts of HIV education where condoms were distributed.[62] In Britain, the 1986 Education Act allowed schools to opt out of sex education altogether, and the

1988 Local Government Act, prohibiting the promotion of homosexuality, discouraged discussion of such matters. During the early 1990s, a Catholic Labour peer sought to remove HIV education from the compulsory part of the curriculum. And the 1993 Education Act shifted HIV education from science to sex education, a subject from which, unlike the former, parents had a right to withdraw their children.[63] In contrast, on the Continent, at least outside the Catholic countries, such disputes were fewer.

Because information was crucial to this new public health strategy, new actors joined the field. The media, including the gay variants, were embraced now as collaborators—and ones that worked for free at that—in the government's information dissemination efforts.[64] In Britain, so close was cooperation with the government that the media began to worry about their independence. Advertising techniques of the sort employed by corporations to introduce new brands were held up as the model to be emulated by public health awareness campaigns.[65] Indeed, a media-saturated landscape, able to deliver the authorities' messages on behavioral change, was a precondition for implementing an approach based on information and education in the first place. The same held, of course, for schools and universities. The higher the average educational level, the more likely the success of an approach based on dissemination of information.[66]

BEHAVIORAL CHANGE

The effectiveness of the voluntary approach, based on education, information, and counseling, depended on what was expected of it. Compared to doing nothing? Compared to possibly effective, but politically intolerable, strictures? Compared to behavioral changes made in the past by other risk groups? And how did you measure the behavior in question? Were condom use and foregoing the pleasures of fisting the only relevant indicators? What about substituting oral for anal sex? How about picking partners more carefully or the so-called negotiated safety strategies: practicing safe sex, though not with a trusted and tested partner?[67]

Within the general population during the 1980s and early 1990s, the average number of sexual partners per person did not change much, but condoms were more frequently used.[68] Among gays, the evidence that AIDS prompted behavioral change was ambiguous.[69] Generally, the average gay man began to behave less riskily during the epidemic's course. Some have claimed that safer conduct predated the epidemic. Perhaps the pleasures of promiscuity had been fading in general; perhaps energies flagged as the gay population grayed. But AIDS clearly encouraged whatever such developments were under way.[70] Some observers maintained that gays' conduct changed unprecedentedly compared to previous attempts at behavioral modification in personal hygiene, smoking, exercise, and diet.[71] Others were content to note that large numbers of gay men began acting more circumspectly.[72]

Nonpenetrative sexual practices proved unappealing. While more esoteric sex play—fisting, water sports, scat, and the like—declined in Australia, casual sex between men remained popular.[73] Not surprisingly, disparities in behavior modification appeared. There was less change toward safer conduct in rural than urban areas, less among minorities than whites in America, less among closeted homosexuals, less among lower classes, less among the young, and less in some nations than others.[74] Claims to practice safer sex were often belied by actual conduct—a disparity that tended to escape the multiple choices of social science questionnaires, and that was uncovered only by in-depth anthropological fieldwork. Among heterosexuals, evidence suggested there was qualified change in sexual behavior. Much lip service was paid to the virtues of safer sex. But there was an equal willingness to make exceptions in the heat of the moment.[75] Timing was also important. Most changes took place during the mid-1980s. A willingness to try riskier behavior reappeared once the epidemic became routinized, once certain well-meant attempts to change practices faded away (making condoms a desirable part of sex play rather than a grudging necessity), and once effective antiretroviral treatments encouraged a smidgen of complacency.[76] Indeed, a small literature appeared on this trend, and one issue in dispute was whether to regard it as a "relapse" and, if so, from what prelapsarian standard of initially safe sex.[77]

Preventive education left personal prophylaxis—behavioral change—as the main means of hampering HIV's spread. Just as depriving yourself of the pleasure of smoking reduced the risk of lung cancer, so abjuring previously possible delights was the key to avoiding HIV. This could mean abstinence altogether. That was, of course, not always popular. "It is important to note," one fine specimen of social science insight revealed, "that celibacy is not the preferred strategy of gay men for dealing with the risk of AIDS."[78] Short of that, behavioral change meant reducing the number of partners or choosing them more carefully. It might also involve avoiding unprotected anal and oral sex, sex during menstruation, or indeed intercourse of any sort without condoms. The preservative became quite literally that. Celebrated in the nineteenth century as an invention on a par with Jenner's smallpox vaccination, it was that thin barrier of linen, bestial ceca, vulcanized rubber, or—eventually—latex that provided the last palisade protecting pleasure from the suppurating world of malevolent microorganisms.

Condoms, in both their venerable form and the new, but much less popular, female version, were the key to epidemiological security. Certainly, they were the single most cost-effective means of reducing risk. Yet they still remained unpopular. Madame de Sévigné's immortal words for them, "as strong as gossamer, as sensual as armor," described them well. Thanks to the general shift of contraception to the pill, condoms had acquired a primary connotation of disease prevention. Because they signaled distrust between sexual partners, they took on negative emotional resonances.[79] Proposed innovations sought to make such barrier methods more reconcilable with instinct and enjoyment: spray-on and peel-off versions, embedded dual-control vibrating chips, female-centered devices, and disease-preventing but not contraceptive condoms for Catholics. Yet little was accomplished other than some playing around with color, shape, and taste.[80]

The Friends of Rajneesh, a religious community once headquartered in Oregon, instituted perhaps the most drastic of safe sex guidelines, including wearing both condoms and rubber gloves and not kissing during lovemaking. Ironically, the message of safe sex and the prophylactic virtues of latex were most known to lesbians, who needed it least. Their eager embrace of latex (condoms even for strap-ons and dildos; dental dams even for rimming; gloves even for solitary masturbation) may have been inspired not just by distaste for the ickier aspects of sex inherited from long antifemale inculcation, nor just by hopes of not being forgotten in the attention lavished on male gays (the so-called AIDS envy, or Munchausen AIDS). It may also have been a way for lesbians, who were now embracing the liberating possibilities of sex long familiar to their male peers, to publicize their pleasure in carnal excess. Lesbians seem to have accomplished what was otherwise regarded as the impossible task of eroticizing latex.[81]

Besides their obvious pleasure-inhibiting effects, condoms were also regarded suspiciously by observers who worried that they were but an amoral technical fix that failed to address the underlying problems of promiscuity and transmissive sexual practices, indeed that they were allowing business to continue as usual.[82] As John Cardinal O'Connor of New York put it in rejecting the use of condoms against AIDS, "The church could not condone the public provision of condoms because the greatest physical harm is less important than the smallest moral harm."[83] Unholy alliances were brokered over such issues between moral conservatives and those who took a broadly social approach to the epidemic, seeing the solution in lifestyle changes. For the first, the answer was suppressing homosexuality and returning to "traditional" family values. For the latter, it was gay marriage and the possibility of homosexual monogamy. Both heralded, as the only true solution, an end to the anonymous promiscuous coupling allegedly characteristic of gay mating behavior.[84] In addition, because of the contraceptive effects of barrier methods, these were also embroiled in ancillary battles over such issues.

Condom use therefore varied with cultural, economic, and religious circumstances. With certain subgroups, like the military, condoms could be almost mandated. French military personnel posted to Africa were issued condoms and encouraged to use them. American soldiers were required to do so.[85] With prisoners, in contrast, distributing condoms was a tacit admission of illegal activity. With still other groups, like prostitutes, the best approach appealed to an enlightened cost-benefit analysis, with their long-term health weighed more heavily than immediate profit. Where religion frowned on contraception, the condom, even if used only to prevent disease, was tainted by association. In France, as in all Catholic countries, the Church had long opposed contraception. Only slowly, in the late 1980s, following a similar process among American Catholics, was it persuaded to accept condoms against disease as the lesser of two evils.[86] Nonetheless, Catholic ethicists, otherwise at pains to sympathize with the afflicted, spent much energy explaining why latex alienated humans from their true sexuality.[87]

Different national styles of contraception were also important.[88] In Japan, where the condom was far more widely used than the pill, unprotected intercourse and sexual transmission were correspondingly infrequent. In the Caribbean, contraceptive habits were the reverse and the problem was much more acute.[89] In Britain and Sweden, condoms were already a common means of contraception. Less was required to encourage their use there than elsewhere, as in France, Lithuania, and Russia, where popular custom was latex-averse.[90] In France, only some 6 to 7 percent of couples used them, compared to 70 percent in Japan and 37 percent in Britain. The condom market was correspondingly small and dominated by imports.[91] Because condoms were unpopular, buying them in pharmacies (as was necessary until 1986) was commonly interpreted as an admission of homosexuality.[92] Besides the Church's influence, the popularity of natalist policies in France made contraception a ticklish issue. Indeed, so deeply rooted were such ideas that, when reformers sought to change the policy on advertising condoms, they argued that limiting HIV's spread through their use in fact stimulated population growth by decreasing mortality.[93]

Even where condoms were broadly accepted, they provoked curious objections. The American sexologists Masters, Johnson, and Kolodny regarded safe sex techniques as no more than a stopgap. Latex gloves worn during sex—testimony perhaps to excessive caution—they condemned as violating human dignity. In the United States, blacks were more reluctant than whites to use condoms. Latino gays hated them so much that some were willing to forego anal sex, if that was the choice.[94] But latextual habits were also flexible, and they changed. Among the youngest consumers in France, condom use grew during the early 1990s. In many nations, sales increased during the epidemic's apex, though flattening thereafter.[95]

Where condoms were already widely available, providing them free or at subsidized cost promised to do little to encourage their use. Conversely, where they were neither available nor much in favor, as in large parts of Africa, the costs of provision were daunting. Giving all sexually active Africans condoms for two to four acts of sex weekly at three or four cents per condom would cost donor agencies up to a billion dollars annually.[96] But shortages were not just a Third World problem. East Germany (the economy that prided itself, as the joke had it, on developing the world's largest microchip) also experienced shortages of condoms and sexual lubricants. In the Soviet Union of the late 1980s, only enough condoms were produced annually to provide each adult male with three. In Spain, too, though the market was large, condoms were in short supply and priced above the European average.[97]

Many questions arose: whether and how to advertise condoms in the popular media, whether to distribute them to minors, whether to admit their presence as evidence of prostitution and thereby discourage their use. New York City blazed the way in America in 1990 when it made condoms available in high schools.[98] Even in Sweden, normally relaxed about such matters, conservatives were upset when schoolchildren received AIDS information and condoms.[99] After long debates in France, sales were finally allowed as of 1986 in vending machines, no longer just in pharmacies. When advertisements were finally permitted the following year, they could tout only the condoms' disease-preventing virtues.[100] In many European nations, however—Britain included—intelligent and witty campaigns promoted condom use. In France and Switzerland, some cafés and bars offered free condoms along with drinks.[101] In America, predictable agonies arose over the issue. In 1986, *USA Today* was first to publish a half-page ad for condoms, one that had been refused by the *New York Times, Time,* and *Newsweek.* Why condom promotion—supported by American agencies in Africa and elsewhere abroad—was verboten at home was a question raised in the House of Representatives.[102]

As during the nineteenth-century battles over syphilis, circumcision was now found (the evidence came from Africa) to be correlated with lower rates of HIV infection.[103] Not surprisingly, when the subject involved both sex and anti-Semitism, the opposite was also argued. The right-wing National Front in France claimed that circumcision helped spread the disease when performed in African conditions of poor hygiene. Therefore, such practices among Jews, even in the First World, were suspect.[104] As in the nineteenth century, too, fears of transmission via the communion cup led to restrictions on this practice.[105] A symbol of the fellowship of believers, the common chalice was now replaced by individual ones, showing how the "socialism of the microbe" isolated humans from each other. As then, too, fears of transmission prompted the sales of disinfective materials promising to sanitize objects of daily use.[106]

NEEDLES

In public health terms, the problem with addicts was not the drugs' effect as such (though the bodily ravages of misuse did not help), it was how they were ingested. While possibly desirable, abstinence was not necessary to hinder the epidemic. But addicts should avoid sharing paraphernalia. To the uninitiated, this might have seemed like a technical issue, involving at most a minor cost. And yet some evidence suggests that addicts in shooting galleries shared works as a form of self-protection (to flush out undercover police unwilling to go that deep) and as a bonding ritual.[107] Others argued more pragmatically, in contrast, that needles were shared simply because they were legally unavailable.[108]

From an epidemiological point of view, ensuring that needles were clean was the equivalent of boiling water in a cholera epidemic or using condoms: an easy and cost-effective means of preventing transmission of microorganisms that entailed few changes in behavior or attitude. In practice, however, providing works to addicts was fraught with political and ethical controversy. The epidemic placed addicts among the most feared and demonized of HIV's victims, along with bisexuals and prisoners, because they threatened to bridge the gap between encapsulated high-risk categories and the mainstream population.[109] (As the exception to this rule, American blacks tended to view drug use as less stigmatizing than homosexuality.)[110] In New York City, for example, addiction was the apparent source of HIV in 87 percent of heterosexually transmitted cases and in 80 percent of perinatal cases.[111]

Nonetheless, the epidemic revealed that even drug addicts, though often regarded as beyond the reach of persuasion, proved to be surprisingly rational interest maximizers.[112] Though it is hard to know precisely how to quantify and compare such matters, addicts arguably did more to alter their conduct than the population at large. In Britain, for example, needle sharing among injectors dropped from 60 to 90 percent in the mid-1980s to some 20 percent a decade later.[113] But while perhaps able to change injection habits, drug users—like others—found it harder to modify their sexual behavior.[114] In some respects, the epidemic helped bring about a social reconceptualization of addicts. Especially in Europe, where injection was less ghettoized in an underclass than in America, users' positive response to the risks of transmission, and the evidence that they were not sociopaths incapable of rational concern for their own health, helped depathologize addicts and humanize their image.[115]

Despite this, rendering needles harmless, either through exchange or disinfection, was among the most controversial public health issues. Against needle exchanges were arguments marshaled from practice: despite their theoretical persuasiveness, such programs often proved ineffective. It was hard to isolate a simple inverse relationship between the availability of sterile syringes and the spread of HIV among addicts. In Edinburgh, high disease prevalence among users correlated with restrictions on the availability of syringes. But in Italy, where needles were easily and widely accessible, HIV had also spread rapidly among addicts.[116] Just as it was argued that, by reducing the consequences of promiscuity, condoms promoted sexual immorality, syringe exchanges were attacked for encouraging or at least implicitly condoning drug use. As with safe sex, Jesse Helms mocked, so there should be safe drug abuse.[117] The difference was one of degree, since promiscuity was no longer illegal and often not even disparaged in most Western nations, while drug abuse remained illicit and addiction a social problem of greater magnitude than irregular sexual relations.[118] Two important policy trajectories intersected and contradicted each other at the point of needle exchanges: fighting drug addiction and rendering injection habits epidemiologically harmless. In many instances, these two aims were entrusted to different government authorities, reinforcing a theoretical distinction with institutional underpinnings. Law enforcement agencies countered drug imports, sales, and consumption. Public health agencies, in turn, were responsible for the epidemiological consequences of drug use.[119] As a result there were at least two sorts of policy, which often ran at cross purposes: drug control and harm minimization.

Syringe exchange policies varied among nations. In response to the epidemic, German federal drug policy slowly changed as of 1987, and the need for exchanges and other forms of risk reduction were discussed.[120] The state health ministers accepted in 1987 that disposable syringes did not add much temptation to the use of drugs and could be accepted as a flanking measure to fight the epidemic.[121] By the early 1990s many German cities had exchange programs and automat dispensers in place. Finally in 1992, the Narcotics Act was changed to allow dispensing disposable syringes to drug addicts.[122]

In Britain, the epidemic helped swing drug policy, which had become increasingly punitive, back toward its traditional pursuit of harm minimization. In 1987, pilot needle-exchange programs were introduced as experiments, and pharmacists were encouraged to sell syringes. Exchanges were quickly established and without much controversy.[123] Reactions were colored by the geographic concentration of drug-related AIDS transmission in Scotland. In 1986, the McClelland Committee's recommendation in favor of exchanges in Scotland provoked a storm in Westminster. Two years later, however, the Runciman Report, which also favored exchanges and pharmacy sales of syringes, marked a change in official attitude.[124] The pressing problems afflicting Scottish cities led to the establishment of the first official schemes there in January of 1987, following unofficial ones in Liverpool and London. Nonetheless, despite the particularly urgent issue in Scotland, needle exchanges were in fact not as widely implemented as they were south of the border.[125]

Though it initially opposed the unrestricted sale of syringes in French pharmacies without prescription or proof of identity, the conservative Chirac government allowed it from 1987.[126] In the mid-1990s, discussion was under way regarding installing syringe dispensers under outlying Parisian bridges. Nonetheless, the presumption of misdemeanor that syringe possession constituted was never explicitly lifted, and the police continued to arrest drug users for such cause.[127] Only a few exchange programs were established—three in 1989, compared to one hundred in Britain. Not until 1995 did they finally become legalized and begin to expand.[128]

In Sweden as well, official resistance to needle exchanges was strong. The government feared the implication that it tolerated drug use. Nations with more liberal policies did not seem to be favored with lower incidence rates. Denmark—ever the Swedish foil—was the obvious example.[129] Needles were available by prescription alone, making Sweden one of the few European nations where they could not be purchased over the counter in pharmacies. But in 1985, a group of physicians began to argue for freer availability.[130] Pilot exchange programs were set up, either independently of official sponsorship or with only grudging approval.[131] In Lund, addicts were required either to cease consumption or to be medically examined for disease quarterly. Only so long as they kept in contact with the drug enforcement authorities did they receive needles in exchange from their physicians.[132] Those in favor of a more liberal approach were disconcerted to find Sweden, like Bavaria, isolated within Europe on such matters.[133] By contrast, in Denmark (which was more liberal on drugs than Sweden or Norway) syringes could be bought from pharmacies and in vending machines and were handed out free to drug addicts.[134] The Dutch were the Continental exception and the most celebrated or infamous example—depending on one's view—of harm minimization. They established widespread needle exchange programs, and the government indirectly supported activities like safe shooting workshops, with no marked public disapproval.[135]

In the United States, a majority of states allowed needles to be sold without prescription. Almost all, however, had drug paraphernalia laws that ruled needle exchanges out of court.[136] Exchange programs were not nearly as popular as in some parts of Europe, and those in existence were sometimes clandestine and illegal, sometimes illegal but tolerated, and, when legal, always bereft of federal funding.[137] The 1990 CARE Act made government funds contingent on their not being used to provide needles or syringes. Because of such political difficulties, American policy was generally to "bleach and teach" rather than to foster exchanges.[138]

Objections to needle exchanges in the United States came not only from the usual variety of social conservatives, who were opposed to the moral neutrality of harm minimization, but also from minorities, blacks above all. New York City's needle exchange program, which lasted from 1988 to 1990, proved hugely controversial, largely because of the opposition from black activists. Exchanges, they charged, represented an abnegation by white public health authorities of their responsibilities to fight addiction. City Councilman Hilton B. Clark of Harlem went so far as to accuse them of genocide. Partly, such protests stemmed from the same religious condemnation of sin as among white conservatives; partly it rested on distrust of any government program that appeared to experiment with blacks, as in the infamous Tuskegee syphilis trials. Drug addiction was also perceived as a bigger problem than AIDS, which was then still regarded primarily as a disease of white homosexuals.[139]

In some cases, the problem was aggravated by enforcement techniques. Prosecuting for drug use on the basis of possession of paraphernalia, for example, as was practice on the eastern seaboard, helped create the shooting parlors—largely unknown on the West Coast—where works were rented or shared. This was also the situation in the Lothian region of Scotland in the early 1980s. In Britain, reforms to the Drug Trafficking Offences Bill on cocaine paraphernalia in 1986 specifically exempted syringes to avoid encouraging their reuse. In Germany, since addicts in possession of several needles were more likely to face charges, most carried only one, with the consequences of reuse and sharing.[140]

Needle exchanges were influenced by the broader question of dealing with drug addiction. Since the beginning of the twentieth century, international attempts to control drug use, spurred in large measure by the United States, had concentrated on limiting production and supply.[141] During the middle years of the century, a more lenient approach was adopted, above all by the British. When drug addiction was medicalized—turned from a crime into an illness—in the 1960s, tensions arose between policies aiming to stamp out drugs and those seeking to guide a residual and unavoidable level of use into the least harmful channels. The epidemic coincided with and partly helped fuel a return to tactics based on the penal code. The approach in most nations to the availability of drugs became increasingly martial and restrictive. Sanctions repressed and punished drug use domestically; the borders were strictly controlled to prevent their ingress; and quasi-military incursions into producer nations sought to quash the supply at its fount. While the United States took the initiative in this, the European nations largely fell into line.

In Germany, drug policy, having headed in this direction already in the mid-1950s, adopted increasingly repressive measures against heroin during the late 1970s and the 1980s, described in terminology that echoed the concurrent fight against terrorism. This set the tone at the beginning of the AIDS epidemic.[142] In Italy, after a liberal phase in the 1970s, drug policies increasingly repressed use during the late 1980s and early 1990s. Only as of the mid-1990s, and then among local administrations, was much attention paid instead to risk reduction strategies.[143]

The Swedes were among those who took the most drastic turn. In 1988, the government criminalized the use of illegal drugs, not just manufacture, sale, or possession, thus expanding the purchase of criminal law on substance abuse. Possession of even the smallest quantity was now considered reason for prosecution, and prisoners jailed for drug offenses were subject to an especially harsh regimen. Only the sentences for murder, aggravated robbery, and aggravated arson were stricter than for serious drug offenses. This set Sweden at odds with the Danes, Germans, and British, among whom possession, but not use, was illegal. The Norwegians, and the Finns, however, joined the Swedes in criminalizing use and in reserving the longest punishments possible for drug offenses. The Norwegians also allowed compulsory institutionalization and treatment of addicts.[144] In France narcotics use was criminalized in 1970. Users of either hard or soft drugs, which in theory included also one-time offenders, could be prosecuted or placed under medical treatment. As in Sweden, addicts could be forcibly treated.[145] Britain, despite its record of a liberal approach during the middle decades of the century, introduced more penal policies during the 1980s. But this was again partly reversed during the mid-1980s with recognition of HIV transmission among addicts and the threat posed to the larger community. Holland too bucked the trend to harsher policies. It refused to criminalize possession of small quantities of soft drugs for personal use and concentrated penal sanctions on hard ones.[146]

Although drug policy generally became more repressive during the AIDS era, another facet of the issue developed less uniformly: the question of whether to aim at a complete weaning of addicts from illegal substances or to settle instead for a substitute dependence on licit and less harmful chemicals. Nations differed starkly. The important distinction lay between a harm minimization approach (analogous to the safer sex techniques prescribed in despair of abstinence) and zero tolerance attitudes. In a thumbnail sketch, the fault line ran between the Continent (excepting the Dutch and partly the Swiss) and the Anglo-American nations. The former were insistent that dependence on hard drugs was not to be tolerated, and that the solution to addiction was complete weaning. The latter—Britain especially, and the United States less consistently—were more willing to try substitution techniques that allowed drug users to live approximately normal lives, even though their addiction remained clinically the same.

Britain had pioneered harm minimization during the 1920s. Medical prescribing of opiates was allowed to keep addicts away from the black market and to reduce the criminality associated with prohibition. Policy here danced to the tune of medical professionals prescribing for a select group of middle-class addicts, and not to that of law enforcement authorities hoping to stamp out a behavioral epidemic. Maintenance was thus possible thanks to the relative unimportance of the problem it sought to solve. Drugs were generally available by prescription, though during the 1960s only doctors authorized by the Home Office could dispense heroin and cocaine.[147] During the 1980s, policy sported a Janus face. The official approach focused on repressing usage, while the drug policy community favored risk reduction tactics. With the disconcerting news from Scotland during the early stages of the epidemic that HIV was widespread among injectors, prevention of transmission was gradually accepted as more important than reduction of drug usage. Though harm minimization was not invented during this time, the epidemic encouraged a reappreciation of its potential virtues. While substitution treatments in the United States and elsewhere primarily used oral methadone, Britain kept open the possibility, though ever less employed, of maintaining users on injectable drugs as well.[148]

In many respects, America took Britain as a model in drug matters. After 1919, the Harrison Act was interpreted to prohibit maintenance of addicts. But some states had already adopted a medical model of addiction. It was seen as a physical disease whose victims were often maintained on opiates. During the interwar years and the 1950s, strict prohibitionism held sway, but starting in the 1960s a more medicalized approach, including maintenance or substitution on the British model, reemerged. Under the Nixon administration, a public drug treatment system, including substitution methods, was developed as part of policies to cut crime. Nonetheless, harm minimization was still being resisted well into the AIDS era. In practical terms, the United States applied contradictory means. Its zero tolerance approach sought to keep drugs illegal and to limit supplies through a war on them. While needle exchanges were not widely adopted, substitution treatment for addicts was more commonly accepted than in most Continental nations.[149]

In France, harm minimization had long been resisted. A complete weaning of addicts, rather than reducing harm to them and society, was the goal. Drug policy was a central element of French conceptions of citizenship. The ideology of republican egalitarianism dictated that no member of the community be abandoned to his own addiction. The addicted citizen was imprisoned in his own private sphere, cut off from participating in public life. Bringing him back into the fold required restoring his faculties to their preaddictive stage. Therefore no compromise was possible with chemical dependency. The choice was binary: between citizenship and dependence. One could emphasize this ideology's universalist egalitarianism, its refusal to consider even the most hopeless addict as lost to the republic of equals. Or one could focus on the way it prescribed a common standard of behavior and conduct to which all were held, regardless of their wishes and abilities to toe the line.[150] In Germany and Sweden similar arguments were heard: substitution programs implied a moral triage—a decision about which addicts could be saved for a normal existence and which thrown into the gutter of continued chemical dependency. While possibly acceptable for the small minority of addicts with no hope of overcoming their thralldom, substitution was seen as unethical if it served simply to shift dependence from one drug to another. Both in Germany and in France, measures undertaken to relieve the addict's suffering were seen as undercutting the incentive to abstain, a remarkably unflinching, not to say cruel, approach.[151]

From this perspective, harm minimization was considered immoral in setting society's interests above those of the afflicted individual. Rather than reclaiming the addict for the community, harm minimization wrote him off as a loss. It sought only to ensure that, if he insisted on hurting himself, at least he did not damage society. In the context of AIDS, critics charged, it was the fear of addicts spreading HIV into the general population that lent harm minimization its sudden popularity. The community's security was to be bought with the sacrifice of addicts who would be rendered harmless but not cured.[152] Risk reduction policies also had implications for conceptions of citizenship insofar as they tacitly accepted divergent behavioral norms among subgroups. Substitution treatment accepted the addict as an addict, rather than as a failed abstinent citizen. Whether one saw this as the bankruptcy of a single, desirable standard for all, or as the flourishing of many parallel ones, depended on much broader views of social cohesion and the potpourri of theories of multiculturalism. But Continental critics were correct that arguments for risk reduction tended to be pragmatic: given the inevitability of addiction and addicts, it was better to limit the harm they did to themselves and others.[153]

Such basic ideological differences colored approaches to substitution programs for addicts. In France, methadone was not even legally on the market until 1995.[154] Starting in 1988, when a health minister was forced to resign in part for having supported substitution treatment, debate over methadone use finally began, now fueled by the risk of HIV transmission.[155] Though two experimental methadone programs had been in place since 1973, they treated very few patients: some forty, compared to two hundred thousand in the United States in 1979. As late as 1993, only three institutions prescribed methadone—to fifty-two addicts.[156] Physicians were also restricted in their ability to prescribe otherwise illegal drugs. In 1992, the government cracked down on doctors for dispensing Temgésic, a painkiller, for substitution purposes.[157] Only in the early 1990s did a modest proposal, the Henrion Plan, remind the French that drug addiction was a real problem requiring solutions. In 1993, the National AIDS Council argued in favor of risk minimization policies and dramatically portrayed France's lag behind her neighbors.[158]

Such arguments helped forge a new consensus in French drug policy, swinging official opinion in favor of harm minimization. Gradually, starting in 1993–94, risk reduction became official policy at the Ministry of Health, and maintenance programs were finally regularized and began to expand.[159] It was now recognized that republican ideology's refusal to distinguish between addicts and others had led not to an impartial and equal treatment of all but to a shortchanging of measures desperately needed by drug users.[160] Centralizing drug policy at the national level had handicapped the policy response by eliminating the local initiatives that proved so fruitful elsewhere.[161] Nor in this land of republican ideology were addicts encouraged to organize on their own behalf, as they did in the Netherlands, because the political formation of groups was resisted on any basis other than abstract, universal citizenship.

The German approach was similar, though the nation began reorienting drug policy toward minimization earlier. Here, too, substitution programs were resisted well into the later phases of the epidemic. Local programs were established in Frankfurt, Hamburg, North Rhine–Westphalia, Bavaria, and Lower Saxony, though they were often opposed by other states and by much of the medical and drug treatment community.[162] In Berlin as of 1987, seven hundred addicts were in substitution therapy, but in Munich five years later only eighty-six were.[163] In 1988, the AIDS Enquête Commission recommended substitution therapy as an additional measure, though not to replace abstinence. In 1991 the Supreme Court allowed physicians slightly more leeway in dispensing substitute drugs.[164] Despite such changes, the abstinence model remained dominant. Prescribing drugs to an addict solely for maintenance continued to be a criminal offense, with physicians prosecuted into the 1980s. Methadone could not be legally given, although codeine-based drugs could be.[165] Even German critics of the abstinence model, whose colleagues elsewhere often favored substitution treatments, here espoused the ideal of freedom from drugs, and offered as an alternative what was known as *Suchtbegleitung*, a program of counseling and help with the everyday practical problems afflicting junkies, but without chemical substitutes.[166]

Within Scandinavia, the differences were stark. While the Danes had extensive methadone substitution programs, their Nordic neighbors failed to follow suit. The Norwegians had none, and the Swedes had only modest experimental schemes, expanded in 1988 to accept some three hundred addicts (compared to the eleven hundred to two thousand who were compulsorily treated for drug abuse).[167] In fact, the tendency in Sweden during the 1980s was toward a more penal approach, reversing the high road to risk minimization followed elsewhere. The goal of Swedish authorities remained a drug-free society, and they saw the epidemic as reason to reinforce, not dilute, this commitment. Because of its peripheral location, Sweden had a fighting chance of keeping drugs at bay by border checks and by discouraging addiction through harsh policies. Narcotics abuse promoted disease transmission, the authorities reasoned, and infected addicts should not be allowed to continue their habits.[168]

The Swedes had long taken a strict and often punitive approach to addiction. Alcoholics were subject to compulsory treatment, and addicts were also included in this regimen as of 1981. Conservatives called for a strengthening of mandatory measures, lengthening the time addicts could be kept for treatment, and ensuring sufficient institutional places for them.[169] In 1986 an institution for the compulsory treatment of drug abusers was opened. Two years later, a new law confirmed Sweden's unusual approach. Covering addicts of both alcohol and drugs, and motivated in part by the threat of seropositive junkies, it brandished the stick of compulsion in hopes of persuading addicts to cooperate voluntarily. It imposed treatment to break addiction at an earlier and less acute stage, extending the duration of compulsory measures and allowing the social authorities, not just the police, to make such decisions.[170] The law was adopted despite the objections of Communists and some Social Democrats, who feared the increased use of compulsion even in the social sector. With Finland, Sweden was now the only Western nation still to compel treatment of abusers.[171]

The epidemic thus wrought changes in approaches to drug policy—and needle exchanges in particular. In those Continental nations where complete abstinence was seen as the solution to addiction, a reconceptualization now allowed more positive evaluations of harm minimization, a pragmatic acceptance of substitution as a lesser evil rather than a Faustian pact.[172] Nonetheless, national differences remained. Britain and the Netherlands led the way in harm minimization, especially in needle exchanges. Other European nations, above all France, followed at some remove. Conversely, the United States and Sweden were among the industrialized nations that most doggedly resisted a liberalization of policy on needle access. In terms of other harm minimization policies, however, especially methadone substitution, Britain, America, and the Netherlands went furthest. The Continental nations, except Switzerland, held fast to the idea of total weaning as the goal. With such mixed motives and behaviors—American strictness on needle exchanges, but not on substitution, and the Continental nations other than Sweden reversing this situation—differing attitudes toward drug use cannot be explained by the obvious whipping boy of puritan attitudes, at least not unless we are willing to admit also Lutheran and Catholic puritanisms—puritanism, then, of a chameleon-like and unilluminating nature.[173]

Differences in the social incidence of drug addiction were also important in explaining variations in approach. Whether addiction seemed more or less pressing than the threat of HIV transmission from users to the general population depended largely on the size of the drug problem. Britain's ability to adopt harm minimization was the result, not the cause, of a drug problem less urgent than elsewhere.[174] In toto, hard drug addiction did not vary dramatically between Europe and the United States. Each had somewhat more than a million users. What did differ was the local and socioeconomic incidence. In America, the majority of intravenous drug abusers were black or Hispanic. Blacks were more likely than whites to be infected via injection or sexual contact with an injector.[175] The fact that addiction and disadvantaged minority status uniquely coincided in the United States doubtless helped undermine attempts to liberalize access to needles.[176] But logically, if the critics of harm minimization were correct as to the motives behind such approaches, then the fact that addicts belonged to an underprivileged class should, if anything, have made needle exchanges—the sacrifice of users on the altar of security for the rest of society—more, not less, likely. This was, after all, precisely what prompted black leaders' charges of genocide: that harm minimization could be construed as public-policy triage practiced on minorities. The attitude of black Americans on this point was part of a broader critique of harm minimization familiar on the Continent, though less present in the Anglo-American world: the insistence that policy should be to wean addicts off drugs, not to make drug use safe for society while it remained dangerous for the individual. In America, this position coincided with an ethnic and social group. In Europe, it remained an abstractly ideological stance.

7. The Polymorphous Politics of Prevention

The developed nations took more divergent approaches to the AIDS epidemic than might have been expected, given the broad similarity of the problem in each and the globalization of scientific and epidemiological knowledge. The British reacted early and effectively, the state taking a leading role and following historical precedents that pointed it in a consensual and voluntaristic direction. A massive public education campaign began in 1986, and a Cabinet committee was established, one that included everyone concerned short of the prime minister herself. A parliamentary select committee and an AIDS unit in the Department of Health were set up; extra funding was granted London hospitals with the heaviest caseloads; and special physicians were appointed by health authorities.[1] But the British passed little legislation to protect the infected from discrimination. Moreover, though they remained largely unused, measures sanctioning drastic actions, such as compulsory removal of recalcitrant seropositives to hospitals, were put on the books.[2] As elsewhere, with more treatments becoming available during the late 1980s, and as victims came to include ethnic minorities and drug addicts without much power to defend civil liberties, traditional public health techniques both made increasing medical and epidemiological sense and were less resisted. This shifted the emphasis away from a consensual approach to one that was more decisively interventionist. On the whole, however, the British, along with the Dutch, were consensual and voluntaristic.[3] Perhaps the phrase *masterly inactivity,* applied to related aspects of British policy like VD legislation, would serve equally well here.[4]

The Swedes reacted early, too, but in a starkly different direction. They followed a *Sonderweg* formulated by the Social Democratic government and welcomed by most parties, with some objections from Liberals and Communists. They were the first European nation to legislate on the epidemic, in March 1983. Two years later, the Swedes decided to treat AIDS as a venereal disease and thus to invoke the inherited public health provisions of the Contagious Disease Law. Since no medical solution was forthcoming, so the government reasoned, recourse to the tried and true methods of prevention was the answer.[5] Applying the Contagious Disease Law allowed a panoply of interventions, many of which would have been politically impossible in other nations.

The Swedes subjected seropositives and AIDS victims to restrictions without compare outside eastern Europe's socialist—and later formerly socialist—nations: compulsory examination, mandatory contact tracing, possibly indefinite quarantine of recalcitrants, as well as extensive monitoring of seropositives' behavior by the police and social authorities. Another Swedish anomaly was to rule out anonymous screening for those who proved to be infected. Gay saunas and bathhouses were closed. Needle exchanges were permitted only within limits, and drug policy remained fixated on abstinence, with little of the harm minimization increasingly in favor elsewhere. The main principle of Swedish epidemic control legislation, as the authorities themselves put it, was to assure the power to compel behavior that citizens might not adopt on their own. It could not be left to individual choice whether to seek medical treatment.[6] Educational efforts were heavily targeted at the average person outside the main risk groups, and a particularly pungent fear of epidemiological outsiders—not just gays, prostitutes, and addicts but also Danes and other foreigners—was given voice.

The French, by contrast, adopted a largely liberal approach—not out of strong conviction so much as an inability to do otherwise. Inaction was dressed up in the vestments of liberalism.[7] Muddling through as always in public health, the French were stronger in theory than action. They staked their hopes on a cure, devoting resources and national prestige to the scientific pursuit of a biomedical solution that, if successful, would have spared them the need for more decisive alternative interventions. Shying away from other forms of prevention, they neither required, nor even encouraged, widespread testing; they failed to act decisively against drug abuse and its dysfunctional habits; and they were hesitant to deal with gays and other victims in terms other than those of abstract citizenship.[8]

Though observers often claim that the United States took a liberal approach, in fact, along with Sweden (and Bavaria), it was one of the developed nations that arguably adopted the most restrictive line. The presidential commission on AIDS, reporting in 1988, put forth a highly interventionist program. If fully implemented, it would have imposed measures without parallel outside of Sweden and Bavaria. It called for nominative reporting of seropositivity, partner notification, and contact tracing. It wanted to permit medical personnel to test patients and wardens to screen prisoners; it sought limited isolation of recalcitrants; and it aimed to criminalize potentially transmissive behavior.[9] Because of the country's federalism, it is hard to generalize from coast to coast. But an interventionist approach was often practiced as well. The federal government imposed HIV screening on many of its subject populations: military personnel, the Foreign Service, and applicants to the Job Corps program. Congress required testing of immigrants and barred the infected. Prisoners in federal, state, and local jails were often screened.

The United States was particularly active in using the penal code against potentially transmissive behavior. Those states with the most restrictive policies instituted measures much like Sweden's. In 1986, Florida, for example, established a broad-gauged system of preventing STDs that forbade the infected from having sex without informing their partners, and required disease reporting, contact tracing, and examination of contacts, as well as treatment—compulsory if necessary—of the infected, quarantine if required, and screening of pregnant women.[10] Except for testing the pregnant and directly compulsory treatment, all other measures were in effect in Sweden and Bavaria as well. On the other hand, the United States had one of the most extensive systems of civil rights protections for the infected and ill. Many of the most drastic interventions were overturned by courts or tempered by experience: Illinois's attempt to mandate premarital screening, Utah's forbidding of marriage for seropositives.[11] It is perhaps most accurate to say that the American response was as hard to characterize in one denominator as that of all Europe, taken together, would have been. Nonetheless, in a comparative perspective, the continued salience of traditional strategies stood out. Screening, reporting, even isolation, and other traditional measures were more prevalent here than in most west European nations.

Germany, finally, was the nation that perhaps most obviously avoided the approach it might have pursued, given its historical proclivities. More drastic measures were taken than advocates of a liberal line often cared to admit: screening of foreigners (including students from abroad), of civil service applicants, and of prisoners. Bavaria demonstrated what the country could have done had it simply, like the Swedes, applied inherited legislation to AIDS. Outside of Bavaria, however, other states rejected this traditional approach for a consensual tack.

Despite such differences in approach, there were clearly common elements to the fight against AIDS and forces that encouraged similarities among nations' policies. Before we turn to divergence, then, a glance at convergence is useful.

THE CIVIL RIGHTS REVOLUTION

One of the most important factors affecting the approach to AIDS was the expansion of individuals' rights across all Western nations during the postwar era. A major political sea change had taken place. Measures once regarded as progressive, democratic, egalitarian, and feminist were now judged to be intolerant, illiberal, invasive, and, indeed, totalitarian.[12] Most traditional public health legislation had been formulated during the late nineteenth century or, by the latest, during the interwar years. Two experiences helped reverse its inherited prioritizing of the community over the individual: first, that of Fascism and then Communism; and second, the wave of postwar civil rights movements that, starting in the United States with blacks, continued with students, women, gays, and the handicapped, and eventually also included animal rights. Such movements emphasized individual rights and the pursuit of happiness, which increasingly became the goal of the social order. During the first half of the twentieth century, syphilis victims were commonly forbidden sexual intercourse. But similar restrictions were impossible for seropositives, not just for the obvious reason that, with AIDS, the prohibition would be for life. Attitudes toward sex had also shifted. It was no longer regarded just as pleasure, much less as merely a happy interlude on the road to reproduction, but was also seen as a fundamental human right.[13]

Eugenics exemplifies this shift. Even into the interwar period, it was considered a progressive, enlightened way to improve the health and well-being of the community, sparing individuals the torments of inherited disease and the stigma of inferiority, and relieving the community of the needless cost of avoidable disability. After the Nazi regime, however, eugenics came to be seen as an unjustified trampling of individual autonomy and inviolability. Subordinating civil liberties to a collective goal was regarded as dictatorial and inhuman. Interwar eugenic policies in the United States and Sweden acquired retrospectively the taint of the Nazi era.[14] More recent controversies over euthanasia resonate equally inescapably with that period. Is euthanasia an enlightened attempt to spare mortals needless suffering at the hands of a technologically enamored but morally blinkered medical establishment? Or does it reveal an overly utilitarian concern with the costs imposed by illness, and a disregard for the absolute value of human life? The strict limits now set on the use of humans in scientific experiments are a result of their grotesque misuse in Dachau and Auschwitz and of the morally careless use of people as guinea pigs—in the investigation of untreated syphilis in blacks in Tuskegee and in Armauer Hansen's attempts to inoculate unknowing Norwegian patients with leprosy.[15] The restrictions increasingly set on the use of laboratory animals extend such lessons across the species line. More generally, the growing emphasis on the claims of patients vis-à-vis their caregivers is part of this overarching civil rights revolution. It supports the right to be told a diagnosis, even a hopeless one, and to participate in decisions on treatment rather than remain subject to paternalist doctors.

And yet neither totalitarianism nor the civil rights movements alone automatically brought about major changes in public health. In the United States, the individualizing turn in jurisprudence that downplayed the community's interest in public health in favor of citizens' rights to bodily autonomy began during the second and third decades of the twentieth century.[16] In other nations, it was not until the 1960s that the wartime and cold war experiences were taken as warning examples. In Germany, traditional contagious disease legislation remained in effect—and indeed was renewed—well into the 1960s. It became politically unfeasible only during the AIDS era. The end of the Second World War did not, as such, clear the decks for a new approach. The Council of Europe's human rights convention of 1950 blithely allowed restrictions on the civil rights of the insane, alcoholics, drug addicts, and vagrants (an ill-defined category that could include, for example, Roma and Sinti), as well as everyone else when preventing the spread of infectious disease.[17]

Many such issues persist today. The advocacy of animal rights, and the dilution of humans into a larger pool of sentient beings with increasingly equal claims to moral consideration, has posed the possibility of utilitarian tradeoffs between intelligent animals and handicapped humans. The absolute moral equality of all human beings is questioned as ethical equivalence is extended across species lines. Genetic testing and therapy raise the question of whether the eugenic impulse, having disappeared as state policy, now reemerges as each parent's individualized desire for perfect babies. It is horrifying for the state to wish for little Aryans. But it is also worrisome that the collective outcome of individual reproductive choices may be a surfeit of males—or blondes, or whatever.

Though individuals' rights have expanded during the postwar period, developments have not run in one direction only. As AIDS, and even more recent epidemics, remind us, the threat of contagious disease remains strong. It is plausible that our present freedoms owe less to an increased veneration of civil liberties than to an insouciance born of antibiotics and their victories—and so those freedoms could quickly vanish with technological setbacks.[18] We venerate the right to individual happiness and self-fulfillment, allowing a hedonistic and benign fragmentation of society into masturbatory monads. But we are pushed in increasingly collectivistic directions as well. As consumers of goods and services, and as workers, we find the state an ever more exclusive caretaker of our interests. John Stuart Mill's notion of the autonomous citizen, acting now as a consumer with responsibility for making the right choices when buying food, now as a worker and operating heavy machinery with only such precautions as we chose, strikes us as hopelessly naive and outmoded. No one but the state can stay abreast of the information required to be well informed.[19] While becoming ever more free in terms of expression, we require salvation from our ignorance. The arena for individualization has become restricted to issues of lifestyle, while we are deprived of autonomy in areas once regarded as crucial—rearing children, say, or entering binding contracts, and assuming individual responsibility for managing risk.

Where the individual was once subordinated to the community in terms of public health, the civil rights sea change has reversed these positions, but to differing degrees in different nations. Though improvements in treatment have shifted tactics back toward more traditional approaches of testing and tracing victims, in many nations AIDS has been dealt with by emphasizing individual rights more than in earlier epidemics. The mantra, repeated endlessly by public health experts, was that, for AIDS, no contradiction separated individual rights and human dignity, on the one hand, from public health and the community's need to protect itself, on the other.[20] Whether this was true depended, obviously, on how both sides of this equation were defined. Neither individual rights nor society's claims on its members are timeless or unchanging. Maintaining the balance between the two presents the classic dilemma of political philosophy, embodied by public health in perhaps its most ubiquitous and concrete form. Down to what level of risk is society justified in demanding an intervention in individual life, an intervention not without its costs or even dangers for the individual? What diseases permit the restriction of infected victims' civil rights?

The line between individual rights and social demands has shifted dramatically over time, as it has varied among nations at any given moment. During the period of Enlightenment absolutism, cameralism and its formulation of a science of policy included public health as one of government's main functions.[21] In this calculus, individual concerns were subordinated to communal goods. With the democratic revolutions of the eighteenth century, in turn, came the idea of a tie between the rule of the people and their health. Thomas Jefferson argued that democratic systems promoted their citizens' health, while autocracies sapped their subjects' strength.[22] With the French Revolution and the beginning of modern democracy, health became both a right and a responsibility of the citizen. The state was to ensure public health, yet it was also the duty of newly empowered burghers to maintain their health and thus the common good of the polity.[23]

The predemocratic state was hampered in demanding limits on its subjects' personal behavior and habits. Why, after all, should they agree to change? But it claimed the right to fight disease, harshly if necessary, by identifying the ill, isolating them in lazarettos, tracing their contacts, and destroying infected possessions. The modern democratic polity, in contrast, leaned less severely on its citizens, but only so long as they conducted themselves responsibly: by adopting habits of personal cleanliness and hygiene, refraining from epidemiologically objectionable customs like indiscriminate spitting or excreting, and avoiding having sex or other contacts likely to transmit disease if infected. The outright and external demands made by the community and state lessened, but only to the extent that individuals imposed controls on themselves. One side of the coin was the democratic expansion of rights; the other was an increase in citizens' responsibilities. External controls were replaced by internal ones—one of the central insights formulated by Norbert Elias and extended by Michel Foucault and other scholars of what has come to be known as governmentality.[24] The modern state enlists its subjects, now elevated to the status of citizens, as participants in their own governance. In the process, it shifts the locus of control to the internal. Although state and civil society, public and private, are now clearly distinguished from each other, they are also more intertwined. Citizens govern themselves not just in terms of politics but also in their own moral, instinctual, and emotional economy. Limiting their actions before the fact, moderating their impulses, and controlling their behavior, they eliminate the need for the harsh early modern state. The modern state no longer instructs, commands, and punishes. It educates, informs, persuades, and discourages.[25]

The internalization of control and its increasing informality in the modern state has continued apace into our own day. The ill or infected are no longer regarded on the analogy of criminals, to be spurned and constrained as though they had committed a crime. Instead, they are treated as partners in the public health effort. On their voluntary behavioral modifications rest the community's hopes to avoid disease and epidemics. Their cooperation required, they must be treated as equals in the preventive enterprise.[26]

But then there are those who do not follow the voluntary prescriptions of healthy living, as defined by the medical science of the day. Those who refuse to be monogamous joggers are spurned in some circles virtually as enemies of the people. Smokers, the overly carnivorous (but also the exclusively vegan, who are blamed for their children's nutritional and developmental deficiencies), the obese, drinkers of more than the occasional glass of Chablis, ingesters of drugs, the promiscuous: these are the new social outcasts, violators of the ethos of democratic restraint. Those who long for the old regime of strict external control, combined with indulgence of pleasurable bad habits, attack this ethos of behavioral auto-limitation as "health fascism."[27] While exaggerating, they are right in pointing out that there has been no overall lessening of control. If anything, bodily discipline and restraint have become more pronounced. Hygiene is our religious tic. No fluid, no odor, no blemish is permitted—increasingly not even hair: the beard has been effectively banished and in another generation female pubic hair will be equally rare.

Public health used to take the community as its patient, subordinating to it the interests of its individual members. The more recent approach has been to reverse these priorities, refusing even the threat of epidemics as prima facie cause to restrict civil liberties.[28] This alteration in public health outlook rested on the epidemiological shift from acute contagious diseases to chronic lifestyle ailments. Epidemiology had moved faster than the law. But traditional public health legislation remained on the books, though it was needed ever less. Not until AIDS struck—the first major epidemic of transmissible disease to arrive after the rights revolution—was it discovered that existing statutes were, in some nations, politically superannuated.[29]

The shifts in what was regarded as acceptable policy were dramatic. Even in Sweden, the developed nation with perhaps the most communal political instincts, the change was marked. In 1936, the Population Commission had caustically dismissed the idea that people should have free disposition of their own bodies as "an extremely individualistic conception." By 1974, however, the Sterilization Commission concluded that in principle all should have the right to decide over their own bodies.[30] In the United States, *Jacobson v. Massachusetts* (1905), which accepted compulsory smallpox vaccination, held the liberty of the individual subordinate to the safety of society.[31] It was considered normal during this period to inspect and quarantine travelers. Prostitutes and persons convicted of adultery and fornication were sometimes detained, especially during wartime. Children with polio were routinely quarantined during epidemics in the early twentieth century. Victims of tuberculosis and leprosy were isolated for indefinite periods.[32]

Such restrictive measures now changed late in the century. When in 1983 Texas overhauled its contagious disease legislation, as one of the first American states to do so, the new version still allowed quarantining those infected with various diseases, but not until they had been instructed to alter their behavior and had refused to comply, and then only after a court appearance. In Los Angeles County, health officers had been able to order confinement of tuberculosis patients without explanation or review. Now, patients could request court hearings, repeated before a jury after sixty days.[33] The individual's claim to bodily autonomy and freedom from communal demands was asserted with increasing fervor. The rights of patients vis-à-vis medical personnel were upheld, and those of the mentally ill expanded, precluding involuntary open-ended commitments. Addicts and alcoholics became regarded as ill rather than as deviants, and the disabled were treated as equal to other citizens.[34]

The sexual revolution of the 1960s and 1970s was a major element of the expansion of civil rights. Antibiotics and trustworthy contraception allowed the free disposition of sexual capital and fostered permissive moral norms. Politics became increasingly sexualized in the definition of individual freedom via the pursuit of erotic gratification. In George Orwell's *1984*, love and its sexual expression were blows against totalitarian tyranny. During the 1960s and especially with the beginnings of the gay movement, the personal became even more the political (though it was tempered by those elements of feminism that rejected sexual abandon as peculiarly male). Sexual pleasure was now constituent of identity.[35] Copulation, the moment of greatest thralldom—however delicious—to the least masterable of our instincts, was seen, ironically, as our highest freedom.

In a more technical sense, the rights revolution required that statutory impositions respect a reasonable relationship between means and ends—the principle of proportionality.[36] Drastic measures were out of court unless more moderately interventionist ones failed to accomplish their purpose. For example, quarantining gays threatened to violate the American Constitution's Fourteenth Amendment on equal protection of the law, since only some would be seropositive and far from all seropositives were gay. In general, quarantine of seropositives was overreaching if chains of transmission could be broken by encouraging behavioral change. Forbidding marriage for the infected threatened more deep-seated rights for no sufficiently redeeming purpose. Many measures allowed in old-style public health statutes were thus ruled out of bounds in most nations by contemporary interpretations of constitutional protections.[37] The 1987 Arline case in the United States nailed fast the emerging principle that public health measures could limit constitutional rights only when medically necessary.[38]

Despite common traits, such tendencies were more pronounced in some nations than others. Battles were perhaps most pointed in America, where two contradictory tendencies intersected. On the one hand was the importance attached to the abstract qualities of the citizen, regardless of gender, race, religion, sexual preference, disability, or other factors that formerly had influenced acceptability, admissibility, or employability. The civil rights legislation of the 1960s and later outlawed discrimination based on ethnicity, religion, gender, and handicap. The focus shifted from group identity to individual merits. On the other hand, positive discrimination meant that being disadvantaged, phrased in terms of group membership, now conferred privileges in employment, education, and other social benefits. Such affirmative action programs were potentially at odds with meritocratic principles; they enjoyed comparatively little public or political support; and they passed into law without great deliberation.[39] Nonetheless, they dovetailed with, and encouraged, the shift from an assimilationist model of national identity to a subcultural balkanization where race, ethnicity, religion, and gender increasingly determined both personhood and politics. On one side, a growing hyperindividualization; on the other, a focus on group identity. So dramatic was this double-barreled change that not only traditional conservatives but also many feminists and old-style leftists feared that the denigration of the community, the fixation on rights rather than responsibilities, and the fracturing of citizenship into multifaceted identity politics had simply gone too far.[40]

The French misleadingly interpreted American political ideology as wholly in debt to the multicultural splintering of identity politics, and they ignored the classic base of universalist meritocracy on which such policies rested. Both French gays and French feminists, for example, rejected subcultural group politics, based on what they interpreted as the American model, in favor of a traditionally republican and universalist definition of citizenship whereby all members of the community were treated as abstract incarnations of the same principles.[41] And yet, more than most other European nations, France followed the American example of formally outlawing discrimination based on race, religion, sexual preference, and handicap.

As part of this focus on individual rights, the dangers of Nazi authoritarianism were invoked in all nations, sometimes quite shamelessly. Ian

Kennedy, professor of medical law and ethics at Kings College, London, and a vociferous opponent of even blinded seroprevalence studies, used the Nazi specter to argue the virtues of epistemological virginity. If the only route to knowledge (such as epidemiological soundings of the spread of AIDS) was unethical, then the lesson to draw from the Nuremberg trials, he claimed, was: better not to know.[42] Among the Germans such admonitory parallels were especially resonant. This Holocaust Effect, as it has been dubbed in another context, came through time and again during debates over public health.[43] Polemicists of every stripe drew parallels between Nazi repression and AIDS regulations: HIV screening was analogous to the proof of Aryan blood required in the Third Reich. Like the public denunciations of totalitarian regimes, testing revealed damning secrets. The Bavarian measures evoked disquieting memories, were experienced by victims as a "final solution," and were seen as leading to a dictatorial, totalitarian Plague State. Anti-AIDS measures persecuted gays, as had the Nazis. Solidarity with seropositives who resisted measures of screening and quarantine conjured up the Danish Gentiles who wore Stars of David during the occupation.[44] Journalists played a sad practical joke on eight mayors of small West German towns in 1987 by persuading them to favor erecting closed institutions for AIDS patients modeled on the plans for the Nazi concentration camp at Sachsenhausen.[45] The German allergy to making the disease reportable, even anonymously, was tied to fears of an authoritarian state.[46]

And yet, in the mechanics of the pertinent legislation, changes from a traditional to a more consensual style of public health were far from obvious during the early post-Nazi era in Germany. Indeed, they were not worked out until the AIDS debate. True, the postwar German constitution, or Basic Law, enshrined the right to bodily autonomy. This was now judged a necessary protection against state violence: the sterilization and murder of citizens judged unworthy of life or reproduction, or the medical experiments of the camps. When contagious disease legislation was discussed after the war, allergies to overpowerful authorities were palpable in attempts to protect individual rights.[47] In the name of fighting epidemic disease, however, the constitution also legitimated restrictions on individual rights, thus justifying already at this level the kind of interventions that other nations left to administrative regulation or local legislation.[48]

The 1961 Contagious Disease Law largely followed its traditional predecessor of 1900. Had it been applied to AIDS, as in Bavaria, it would have allowed drastic interventions against anyone with even a theoretical chance of infection. The untenability of the 1961 law, with its categories of victims taken largely unchanged from the earlier act, meant that only political extremists proposed its undiluted application. Indeed, the AIDS Enquête Commission's investigations, spelling out the law's implications if applied to AIDS, may have been motivated by hopes of undermining support for any such course of action.[49] The debate in Germany was fought between (mainly Bavarian) adherents of traditional public health tactics and those who supported a voluntary approach. In the event, not only did the moderates triumph, but, in testing and reporting, Germany was even more cautious than most other nations.

In Sweden, by contrast, even the growth of formalized civil rights did not change the traditional approach to epidemic disease. The new constitution, first implemented six years after the 1968 Contagious Disease Law, explicitly protected fundamental civil rights. Limiting them could be undertaken only by law, only in pursuit of acceptable democratic goals, and only via means proportional to the aims. Nonetheless, when the Contagious Disease Law applied traditional instruments of public health control to AIDS, the Ministry of Social Affairs argued that society must retain effective measures against common threats.[50] Alone among European nations outside Bavaria and Austria, and paralleled to some degree only by the United States, Sweden followed a traditional approach to this epidemic. Earlier, Sweden had been admired as progressive for treating VD like other contagious diseases and subjecting all victims of the ailment—not just prostitutes—to prophylactic measures. During the 1940s, such evenhandedness had been lauded as emblematic of Sweden's Social Democratic, egalitarian approach to public health.[51] The rest of the world had changed, however, in the meantime, while Sweden had not. It rested on the laurels it had won during the 1930s and 1940s and saw no reason to change. What had once seemed evenhanded now struck others as heavy-handed.

The civil rights revolution encouraged a more consensual approach to public health. So did the particularities of AIDS as a disease. Nonetheless, despite such pressures in a common direction, nations took surprisingly different approaches to the epidemic. The question we must now turn to is, why?

8. To Die Laughing

Gays and Other Interest Groups

For diseases, the interest group most concerned should—in theory—be easy to identify. In large measure, it is created by the affliction. The (potentially) ill have obvious interests in research, in treatment, and in compensation for damages. And, in fact, political mobilization on this basis takes place. This explains, for example, why breast cancer has gone from being underresearched to receiving a generous share of resources—but not perhaps why it has taken longer for prostate cancer. It accounts for why a problem like Lyme disease, afflicting suburban commuters, receives attention, while the all-too-common and preventable diseases that kill most people, but alas mostly in the Third World, remain like poor relations.[1] But being ill can also impart stigma, which may discourage a group from mobilizing even on behalf of its own medical interests. During the 1970s, when hepatitis B spread among them, gays had little interest in organizing to counter a disease that threatened to draw unwelcome attention to their changing sexual mores. Nor were physicians—also particularly exposed—eager to publicize the dangers they thus posed to their patients.[2]

For AIDS, those people most obviously interested in more research, subsidized care, and preventive measures respectful of individual liberties were seropositives and the uninfected who were most at risk.[3] Intravenous drug users, hemophiliacs, and blood transfusion recipients, as well as gays and straights who practiced unprotected anal sodomy with multiple partners, were among the members of this group. Did they share any basis on which to mobilize, other than their potential risk? In the past, some diseases have sparked action, even when possible victims had little in common besides their susceptibility to the ailment and to the strictures targeting it. Compulsory smallpox vaccination prompted massive, now largely forgotten, protest campaigns during the late nineteenth century. Women organized against regulating prostitution to solve the syphilis problem. Their activism was among the first causes—earlier even than the vote—of the feminist movement, and a self-conscious act of gendered solidarity across class lines.[4] Mobilization by potential patients was thus not unprecedented. But partly because it was incurable, and partly because we can now define ourselves through disease (a tendency pioneered by Alcoholics Anonymous), AIDS was the first affliction in whose terms both an identity and a new moniker were formulated: Persons with AIDS (PWA) and its variants.[5]

One epidemiologically exposed group, American and European gay men, were self-conscious, articulate, socially well endowed, and politically effective. They were able to demand attention and resources and to provide self-help. As a result, the response to this epidemic was initially different from what it might have been if, for example, it had struck drug users and ethnic minorities alone. Syphilis afflicted a broad range of victims with no unifying characteristic. In developed nations, because AIDS first spread within an organized, mobilized group, the epidemic was unprecedentedly politicized. In those (mainly developing) countries where HIV was transmitted largely heterosexually, it was more like syphilis—without a focused, politically active group to take up the cause.[6]

The remarkable and—in time—generously financed public response to the epidemic helped create an entire industry of biomedical researchers, social science investigators, social workers, physicians, and other caregivers. They all had a professional and personal stake in the epidemic, whether within the state's apparatus or the extensive voluntary sector that arose to meet the challenge. More people lived from AIDS than died of it, as the most acerbic observers complained.[7] Public health experts, once shunted aside as the microbiological and virological revolutions elevated cure over prevention, now won a new lease on life and prestige. For them, the absence of a biomedical solution was an inadvertent blessing. It shifted the focus to their armamentarium of preventive tactics. Their colleagues in genitourinary medicine were lifted out of obscurity and back into the limelight formerly reserved for those specializing in less embarrassing body parts. CDC suddenly became an acronym recognized around the world, and the Centers for Disease Control, having stumbled in the mid-1970s, and especially during the false alarm of swine flu immunization, rehabilitated itself with aplomb. The epidemic saved its British equivalent, the Communicable Disease Surveillance Centre, from an uncertain future.[8] With other "emerging" infectious diseases as well, and the renewed fear of contagion during the AIDS era, epidemiology became the stuff of thrillers, the CDC the new CIA, and microbes a hot topic in the post–cold war and pre–September 11 search for plausible enemies.[9]

Pharmaceutical companies made fortunes on AIDS drugs and were damned accordingly—as have physicians since the first ointment was mixed—for turning plague into profit. In the absence of an orthodox biomedical cure, alternative approaches flourished. The usual band of quacks reappeared—ever happy to peddle their nostrums to the desperate, and now with loins girded by postmodern suspicions of biomedicine.[10] The Germans—heirs of Ignaz Semmelweis, Robert Koch, and Wilhelm Röntgen, yet curiously partial to alternative medicine—allowed so-called *Heilkündler* an official role in treating AIDS patients.[11] The argument was that, since orthodox medicine had little to offer victims, what was the harm in letting the heterodox at them?[12] Given biomedicine's inability to help victims and the noxious effects of the few effective drugs, sympathy came naturally for those poor souls who preferred to let nature take its course, unaided by human ingenuity.[13] The self-proclaimed AIDS dissidents, for whom the disease was prompted by all manner of cofactors, broadened this unorthodox deviation from scientific opinion.[14]

How nations responded to the epidemic depended on the reactions of the affected—both negatively (gays, but also various ethnic minorities, prostitutes, intravenous drug addicts, and hemophiliacs) and positively (public health experts, pharmaceutical researchers and companies, scientists, and physicians). Oftentimes these groups interacted harmoniously, coordinating interests. Scientists discovered, for example, that gay activists could help force health insurance companies to reimburse experimental drugs, whose cost would otherwise come from research budgets.[15]

At other times, the afflicted were at cross-purposes. The infected had a stake in treatment and cure, while prevention seemed more promising to those at one remove from the epidemiological front lines.[16] Gays and hemophiliacs clashed over whether homosexuals who did not act transmissively should be allowed to donate blood. Hemophiliacs, who eventually won compensation from governments and institutions in many countries, had little interest in organizing with more stigmatized groups on the basis of joint seropositivity. For obvious reasons, they were initially tempted to draw lines between innocent and culpable victims.[17] Indeed, the fact that they were in some nations the only ones compensated for their injuries put a price on the distinction between supposed innocence and guilt.[18] British feminists, seeking to portray women as among the primary victims of the epidemic, downplayed the extent to which most seropositive females were Africans. First

World homosexuals resented attention to the Third World epidemic as a "degaying" of efforts. Blacks attacked gays' susceptibility to arguments on the African origins of the disease. Homosexuals refused to accept arguments by ethnic minorities that men who have sex with men (MSM) in their communities did not identify as gay in the "Western" sense. Gays resented having nonpenetrative sexual practices recommended to them but never to straights.[19] Lesbians lamented the money spent on a largely male ailment at the expense of women's problems. In quarrels over how much at risk women who have sex with women (WSW) were, lesbians were accused of AIDS envy, of feeling left out as attention focused on a disease from which they suffered mainly as members of other risk groups: their primary risk was anal intercourse with men.[20]

American gays and ethnic minorities fought one another repeatedly—in Washington, D.C., for example, where their accusations of racism and homophobia lent an air of undignified one-downmanship to both these dispossessed groups.[21] Residual tensions between the women's and the gay movements were heard in arguments that homosexual men were acting according to conventional male norms—with their pleasure in promiscuity, anonymous copulation, insistence on the primacy of penetration, and belief that restraint was repression. From the vantage of lesbian separatists, gays—and especially leathermen and their ritualized macho swagger— were worse than straights, with their immodest consumption of pornography, their fixation on youth, beauty, and the dimensions of certain body parts, and their stylized power hierarchy in sex. At least straight men, hardwired with carnal desire for the objects of their supposed contempt, might be expected to make the occasional concession. Conversely, in the name of homosexual solidarity, other lesbians rejected attacks on male gays. Antiporn feminists did battle with their anticensorship sisters over explicit and therefore often phallic, if not patriarchal, anti-AIDS propaganda.[22]

Old battles between the sexes flared up once again. Did sex mean penetration—now feared as epidemiologically pernicious as well as patriarchal? Or was there equally enjoyable and valid noninsertive sex (the felicitously named outercourse), less focused on the penis and the alleged submission of the vagina to its ministrations? Sociobiological arguments were heard not just from conservative moralists but also from feminists who otherwise claimed to know that sexual behavior was socially constructed, not biologically given: that the epidemic was due to male promiscuity, for example, while women were more likely to keep their end of the monogamy bargain.[23]

Nor were gays a homogeneous group. White middle-class homosexuals differed from gays of color.[24] Generations separated older gays, who had experienced the closing of the era of insouciant sexual abandon, from subsequent cohorts who had known only the tyranny of safer sex. There were contrasts between closeted and open gays, between those who snuck off for the occasional furtive encounter and regulars at the baths' Dionysian possibilities. Pre-AIDS gay political organizers feared that the public-health attention paid to the epidemic might undermine broader claims, such as legal equality for homosexuals.[25] Though it was rarely acknowledged or discussed, seropositive and uninfected gays had different stakes in prevention, testing, and, above all, obligatory condom use.[26]

The classic dilemma posed for any liminal group flared up too: whether to cooperate with established authority or persist with a parallel universe of autonomous organizations. Battles were fought over when cooperation became cooptation, and where authorities crossed the line between benevolence and imposition. Were gays relieving the state of its responsibilities when they helped themselves? Or were they claiming an authority-free space authentically their own? Was the "queer corporatism" of the AIDS organizations a grassroots delivery of services or a sign of the welfare state's bankruptcy? At what point did social movements become institutions? Were the self-help organizations death camps where those marked to die were sent to perish, as the AIDS activist Larry Kramer put it with his usual hyperbole?[27] Despite its studied anarchist pose, was the AIDS Coalition to Unleash Power (ACT UP) in fact venerating the state by demanding its initiatives? Was AZT a poison being pushed aggressively by the pharmaceutical industry, or a legitimate treatment, however imperfect?[28]

THE MACHINERY OF RESPONSE

None of these groups, of course, influenced decisions alone. The response to the epidemic evolved out of a triangular relationship among (1) victims and their allies, (2) the medical community, including public health authorities, and (3) the statutory powers, including not just public health but also the military, penal, and foreign services. Each member of this triangle had different interests and ambitions, sometimes contradicting the others'. The victims wished for resources poured into research, care, and treatment. They were also averse to meddling by the authorities, and their eagerness for immediate results sometimes contradicted established scientific procedure. The medical and public health establishments longed for the resources, prestige, and power that came with effectively tackling an important social issue. But they also wanted to accomplish the task on their own terms, untroubled by popular and political opinion. The authorities and politicians wished to be seen as effectively tackling a major problem, yet not as pandering to victims whose lifestyles struck many voters as reprehensible. Different legs of this triangle had different strengths in different nations, depending on their political and governmental systems.

In all developed nations, the epidemic's victims—gays especially, but other affected groups as well—formally participated in policy decisions. Specific AIDS institutions were set up in the government to coordinate and plan the response. In Britain, the National AIDS Trust was established with official support to fund voluntary bodies and coordinate their activities. In France, the National AIDS Council advised the government.[29] Self-help organizations mobilized by the most affected constituencies—again above all gays—were relied on, indeed encouraged and subsidized, to accomplish much of the work. Gays and their organizations were integrated into the policy-making machinery. Both private, grassroots voluntary associations and international nongovernmental health organizations played a remarkable role in the epidemic.[30] In the United States alone, some eighteen thousand AIDS service organizations were registered in 1994 with the National AIDS Clearinghouse. So important was volunteerism in the fight, it has been argued, that the largest resource invested was unpaid labor. The Gay Men's Health Crisis (GMHC) budget in 1988 of $7 million would have topped $30 million, it was calculated, if the worth of its fourteen hundred volunteers' labor were counted.[31] Even on the Continent, which traditionally relied more on statutory initiative and less on civil society's own organization, the epidemic roused a different response. The Germans, federalist in their instincts, counted more on voluntary organizations than did the French, who regarded them with suspicion, as incompatible with native traditions of centralized statutory action and leadership.

In Germany, the Deutsche AIDS-Hilfe and, in France, AIDES were encouraged and in large measure financed by authorities, who wanted a single main organization to coordinate relations with gays and other victims. In federalized America, in contrast, such centralization was both less practicable and less necessary. The most comparable organization was the AIDS Action Council, which enlisted some eleven hundred member organizations to act as a national lobby and resource group. Even in France, where such intermixture of private and public remained more of a novelty, the agency for AIDS prevention, established in 1989 and attached to the Health Ministry, was a private organization—so structured in hopes of obscuring its relationship to the government. In Britain, government-funded voluntary organizations, like the National AIDS Trust, tended to displace more purely private, though still officially supported, organizations like the Terence Higgins Trust.[32] Northern European gay self-help organizations were heavily subsidized. In Germany and Scandinavia, the lion's share of their budgets came from the state, while in Britain and France public financing accounted for only some 30 to 40 percent. In the United States, public subsidies were naturally smaller. But even so, half of the GMHC 1986 budget came from sources other than donations, and the Shanti Project received 40 percent of its 1988 funding from the San Francisco municipality.[33]

Indeed, the nature of the epidemic, afflicting despised and alienated groups with no fondness for the state, put a premium on self-organized intermediary bodies with autonomy and distance from the central powers. The authorities, in turn, learned to encourage voluntary initiatives that were direct, effective, and politically acceptable when faced with this morally charged epidemic intimately caught up with sex, drugs, and death. Such organizations were employed to further policies and conduct discussions on subjects the authorities preferred to keep at arm's length—what to average citizens were the ickier aspects of gay sex, say, or the risk-embracing elements of homosexual conduct. They sought to avoid moralistic backlashes by seeming too beholden to gay interests, as well as avoid resistance by homosexuals who thought decisions were coming from distant, unconcerned sources.[34] On the other hand, the informal, grassroots nature of AIDS organizations created difficulties when a more bureaucratized structure was later required, or when organizations catering primarily to gays sought to reach beyond the clientele of the first hour.[35]

Devolving responsibilities to intermediary organizations beyond the authorities' immediate control occasionally led to conflicts—as when the French AIDES insisted on its role for all AIDS victims, not just gays, thereby competing with the central authorities, or when the Deutsche AIDS-Hilfe contradicted official opinion by recommending against voluntary HIV testing. Grassroots input did not mean that local interests saw things the same way that experts did.[36] The value attached to such voluntary mobilization depended on national and ideological context. One could view it as a welcome resurgence of civil society, empowering disenfranchised marginal groups in the face of distant medical and scientific expertise. Or one could see it as a stopgap measure, made necessary by the incompetence of the authorities, who should have led the way.[37]

The success of voluntary organizations did, on occasion, give the authorities an excuse for inaction. The symbiosis between voluntary and statutory efforts was not only a radical, ad hoc response to a pressing problem but also an aspect of the ideology of privatization by conservative governments when the epidemic struck.[38] This was more characteristic of the Reagan and Thatcher administrations, with their efforts to roll back the welfare state, than Continental governments. But the effect was felt also there. In Hamburg, otherwise a fortress of Social Democracy, so successfully did gays organize measures themselves that the municipal authorities were tempted to regard the problem as already addressed and ignore it.[39] With such diametrically opposed views, unholy political alliances were sometimes brokered—above all between Anglo-American conservatives, who aimed to cut the state in size and scope, and radical libertarians, inspired by Gramsci, who sought release from the state Moloch, not action through it.

Balancing integration and resistance by the epidemic's initial victims led in at least two directions. On the one hand, as impatience with medical researchers' inability to produce a cure took its toll, more radical tactics found favor. Dovetailing with this was the question of "degaying" the epidemic. Encouraged by some in the gay movement, resisted by others, degaying meant that, during the late 1980s and early 1990s, initiatives were increasingly shifted out of homosexual self-help groups and into the growing AIDS establishment of public health experts.[40] Closely related to this was the epidemiological displacement, especially in the United States, from gays to ethnic minorities, who were most commonly infected via drug injection or heterosexual transmission. As gays were diluted into a larger pool of victims, and as more effective treatments became available during the early 1990s, the consensual, exceptionalist approach to AIDS gave way to more traditional public health tactics.[41] A resurgence of gay militancy was the result, which rejected unquestioning cooperation with the authorities and cultivated provocative political tactics, designed to grab media attention, embarrass the AIDS establishment, and out prominent closeted homosexuals. Organizations like the Body Positive Group and OutRage in Britain, or ACT UP and Queer Nation in America and other countries, pushed such tactics of making the private political.[42]

Yet gay organizations also found themselves caught in the iron logic of bureaucratization. Even groups set up to oppose a business-as-usual approach to the epidemic were drawn into the maw of established institutions. In Denmark, the main gay AIDS group became a mainstream interest organization intimately connected to political parties and the civil service. Even ACT UP, debuting as a self-consciously alternative group in 1987, did not remain wholly oppositional for long. It quickly learned how to coordinate its "spontaneous" interjections with the organizers of scientific conferences, minimizing disruption and maximizing press coverage. Activists also appeared in Burroughs-Wellcome advertisements to advocate early testing and the like.[43]

Though common traits could be found, countries varied in terms of how gays organized, mobilized, and integrated into the machinery of policy making. Federalized governmental systems, like the United States and to a lesser extent Germany and Switzerland, were more responsive to grassroots organizations than were centralized structures like Sweden and France.[44] In America, input from the affected communities was institutionalized in the policy process: first with the CDC's funding of community-based organizations in the late 1980s, and then, early in 1990s, when the CARE Act funneled funds via planning councils that included representatives of many distinct groups.[45] In the Netherlands, gays were included in policy making from the very start. In Germany, parliamentary commissions set precedents by inviting gay organizations to hearings on AIDS in 1986. The Deutsche AIDS-Hilfe became a quasi-public element of the administration, with a seat in the national AIDS Council and on government commissions of inquiry.[46] In Australia, the federalized nature of the health care system encouraged early cooperation with gay organizations, which were already organized, knowledgeable, and active on the ground.[47]

In Britain, in contrast, with its more monolithic and centralized parties and political institutions, divergent interests won less of a toehold. Gay organizations were given a role early in the epidemic, and the gay lobby had reasonably good access to the public health administration. But the formation of a cabinet committee to deal with AIDS in 1986 shifted power away from the Department of Health and Social Services. As of the mid-1980s, the initiative fell increasingly into the hands of the established policy-making elite among medical and public health authorities, with diminishing input from the grassroots.[48] In Britain, neither gay and other victim organizations nor the conservative religious groups that were active and influential elsewhere had much say. In Scandinavia, special AIDS directorates were established, connected to the government's public health agencies. The active inclusion of gay organizations in these was a novelty. Otherwise, a formal means of cooperation with patients was not developed. French civil servants, in turn, resisted any abandonment of direct control over prevention and education work and hesitated in cooperating with intermediary gay and AIDS organizations. As elsewhere, self-help groups, like AIDES, were represented on the National AIDS Council. Yet French interest groups were not as integrated in decision making as elsewhere and tended to articulate their positions in conflicting fashion. Insisting that it represented all victims of the disease, not just gays, AIDES competed, rather than cooperated, with the state.[49]

THE VARIETY OF GAYNESS

Upon hearing the news from America of a new cancer that struck only gays, Muzil, the character based on Michel Foucault in Hervé Guibert's autobiographical novel, *To the Friend Who Did Not Save My Life*, exclaims, "That's too good to be true, I could die laughing." Only a guffaw did justice to such a grotesquerie. Though a persecuted minority, gays had finally managed to cast off the fetters of millennia before the epidemic hit, revolutionizing in the process Western society's views of the body and sexuality, reclaiming the polymorphous perversity, the *gesamtkörperliche* tactility we enjoy as infants but find increasingly repressed, focused, and genitalized as adults. They had exploded the Protestant belief in sublimation as the key to worldly success by combining above-average socioeconomic indicators with libidinous abandon, experimentation, and innovation of an intensity undreamt of in the heterosexual imagination. But now, gays in the Western world were to be punished with a miserable fate that awaited them alone— transmitted, with the kind of petty predictability one might expect of a spiteful minor deity, by the very acts with which they had dared defy nature and morality. The Promethean myth had rarely seemed more appropriate. Conversely, from the vantage of conservative moralists, gays fucked like bunnies and were now dropping like flies, and these two observations were not unrelated.

Understanding the response to the epidemic means looking at the gay community in each nation and its organization, mobilization, and political clout.[50] Germany's gay movement was among the oldest and most venerable, dating back to the nineteenth century and equipped with impeccable intellectual and scholarly credentials. Homosexuality was decriminalized in 1969. Yet the precedent set by the treatment of gays during the Nazi regime lasted into the postwar period; indeed rates of prosecution increased after 1945.[51] In France, the law was more liberal. Homosexuality was not criminalized in the Napoleonic Code, though the Pétain government introduced a differential age of consent, twenty-one for homosexuals, fifteen for straights. Such comparative lenience may have helped delay the development of a gay movement there. Nonetheless, homosexuality remained more stigmatized than was common in northern Europe. Similarly, for Italy it has been argued that, because homosexuality was not criminalized in the first national penal code in 1889, the gay movement was weakened by not having discriminatory laws to contest.[52] In Finland harshly antigay attitudes prevailed. Though homosexuality had been decriminalized in 1971, the law still prohibited disseminating positive information about it.[53]

British attitudes toward homosexuality had long been more censorious than on the Continent. The middle classes battled aristocratic tolerance of such sins of the flesh. Workers regarded homosexuality as upper-class decadence, with randy nobs preying on the sons of the proletariat. Private homosexual sex above age twenty-one had been decriminalized in 1967 (while the age of consent for heterosexuals was sixteen). But buggery in public, including a provision defining public as more than two participants, remained an offense, and in 1989, 178 men were imprisoned for the act. The legal restrictions on homosexuality were harsher than in most Continental nations, including barring gays from the military and criminalizing homosexuality in it (until 2000). The passage of the Local Government Act of 1988, which included a clause prohibiting local authorities from promoting homosexuality, revived bitter debates. On the other hand, the age of consent was finally equalized at sixteen, over objections from the House of Lords, in 2000.[54]

The American situation was, as always, complicated by the country's vast scale and heterogeneity. Attitudes toward sex of any sort remained more conservative than in northern Europe. Starting inauspiciously during the nineteenth century, the gay movement did not gain momentum until the 1950s. Gay sex remained theoretically illegal in a number of states. As late as 1986, in *Bowers v. Hardwick*, the Supreme Court refused to extend privacy protections to consensual sodomy between same-sex partners, though this was overturned finally in 2003. Fundamentalist Christians helped condemn homosexuality to opprobrium at the same time as the best-organized and most visible gay movement in the world made it increasingly public. President Bill Clinton's inability to make good on his promise to end the military ban on homosexuality in the ranks demonstrated how polarized attitudes remained.[55]

Added to national differences were the multiple ways in which homosexuality was understood across cultural blocs. In the recently evolved northern European and (white) American approach, the sex of the partner in intercourse was the crucial determinant of gayness, while in the more traditional view of homosexuality—widespread around the Mediterranean and in Latin America and shared by many American blacks—the action in intercourse was what counted.[56] In the first case, men who had sex with men usually varied positions and were sometimes receptive, sometimes insertive. In the second case, those who were consistently penetrated were considered gay, while the penetrators of other men were often still seen as heterosexual, so long as their behavior remained "active" in this sense. Indeed, in some cultures having sex with both men and women was considered especially manly (though the evidence about this view is, not surprisingly, contradictory).[57] The traditional approach sprang from a more patriarchal division between the sexes. The "true" gays—the receptive ones—were classified as like women, and the active ones were considered men, so long as their sexual activity and position remained constant.[58] The northern approach, in turn, was consonant with a greater equality of relations between the sexes, institutionalized in companionate marriages, and it was applied to both men and women, regardless of the gender of their partners.

The implications of such differences were important. In the traditional approach, the numbers of gays in the strict sense would, by definition, be smaller. To the extent that insertive anal intercourse was less risky than receptive lovemaking, transmission was hampered so long as each partner stuck to his role. Gays did not exist as a socially identifiable subgroup, living apart from the straight mainstream, to nearly the same extent as further north for reasons that included not just cultural preference but also such mundane considerations as tight housing markets and the inviolability of family life, broken for adult children only upon marriage. The egalitarian behavior of role switching and sexual versatility of northern gays—sometimes penetrating, sometimes receiving—involved a reciprocity that allowed both partners to know the other's experience. It made gay sex more a meeting of the twain than its straight—or lesbian—variations could aspire to (though increasing numbers of straights have also sought similar experiences, making strap-on dildos an item no longer only for lesbians but also for heterosexual role-reversal). The northern approach was also the most dangerous epidemiologically, leaving all partners, and not just at most half, susceptible to infection and more likely to pass it along.[59]

In southern nations, both the overall number of cases and their localization among gays were therefore limited, reducing the salience of the issue. Conversely, the likelihood of transmission through what, from a northern point of view, was bisexual behavior was greater. Men who, to the north, would tend to act exclusively as gays, swung both ways in Latin and Mediterranean cultures—and the same occurred among American blacks, where bisexuality, or covert gayness (depending on how one judged it), was higher than among whites. The same, obviously, held for North American Latinos.[60] Because of the denial of what, from another perspective, was gay sexual behavior, HIV transmission via drug use appeared to be more important among such nations, and sexual transmission less so, than was actually true. Thanks to role separation, the penetrators were often hard to convince that they were at risk and should use condoms.[61] Conversely, the rigid role differentiation characteristic of the southern approach may have been partly effaced by the AIDS epidemic and the attendant shift to safer sex. As one Costa Rican sex worker complained, with all this masturbation, it was hard to tell who was active and who was passive.[62]

The relationship between gays and AIDS must, of course, be a leitmotif of any attempt to understand the epidemic. In the West, gays were among the groups first and hardest hit. A self-consciously gay community had evolved, with common patterns of residence and recreation, in sexual and social self-isolation. Homosexuals' socioepidemiological behavior at this moment in history gave HIV its perversely favorable ecological niche. Once the mechanism of transmission was known, it became clear that the problem was not gayness, in some vague and mysterious manner, but certain practices—above all promiscuous anal sex. It was no more the homosexuality of gays that facilitated HIV transmission than it was the femaleness of prostitutes that made them a crossroads for syphilis in the nineteenth century, or the Hinduism of Indians who excreted in, bathed in, and drank from the Ganges that left them perfect vectors of cholera.[63] Needless to say, anal sex and promiscuity were not exclusive to gays. But such behavior did remain characteristic especially of male-to-male intercourse. This helped underpin the more generalized antigay sentiments common among the straight population.[64] Already in the winter of 1982, when Representative Robert K. Dornan first raised the issue in the House, he called attention to gay sexual practices (one thousand to fifteen hundred annual contacts per person was his statistic) as the reason for their susceptibility. "We learned," Surgeon General Everett Koop said, "of homosexual practices that were hitherto barely mentioned, and we understood, perhaps for the first time, the extent of homosexual promiscuity."[65] Although the seropositive basketball star Magic Johnson did gays no favor in terms of the enthusiasm with which he vaunted his heterosexuality (while also confirming white stereotypes of black male hypersexuality and blacks as carriers of VD), he at least helped even the playing field of promiscuity.[66]

The gay behaviors that proved epidemiologically risky had become common in Western culture during the decades preceding the epidemic. As a socially stable gay identity coalesced during the middle years of the century, new sexual behavior was part of it. Earlier in the century, gay relations had tended to involve encounters with men who could pass as straight because they were only the passive recipients of oral sex—rough trade. Now, male homosexuality became spectacularly Dionysian: multiple partners, group sex, anal sodomy, sadomasochism, rimming, scat, water sports, fisting. In epidemiological hindsight, such behaviors seem to have been designed to promote easy and efficient transfer of microorganisms.[67] Also crucial for the epidemic's spread was the way that gays with different sexual habits interacted—from the core of hyperpromiscuous bathhouse regulars, through the middle range of averagely libidinous MSM, to the fringe of closeted homosexuals, sometimes bisexual, often married, and furtively engaging in the occasional dalliance. The spread of disease was accelerated by average gays making occasional forays into the gay ghettos, whose institutions of erotic recreation were among the most effective loci of transmission—barring perhaps the shooting galleries with their direct blood-to-blood avenues of viral peregrination.[68]

Gays happened to practice behavior—and to have begun it in the era preceding the epidemic—that laid down well-paved routes of transmission. They also formed a largely isolated community, so that HIV spread quickly within, but only slowly beyond, it. It was precisely those aspects of northern homosexual behavior that defined the modern gay identity (self-chosen isolation, anal sex, role switching, and promiscuity) which posed such risks. Had gays lived as they did earlier in the century, or as they continued to in Mediterranean and Latin cultures—covertly and bisexually, with clear role separation in sex—the epidemic would have wrought less damage among them. Conversely, the fact that AIDS was identified early on, rather than spreading slowly into the heterosexual population and being conceptualized as a separate disease only when it had ravaged more widely, as in Africa, resulted largely from the sociosexual visibility and encapsulation of the gay community. Gays sought treatment early from sympathetic physicians, who were attentive to their problems. It was not until later, in the mid-1980s, that epidemiologists retrospectively identified a similar mortality increase among drug addicts. Gays were like the canary in the coal mine. They gave the first warning of a danger that would otherwise have remained invisible far longer.[69]

Since the disease first struck and ravaged gays, the initial public response was miserly at best and often punitive. Little research money was forthcoming, and harsh sanctions were at first imposed on the infected and at-risk. AIDS was pounced on to justify continued prejudices against loathed ethnic and especially sexual minorities. The public health response to the epidemic, in this view, was influenced as much by such dislikes as by any medical understanding of the disease. Traditional precautions against epidemics simply continued the social ostracism to which gays were otherwise subject.[70] That such widespread antipathy played a role in the response to the disease is too obvious to require elaboration. Popular opinion everywhere was at first happy to accept more drastic restrictions on the infected than if they had sported a mainstream social identity. Recriminalizing homosexuality was proposed, as were quarantines of the sick and infected; tattooing seropositives to warn prospective sexual partners was a common idea. That drug addicts and "sexual perverts" were the cause of the epidemic was widely argued.[71]

Antigay sentiments may also have been stoked not just by standard-issue homophobia but equally by subterranean jealousy among straight men for a lifestyle of sensual abandon that they could never hope for—burdened with the obligations of the courtship ritual, monogamy and fidelity, family life and child rearing.[72] The hostility of straight males to their gay brethren may have been reinforced by a psychological backlash against the women's movement and its success in ending double standards and the acceptability of commercial sex, elements that had earlier lubricated gender relations. The heroic feats of gay promiscuity, elevated from urban myth by the unflinching efforts of social science surveys, appeared to confirm the insights of sociobiology. Gays—mobile, sexually restless, and spectacularly disseminatory—seemed to incarnate the Y chromosome's sexual imperative.[73] They were Lotharios whose conquests made the most active straight Don Juan seem monastic in comparison. Lesbians, in turn, were revealed to be among the epidemiologically safest of groups because of their quintessential female virtues of bonding, abstinence, monogamy, and nesting. Everyone else, male and female, found themselves accommodated willy-nilly like passengers in tourist class—uncomfortable but there—between these conceptual extremes. (One day, an account of attitudes toward AIDS will also take measure of the way white men, implicitly supported by their monogamous female mates, looked with a volatile mixture of contempt, envy, and desire upon what seemed the polygamous abandon of their African brothers, and how this motivated their indifference to the ravages of that continent.)

On the other hand, a great deal of mythmaking, much of it heterosexual fantasizing, was cooked up regarding gay sexuality and its intensity. Every despised group is regarded by its self-perceived superiors as hypersexualized—whether blacks in America or Jews in Nazi Germany (portrayed in *Mein Kampf* as lustful despoilers of Aryan maidens). Consider, too, the Orientalist fantasies of the East as a fount of sexual excess and exoticism, the same view of the West found among believing Muslims, and (perhaps oddest of all) the Soviet bloc view (shared by many Africans) of the capitalist West as sexually promiscuous and decadent, especially in its homosexuality.[74] Leaving aside the small core of satyric bathhouse habitués, the average gay man may have had more orgasms than his heterosexual brothers. But if pressed about details by the infallible methods of empirical social science, he revealed that the bulk of such licentiousness took the form of solitary masturbation—nice perhaps, doubtless underrated, but hardly something unavailable to the average Joe.[75]

In one view, the response to the epidemic was neither vigorous nor generous, because of its victims' stigma. At the other extreme were those who resented the ability of gays, as a well-organized interest group, to win privileged treatment: exemptions, for example, from the strictures applied to other diseases, and massive government funding for research, education, and treatment in disproportion to the epidemic's mortality.[76] Observers in Germany credited the consensual approach taken there to the gayness of key government advisors. Swiss physicians complained that the gay lobby hampered the use of traditional measures against AIDS.[77] John Searle, a prominent British physician, went so far as to testify before a parliamentary committee that gays formed a hidden conspiracy, identifiable only to each other, hidden from even their wives (!), unwilling to change their risky habits, and now seeking to bring the rest of society down with them.[78] AIDS, some claimed, was the first epidemic to enjoy political protection.[79] Were they not so uncharitable, one might even take conservative complaints about the gay lobby's power and influence as a backhanded compliment to its prowess.[80]

Whatever one may think of the motivations behind such observations, they did contain a barb of truth. Unlike others of the epidemic's victims, gays were effective actors.[81] Though not held in esteem, they enjoyed above-average levels of education and income. When stricken as a group, they were in a position to act.[82] Gays in America, and therefore the initial cohorts of AIDS victims, were clustered in the two states with the most electoral votes and corresponding congressional clout, New York and California. The beginnings of increased federal funding for AIDS research began as a result of 1983 congressional hearings chaired by Henry Waxman and Theodore Weiss, representatives whose constituencies included large and visible gay communities.[83] Gays also influenced procedures for conducting clinical trials, helping undercut double-blind studies and streamlining the route from test to market. The reorganization of American research efforts, as the National Institute of Health's Office of AIDS Research was set up in 1993, owed much to pressure from ACT UP and the AIDS Action Council.[84]

The public health restrictions imposed on seropositives, even at their most draconian, rarely approximated those required for other contagious diseases. Compulsory examination and isolation of tuberculosis victims, for example, were far stricter than impositions in Southern California on seropositives.[85] However inadequate when measured against some theoretical standard, biomedical research and treatment were eventually more generously funded for AIDS than for most other diseases. That the federal budget for AIDS research and treatment increased fiftyfold during the first decade of the epidemic is hard to correlate with supposed antagonism toward gays and neglect of their problems. Indeed, recent and nuanced examinations conclude that neither antagonism, nor even indifference, toward gays characterized much of the official response to the epidemic.[86] To claim that there was a genocide or holocaust—a deliberate killing, or even letting die, of any of the epidemic's victims—is an unpardonable exaggeration.[87]

If there is a silver lining, it may perhaps be found in the way the epidemic helped integrate gays into society, putting their problems on the quotidian political agenda and normalizing relations with the straight majority—legitimating them through disaster.[88] The epidemic may have transformed gays, as the most optimistic observer put it, from "a disorganized collection of despised individuals into a self-affirming community and a full-fledged civil rights movement."[89] Public opinion, which might have become more homophobic during the epidemic, in fact moved in the other direction. Perhaps it is cynical, as some have suggested, to say that AIDS enhanced the visibility of gays, but no more, surely, than to observe that, without the Holocaust, the state of Israel would not have been.[90]

At the beginning of the epidemic, gays were still stigmatized and marginalized (and of course they remain so) not just by the mainstream's generalized distaste but also in precise legal terms. Unable to marry, even stable gay couples had few of the rights taken for granted by heterosexuals. In some states, gay sex was illegal and, when not, the age of consent was often higher.[91] But in tandem with, and sometimes as a result of, the epidemic, many things changed. Homosexuality was no longer classified as a mental illness. Gay marriage became a hotly debated topic, nowhere more so than among homosexuals themselves: would it mean gays imitating heterosexual mores, or recognizing all couples legally and institutionally?[92] Some countries (Belgium, Denmark, the Netherlands, Iceland, Sweden, and France in 2000) formalized gay unions, though usually short of marriage.[93] Though almost half of American states outlawed same-sex unions in 1997, some allowed gay partnerships that conferred at least partial legal benefits. In 2004 gays were married in Massachusetts. Gay sex was more rarely pursued in

legal terms. In the 1986 *Bowers v. Hardwick* case, the Supreme Court refused to protect private, consensual homosexual acts. This was overturned in
2003. And in any case, only seven states retained sodomy laws pertaining to
gays, and none reinstated a sodomy law as a result of Bowers. In many countries, the age of consent was equalized, or at least the disparity was reduced.[94] Same-sex benefits became an increasingly common feature in social
insurance provision, too.

Although gays mobilized in response to the epidemic, significant differences of opinion divided them. Was promiscuous sex a key element of gay
identity or foolhardy behavior in the face of a lethal disease? Gays split between technocrats, hoping for biomedical cures that promised to sidestep
further behavioral impositions, and moralizers who sought a move away
from allegedly self-destructive habits toward "healthier" pursuits. The first
group became allies of the medical establishment, which had earlier been regarded as a chief regulator of homosexuality and an enemy.[95] The latter
found themselves on occasion rubbing shoulders with conservative heterosexual moralists, convinced that gay culture had its pathogenic aspects. Tactical differences separated urban gays from their rural cousins, many of
whom were married and feared publicity. Gays in low-incidence areas
sometimes saw AIDS as a problem of big cities and sought epidemiological
security in avoiding their peers from elsewhere: Europeans meeting Americans, Oxford men meeting Londoners.[96] There were local differences, too:
between San Francisco's largely white, middle-class, and well-organized
community and New York's variegated and fragmented conglomeration,
hobbled in its organization and politics.[97]

Gay communities varied across national borders, too. Besides the north-
south split, the main distinction was between the subcultural approach of
American homosexuals—with their voluntarist, self-help organizations;
flamboyant residential ghettos; and identities formulated in terms of sexual
practices, patterns of consumption, residence, modes of behavior, and
dress—and the nations of central and northern Europe. Here, gays were a
self-conscious, organized, and recognizable social force, unlike their brothers in the Mediterranean region or eastern Europe. Yet, though pursuing the
same sexual practices as their American peers, they remained more integrated into society and less stratified by consumption or residence. In sum,
they were less a subculture.[98] Within such broad distinctions, however, the
variations were nearly as great. The English, German, and Scandinavian gay
movements were more akin to the American, while the French, with their
partly republican, partly Mediterranean insistence on effacing differences,
stood apart. Endless political debates resulted, concerning above all whether

to emphasize a universalist civil rights approach that sought equal treatment for gays, or whether to accentuate the differences, celebrating what set homosexuals apart from mainstream society.

The organizational skill of gay movements and their capacity for self-help also varied. At one end of the spectrum lay nations like the United States, Scandinavia, and the Netherlands. A middle position was occupied by central Europe: Germany, Switzerland, Austria, Belgium, and the United Kingdom. Then came a caboose made up of the Mediterranean and Catholic nations: France, Italy, Spain, Ireland, Greece, and Portugal.[99] The first had long traditions of gay organization, dating back to the 1940s and 1950s. In central Europe, with the exception perhaps of Germany, little gay infrastructure predated the 1970s. The movement had been radical in Britain and especially France during the 1970s but had largely collapsed thereafter, offering little institutional continuity on which to build during the epidemic. The Catholic nations, finally, had fragmented gay organizations and little public funding. The United States stood between and betwixt: it could boast a strong movement with a reasonably venerable past, but less ideological proclivity to take strong public health intervention for granted, and less reliance on the state.

Gays mobilized in response to AIDS first in America, where an organized movement had developed after the Stonewall riots of 1969 in New York City. The precedent set here was then emulated in Canada, Australia, and northern Europe.[100] The Gay Men's Health Crisis in New York was established already in 1982. It was followed closely by the AIDS Foundation in Los Angeles and the Shanti Project in San Francisco, the latter of which, though not originating expressly for homosexuals, came to devote itself to the care of the infected.[101] San Francisco had the best-organized and politically most powerful gay community. Especially at first, the epidemic here was almost exclusively homosexual and was complicated by few problems associated with an urban underclass, ethnic minorities, or dysfunctional drug usage. Excepting the battle over the bathhouses, the city exemplified gay mobilization's ambitions for a consensual, voluntarist approach.[102] San Francisco's self-help organizations, emphasizing buddy systems, outpatient care, and hospices, but also other American programs, were widely admired in Europe.[103]

In Scandinavia and the United States, gay organizations predated the epidemic and marshalled the response on their terms. In other nations, like Britain and Germany, cart and horse were reversed. The epidemic and the quasi-governmental organizations that emerged in response were also vehicles to organize gays. The British gay movement, flourishing during the

1970s, had since declined. It was revived by the epidemic, especially in protest against the 1988 Local Government Act, which forbade the promotion of homosexuality. Stonewall, an important gay rights group, was founded the same year. The *Pink Paper*, a major national gay newspaper, was not founded until 1987, deep into the epidemic.[104] Mobilization in France also came late and ineffectively. Groups founded during the 1970s, like the Front homosexuel d'action révolutionnaire and the Comité d'urgence antirépression homosexuelle, saw themselves as part of the left. Starting in the mid-1980s, more lasting and less partisan organizations were established.[105] Yet French gays remained suspicious of governmental authority. In Sweden and Britain, gay groups cooperated with public health officials, seeking, for example, to persuade their members not to donate blood. The French, in contrast, considered such recommendations discriminatory and adopted a more confrontational approach.[106]

The gayness of the AIDS organizations also varied. In Scandinavia, the Netherlands, and America, though less clearly in the United Kingdom, the main AIDS organizations were tied closely to the gay community and spoke mostly—though not exclusively—for homosexuals. On the Continent, and especially in France, such organizations aimed to represent all the epidemic's victims, though in fact homosexuals were their workhorses. The Gay Men's Health Crisis in America focused, not surprisingly, on gays; the Swedish Association for Sexual Equality remained a self-consciously gay organization, as did the Gay Health Action Dublin. In France, in contrast, AIDES defined itself as a general interest organization and formulated its mandate in universal terms. Here and in Germany, Britain, and Switzerland, AIDS organizations sought to appeal to more than just gays. They separated mobilization around homosexual identity issues from organization to counter the epidemic.[107]

France was an outsider in its refusal to countenance specifically gay organizations against the epidemic. The Enlightenment ideology of universalist citizenship saw humanity in the abstract and claimed indifference to distinctions of race, religion, sex, or sexual preference. This discouraged the formation of a gay identity, as well as political mobilization on that basis, just as it had undercut a women's movement on the Anglo-Saxon model. It also dovetailed with French preferences for radically assimilating immigrants into mainstream French society rather than allowing them to retain the culture of their origin. Gays were now treated according to the principle enunciated by Count Stanislas de Clermont-Tonnerre for emancipating Jews during the Revolution: give them everything as individuals, and nothing as a community.[108] The French saw their position as the counterbalance to what they regarded as the balkanization and tribalization of the Anglo-Saxon, and especially American, world.[109]

The arguments of Michel Foucault, Guy Hocquenghem, and other post-modernist philosophers against essentialism also influenced French politics. They undergirded the reluctance of French gays to take on an identity whose parameters had, in some measure, been staked out by their enemies. Instead, the French sought to undermine all definitions of identity.[110] With the coming of Queer Theory, early in the 1990s, such ideas began to have an influence. They questioned the Anglo-Saxon approach by exposing the essentialism of identity formation on a sexual basis. When not just motivated by standard-issue homophobia, the traditional left had rejected homosexuals' claims to recognition because gays appeared to accept uncritically the dichotomy of sexual preference structured by bourgeois morality. Queer Theory, after the interlude when gays merely upended valuations by celebrating what had once been castigated, now questioned the very existence of binary sexual proclivities.[111] But if the notion of fixed sexual identities was rejected for the polymorphous perversity of us all—whether Rambo, bimbo, or something in between—then forming political interests on the basis of what was once quaintly called inverted sexual proclivity was of necessity undermined. Postmodernism came up against its own internal contradiction between an individual epistemology that denied the existence of coherent subjects with consistent identities, and a political mobilization that happily accepted cohesive, indeed reductionist and essentialist, identities, the better to arm their group for political battle.[112]

The study of French political culture has moved beyond the traditional claim that society here, unlike that of Anglo-Saxons, was weak at organizing itself.[113] But France's response to the AIDS epidemic was often seen through the lens of such historiography, and a grain of truth remained. French social movements—ethnic and sexual—remained weaker and more universalist than elsewhere, especially in the United States. The Comité d'urgence antirépression homosexuelle, founded in 1979, focused more on politics than lifestyle. It was willing to cut deals with unions and parties, and it pressed for reforms once François Mitterrand had been elected president. Before AIDS, a separate gay subculture on the American model was rejected in favor of a pan-homo-hetero movement of sexual liberation founded on the alleged universality of homoerotic desires and the polymorphously perverse and multiplicitous inclinations of everyone—a kind of political Freudianism.[114]

France had been a land of "new social movements" up through the 1970s. But by the AIDS era, while the ecology, animal rights, women's, and peace movements had established and institutionalized themselves elsewhere, especially across the Rhine and the Channel, here they faded. In part, the old-fashioned left remained dominant, smothering competitors. Its parties and organizations were able to deliver a victory in the form of Mitterrand's presidency in 1981. The Socialist Party, when it came to power, did accede to gay claims and ended various forms of discrimination. But a fondness on the left, either old or new, for gay themes was far from self-evident.[115] The radical left-wing Lutte ouvrière regarded the issue as a petty bourgeois diversion from proletarian heterosexuality. It thought that—come the revolution—gays, like prostitutes, would disappear, and it saw no point in enlightening a prejudiced working class. During the early years of the century, feminism in France had been hampered not only by conservatives but also by the left, fearing that enfranchising women (those notorious clericalists) would boost the right. So too homosexuality, viewed by many leftists during the 1930s as politically in bed with Fascism, now won little support from radicals.[116] Because the right had monopolized abortion and contraception as issues, however, the Socialists had tactical reasons to take up homosexuality, the main subject remaining on which it could strike a stance in such matters. The homosexual vote was also now recognized as a political force. After Mitterrand's victory, police were stopped from harassing gays and haunting their meeting places. Homosexuality was no longer regarded as a mental illness, and the age of consent was equalized at fifteen. Within a year, quickly but belatedly the Socialist Party had purged French law of most of its archaic antigay elements.[117]

Then AIDS struck. Gay organizations had a hard time, with sexuality regarded as a purely individual and personal choice, with subcultural groupings seen as an illegitimate interposition between state and citizen, and with strong old-style leftist parties and organizations cluttering one field where new social movements (now relegated to the right) might otherwise have played.[118] The gay movement was saturated by American habits—a result of sexual globalization, as it were—and a homosexual subculture was regarded suspiciously in France, where losing national identity was a widespread fear.[119] Given the Mediterranean penchant for defining gayness by the role taken in intercourse, rather than by the gender of the partner, many men who would elsewhere be identified as gay were not—to the detriment of homosexual organization. Because in the Mediterranean gays were not a group as clearly victimized by the epidemic, compared to intravenous drug addicts, the stimulus thus offered by AIDS to homosexual mobilization was also absent.[120] The hypernatalist attitude taken by the French even into the twentieth century also made things harder for nonbreeders.[121] Resistance in

France to measures focused on homosexuals and to gay mobilization was also encouraged by the strength of the extreme right. The National Front blamed gays and immigrants for infecting French society, and it advocated drastic measures against both. In response, public health authorities sought to avoid calling attention to high-risk groups. Eager to portray the disease as one that threatened all French, they were loath to insist on measures possibly within the pale, like criminalizing transmission.[122]

It has been suggested that, where gay movements were well organized, strong, and confident, and where social stigmatization was not a dominant concern, gays worried less about the state intervening and welcomed rather than feared new statutory actions.[123] But that cannot be the whole story. Gays' attitude to the state differed even among those nations in which their movement was strongest, the United States, Scandinavia, and the Netherlands, say. The organizational muscle and competence of gay organizations varied across countries. But so too did their basic political instincts, leaving them more American, or German, or French, than gay—if there is such a thing in any political sense. All gay movements, regardless of their national setting, distrusted statutory authority, remembering years of laws forbidding their sexual habits, closing down their meeting places, and generally harassing them. The German movement was especially wary of officials and suspicious of the motives of a medical profession considered unusually conservative.[124]

The American gay movement, populated by middle-class whites able to care for themselves and distrustful of authority, defended the right to privacy and to exclude the state from civil society.[125] It was thus in a slightly peculiar situation. Although it was among the best-organized and most powerful gay movements, its basic political inflection was liberalist. In distinction to the civil rights and ethnic minority movements, American gays were less inclined to seek redress through the state, less concerned to have the authorities remedy past neglect, and more interested in being spared further statutory attention. True, gay organizations sought government support for research and treatment. But otherwise, the ethos was one of autonomous subgroup organization and self-provision of basic services. Gay volunteering, though sometimes damned as letting the government off the hook, was mostly praised as part of a distinctive American tradition. It also inspired a sense of gay community and solidarity, sometimes verging on pantheistic mysticism.[126]

And yet the general rule of thumb for all gay movements, even in America, was that, during the epidemic, they gradually overcame their distrust and sought a more active response from the state.[127] How national gay movements differed had implications for AIDS work. Statutory and gay initiatives were symbiotic. Where homosexuals organized only little, as in France, public health authorities had to fill the vacuum. Conversely, where gays stepped into the breach, others did not have to follow. In more specific instances, too, differences played a role. The battles over bathhouses depended largely on the nature of these institutions. In Britain, where bathhouses had been shut already during the 1970s, the fierce battles of San Francisco or New York, where the baths were a focal point of gay identity and practice, were not fought.[128] In Berlin, bathhouses were not shut, but a third of them closed their doors in the mid-1980s for lack of business; leather-bar back rooms were shut voluntarily for a while. In France, on the assumption that gays would practice safe sex, bathhouses and back rooms remained open.[129] At the same time, the French did not have as extensive a bathhouse scene as North America until well into the 1990s.[130] Foucault's experiences in San Francisco in 1975 suggest that, at the time, his Parisian forays to Le Keller paled in comparison to what he found in California.[131]

Convinced that the squeaky wheel gets the oil, gay political organizations everywhere used new, high-profile tactics: die-ins, memorial quilts, blood splashings, outings. Their spirit was well known from the 1960s—Abbie Hoffman and the Yippie movement had been pioneers—but the specifics were new and often resented by more traditional political activists. Gay political movements deliberately flouted the rules of standard lobbying, not to mention those of good taste and conventional behavior. The Yippies had thrown dollars onto the New York Stock Exchange trading floor; ACT UP splashed pharmaceutical manufacturers with blood. Blacks had called themselves niggers in defiance of the linguistic discretion of their white liberal allies. Gays now became queers and faggots again, or *Schwul* or *pedé*—depriving foul-mouthed bigots of their epithets. In Germany, all citizens were declared *Uneinsichtigen*, or Recalcitrants, to show their solidarity even with the most uncooperative of seropositives.[132]

To many gays, such movements were politically immature and interested more in spectacle than the hard work of lobbying, advocacy, and persuasion. A lifetime of disco music, as Quentin Crisp once remarked, is a steep price to pay for one's sexual preference. In America, Barney Frank, the first voluntarily open homosexual congressman, unfavorably contrasted gay political excess with the discipline and rigor of the civil rights movement.[133] In France, the powerful traditional left-wing parties that might have been allies disapproved of such tactics of cultural provocation. When the Front homosexuel d'action révolutionnaire sought to emulate the American gay pride movement and joined in the 1971 May Day parade, it was sandwiched between the Mouvement de libération des femmes and a high school action committee. With its banners proclaiming slogans like "Revolutionary Homosexuality," "Down with the Dictatorship of the Normal," and "High School Students Are Cute," it scandalized left-wing associates perhaps more than anyone else. The trade union militants of the Lutte ouvrière criticized it for implicitly accepting bourgeois society's definition of gays as marginal by behaving in an infantile manner, and they rejected any organization on the basis of sexuality rather than the "objective" categories of socioeconomic status.[134]

BUT IS IT GOOD FOR THE GAYS?

Gay self-definition via sexual identity does not necessarily impose a particular political persuasion any more than, say, the religion of the Jews. But gays' experience as a persecuted and despised minority has inclined them toward tolerance and equality. In the AIDS era, gays sought to walk a line between asking for help from the broader community and avoiding unwanted impositions by the authorities. In all countries, they hoped for generous resources for research, treatment, and care, and an unpunitive public health campaign against the epidemic.

Like other victims of the epidemic, gays sought to reconcile prestigious basic research on the disease's cause and more mundane attempts to assuage HIV's worst symptoms. Technical aspects of conducting clinical trials laid bare the tensions between scientists' long-term work for knowledge and the desperate hopes of the ill for an effect now. With AZT in 1985–86 and the first hopes—however disappointing in this case—of treatment, the issue became anything but academic. Double-blinded testing, with one group receiving placebos and no one knowing which was which, proved ethically troublesome. The scientist's desire to know whether a drug was effective contradicted the physician's duty to provide effective care to all mortally ill patients.[135] No one wanted to be in the placebo group, to be one of the guinea pigs on whose suffering future treatment rested. Despite researchers' objections that breaking down experimental protocols would lead to bad science, ineffective medicine, and more suffering, standard research procedures proved politically difficult to fulfill given the hopes of the ill and the political will of groups like ACT UP. Drugs not approved for the American market, like ribavirin or dextran sulfate, were obtained in Mexico or Japan and smuggled in.[136]

One result of gay lobbying was to relax stringent Food and Drug Administration safety procedures, abbreviating the testing phases, making experimental drugs available earlier through fast track studies, and allowing imports of foreign drugs for personal use and "parallel track" access for the mortally ill.[137] While welcome, this was not without consequences. Shortening testing times and trying out experimental drugs on the ill held out the danger of administering toxic substances to the already stricken. Lessening liability obstacles to new drugs, as recommended in both the United States and Germany, meant reducing pharmaceutical companies' legal responsibility for iatrogenic effects. A narrow course had to be steered between protecting the ill and letting them suffer needlessly. In the same way, delicate political footwork was needed for gays to partner tactically with conservatives, who were interested not in speeding effective medicine to homosexuals but in cutting back statutory regulation.[138] More generally, the epidemic helped accelerate a larger movement of consumer and patient power. During the AIDS era, streamlined trials of experimental drugs were extended also to cancer, Alzheimer's, and advanced multiple sclerosis. The days when physicians' pronouncements were accepted without question faded now that every home computer could access Medline and a thousand other sources of information.[139]

The resources eventually devoted to the epidemic testified to gays' organizational prowess and contradicted the common argument that marginal groups could command only marginal attention.[140] Indeed, a minor literature on whether monies spent for AIDS were disproportional to the suffering concerned—the cost-benefit analysis that only economists of the most dismal sort can do—backhandedly acknowledged gays' power to bend the public ear. Conservatives argued that this disease received more than its fair share.[141] In the early 1980s, American spending on AIDS research per death compared unfavorably to other recent ailments, such as toxic shock syndrome or Legionnaires' disease. By the end of the decade, however, AIDS was receiving at least its due of research funds. Federal spending on AIDS reached $1.6 billion in 1990, a year after 40,000 Americans had died of the disease. At same time, spending on cancer, which killed half a million in 1989, was $1.5 billion. For heart disease (mortality 750,000), it was less than $1 billion. AIDS spending was four times that on diabetes, which killed 36,000 annually, and it far outstripped more transient illnesses like Legionnaires' disease.[142] Other measures, however, accounted for spending not just per death but in more nuanced terms, including early demise and life quality impairment, which were higher for AIDS, since it struck especially the young. In these terms, spending was comparable to that for heart disease and cancer. There was no imbalance in favor of AIDS. But there was funding equity within a decade of the epidemic's onset. Internationally as well, spending on HIV has been comparable to that on other diseases. Only the international campaign to eradicate smallpox in the 1970s was funded on a similar scale.[143]

Positive discrimination, however, was only half the gay agenda. Avoiding negative discrimination was equally important, whether the exclusion of seropositives from benefits or the imposition of traditional public health strategies. For obvious reasons, gays favored a voluntarist, consensual approach, not subjecting AIDS to the measures commonplace for earlier epidemics. That much needs no elaboration. And yet there were ambiguities.

One concerned how gays related to the medical establishment. It had been a victory when homosexuality was no longer treated as an illness, as occurred in 1973 in the United States and during the 1980s in France and elsewhere. Ironically, AIDS now gave doctors a role again in dealing with homosexuality, but this time a welcome one.[144] Gays had a stake in the medicalization of AIDS—that is, in its treatment not as an outcome of lifestyle choices and personal habits for which the individual was responsible but as the result of morally indifferent encounters with malevolent microorganisms.[145] Attempts had long been made to treat diseases as ethically neutral. In the late eighteenth century, Johann Valentin Müller had argued that if God punished humans via syphilis He was an inconsistent disciplinarian, since it could be caught innocently and He neglected the worse sins of masturbation and sodomy. The concern of nineteenth-century reformers with syphilis insontium (syphilis caught by means other than illicit intercourse—including, for example, the irreproachable banker who acquired a syphilitic sore on his lip from having counted with a moistened finger the wages of sin that a prostitute had hidden in her genitals) was an attempt to lessen the moral freight of the disease.[146] The focus of the bacteriological revolution on the specific microbial causes of illness, rather than on allegedly noxious habits, promised to free patients from stigma. Escaping the stain of personal responsibility for AIDS meant continuing this tradition of seeing illness as a medical and biological phenomenon with few, if any, moral or ethical overtones. It followed that this meant entrusting matters to the medical establishment.

Another ambiguity concerned the alternatives to traditional contain-and-control tactics. The voluntaristic, consensual approach to public health focused on information, counseling, and behavioral change. But there was the rub. What did altering their conduct mean for gays? Gays resisted, of course, reimposing old-fashioned sodomy laws and other legal restrictions on homosexuality. Beyond this, behavioral change meant abandoning the practices that, in the 1960s and 1970s, gays had crafted as their own approach to sexuality. Gay sex, many argued, was distinct from straight sex not just in the object of its desire but also in the nature, variety, intensity, and frequency of its expression. If reducing risk implied abstinence and monogamy or foreswearing the wilder practices, it meant curtailing gay sex. If gay sex transgressed straight norms, then safe sex was no sex.[147] And if gay behavior aimed to undermine inherited concepts of sexuality and pleasure altogether—as Foucault and Hocquenghem argued—then safe sex was the erotic equivalent of the German Socialists buying railway platform tickets when sending their leaders off to fight for the revolution. Others, however, held that the contemporary expression of gay (male) sex, in its multiplicity and promiscuity, was only one resolution of such matters. It was the creation of certain historical circumstances, a particular venereal ideology, and therefore, was as subject to change as anything else.

The question of behavioral change was thus part of larger debates on the nature of gay sex and homosexual identity. Among the issues was promiscuity. Was this the core of gay sexual practice, the "righteous form of revolution" that made gays sexual outlaws, in the words of the writer John Rechy?[148] Or was it self-destructive—however pleasurable—behavior that should be changed in the face of the epidemic? This opened the question of anal sex. Even before the nature of HIV was understood, anal penetration had been identified as an epidemiologically risky practice. Was anal sex the obvious goal of gay couplings? Anal sodomy (along with role switching) was often portrayed as the crucial element of gay sex. It allowed homosexual men to experience true mutuality, each partner both penetrating and being penetrated, in a way that was ruled out for both straight and lesbian couples. It undermined classic gendered stereotypes of the active and passive roles in intercourse.[149] Others argued, in contrast, that anal intercourse was but an inverted homage paid by gays to the primacy of penetration in straight sex, and that it was thus indicative of their inability to imagine new forms of lovemaking. A practice that became popular among gays during the homosexual revolution of the postwar period was now revealed as among the riskiest of acts. It was part of a tricky intersection of conflicting tendencies. Many foreswore anal penetration altogether. Those who did not, especially if they dallied without condoms, had to accept the judgment of even their peers that they were taking excessive risks by indulging in immoderate and misplaced pleasure.[150]

What to do about bathhouses, back rooms, and saunas, where transmissive risks were legion, provoked major debates. Was anonymous, multiple, serial, and sometimes group sex an essential element of gay identity? Or was promiscuity a self-destructive conduct, avoided by sensible people confronting a lethal disease?[151] Supporters of closing argued that public health was the weightiest consideration. Since the baths were commercial establishments, the sex was public and under official purview. Those against closing claimed that this would alienate precisely those who needed to change their habits, would force risky behavior back into the closet and eliminate a key venue for promoting safe sex.[152] Beyond narrow public health rationales lay more transcendent concerns. When heterosexual brothels were defended—which was not often—it was as a necessary evil catering to the sexual needs of the erotically dispossessed: the handicapped, shy, deformed, and others who could not satisfy their needs on the open carnal market. Rarely, if ever, were they supported as good in their own right. The bathhouses, in contrast, were not just like brothels, a place where sex of the usual sort was consumed in unusual settings. They were the venue of sex without par in private, and they thus emblematized gaydom's rejection of received erotic values.[153] Shutting them was therefore more than a public health measure. It attacked the heart of gay identity, much as though marriage had been forbidden in order to fight venereal disease or as if *mikhvas* were closed—as one enterprising rabbi in Posen ordered during the 1832 cholera epidemic—to keep orthodox Jewish women impure after menstruation and thus incapable of relations with their husbands.[154]

Many American gays objected to attempts in San Francisco and New York to shut bathhouses, attacking the closers as "Nazi Fascists"—a pejorative redundancy if ever there was one.[155] Randy Shilts, author of the first popular history of the epidemic, *And the Band Played On*, was spat on by strangers in the Castro for arguing that gay sexual behavior was part of the problem. Larry Kramer caused controversy for criticizing gay sexual excess. Richard Berkowitz and Michael Callen's 1982 article "We Know Who We Are: Two Gay Men Declare War on Promiscuity" provoked an enormously vituperative response.[156] In Germany the filmmaker Rosa von Praunheim played a similar role as a homosexual Savonarola. In France, gay self-criticism was not readily forthcoming. When it did emerge, it was directed—like much cultural criticism in this increasingly insecure nation—outward, against the United States, as the claim that safe sex was but a puritanical American invention to undermine pleasure.[157]

Noted gay sexologists like Martin Dannecker argued that the separation between love and sex characteristic of the sexual revolution—straight and gay alike—had gone too far, and that gays had been ready, even before the epidemic made it a necessity, to link the two more closely. The Swedish government gave official imprimatur to this logic, that gay sex divorced carnal from emotional contact, in defending its closure of the bathhouses. In a closely argued book, Gabriel Rotello claimed that aspects of the homosexual lifestyle, its sexual ecology, left gays the primary victims of the epidemic.[158] Conversely, critics of the new chastity argued—predictably—that only self-hating gays critiqued promiscuity, psychologically identifying with the straight oppressor and accepting heterosexual ideals of monogamy, fidelity, and sexual parsimoniousness. Public sex and public health found themselves at loggerheads.[159] The French slogan was, Better to die of AIDS than boredom.

Bathhouses in the United States were ordered shut in Georgia, New York City, and elsewhere and were closely regulated before being shut in San Francisco, though they remained open (at least longer) in Los Angeles and smaller cities in the San Francisco Bay Area.[160] Though Sweden's gay organizations at first attempted to implement safe sex guidelines for conduct in bathhouses (bright lights, doorless contact rooms, plugged glory holes), the authorities rejected such stopgap measures. Almost alone in Europe—except for its usual ally Bavaria—Sweden shut establishments that allowed anonymous genital contact between visitors, whether gay or straight, and thus the bathhouses, in 1987.[161] During the winter of 1984–85, the police closed back rooms in Paris and the provinces, using the penal code's provisions against public debauch.[162] But otherwise French gays were largely left alone, as gays were in the Netherlands.

The question of safe sex, otherwise the gold standard of voluntary behavioral change, was also controversial. Safe sex meant, above all, using condoms during anal intercourse. Perhaps not the most enticing addition to sex play, it was widely considered a small price to pay for comparatively risk-free pleasure. Supporters argued that safe sex was a solution that sidestepped the need for more drastic behavioral changes, like limiting the number of partners: condoms, not chastity. By obliging each person to act as though he and everyone else were seropositive, other interventions or changes in conduct were unnecessary.[163] Others, taking a broader approach to gay sex, saw this as precisely the problem. The technical fix of latex allowed continuation of the behavior that had gotten gays into trouble in the first place. Condom use was not promoted by Dutch public health authorities, who sought instead to discourage anal sex altogether as an inherently risky practice. Safe sex was criticized, too, by those who rejected the primacy of penetration in gay lovemaking. Why, they asked, must ejaculation within the body of the lover be the goal? Why should other (nonpenetrative) techniques and practices be marginalized as mere foreplay and substitution?[164]

The bathhouses, promiscuity, and safe sex illustrated a larger issue at the heart of gay mobilization: liberation or legitimation. Was the goal to carve out a separate identity challenging the hetero status quo, or to assimilate on terms dictated by the majority culture?[165] Gay marriage posed the dilemma clearly. Besides the question of equal treatment before the law, gay marriage was a practical and technical issue involving inheritance, immigration, insurance coverage, rent control, hospital visiting rights, adoption, and other matters that became tragically salient as large numbers of gays began dying and discovered that they were unable to enforce their last wishes for their partners.[166] At another level, however, the question was less about property and other nuptial rights than about monogamy and fidelity. Would marriage for same-sex couples help gays be accepted as fellow citizens with the same rights and responsibilities as straights? Or was it a misguided attempt to impose the norms of bourgeois propriety on a group that defined itself by stepping outside mainstream society?[167] This debate, in turn, was an instance of the general problem of multiculturalism. Does multiculturalism mean assimilating increasingly homogenized groups, struggling fruitlessly to assert ever less important differences: the garlic in the sauce, the banda music on the radio dial, the faint whiff of folklore in an otherwise bland culture of English-speaking, Disneyland-going, secularized, public-schooled citizens? Or is multiculturalism a clash of divergent tribes whose customs and habits are actually different and often mutually repulsive? Is Kwanzaa just Christmas in a kente cloth? Is Hanukkah yuletide with a yarmulke? Is gay sex the same as straight, merely targeting a different orifice? Or is it something altogether different?

Such debates also raised issues about the nature of the gay community. Epidemiologically speaking, it was not, of course, a passion for disco music, drag shows, or button-fly Levis that put men at risk. Risky behaviors were pursued by more than just those who identified outwardly as gay. Though it might start with the gay community, spreading the message of behavioral change was a task that could not end there. Indeed, if closeted homosexuals consciously avoided being identified, precautions channeled only through gay organizations might be counterproductive. To broaden the reach to all men who had sex with other men, the most narrowly focused American gay groups were increasingly bypassed, as of the mid-1980s, in favor of assimilating activists from a variety of backgrounds into a broader AIDS service industry.[168] Elsewhere, AIDS organizations, though often based on a core of gay activists, included others as well.

If behavioral change—aligning gays to more mainstream sexual practices—was the quid for the quo of a nonpunitive public health strategy, was it worth the price? Implicitly, gays were being asked to rein in their animal spirits in return for a consensual preventive approach. Involving gays in policy making and behavior enforcement empowered them as partners in making such decisions—or it made them complicitous. Was the inclusion of gays in decision making even under conservative administrations a sign of newfound power or of cooptation? While the moralistic right fulminated about sodomy and other allegedly unnatural practices, the public health establishment, in the guise of enlightened liberality, also sought to discourage such practices or at least to belatex them. The old-fashioned approach would have sought to force gays to act in nonrisky ways. Modern consensual public health, in contrast, included gays voluntarily. At the moment of their incipient incorporation into mainstream society, gays were asked to make the choice that had been posed to all citizens with the start of democratic politics: be healthy or be a pariah. When the French revolutionaries made a healthy lifestyle a precondition of democratic citizenship, they were formulating the reciprocal relations of duties and rights. Universal conscription and health were the exchange for suffrage and citizenship. Sobriety, abstinence, and moderation: these were the watchwords of democratic citizenship, the leitmotifs of informal control that obviated the need for the external restraints of the predemocratic, absolutist polity. Excess, whether gustatory or sexual, became the ultimate sin. Were male gays now willing to adopt the straight (and lesbian) virtues of fidelity and sexual restraint? For many gays, epidemiological bad habits were also civil and personal liberties. For others, such change was worth the price of full membership in the larger community.

Such ambiguities help explain why the gay community's response to AIDS was not—from a public health point of view—as clear-sighted and rational as it might have been. In each nation, gays naturally regarded first attempts to contain the epidemic as an excuse to push them back into the closet. The dangers of the new threat were underestimated by many gays, as indeed by most others, and some gays saw no reason to act prudently to curb risky behavior.[169] Since gay identity was tied up with its sexual behavior, the attempt to change such conduct was not just cautious advice on avoiding risk but also a demand to alter the very nature of the homosexual.[170] Michel Foucault's existential wager embodied the dilemma: whether to surrender to the Dionysian rush of earthly pleasure or to postpone death by adopting the bourgeois virtues of prudence, risk-avoidance, and abstinence.[171] The very foundations of modern, self-abnegating, bourgeois life had been challenged by the homosexual revolution; it was not just gays getting their rocks off.

DEGAYING THE EPIDEMIC

The epidemic struck a particular group first, spreading from there. This meant that precautions, even if they initially concerned gays, would eventually have to be taken further. But what did "degaying" the epidemic mean?

From one vantage, it meant normalizing, heterosexualizing, and universalizing the epidemic, striking fear in the hearts of average citizens and thereby encouraging sympathy with an otherwise despised minority; ensuring more support for care, treatment, and research; lessening the threat that unpopular groups would be treated harshly; and allowing governments to sidestep embarrassingly specific stances on gay sexual practices. The button to push for more money, as one observer cynically put it, was labeled "Everyone is at risk."[172] In Britain, the public education campaign of 1986 deliberately sought to universalize the epidemic in hopes of heading off a backlash against high-risk groups. In Sweden, there was wide support for extending testing to include not only high-risk groups but also others, like pregnant women and military personnel, in hopes of dedramatizing it and lessening its stigma. This was the public health version of what has been called the Struwwelpeter effect, extending measures to all in order to dilute negative associations.[173]

But degaying was also seen as deflecting attention from the epidemic's primary victims, squandering resources on the worried well or on education campaigns that preached to the converted and least threatened.[174] In Britain, for example, little educational work was targeted at gays, though they made up 80 percent of reported AIDS cases.[175] In Sweden, where education campaigns hardly targeted high-risk groups, the massive voluntary testing program was taken up especially by social groups in least danger. In the United States, $100 million was spent trying to educate groups at very low risk.[176] The classic dilemma of universalizing social policy played itself out here too: building political support for measures through spreading them widely would undercut the effectiveness of targeting.[177]

Nor were the political implications and valences of degaying clear cut. Degaying the epidemic might increase the resources dedicated to it. But it could also focus hatred on gays, now seen as the "rats and fleas of the new plague" that threatened all.[178] In Britain, the backlash during the late 1980s against universalizing the epidemic's threat was launched by those who suspected that gays were seeking to continue accustomed behaviors. In France, the government declared AIDS a national cause in 1986 in response to the politicization of the epidemic by the extreme right wing.[179] Those who saw the disease as transmitted through ordinary contacts, and thus threatening all, could plausibly argue for strict precautions. Mainstreaming the epidemic also at times forged odd alliances, between a conservative, and often Christian, right and gay radicals.[180] To conservatives, universalizing the threat was a weighty moral cudgel with which to lambaste those responsible for the decline of modern society. The wages of sin afflicted not just the irremediably wicked but also average citizens and encouraged them to toe the line.

In the Western world, gays were thus the most important interest group concerned with the epidemic. In contrast to the ethnic minorities also ravaged by the epidemic, they could flex their political muscle. In Europe, ethnic minorities were fewer and immigrants were often suspended in citizenship limbo. Little was to be expected, and less was forthcoming, from this politically unorganized quarter. But even in the United States, where such inaction was not necessarily predictable, the disparity between gays and other groups was stark. For ethnic minorities, above all blacks and Hispanics, AIDS was not an issue around which to organize. It was only another hue in a full palette of misery. Moreover, the epidemic's homosexual overtones left the instincts—political, social, and sexual—of these groups in conflict. Blacks suffered from the image of hypersexuality that oppressors typically attach to subordinate groups. They were whiplashed between denial and celebration of traits, especially prowess and physical endowment, that—though earlier denigrated—were increasingly admired by an ever more eroticized culture. Mainstream black community leaders responded allergically to suggestions that their constituencies were especially afflicted by a venereal epidemic.

Blacks, and even more so Hispanics, felt ambivalent about the homosexuals in their midst. To some extent, both cultures shared the traditional approach to such matters; gayness fit into more broadly gendered roles based on male machismo and insertiveness and female passivity. Blacks and Hispanics who had been infected by sex with men were many times more likely to consider themselves heterosexual than were whites.[181] For mainstream homosexuals, blacks and Hispanics seemed even more antigay than whites.[182] Conversely, minority organizers noted that well-financed gay groups had apparently little interest in their constituency. Hopes of cross-group alliances on the basis of common epidemiological concerns proved unrealistic. A group of six hundred black fundamentalist ministers in Washington, D.C., for example, happily opposed attempts to outlaw underwriting in the insurance industry on the basis of seropositivity.[183]

Added to this was the neuralgenic issue of intravenous drug use, which especially afflicted minority communities. The connection between AIDS and drugs was fraught with potential misunderstanding. Needle exchanges sought to reduce harm to addicts and those in contact with them. At the same time, by allowing addicts to continue their habits, these programs could be seen as uncommitted to weaning addicts off their self-destructive habit. Such tacit acceptance of addiction was often portrayed by black and Hispanic leaders as exemplary of society's studied indifference to minorities. Most extremely, needle-exchange programs were regarded as a form of genocide, tolerating the death of minority addicts so long as they stayed harmlessly within their community. Even moderate minority leaders understandably regarded the authorities' sudden concern with drug addicts' problems as motivated by something other than fresh altruism.[184]

One hardly expected rational interest maximization, much less organizational skills, from drug addicts. Would needle exchanges have otherwise remained controversial?[185] Yet, to some extent, addicts—usually together with the professionals treating and counseling them—organized to pursue their own concerns. The earliest addict organizations were established in the Netherlands during the 1970s, in conjunction with substitution treatments. Germany and Australia also developed strong addicts' organizations, and less powerful ones existed in France. Even the United States had such organizations, as in Baltimore with its Street Voice, and New York, where the Association for Drug Abuse Prevention and Treatment was established by former users and sympathetic health professionals to educate about AIDS and provide a voice in policy discussions. The European Interest Group of Drug Users was set up, and even a worldwide federation, the International Drug Users Network, was formed in 1992.[186]

Hemophiliacs also organized, especially in response to the scandal of receiving tainted blood after it could have been tested. And yet, as with gays, there were ambiguities. Like gays, they sought to preserve a prized form of behavior in the face of mounting evidence of its toxicity. Hemophiliacs had to digest the crushing news that precisely the technique—the use of factors VIII and IX and other plasma concentrates—that had promised them freedom from the inconvenience of cryoprecipitates, not to mention whole blood transfusions, and thereby held out hopes of a quasi-normal life, was also that which increased their exposure to risk a thousandfold. Epidemiologically speaking, they were the most sanguinarily promiscuous of all risk groups. In 1982, American hemophiliac organizations rejected evidence from the CDC that the new disease was blood-borne in fear that this meant returning to earlier, primitive methods of treatment. In France and Germany, hemophiliacs' associations pressed for the broad use of concentrates as the modern treatment that victims of this disease deserved, precisely at the time that the first intimations of risk were heard. For political reasons, they were taking a stand that proved to be an epidemiological disaster.[187]

Hemophiliac organizations were also hobbled in their potential radicalism by close links to the medical establishment on which they depended, as well as by their fear of being classified together with other, socially less respectable groups of victims. The retardation of a consumer rights mentality in certain nations, like France, also influenced hemophiliacs, who felt unprepared to insist on beneficial changes. While hemophiliac organizations in the West pressed for collective litigation for transfusion damages, they did not serve as a vehicle for any broader mobilization around AIDS. In Japan, however, where hemophiliacs made up the bulk of victims, their organizations powerfully influenced the government response. In other countries, more radical groups eventually emerged, venting their anger at medical corporations and at the profession that had betrayed their interests.[188]

During the AIDS era, prostitutes were increasingly prompted to explore the possibilities of professional representation, both in nations where sex work was legal and regulated, as in the Netherlands and Germany, and where it was largely banned, as in America and Sweden. Prostitutes rejected the idea that they especially were carriers of the disease and that they should be particularly restricted. Clients who paid extra for unprotected sex, and the swingers who copulated right and left on an unmercenary basis, were vectors as much as they.[189] The epidemic served as the occasion to reiterate long-standing demands: to be left alone by the police and to be recognized as an ordinary profession, with rights to social insurance benefits (and obligations to pay taxes).

Women as such were also affected by the epidemic in ways that were potentially a basis for mobilization. They were often blamed for the epidemic as it came to be seen as a threat to all, and especially in those parts of the—largely—underdeveloped world where transmission was commonly heterosexual and where patriarchal mores still prevailed.[190] Females' oppression was a factor in their vulnerability to infection. Their poverty tempted them to trade erotic favors for financial gain.[191] Often they could not control their mates' sexual behavior or even deny them access if they feared becoming ill. Unless men could be forced to be faithful, women needed their partners to use condoms, however difficult it might be to require them. One goal, therefore, was new preventive techniques (female barrier devices or microbicidal vaginal products) that, unlike the condom, were under female control.[192] Contact tracing was also seen as a women's issue. Gays and addicts quickly

learned that they were high-risk groups. Women, endangered by their partners, were the last ignorant risk category, and therefore most likely to benefit from partner notification.[193] When infected, women suffered from severe
opportunistic gynecological infections. They were often excluded from experimental drug trials for fear of liability with respect to childbearing. Because research concentrated on AIDS in men, women's symptoms were long
ignored or downplayed. Social insurance benefits were even sometimes denied, since these were based on male symptomology.[194] Safe sex campaigns
aimed at women lacked the edge and erotic daring of those addressed to
gays—though it remains an open question whether this was the result of
their formulators' timidity and sexism, women's disinterest in sexual im-
agery, or fears of provoking a backlash from antiporn feminists and their
conservative allies.[195] And, of course, perinatal transmission, discussed in
chapter 4, tragically affected women.

9. Vox Populi Suprema Lex Est

Expertise, Authority, and Democracy

Public opinion influenced responses to the epidemic. Yet opinion's effect was in turn shaped by the nature of the state. How permeable to grassroots fears was it? How able to resist easy but vindictive solutions at the expense of vulnerable minorities?

Faced with past epidemics, the public had—not surprisingly—been fearful and anxious. It often clamored for the authorities to take decisive, even harsh, actions, and was willing to blame scapegoats: Jews during the plague of the Middle Ages; Germans in Philadelphia for yellow fever in the 1790s; the poor, Jesuits, and physicians for cholera in the 1830s; the Chinese for smallpox in Australia and California in the 1890s; Italians in America for polio in 1914; and prostitutes everywhere for syphilis.[1] In the AIDS era, foreigners, blacks, gays, Haitians, prostitutes, bisexuals, drug addicts, and other Others were blamed. That AIDS was initially of unknown provenance, and that it proved to be lethal, only made matters worse. The cruel association between the epidemic and groups at the bottom of the social totem pole helped fan the fires of prejudice and stigma. So did the connection between AIDS and behaviors commonly regarded as reprehensible and sometimes illegal: anal sodomy, prostitution, drug use. Hemophilia had long been a stigmatized disease. This new, unelective affinity did not lessen that. As one observer put it, many illnesses have transformed their victims into a stigmatized class, but AIDS was the first epidemic to single out already stigmatized groups to make them victims.[2]

Conspiracy theories offered their usual tempting and pat yet wholly unprovable answers. If the extreme right wing saw the epidemic as the outcome of gays' nasty habits or the general decadence of modern life, the lunatic left believed that the virus had been engineered in CIA or Pentagon labs for biological warfare, that the epidemic was a deliberate act of genocide against gays or Africans, that officials consciously spread it among prisoners to trim their costs, or that it had been invented by drug companies in search of new markets.[3] Republican Congressman William Dannemeyer claimed in 1985 that gays donated blood to contaminate the supply in protest that the crisis remained unsolved. Such far-fetched accusations were lent a grain of plausibility by threats of "blood terrorism" from at least one gay leader. The German terrorist group New Cancer Power sought to use HIV against prominent politicians.[4] God, too, figured in such explanations. Each nation had its religious fundamentalists convinced that AIDS was a divine sign that immoral behavior deserved punishment. Jerry Falwell and the Moral Majority in the United States, the Inner Mission in Denmark, the chief rabbi in Britain, the Catholic Church everywhere: all claimed that AIDS demonstrated the fundamental rot of the modern values of individual self-realization.[5]

Each country blamed its own scapegoats, much as syphilis had once been defined in national terms. In North America, AIDS was at first a disease of Haitians; in the Soviet Union, of the West and capitalism; in India, of Africans; in Japan, of all foreigners. The Swedes worried about the loose-living denizens of Copenhagen, that Nordic Sodom. In eastern Europe and Iceland, natives were warned against sex with foreigners. Norwegian women were cautioned against intercourse with Africans.[6] At least there was a poetic justice to such scapegoating: Americans, eagerly screening foreigners to exclude the epidemic, were in fact net exporters of HIV and were themselves regarded in much of the great abroad as dangerous vectors. American homosexuals were shunned in Europe's gay bars, American travelers to Saudi Arabia were screened, and public health officials in Rio worried about the dangers of carnival visitors from the United States.[7] For whatever it is worth, AIDS revealed humans to be equal opportunity bigots. It was not just whites fearing blacks, or the First World the Third. Westerners were stigmatized in Asia, Africans in India, Third Worlders in the Second World.[8] Africans and South Americans gave as well as they received. For every Western tale of Africans sodomizing green monkeys, there were speculations about whether Robert Gallo, codiscoverer of HIV, was gay and therefore eager to subjugate Africans, or accounts of perverse Westerners who spread the epidemic by paying local prostitutes to have sex with their AIDS-infected dogs.[9]

As in previous epidemics, the public first likened AIDS to the plague, transmittable by casual contacts and requiring draconian precautions. Surveys everywhere uncovered fear and distrust of the infected, and a willingness to impose harsh measures.[10] Lyndon LaRouche's ballot in California in

1986 showed that sizable numbers of voters (29 percent) favored strict controls of risk groups. Similar fears made themselves felt elsewhere in the United States.[11] In Germany, large majorities supported restrictions on risk groups, beefed-up immigration controls, punishment of transmissive behavior, and mandatory reporting.[12] In Britain in 1987, polls revealed broad backing for criminalizing homosexuality, sterilizing AIDS victims, screening unfaithful sex partners, quarantining seropositives, requiring seronegativity as a condition of admitting foreigners, and allowing the healthy to refuse to work with the infected.[13] In France, there was widespread acceptance of compulsory screening for risk groups, for those about to wed, and even for the population as a whole.[14] The Danish Progress Party sought to include AIDS in the old venereal disease law, with its promise of testing, internment, and the like. In Sweden, conservatives advocated a national registry of the infected, screening of all citizens, and a reemphasis on classical humanism, offsetting the free love, drug, and rock culture so pervasive in modern life.[15] The Ministry of Social Affairs was convinced that the public supported imposing drastic limitations on disease carriers.[16]

European observers, especially on the left, typically congratulated themselves on how balanced and unhysterical an approach their nations took compared to the excesses of American puritans.[17] In fact, extreme positions were much the same everywhere. Australian states like Queensland and New South Wales imposed stringent measures without compare except in Sweden, Bavaria, a few Canadian provinces, and certain American states.[18] Every nation had people who thought that seropositives should be tattooed and the infected quarantined.[19] (Indeed, surprisingly many Africans thought that AIDS victims should be killed to prevent transmission, as did a fundamentalist preacher in Reno in 1983, a politician from Houston two years later, and reportedly Representative William Dannemeyer from California.)[20] To her credit, Rita Süssmuth, the German minister of health, made the obvious point that, since Germany had earlier tattooed concentration camp inmates, such tactics were now impossible. In Finland, with one of the lowest incidence rates in the industrialized world, a professor of virology proposed detaining seropositives on a deserted island, once home to a leper colony. In Boston, a Harvard neurosurgeon proposed similar plans for an island in Buzzards Bay.[21] In Switzerland, outrage bubbled over in Parliament at the allegedly lascivious details of publicly funded safe sex propaganda, in this case aimed at leathermen.[22] In 1987, the Helms Amendment (overturned in 1992) prohibited funds for organizations that could be said to promote homosexuality or promiscuity. A year later in Britain, the Local Government Act followed suit, and a year after that, the Kent County Council bravely faced up to its responsibilities by banning a school performance of Benjamin Britten's opera *Death in Venice*.[23]

The most extreme opinions were arguably to be found in France. Racism against blacks and other foreigners and homophobia were mingled with deep-rooted anti-Semitism.[24] That Haitians, Africans, and—outside the United States—Americans should be seen as special threats is hardly surprising. That the Jews, who are apparently ever useful for a spot of scapegoating however implausible the connections, should also have been regarded as a danger is more startling. François Bachelot, physician and National Front deputy, argued that circumcision could transmit AIDS, that it was no coincidence that Kaposi's sarcoma was found especially among elderly Jews and AIDS victims, and that many in the Parisian Jewish community were seropositive.[25] The National Front articulated consistently outré opinions. It not only fomented a hatred of outsiders, especially Africans and Jews, but also advocated screening and restrictions on both risk groups and many average French: pregnant and married women, recipients of blood transfusions, health care workers, and military personnel with African experience. Perhaps unexpectedly, its venom was reserved more for foreigners than gays.[26] It was also in France that extreme opinions, suppressed elsewhere by political correctness or residual civility, were heard most unabashedly: that AIDS resulted from the sodomization by Africans of green monkeys, say, or that the epidemic at least promised a brisk eugenic spring cleaning.[27]

Examples of first reactions that, in retrospect, proved to have been exaggerated and sometimes hysterical were found everywhere: parents held their children out of school if they had ill classmates; medical personnel refused to treat the infected; police and firefighters donned protective clothing for routine encounters with suspected seropositives; mail carriers would not deliver to the ill. The Scandinavian airline SAS refused to fly an AIDS victim; Delta Airlines proposed excluding sufferers from flights; and Swedish boxers would not spar with their Kenyan colleagues. The head of an Edinburgh primary school issued gloves to his teaching staff to protect them from pupils.[28] Worries were rife that, with condoms flushed down the sewers, HIV might spread through the water system. In West Virginia, stories persisted of a vengeful seropositive infecting farm produce by licking and reshelving it. In Berlin, junkies were said to disinfect syringes by sticking them into lemons in the supermarket. Somewhere a hysteric advocated castrating risk groups.[29] Everywhere, the yellow media inflamed fears and phobias. Even serious journalism was not immune to the temptations of gay bashing. The intermittently respectable German news magazine *Der Spiegel*, for example, pruriently fixated on homosexual promiscuity.[30]

The average citizen, then, was ignorant of epidemiology, fearful of contagion, and repelled by the most common means of transmission. Those who favored harsh, restrictive policies were typically poor and uneducated. Usually those who took an enlightened, moderate, and voluntary approach were middle-class. Superannuated sociological stalking horses reappeared for an encore. European social science found itself wrestling with ancient demons as the petty bourgeoisie, that classic social base of Fascism, once more reared its ugly head. The so-called AIDS intolerants uncovered by surveys were surprisingly reminiscent of Seymour Martin Lipset's declining middle classes, the extremists of the center, who, according to a long-venerated but increasingly challenged theory, provided the sociological basis of Nazism.[31] They included socioeconomically challenged fractions of the middle class and elements of the blue-collar proletariat, those who lived in small communities, the less educated, and the old. These were the social categories who overestimated the dangers of AIDS, the possibilities of casual transmission, and the epidemic's effects on social and economic equilibrium, and who feared contact with immigrants and other foreigners. As a result, they tended to support coercive measures. On the other side of this Manichaean apportionment of blame were the libertarians, who tended to be highly educated single students and professionals, people who often knew victims personally and who rejected all preventive strategies other than information and education.[32] Even the venerable theory that there exists a specifically authoritarian personality—long out to pasture if not already at the glue factory—was resurrected in the finding that such people were more likely to discriminate against cancer and AIDS patients.[33]

Informed public health and medical attitudes provided the counterweight to popular opinion. True, certain radical advocates of victims saw the experts as being in cahoots with conservative forces, seeking to impose technocratic and restrictive solutions rather than respecting patients' rights and liberties.[34] Generally, however, those rallying in serried ranks behind a consensual, voluntary strategy were public health experts (who knew how difficult HIV was to transmit, how important it was to elicit cooperation from the most grievously afflicted groups, and how unsuccessful draconian strategies had proven in the past).[35]

If one distinguishes between medical opinion's trade unionist mentality and its more general inclinations, it tended to take a liberal approach, seeing itself as an antidote to the fears that gripped popular feeling early in the epidemic. There was, of course, medical opinion in favor of strict precautions.[36] Some of the most extreme proposals came from bona fide medical personnel: John Searle in Britain and the Finnish professor of virology and Harvard neurosurgeon mentioned above. But they were not typical. Since physicians could not yet offer much in the way of treatment, much less cure, this limited their desire to press for testing or more drastic strictures.[37] The ethos of professional confidentiality also inclined them in laissez-faire directions. Since the nineteenth century, when public health officials began recruiting them as information gatherers, physicians had been hamstrung between a concern to protect their patients and the responsibility to preserve the *salus populi*. Their instincts had generally been to resist official demands, such as that to report patients struck by contagious diseases.[38] Especially in France, where medical confidentiality remained dogma, but also in Britain, the reluctance to report seropositives to the authorities had less to do with liberal political instinct than with physicians' insistence on their traditional prerogatives. When home HIV tests were developed, resistance and bans followed in Europe.[39] The arguments advanced against home screening invoked concern for the well-being of those testing themselves (such tests could be inexpertly administered, and it would be irresponsible to allow a discovery of such import without counseling). But there was more than a touch of professional territoriality as the medical establishment snatched a diagnostic tool from the hands of consumers, who were presumed incapable of dealing with what they had, by their purchases, shown they wanted.[40]

On the other hand, physicians also had interests in measures that did not fit the liberal mold. In intimate bodily contact with their patients, they would naturally have preferred to know who was infected, however effective in theory were universal barrier precautions. But such preferences cut two ways. To the extent that physicians sought to test patients, patients could demand to know the serostatus of caregivers. A fine line had to be walked. The British Medical Association, for example, rejected applying traditional precautions to seropositives. But it would have liked patients undergoing surgery to inform physicians of their status. It argued for precautions against high-risk patients who rejected testing and were undergoing tricky procedures (placing them at the end of the operating list to allow for extra sterilization thereafter, and informing operating room staff of their refusal). The German Society for Internal Medicine sought to institute the most widespread and frequent testing possible.[41] This delicate epidemiological tango between medical caregivers and their patients, each wishing to know more than the other would reveal, is discussed in chapter 5.

POLITICIZING THE EPIDEMIC

Invariably, epidemics are more than just that. Though they are obviously medical events, they also resonate with unresolved political and social tensions. They reveal fault lines that might have remained covered, aggravate dormant problems, and expose otherwise accepted hypocrisies. This was especially true for the AIDS epidemic. And yet not every nation fought heated political battles over how to approach matters, and in those that did, the tenor and pitch of the confrontations varied. Disputes were intense in certain Australian and American states and German *Länder*. So, too, in France, during the second half of the 1980s, where the extreme right polarized the issue and managed to forge an otherwise improbable consensus among the moderate parties. In Scandinavia, as so often, consensus ruled, whether its outcome was a liberal approach, as in Denmark, or severe interventions, as in Sweden.

All nations suffered a basic tension between public opinion, especially in its initially fearful willingness to impose strict precautions, and public health and medical expertise, which resisted such visceral and immediate reactions. Who determined the response? The political and medical elites attempted to head off popular opinion, shifting decision making out of the public eye, out of Parliament, away from politicians, and into the offices and committees of an appointed, professional, and less accountable vanguard of policy makers. As a rule of thumb, the more that popular opinion made itself heard, the more likely drastic interventions were. A liberal approach was inversely proportional to democratic decision making. Of course, AIDS was far from the only issue where this was so: capital punishment, homosexuality, and abortion were others where liberal elites sought to ignore harsher public opinion.[42]

The AIDS debate was intensely politicized from the start. Those who called for drastic precautions confronted the defense of civil rights by recently mobilized sexual and ethnic minorities. No wonder experts and policy makers sought to shift the issue from the glare and heat of public dispute to the more temperate clime of bureaucracy. In some nations, AIDS policy was almost wholly removed from the parliamentary arena. Referenda, tapping directly into popular fears, were threatened in France (by the National Front) and put on the ballot in California (by Lyndon LaRouche): another reason for the forces of expertise to retire the issue from public.[43] Partly because public health was generally delegated to the proper authorities, who took decisions through administrative means (rather than as a matter of high politics and its legislative expression), and partly in hopes of shifting policy making out of the limelight, most legal instruments dealing with AIDS were not laws, debated in Parliament or Congress and open to political grandstanding, but decrees, ministerial orders, and circulars, issued by officials without consultation or input from elected representatives.[44]

Decisions on AIDS were shifted off the political stage especially in Britain and even more so in France and Switzerland.[45] In Britain, in order to avoid witch-hunts against gays and blacks, education campaigns aimed to convince average citizens that the issue concerned them too.[46] The traditional policy-making elite of moderately liberal mandarins, though challenged by Margaret Thatcher's populist conservative groundswell as of 1979, still managed to determine the response to the epidemic. Thatcher did influence some AIDS policies. She undermined a proposed national survey of sexual habits and so rendered health education campaigns cautiously inexplicit. But on the whole she preferred not to meddle in these matters. She left the special cabinet committee on AIDS to be chaired by others, allowing the Department of Health's more liberal tendencies the upper hand. Decisions were given to health policy bureaucrats, with little input from grassroots organizations—whether victims and their allies, or the fearful man on the Clapham omnibus. Policy making was insulated from populist forces. Though rabid opinions could be heard, they exerted little influence.[47] The relative lack of a hearing for gay organizations was paralleled by deafness to populist and conservative opinion.

In France, a coercive approach was taken up by, above all, the right-wing National Front. In June 1987, the party proposed establishing a register of AIDS patients and possibly seropositives. In some departments, supporters in local office encouraged this. In the National Assembly, Front deputies supported a unified plan against AIDS to screen risk groups, isolate the ill, and watch the borders.[48] For its pains, however, the Front managed to unite the parties of the moderate right, especially the neo-Gaullists, the Rassemblement pour la Republique, which might otherwise have been sympathetic to such ideas, with their opponents left of center to counter the extremists' hopes of whipping up support. Once policies like testing high-risk groups (which had been under consideration) were taken up by the Front, they were tainted by association.[49] Leon Schwarzenberg, minister of health in the new Socialist government as of July 1988, had the audacity to propose (without consultation) the mandatory screening of pregnant women and surgical patients. In return for advocating measures reminiscent of the National Front's, he was dismissed nine days later. Screening, the government decided later that year, would not be obligatory but only proposed to groups potentially at risk.[50] In June 1987, an act was passed that removed AIDS from the bailiwick of local authorities, into which the policies against STDs otherwise fell. Instead, the power to define AIDS policy was reserved for the central government, thus taking matters out of local fora—susceptible to public opinion, where the National Front had or might gain influence—and into the back rooms. As a result, in public AIDS was left to the less tender mercies of the press alone and rarely debated in the National Assembly (while in Germany and even Britain, parliamentary participation was marked).[51]

In Germany, a similar, though less pronounced effect was achieved by the Bavarians' insistence on their own *Sonderweg*. The Bundestag's Social Democrats, Christian Democrats, Liberals, and sometimes even Greens were thereby convinced to cooperate on a consensual approach. Fears were rife that right-wing populism might encourage a return to the Third Reich's penalizing public-health tactics.[52] The Bavarians were seen as having taken a clear and simple, but unrealistic and highly populist, approach to complex problems. Responsible action, a Social Democrat noted, had to resist the temptations of populist decisions based on public opinion surveys.[53]

In contrast, American politicians were suspended more awkwardly between the experts' insistence on a consensual approach and the grassroots clamor for decisive and not necessarily gentle action.[54] The debate over screening foreigners illustrates the point. In the early 1990s, it was proposed to eliminate seropositivity as a bar to entry of foreigners. In 1990–91, the CDC and Department of Health and Social Services agreed to remove HIV and all diseases other than infectious tuberculosis as reason to deny admission. During the public comment phase of the legislation, however, forty thousand protest letters flooded Washington, D.C., elicited by Republican Congressmen William Dannemeyer and Dana Rohrabacher with the aid of TV evangelists. Removing HIV, in turn, had been in part a response to demonstrations at the 1990 AIDS conference in San Francisco. When, after conservative counterprotest, HIV was retained and the comment period extended, gay activists managed to send more than one hundred thousand pieces of mail to the CDC.[55] Screening foreigners got the United States into more hot water with its allies than any other single matter. It led directly to the partial abstention by non-American participants from the San Francisco conference and the complete boycott of the planned meeting in Cambridge, Massachusetts, two years later (it met instead in

Amsterdam). The administration and the political elites would have preferred to avoid the issue, but it was forced on them by grassroots mobilization from both sides. Those who wished to allow entry to seropositive foreigners sought to shift the decision from the political process to public health authorities. Their opponents argued that public opinion favored such exclusion and should be respected.[56]

In a similar way, school officials openly took decisions about whether to keep infected children in school, pressured by meetings of anxious parents. "We wouldn't have dared to hide what we were doing from the parents. Imagine the firestorm if they had found out," one public school official in Chicago remarked of the public nature of admitting a seropositive child.[57] In Britain, by contrast, parents' worries were assuaged less confrontationally by officials sent out from London. In France, the Minister of Education admonished all school administrators to do what was necessary to protect infected pupils from discriminatory reactions.[58] Zoning and land use decisions, too, were more democratically malleable in the United States. A long tradition of popular control over municipal politics had left cities in the grip of Tammany Hall politics during the nineteenth century. Their European peers were governed sometimes through national control, sometimes by appointed authorities, but usually by institutions less subject to common passions. Ever since 1858—at the latest—when the residents of Staten Island invaded the local quarantine station, brought out the inmates, and burned the buildings, NIMBYism (not-in-my-back-yard) had been an American tradition.[59] During the AIDS epidemic, locals vehemently resisted siting housing and treatment facilities for the stricken nearby.[60] In Europe, such disputes were rarely voiced publicly.[61]

With little compare in Europe, public mobilizations on both sides of the issue helped exacerbate the erratic locomotion of the policy process in the United States. Like weathervanes, politicians swung with the strength and direction of the prevailing ideological winds. Grassroots mobilization was more prevalent here not just because the epidemic first hit America and remained an especially pressing problem but also because of the more open and permeable political system. Extreme opinions on both sides, from conservative moralists and gay activists alike, could leave their mark. And yet, in America too, the power of the professionals and even politicians over ideology was marked. The 1988 presidential commission on AIDS, widely perceived at first to be a patsy of the Reagan administration, in fact delivered a blistering critique of policy and advocated a mostly liberal line. Surgeon General Everett Koop, at first a supporter of the moralistic right, came during the epidemic to favor a consensual approach. More often than not, politicians managed to direct measures that pandered to extreme popular opinion into the byways and dead ends of committees.[62]

THE STATE AND ITS RESPONSE

The political institutions of each state also played a role. The actors and interest groups with a stake in different approaches were important. But equally crucial were the institutions through which these social forces worked. A large literature, which needs no rehearsal here, has arisen to assert the importance of analyzing governmental institutions to understand policy making, an approach often dubbed the New Institutionalism.[63] Because academic dialogue is inevitably fratricidal, such institutional accounts claim to offer an alternative to "social" explanations, which focus on the societal groups that stand to gain or lose from policies, and allegedly treat the state and its institutions as though a neutral and transparent medium through which such actors seek their goals.

There is no reason, however, to be backed into this false dichotomy. Were unitary, centralized states able to take action on AIDS quickly, while federalized, decentralized ones were less nimble? The former included Italy, Norway, and Austria, the latter, Switzerland, Denmark, and the United States. But what meaningful commonalities unite Norway and Italy while separating Denmark from its Scandinavian neighbor?[64] Do institutional differences between Bavaria and the rest of Germany explain their divergent approaches? If the British could not screen soldiers because their voluntary, professional armed forces were seen as analogous to private market employees who were also not tested, why could the Americans?[65] Clearly, there was no automatic institutional lockstep. And yet, for our purposes here, whatever the methodological dogfights, there need be no mutual contradiction. Self-evidently, social groups played a role in formulating the public health response of each nation. Equally obviously, they acted within given institutional frameworks. The nature of the respective states is part of any explanation for the varying responses. The subject is amorphous; the literature is often contradictory and allusive. It is, in short, one of the most difficult aspects of the story.

A distinction relevant here separates centralized from federal states. Among the nations under scrutiny, Sweden, France, and Britain tended toward centralization, the United States and Germany in the opposite direction. Whether this distinction, as was sometimes claimed, consistently influenced the timing of the response is doubtful. It would seem intuitively persuasive that centralized systems take initiatives earlier than federalized ones. Yet Sweden intervened when the epidemic was scarcely present at home. France, though facing a much greater threat, was a belated responder. Centralized Britain and federal Australia both reacted more quickly than the United States.[66]

When turning from timing to the nature of the response, however, such differences may have left more of a mark. The federalized and decentralized systems, while they perhaps took longer to act, often responded more effectively. Decisions rested with local authorities who sought solutions to pressing issues, while those at the center, at a remove, were often content with symbols and posturing.[67] The history of public health has many examples of locally empowered authorities acting more nimbly than those dependent on directives from distant centers. During the early modern plague epidemics, absolutist regimes often responded ineffectively for this reason. In the face of cholera in the early nineteenth century, fragmented and locally permeable systems, like those of Germany, were able to wheel their policy machinery around in response to changing circumstances with surprising alacrity.[68] So, too, in the AIDS era, the most effective and novel measures often evolved at the local level, only then percolating upward through the policy hierarchy.

Needle exchanges were a good example. They were often set up at local behest, independently and despite rules and directives emanating from the center: in Barcelona and Frankfurt, for example. The reorientation of drug policy on the Continent, emphasizing harm minimization on the Anglo-American model, was instituted largely by municipalities, which then coordinated their policies.[69] In the United States, the centralized war against drugs prevented Washington from favoring needle exchanges. Local initiatives were the rule here, at best tolerated by the higher authorities and often in defiance of them. Even in Britain, while the central authorities endorsed and issued guidelines for exchanges, initiative and implementation were strictly local matters.[70] The establishment of exchanges in Wales exemplified this percolation from below. Similarly, the serious local problem with intravenous drug use faced in Scotland helped liberalize British tactics.[71] Conversely, when the local council of the Alpes-Maritime province in France announced plans to register seropositives, a stop was issued at once by the minister of health. Divergence from the liberal Parisian line was immediately quashed: no local initiative, but also no local extremism.[72] California's creation in 1987 of its own version of the Food and Drug Administration, allowing local pharmaceutical companies to market AIDS drugs more quickly than did the overly cautious federal machinery, was another local initiative.[73]

The regional variations of federal systems limited the strictness of measures that could be imposed within a country. As the speed of a convoy is that of the slowest ship, the degree of public health intervention in a federal system is that of its most liberal entity. When Illinois introduced prenuptial HIV screening in 1988, the local marriage rate plummeted as residents tied the knot in neighboring states.[74] Similarly, once the Bavarians implemented strict precautions, locals began visiting other German states, in a form of HIV tourism, for testing and consultation without harsh consequences.[75] In contrast, the Swedes were subject to a uniform health care system. They could not avoid the requirement that, in transferring between physicians, their serostatus, or suspected status, be communicated in their files. The logic of legislative consistency over mutually permeable territories could also, however, dictate more, rather than less, stringent conclusions. Thus, the French insurance industry feared that, were it not allowed to screen applicants, it would be unable to find reinsurance—today a trans-national market—for its risks. Similarly, when Washington, D.C., sought to prevent insurance firms from excluding AIDS, the companies boycotted the local market and eventually won the right to underwrite as they saw fit.[76]

Federalist systems were better able to customize measures for different afflicted subgroups, while centralized states preferred a unified, universal approach. In the United States, Germany, and Australia, gays had more influence on decisions than in France, Sweden, and Britain.[77] The French case illustrates the point. Their centralized approach fit hand in glove with the reigning ideology of republican universalism, undermining pleas to pay special attention to the most afflicted groups or to include their representatives in policy making. The central state resisted ceding initiative to gay and AIDS organizations, while in other nations such intermediary groups were encouraged to assume important roles. The German principle of *Subsidiarität*, that tasks be devolved to the level of administration best able to deal with them, starkly contrasted with the French preference for keeping the reins in Parisian hands. In the United States, it was a leitmotif of congressional discussion that initiative was best left to local entities, which were more attuned to ground-level variations. Indeed, for some, the hope here was that local decision making would sidestep the conservatism of national policy.[78]

Matters were most fragmented in the United States. The constitution reserved for the states the responsibility for public health, and each had different regulations. Especially early in the epidemic, policy was formulated mainly at the state and local levels, not the federal.[79] The national entities, the Department of Health and Social Services and the Public Health Service, helped coordinate and finance efforts that were largely carried out locally. Whether to make AIDS reportable, for example, was a decision that could be taken only on the recommendation of the Conference of State and Territorial Epidemiologists. But once made, the states enforced the decision in fifty different ways.[80] The geographical variation of the epidemic's incidence combined at first with the federalized allocation of responsibility to discourage national action. Not until the 1990 CARE Act did Washington seriously begin shaping the states' approach—by tying resources to certain conditions.[81] The act, which by 1996 disbursed over $700 million annually, made its generosity contingent on states adopting certain policies, including notifying partners, criminalizing sex while infected, testing prisoners, and not using funds to provide needles.

The result was decisive action and uniform rules on certain matters, with delay, fragmentation, and a potpourri of different approaches on others. Relatively liberal stances—the lack of a uniform reporting requirement for seropositivity, for example—can be explained in part by the decentralized nature of the public health machinery.[82] Similarly, medical confidentiality (disregarding the relative unconcern for this in Anglo-American law) was less pronounced in the United States than elsewhere perhaps because it was federalized, varying by state. The central authorities in America took direct action only on turf they controlled. In the case of AIDS, that meant the military, foreign service, Job Corps, and immigration policy. Here they required measures, like screening applicants, that the courts and the CDC had rejected for private employers.[83] There was a parallel to the direct public health actions taken earlier by the federal authorities with respect to merchant seamen, military personnel, inhabitants of dependent territories, war veterans, and Native Americans—all of whom came, or could come, under Washington's direct authority. More generally, the federal authorities acted here as they had throughout the development of American public health policy. They bridged together those arenas where efforts on a larger-than-local scale were imperative: fighting yellow fever and imposing quarantines during the nineteenth century, combating venereal disease during the early part of the twentieth.[84]

The German system was, in certain respects, even more decentralized. One of the few measures taken at the national level was the *Labors-*

berichtverordnung, the anemic version of reporting. Initially, even that was intended to be a local initiative.[85] Policies on screening foreign applicants for residence permits were the remit of the federal states, which often enforced national laws in different ways. Matters like regulating prostitution were decided locally. Attempts to reform policies were frustrated by the national authorities' tendency to shrug off such issues as not their concern or province.[86] Many of the federal initiatives on AIDS, relatively well financed at first, were seed programs. Intended to elicit substitute funding from the states, which were responsible for public health, they died an inevitable death by the mid-1990s as money from Bonn and then Berlin dried up.[87]

In Sweden, in contrast, national legislation made measures the same throughout the country. Health care and insurance had been localized, but the government maintained central control and thus uniformity.[88] The French, in turn, switched horses in midepidemic. Though traditionally centralized, France had dispersed aspects of public health, including control of STDs, to the departmental authorities starting in 1984—part of a more general attempt to spread responsibilities away from Paris.[89] Classifying AIDS as an STD would have made it a departmental matter, subject to precautions like obligatory treatment, notification, and screening. It was precisely to avoid this, and the politicizing of the issue in southern regions where the National Front and other right-wing movements held sway (departments like the Bouches-du-Rhône), that the government took back the power to act against AIDS in 1987.[90]

Nonetheless, the contrasts should not be overdrawn. Measures in France and Sweden were largely uniform across the nation. Compared to this, the American response seemed at times directionless. With little central initiative, it was shot through by contradictory forces. Such fragmentation, however, was also found in Europe, especially the Mediterranean—in Italy, for example. In Germany, the Bavarian measures applied only to the happy land of laptops and lederhosen. Even in centralized nations, there were regional variations. In Britain, the Public Health (Infectious Diseases) Regulations of 1985 did not extend to Scotland, for example, because the authorities there already had powers covering infectious diseases.[91]

Differences in subsectors of the state apparatus also had an influence. Which branch of government took responsibility for the epidemic was important. Public health ministries tended to favor a liberal approach, while interior ministries, accountable for immigration and policing the borders, often took a harder line. In Bavaria, an old-fashioned approach was encouraged when AIDS was made a matter for the Interior Ministry, concerned with public order, rather than the Ministry of Social Affairs. Public health authorities often supported needle exchanges, while justice departments re-sisted policy liberalization that encroached on their drug-enforcement ter-ritory. In France, under the Gaullist administration, the health minister, Michèle Barzach, sought to encourage condom use and needle exchanges, while the minister of the interior, Charles Pasqua, attacked gay periodicals even though they usefully disseminated public health information.[92]

Variations in administration also had implications for preventive mea-sures. On the Continent, testing civil servants had different ramifications than in the United States. Screening applicants for such positions was a form of indirect compulsion. There was generally no requirement to be tested, but the job could not otherwise be yours. Despite some privatizations, the public sector on the Continent still remained an employer of a size and scope unknown in the Anglo-American world. This meant potential exclu-sion from a broad range of work—from teaching in the (all-but monopolis-tic) state system to punching tickets on the railroads. In the United States, the civil service was a more narrowly defined concept, and tests were given only to those, especially in the foreign service, subject to specific functional realities. A simple matter like tracking seropositives was quite different in nations with identification cards, and those, like Britain and America, with-out. The U.S. presidential commission's recommendation that changes of address of recalcitrant seropositives be recorded would have represented a major change here if carried out, while easily fitting into standard operating procedure on the Continent.[93] Locating any citizen, seropositive or not, was far more easily accomplished in Europe than the Anglo-Saxon realm. As one observer put it, so long as the same strictures were imposed throughout Germany, the danger of many citizens disappearing underground was not urgent.[94]

The varied role of courts, law, and litigation also helped shape the re-sponse. In the United States, and to a lesser extent in Germany, courts were active in formulating policy. In Britain, where Parliament reigned supreme, there were few judicial challenges to the wisdom of the legislator and no written constitution against which to judge measures.[95] In America, courts had long been important players in public health. By broad constitutional interpretation, they had created many of the national powers of public health that otherwise—given that the constitution was crafted for an era largely innocent of metropolitan problems and the need for national re-sponses to them—were left to the increasingly hapless individual states. With notorious exceptions (like *Bowers v. Hardwick*, where privacy protec-tions were not extended to homosexual sodomy), American courts gener-ally defended the rights of individuals during the epidemic. They upheld the claims of seropositive children to be educated with their cohorts, and those of the infected not to be detained without good cause or due process. They also helped overturn decisions excluding unpopular treatment centers or housing facilities from resistant neighborhoods. Courts countered populist pressure for quick, easy, and unfair solutions, as well as actively formulated policy. The construction of HIV infection as a disability, for example, was the work of the judiciary interpreting statutes written before AIDS.[96] In the United States and Germany, cases involving legal liability for transmission were hashed out both in courts and jurisprudential theory, nowhere with finer hairsplitting than among the Germans.[97]

The role of liability law also varied. Medical malpractice in America was dealt with largely through the courts, as the injured sued their doctors. In Europe, in contrast, self- or state regulation of the profession became the norm.[98] Compensation for harm tended here to be resolved through the social insurance system. Starting in the 1950s, American tort liability burgeoned, imposing through litigation a hidden tax on manufactured products to compensate victims and encourage safer design. Covertly, it accomplished what the welfare states of Europe did more explicitly, with their universal health care and disability pensions. The United States tended to rely on strict liability imposed on manufacturers, rather than accident insurance— on risk shifting, rather than risk spreading.[99]

On the other hand, as everyday liability exposure expanded and the insurance industry retreated, even the United States turned to government compensation for victims of injury. The swine flu episode in 1976 was followed a decade later by the National Childhood Vaccine Injury Act.[100] In Britain as well, the state did not compensate those harmed by medical procedures, leaving negligence to be regulated through the courts. Sweden, in contrast, following the example of New Zealand in 1975, had a system of no-fault insurance that compensated the injured with publicly funded payments, relieving physicians of liability.[101] The Anglo-American reliance on liability law, assessing financial responsibility for tainted products or broken promises, was thus partly caused by the spottiness not only of health coverage but also of maintenance for disability.[102] Continental nations guaranteed citizens medical treatment and subsistence coverage in case of sickness and inability to work. This rendered less necessary any recourse to liability and an assessment of fault, blame, and responsibility. In the United States such legal maneuverings were often the stricken's best hope of avoiding poverty. In Sweden claims for economic losses from faulty medical treatment were indemnified through social insurance, and liability law played a role only in compensating for bodily damage.[103] The German case, in contrast, came closer to the American one. Courts often ordered responsible entities (for example, the city of Hamburg as liable for municipal hospitals) to pay compensation for transfusions of infected blood.[104]

The divergence can be seen in the case of hemophiliacs infected by contaminated blood. Though the Swedish state compensated them earlier than other nations, restitution, it was charged, was modest compared to elsewhere. The authorities, in defense, argued that Swedes were provided for by the welfare net. What afflicted infected hemophiliacs—sickness, unemployment, disability, and so forth—was also covered in that way.[105] In some nations, above all France, the state directly negotiated compensation for the victims of transfusional transmission, though mostly the sums were paid both by the state and other involved organizations—insurance companies, pharmaceutical manufacturers, and blood collectors. Infected German hemophiliacs received compensation directly from the pharmaceutical industry.[106] In contrast, the United States long had no national compensation program. Civil litigation bore the brunt until a compensation act was adopted in 1998.[107]

Nonetheless, there were ambiguities. In both America and Germany, government commissions recommended lessening liability obstacles to developing and testing drugs. In California, the developers of HIV vaccine were offered legal protection against litigation.[108] American courts and legislatures, seeking to ensure supplies of blood, and therefore putting the community's interests above those of the damaged individual, restricted the ability of seropositive hemophiliacs and others to sue for infection via contaminated blood. They regarded blood as a service and not a product and, thereby, not subject to the laws of sale and warranty.[109] Most states enacted "blood shield statutes" to nail this fast in law. In contrast, German courts regarded blood as a product, allowing plaintiffs to pursue actions against suppliers under product liability laws.[110] In France, blood was considered an industrial, not a pharmaceutical, product. A 1992 lawsuit on the issue had to frame its arguments accordingly, in terms of damaged goods rather than harm caused.[111]

Legislative consistency also influenced responses. Nations that uniformly curtailed individuals' rights had logic on their side. The strict drunk driving policies of northern Europe, or seat belt laws, supported those who saw no principled difference between enforcing such measures and asking for broad screening for HIV.[112] A nation that prohibited brothels, like the United States, could more easily shut gay bathhouses. Those that did not had to face questions about sex preference equity. In Bavaria, brothels, sauna clubs, and other venues conducive to HIV transmission—gay or straight—could be closed.[113] Such measures at least were impartially heavy-handed. In a similar way, where harm minimization for drug addiction and needle exchanges were resisted, even the new threat of AIDS often did not change attitudes.

Moreover, there were symbiotic, and sometimes inconsistent, effects from various forms of legislation. Blood donation systems, for example, had implications for other aspects of public health policy. The British prided themselves on their voluntary system of blood collection, as they had since the days when Richard Titmuss, in an influential book, had told them that it embodied the civil solidarity of the nation.[114] The British authorities argued early in the epidemic that, with no financial incentive for donors to give, there was also no reason to legislate to deter high-risk groups from donating.[115] But if there were no mercenary motive behind giving, high-risk groups would presumably donate for the same altruistic reasons as all others, leaving the problem unresolved. A strictly voluntary system of donation did, however, lessen the need for laws of the sort passed in the United States (as well as Canada and Australia), making it a crime to give blood knowing that one was infected. Drug addicts often earned their keep selling blood to commercial operations, and a legislative stick to threaten them with was therefore useful.[116] Other examples of cross-influencing among policy areas included the vested interest that American states were given in nominative reporting of seropositivity after 1993, when the definition of AIDS used by the federal government to allocate monies was shifted from physical symptoms to include a positive HIV status and T cell counts below two hundred. The more such cases, the more federal resources to be spent.[117]

WELFARE STATES

Social policy systems also significantly determined the institutional parameters of the response. In all nations the regional specificity of the epidemic, striking urban gays and minorities, meant that central powers needed to redistribute resources geographically. In most nations, the epicenters demanded and received extra resources: Stockholm, Gothenburg and Malmö in Sweden, for example, and the Thames region in Britain.[118] In the United States, the CARE Act distributed monies according to incidence. But by using the gauge of the total number of victims since the epidemic's onset, many of whom had already perished, it skewed funds disproportionally to initially hard-hit areas, not emerging nodes of infection.[119]

Health care systems varied markedly. Europe had either national health care, as in Britain and Scandinavia, or largely mandatory insurance options, as in France and Germany. The United States, by contrast, had a fragmented system: patchwork statutory provision for the old, the poor, and veterans, and voluntary private arrangements for everyone else. This left uncovered a significant and growing fraction of the population, dependent on the last resort of public hospitals and charity.[120] The epidemic prompted calls for wide-ranging reform of the health insurance system, including ambitious visions of universal coverage.[121] Few were pursued. When the epidemic turned out to be less apocalyptic than initially feared, hopes of harnessing it to major change evaporated. The 1990 CARE Act dealt with the problems of the uninsured. It maintained private health insurance coverage for the poor, supported health care centers serving the homeless and migrants, and provided treatment for those not covered by Medicaid.[122]

America's fragmented health and disability insurance meant that solutions were ad hoc. The merely infected were sometimes classified as ill or disabled in order to qualify them for benefits, leading on occasion to definitions of the disease that differed from those in Europe—for reasons driven by the social insurance system rather than medical knowledge. When the CDC proposed to add low CD4 cell counts to its definition of AIDS in 1991, the Social Security Administration objected, since this more expansive diagnosis threatened it with a heavier case load and increased costs.[123] Because of the employment focus of health insurance, stopgap measures were required that were not specific to the epidemic, but that often gained particular urgency from it. As of 1985, the Consolidated Omnibus Budget Reconciliation Act (COBRA) obligated employers to offer departing employees continued health insurance. In the early 1990s, the CARE Act required Medicaid to pay COBRA continuation coverage premiums, thus making the statutory system support private insurance. Introducing employment-related coverage for same sex partners was characteristic of American debates, since job-related benefits were crucial and gay couples were otherwise excluded. The AIDS Drug Assistance Program of 1987 provided monies to states to pay for medicine for the poor. Many states also assisted the indigent without medical care, and the CARE Act helped public hospitals treat poor AIDS patients.[124]

Since many of the ill lost their jobs and thus private health coverage, burdens fell during the 1980s increasingly on Medicaid, the state-federal system of financing care for the indigent. Medicaid (and to a much lesser extent

Medicare for the disabled) in effect became the national health service for AIDS victims. Bereft of other coverage, even those who had been employed and covered by private health insurance spent down their resources to pass the means test.[125] This dysfunctional outcome reduced even further the few resources available to the already deprived. As private health insurance shunned high-risk groups, more of the ill turned to government programs or charity.[126] Insurance companies competed for the most lucrative pickings, while tax-financed systems of last resort were obliged to take up the cases rejected by the market. Eventually, laws limited the risks that insurance companies could exclude, thus forbidding, or at least regulating, discrimination. But a fifth of American employees worked for firms that, because they insured their employees themselves without using health insurance companies, were exempt from restrictions on risk discrimination.[127] In essence, the authorities had created the worst of all possible worlds—leaving the choicest candidates to the private market, while assuring the riskiest for themselves.

The balkanization of the American system led to stark examples of risk skimming and shunning. The prison systems, for example, had a vested interest in releasing AIDS victims early. Ill prisoners were cared for by the Public Health Service. Ineligible for Medicaid or Social Security disability, their numbers mushroomed as a massive increase in incarceration coincided with the epidemic.[128] Such problems were largely avoided in the European systems, where prisoners were treated like other citizens. In France, prisons contracted with hospitals to pay for care, and inmates received the same health benefits as free people.[129] More generally, such issues of selection against the fund were much less troublesome in Europe. In national health systems, private insurance provided mainly special services, incidental to the basic question of treating all AIDS victims.[130] Even when private and public systems competed, as in Germany, the terms of the battle were heavily regulated and costs and benefits were largely comparable in each. Thus, if the private companies too selectively winnowed members, they risked driving potential customers to the statutory plans.[131]

But even in Europe, questions of access could be troublesome. Some countries, like Britain and Sweden, had national health care systems, willing to treat all who were physically present. Determining access was here left to the immigration and border control authorities.[132] In countries with compulsory insurance, with their premium payment and membership requirements (Germany and France, for example), some groups fell through the mesh. Prostitutes were often not insured, at least not in that capacity. A third of French drug addicts were bereft of claims to health insurance. Illegal aliens and various immigrants were often not included.[133] In the United States, where entitlement to all but emergency care at public hospitals was contingent on membership in one group or another, admitting infected foreigners was thought to impose costs on taxpayers, through their eventual eligibility for Medicaid.[134] Such eligibility, in turn, also raised issues of basic equity in a nation where a tenth of citizens were not covered. As one congressman—himself an immigrant—put it, how could one justify paying for the treatment of aliens when coverage was not guaranteed to all citizens?[135] The issue of caring for stricken foreigners, however limited by the general immigration provisos against those likely to become public charges, was aggravated by its coincidence with the Clinton administration's attempt to reform health insurance, which called attention to the many who remained uncovered.

In a more general sense, too, the nature of the respective welfare states influenced national divergences in response. The basic rule of thumb for the interaction between social and AIDS policy was, the more generous the benefits promised, the more those who paid the costs—the state or others (like employers)—claimed the right to minimize risk by investigating potential recipients. The state's generosity and its right to intervene went hand in hand, much as sterilization policies had been motivated in interwar Sweden with the argument that munificent maternity and child benefits gave the community a say in its citizens' reproductive habits.[136] This meant, as mentioned earlier, that European employers had greater rights than their American peers to ask questions and to exclude potential benefit recipients. German civil servants' health was thoroughly investigated to ensure that they would not become disabled before retiring. Obese applicants, or those with high blood pressure, could, for example, be refused employment as university professors. Though there were dissenting opinions, and procedures varied by federal state, the common assumption was that seropositivity precluded employment as a civil servant.[137]

In Europe many social benefits were related to employment: vacation and sickness pay, maternity benefits, and of course job security. European employers had broad rights to test and scrutinize job applicants. In Denmark, job applicants had to inform employers of an AIDS diagnosis (though not seropositivity). Otherwise, they forfeited the right to sick pay and were liable to termination without the usual period of notification.[138] In Germany, employees' claim to pay when sick was contingent on not having caused their own incapacity. An employee who fell ill because of promiscuous unprotected sex might lose this right. Employees were obliged to inform employers of the circumstances of their sickness and to forfeit their medical confidentiality.[139]

The greater ability of American bosses to hire and fire at will, in contrast, meant that less was at stake in an employment relationship. Consequently, limiting employers' rights to investigate potential liabilities—as antidiscrimination legislation effectually did—mattered less, since they retained greater final authority on firing workers. In this sense, antidiscrimination legislation patched holes in American employment security that, in Europe, required less filling in the first place. Without such protection, seropositives in the United States would have been less able to work and, thus, to care for themselves. In the absence of other welfare provision, continued employment was a necessity. This, at least, was the concern voiced by the congressman from Los Angeles, Henry Waxman.[140] The same logic had prompted the extension of antidiscrimination legislation to the handicapped. Keeping the moderately disabled out of the job market not only undercut labor policy and drained the pool of taxable incomes but also meant that more money had to be spent caring for those who could, in fact, be gainfully at work.[141] In the United States, battles over benefits contingent on employment focused on health insurance, a matter that in Europe tended to be independent of job status. Employment-related screening was widespread and easier to accept in Europe since, even in the worst case, a seropositive was not, as in America, deprived of health care. Organizing health insurance through the job also meant employers were more likely to know about employees' illnesses. Protecting privacy was thus important in the United States in a manner not always true in Europe.[142]

In a broader sense, there were tradeoffs between generous social policies and public health regulations. The Swedes isolated recalcitrant seropositives, but they also paid these prisoners standard sick pay. In Germany, had the Contagious Disease Law ever been applied to AIDS victims, similar compensation would have been due.[143] Such trade-offs, however, threw up problems that did not plague American authorities. Did European prostitutes, with theoretically taxable earnings, who were not enrolled in the health insurance system, have a right to compensation when public health statutes prevented them from working?[144] Hopes of allocating scarce resources effectively meant that some social programs were made contingent on seronegativity, whether scholarships for African students in Germany or costly drug abstinence programs that seropositives were unlikely to live long enough to benefit from.[145] A similar logic informed French authorities' insistence on strict abstinence as the goal of drug policy, and their consequent reluctance to institute needle exchanges. In return for publicly financed treatment, addicts were expected to surrender their bodily autonomy.[146] In the United States, conversely, the authorities' inability to guarantee access to medical treatment undercut hopes of mandating interventions. How could one require testing of at-risk pregnant women or their infants if many of them were cut off from medical care?[147]

The tit-for-tat logic of social policy also implied that citizens covered at public expense owed the community a sacrifice of their privacy rights. The growing importance of third-party payers in health care meant that medical confidentiality was looser than in the nineteenth century. Then, physicians owed allegiance foremost to their patients, the source of their fees. Today, even millionaires are unwilling to face the vagaries of mortality without the risk averaging of insurance. At a minimum, confidentiality was breached in that third-party payers wanted to know what they were reimbursing for. Patients increasingly executed routine privacy waivers.[148] Beyond this residual level, however, there were differences across nations.

In national health systems, where all citizens were entitled to publicly financed care, confidentiality was most eroded. Swedish patients who refused their dentist's request for a HIV test had this noted in their file, for the information of future caregivers, and were treated as though infected.[149] Sometimes transparency was achieved inadvertently. In France as of 1986, AIDS was one of the few diseases fully reimbursed by the health insurance system. Those thus entitled presented a special mauve-colored social security card to the attending physician. Banks and employers, who often asked to see these cards, could easily guess the nature of the illness.[150] And yet there was no functionalist lockstep by which more generous social provision gave the authorities greater control over their subjects' lives. Other factors, like legal traditions and political ideology, also played a role. The Anglo-American nations were not as meticulously protective of confidentiality, despite less generous social insurance than, say, France, where confidentiality was jealously guarded as a citizen's prerogative against an overweening state.

When general social measures were sufficiently elaborate, particular protection of AIDS victims was obviated. In the United States, handicap discrimination laws were seamlessly extended to seropositives. In Germany and Sweden, special legislation guarding seropositives and AIDS patients against dismissal was regarded as needless, given that any employee could be fired only with justified cause.[151] German employers had both greater abilities to scrutinize the health of potential employees than their American colleagues and a harder time dismissing their workers. The same held in housing legislation. Little prevented landlords from discriminating against seropositive prospective tenants. But once installed, tenants were hard to remove for that reason alone.[152] Swedish employers, however, were allowed to refuse to employ seropositives. In turn, the social security system covered those who were not hired for such reasons.[153] Abrogation of a civil right was compensated for with provision of a social right.

Another issue was whether social benefits were to be provided by the state or voluntary self-help organizations. Voluntarism was a distinguishing feature of the response to the epidemic. But it, too, varied across nations. Partly, this was a response to the failure of statutory organizations to take the initiative. Partly, it was an adaptation, in collaboration with the state, to the novel aspects of the epidemic, especially the marginalization of its victims. Odd coalitions of political groups were brokered. Conservatives, interested in cutting back the state, agreed with gays who sought to devolve care responsibilities to their own communities. In America, where volunteering was prominent, the results were prodigious. In Europe, where more was expected of the state, less happened. Voluntary self-help was notable, however, in Britain, the Netherlands, and Germany, though much less prominent in France. Sometimes there were negative symbiotic effects, as in Hamburg, when gays' voluntary work allowed the authorities to rest on others' laurels and provided an excuse for inaction.[154] In all cases, the voluntary and statutory were closely intertwined.

10. Clio Intervenes

The Effect of the Past on Public Health

The nations under the glass here approached an epidemiologically similar problem in quite different ways, and did so for many different reasons. Yet the multiple causal roots of policy divergence must not obscure this book's central observation: national public health strategies adopted during the AIDS era were remarkably similar to those that had governed contagious disease for at least the last century. Like generals fighting the previous war, surgeons general and their counterparts wheeled out the inherited preventive artillery when faced with a new disease. Even the novelties introduced to account for the unusual characteristics of the AIDS epidemic could not obscure the fundamental continuity with past tactics. The one nation that set off in a significantly novel direction was non-Bavarian Germany. In all others, the tried and true held sway.

Sweden had been one of the most drastic interventionists during the cholera epidemics of the nineteenth century, imposing traditionally quarantinist measures—inspecting travelers, disinfecting goods, isolating the ill, and fumigating dwellings—well into the latter part of the era, and long after more lenient methods had been implemented in most other nations.[1] For syphilis, the Swedes had invented the widely imitated system of sanitary statism, which subjected all citizens to much the same restrictions as were elsewhere imposed only on prostitutes: medical inspection, compulsory treatment if ill, reporting of disease to the authorities and to sexual contacts, strictures on potentially transmissive behavior, and incarceration for recalcitrants. Into the AIDS era, Sweden remained among the harshest interveners, imposing much the same measures on the new epidemic's victims as it once had on those with syphilis. Its state elites were firmly convinced that, though Sweden's approach might be drastic, it was also effective and equitable in treating all citizens as equally dangerous and culpable. While other

227

nations had to develop a means of responding to AIDS, Swedish officials congratulated themselves on already having their procedures in place. With a venerable system for VD ready to go, it would have been ridiculous not to apply it to HIV.[2]

The British were different. Despite having a small state with a reputation for laissez-faire government, they were, in terms of public health, among the administratively best equipped of European polities. Although central control of public health had stumbled during the middle of the nineteenth century when the reach of the sanitary reformer Edwin Chadwick turned out to have exceeded his grasp, it was a recognized English principle by the end of the century.[3] With their administrative machinery in place, the British took a distinctive approach to public health. They were among the first to abandon quarantinist precautions against cholera, preferring instead a sanitationist improvement of the environment to lessen the disease's ability to take hold and spread. Though it was inaccurate, the sanitationist etiology—seeing contagious illness as caused in large measure by insalubrious surroundings—carried enormous influence. British cities, then the largest and densest in the West, were also the smelliest and filthiest. The ancient intuition that stench and illness were related was encouraged by a walk in a slum. These ideas of disease causation implied that public health should be pursued through public works—by providing sanitary infrastructure, and regulations to ensure decent housing, food, and so on. Such hopes of improving the lives of the poor, though admittedly far from revolutionary, still represented an attempt to deal with the social problem of the working classes by means of public health projects.[4]

In this way, the British took a broader and more socially reformist approach to public health than did Continental reformers. There, old-fashioned, quarantinist attempts to contain the spread of disease were pursued throughout the nineteenth century. For syphilis, the English abolished their quasi-regulationist system to institute venereal precautions based largely on education and behavioral change, buttressed by universal and free medical treatment. While the Continent either firmly stuck to regulating prostitution or followed the Swedish example of instituting similar precautions for all citizens, the British had their system of VD education and treatment in place by the First World War.[5] Their sanitationist and voluntarist bent continued into the AIDS epidemic. With the exception of a few laws with more tongue than teeth—threatening the isolation of recalcitrants, for example—and some initial restrictions at the borders, the English continued their largely consensual approach, outflanked perhaps only by the Dutch and the Danes. The British saw their laissez-faire tactics for AIDS as continuing the tradition (after repeal of the Contagious Disease Acts in 1886) of a voluntarist response to venereal disease. Lessons were consciously drawn from the past to cement support for a liberal, consensual strategy.[6] The STD clinic system, for example, proved useful during the AIDS epidemic to reach and help gays.[7] The British Medical Association, testifying before a parliamentary committee, invoked domestic traditions of VD control based not, as on the Continent, on compulsion, registration, and control of certain social groups but on voluntary treatment and education. This was the precedent to follow for AIDS.[8] Similarly, when the British debated whether to make AIDS notifiable, they concluded that earlier experience with STDs suggested that sufferers would thereby be driven into the epidemiological underground.[9] Even critical observers agreed that this voluntary strategy, pursued on the analogy of battles against VD a century earlier, was the right one, the result of a "rare flash of moral enlightenment."[10]

While having perfected the system of regulating prostitution, the French were notable during the nineteenth century for their inability to take firm measures, or chart a clear course, in public health. France straddled geoepidemiologically unstable territory. It perched on a fault line between two epidemiological worldviews: On the one hand were the Mediterranean nations, which feared the import of contagion from the Orient, Caribbean, and elsewhere and therefore accepted harsh quarantinist measures. On the other were the North Atlantic nations, typically struck by the classic epidemic diseases only once they had penetrated Europe and, hence, able to take a more lenient approach. As so often, the French were strong on theory, weak in practice. They had commanded the front line of public health prevention during the seventeenth and early eighteenth centuries and may have been forerunners in developing the principles of modern public health during the nineteenth.[11] But at the same time, they were tardy in putting their intellectual achievements to practical use. Cartesians, they focused on basic research and scientific certainty, rather than on the ambiguities and probabilities of public health.[12]

In contrast to Chadwick's insistence on strong action by the central state in Britain, however unsuccessful in the short run, the French sanitary reformer Louis-René Villermé feared the threat thereby posed to individual liberty and sought statutory intervention only piecemeal. His analysis of the poor health of the destitute concentrated on their individual failings, rather than the social problems they faced as a class.[13] The public health law of 1902 was a belated attempt to emulate the developments under way for well over a half century in Britain. Down to today, the machinery of French public health remains weak, fragmented, and unable to hold its own within the structure of government.[14] Such ambiguities persisted into the AIDS epidemic. Extremist political opinion demanded drastic action. The government, shying back from strict interventions, was happy to portray its indecisiveness as liberality.

The American approach to public health, in turn, was complicated. It is worth pursuing in some detail here because of the assumption prevalent in the AIDS literature that the United States' liberalist traditions and its laissez-faire attitudes to government were somehow directly reflected in its consensualist handling of the epidemic. As one observer put it, the voluntary approach to AIDS, based on education and behavioral change, was considered "compatible with our deepest values of civil liberties, privacy, and volunteerism."[15] But the opposite approach was equally reconcilable with long American traditions of public health control, and therein lies the contradiction. Indeed, the idea that the United States consistently pursued laissez-faire tactics in public health is largely an illusion. Though procedures were implemented more by local and state authorities than national ones—not surprising in so vast and geographically fragmented a polity—the American state was as eager to interpose its powers to assure the health of the community as most European ones. In the nineteenth century, interventions to assure the public's health were broad, compelling, compulsive, and sometimes even effective.[16] When it came to public health, the United States was one of the nations that intervened most drastically. Hermann Biggs of the New York City Department of Health described his strict attempts to fight tuberculosis among tenement immigrants in lower Manhattan by removing children and isolating the sick from uncooperative families: "The government of the United States is democratic, but the sanitary measures adopted are sometimes autocratic, and the functions performed by sanitary authorities paternal in character."[17] Biggs himself represented Progressive Era American reformers who believed in the power and responsibility of the state perhaps even more than their European colleagues did.[18]

Historically, the United States took a quarantinist approach to epidemic disease, and did so for a number of reasons. Immigrants, bringing with them diseases from the European and Asian Old Worlds, could be—and were—stopped, inspected, and controlled at nodal points of access. The national topography, with wide spaces separating densely settled regions, allowed a similar logic to hold true within the nation. The weak governmental machinery, with its federal fragmentation and relatively impotent central administration, meant that if anything were done to arrest the progress of disease it would have to be at the borders, points of ingress, and those other few spots where authority's powers of inspection, isolation, and quarantine could be brought to bear. When bacteriology became scientific orthodoxy in the last decades of the nineteenth century, it pushed public health even further in this direction. Bacteriology, with its attendant prophylactic shift away from sanitationist improvements toward the control of individually transmissive behavior, had major consequences for American preventive strategies.[19] Nowhere were the bacteriological revolution's implications for public health more fervently embraced than here. American physicians and public health authorities, especially from New York, learned their bacteriology in Berlin from the great biologist Robert Koch. They thus imbibed what has been described as a purer version of the doctrine, uncorrupted by the environmentalist approach—focusing as much on the soil as the seed—of Louis Pasteur and the Parisian school.[20]

Yet the United States had struck out in this direction already during the colonial era.[21] A nation of homesteaders, America was distant from other countries and lacked decent roads between its few towns, which were generally too small to sustain crowd diseases. This meant that illnesses like smallpox or measles, which were largely endemic in European cities—taking a high and steady toll—in American towns erupted only sporadically, but the more horrifyingly.[22] There was a certain logic and experience behind the colonists' intuition that their country was untainted by Old World corruptions and decay, whether political, moral, or epidemiological, and that it consequently had to be defended against outsiders.[23] The very geography of the colonies lent persuasiveness to a quarantinist response. Because roads were mere tracks—for ox carts at most—merchants and migrants sailed instead. No wonder that port quarantines seemed effective.[24] During the eighteenth century, towns commonly sealed themselves off from each other in hopes of being spared the ravages of disease—smallpox and especially yellow fever. In 1793–94, for example, New York cut off all intercourse with stricken Philadelphia, a citizens' committee establishing itself for this purpose when the authorities were judged insufficiently decisive.[25] In the South, yellow fever raged, and once it began, during the mid-1900s, to be understood as transmissible, an elaborate system of quarantines and disinfections was established. The South, in this sense, played a role within the United States much as the Mediterranean nations did in Europe.[26]

The style of the American administrative system also favored a quarantinist approach. The vast territory and decentralized nature of government stymied attempts to impose public health strictures anywhere other than at a few points of ingress. The statutory powers pertaining to external threats were greater than those to internal ones. Indeed, to the current day, the civil rights and due process restrictions that limit searches and seizures within the nation do not apply to measures imposed at the borders.[27] Public health was long hamstrung, too, by the constitutional division of powers between the national and state governments. Federal powers of public health, based on the constitutional reservation of authority to regulate commerce to the national government, were stronger with respect to foreign than to interstate commerce. Formulated for an eighteenth-century world of limited commercial intercourse and restricted means of assuring public health, police powers had been reserved for the states. But the need was becoming clear for broader and ultimately national legislation to deal with what were no longer just local problems; thus, sometimes extraordinary feats of constitutional legerdemain gave Washington authority to maintain the public's health as part of its power to regulate commerce or to tax.[28] Indeed, the fragmented, spotty, and consequently ineffective local public health systems eventually came, in the case of quarantine, for example, to fuel demands for a national structure of uniform and incorruptible procedures. This gave birth in 1879 to the National Board of Health, which administered national quarantine.[29] Similarly, the comparatively drastic syphilis control system (widespread premarital and prenatal testing, and occasional use of universal adult screening) was largely made necessary by the lack of a broadly inclusive national health care system and the wide disparities in education and medical treatment. The authorities were forced to screen and treat at the bottlenecks at their disposal (marriage, birth).[30]

Most obviously, the United States received vast numbers of immigrants in the nineteenth century. This explained its fixation on screening foreigners as possible vectors of disease.[31] All nations have dealt with the public health implications of acculturation: transforming peasants with the sanitary habits encouraged by wide open spaces and few modern conveniences into urban dwellers living in denser webs of interconnectedness—microbiological, olfactory, and otherwise. But not all have had to deal with the same problems to same extent in terms of immigrants. The fears, phobias, and revulsions that in western Europe attached themselves to the lower classes of big cities—the huddled slum dwellers and lumpenproletariat—that were, in other words, focused through the lens of class, in the United States were also diffracted through that of foreignness. Immigrants were the concern here. Obviously, they were elsewhere, too, but in smaller numbers: the Irish in Britain, Jews in the Austro-Hungarian Empire and Poland, Slavs in Germany, and later on, North Africans in France.

To this, of course, was added the factor of race within the United States.

The variations in morbidity between blacks and whites, especially for diseases like syphilis and tuberculosis, were often attributed to racial and genetic differences. Sometimes environmental and socioeconomic factors were mentioned, but only too often as the noxious traits that Southern and rural blacks brought with them as they migrated to Northern cities—a continued belief in folk remedies, a distrust of orthodox medicine, and an alleged inability to control sexual urges. The Chinese, Japanese, and other Asians were at first regarded as carriers of disease and only slowly became model citizens in the hygienic sense, as in every other one.[32]

The epidemiological targeting of immigrants started at least as early as the nineteenth century. During the 1840s, Lemuel Shattuck's reports to the Boston City Council highlighted how the dangerously unsanitary habits of recent immigrants affected public health. Most immigrants were country folk with customs hard to reconcile with the sanitary necessities of tenements.[33] In 1876 the federal government had been entrusted with sole authority over immigration. As of 1879 aliens could be excluded for health reasons. In 1891, the inspection of immigrants was instituted to uncover those suffering from "a loathsome or dangerous contagious disease" (loaded terminology that was made more neutral only in 1961) or other infirmities that might make them public charges and thus ineligible for residence.[34] During the late nineteenth century and into the early part of the next, immigrants were inspected for cholera, plague, and other diseases. Ellis Island and its medical inspections became iconic in American history. Less well known were the even more drastic examinations—stripping, showering, disinfecting—imposed in the West and Southwest.[35] For intra-European travel, in contrast, similar inspections had largely been abandoned as impractical when applied to the random, Brownian motion of such peregrinations, though they more often remained in practice among the Mediterranean nations.

The bottlenecked nature of arrivals to America, however, allowed such inspections to continue. The most analogous actions taken in Europe were the disinfections, isolations, and sequestered travel arrangements imposed on eastern Europeans, in large measure Jews, making their way across the Continent, especially Germany, for passage from Hamburg and Bremen. The strictures imposed here were largely dictated by the American immigration authorities, who insisted, as of 1891, that the shipping lines make efforts at the ports of departure to reject diseased travelers.[36] The Americans sought to convince the Europeans to allow their representatives to inspect immigrant ships before departure for the New World, in essence overriding national sovereignty in the name of public health.[37] As the Americans saw it, insalubrious European immigrants were the same sort of epidemiological threat that the Europeans feared in Muslim pilgrims, journeying from all points on the compass to Mecca annually, dispersing afterward to carry disease back home.[38] Just as the French had established a system of sanitary surveillance in the Mideast in the 1860s to report back on outbreaks of contagious disease there, so too the Americans sought to train similar prophylactic cannons on the Europeans. Because of their special concern with immigration, consular officials were asked as of 1878 to provide weekly reports on local sanitary conditions. The following year, bills of health for each vessel sailing for American ports were required. Though the Americans failed at the International Sanitary Conference of 1881 to convince the Europeans to join them in a structure of international notification, they did gain cooperation for this bill-of-health system.[39] After the end of the First World War, such precautions were continued. To prevent import of typhus fever, the United States required delousing of passengers before they left Europe.

In Europe, the epidemiological Other tended to reside beyond the national boundaries, and the quarantinist impulse could be entrusted to the authorities at the frontiers. America lived with foreignness, both cultural and epidemiological. It interwove into the very warp of the social fabric, rather than just at its edges, the quarantinist attempts to shut both in and out. In 1900, when the plague appeared in San Francisco's Chinatown, the entire neighborhood was quarantined and roped off with a police guard.[40] When the quarantinist impulse did turn outward, it often served as an excuse to block access altogether. During the 1892 cholera epidemic, in the midst of a new wave of immigrants from southern and eastern Europe, including many Jews, nativists seized on the epidemiological excuse to shut down all immigration for several months.[41]

The unwillingness of American officials to rely on the hygienic habits of foreigners legitimized the state's strong powers to regulate public health. The Americans removed cases of contagious disease to the hospital in part because the tenements of the poor and recent immigrants made isolation at home impossible.[42] As early as the mid–nineteenth century, reformers like Lemuel Shattuck in Boston and John H. Griscom in New York advocated active state intervention to assure private cleanliness and public health. As they saw it, the immigrant poor could not be counted on to adopt habits of propriety on their own.[43] Such concerns also encouraged American public health to focus on controlling and channeling individual behaviors. Venerable traditions spoke for identifying the source of disease in individual conduct rather than social conditions. Mid-nineteenth-century American public health reformers did not share their British colleagues' belief that poverty determined disease and mortality. They saw this more as the result of negligent habits that misery could not excuse.[44] In a society undergoing enormous economic growth, with an unparalleled influx of foreigners, the deep cultural scars of slavery and racism, and an ideology of political democracy and social egalitarianism, an ethos of behavioral self-restraint developed to separate the respectable ins from the disreputable outs. Self-restraint, personal hygiene, and moderation became crucial to American social stratification. To teach immigrants to be clean, sober, and provident was to make them American.[45] But before the American ethos could be imparted to new arrivals, the nation had to defend its borders against the unwashed hordes.

Topographical, administrative, and immigration-related factors thus coalesced during the last years of the nineteenth century to favor border control—rather than internal measures of domestic sanitation, surveillance, and prophylaxis—as a major element of epidemic disease prevention. Edward O. Shakespeare, representing the United States at the 1894 International Sanitary Conference, laid out the choices faced by his country's administration. Four hundred thousand immigrants arrived annually, posing a problem of dimensions unknown to Europeans. These potential disease-carriers dispersed with particular rapidity thanks to America's well-developed railroads, its lack of internal barriers to mobility, and its intense domestic commerce. Many cities had only rudimentary hygienic organization, though some, like New York and Jersey City, were well equipped. Only very recently, during the early 1890s, had the federal authorities won powers to impose sanitary regulations at the borders of the nation and its states. Sanitary matters internal to each state still remained a local responsibility. Techniques possible in Britain, like house-to-house visitations, were thus largely ruled out in the United States. If precautions at the borders were eliminated, trade might thrive but the nation would succumb to cholera from Europe.[46] Just as the Mediterranean countries saw quarantinism and border controls as the poor nation's best prophylaxis—not requiring the administrative and financial muscle of domestic sanitation and internal disease surveillance—so too the United States, as opposed to Britain, rejected sanitation at home in favor of outward restrictions.

For such reasons, the United States was strictly quarantinist in its approach to cholera.[47] The Americans also took more drastic measures to control other transmissible diseases than did the British. The fear of immigrants and their unhygienic personal habits remained paramount. For diphtheria in the 1890s, New York City authorities insisted that children with sore throats, their families, and other contacts undergo throat cultures. They quarantined (by force if necessary) those who tested positive, and required two negative cultures twenty-four hours apart before release. By the early years of the following century, preschool immunization was compulsory. Baltimore and Providence instituted isolation of otherwise healthy diphtheria carriers. In contrast, the British did not take decisive action and suffered much higher incidence rates.[48] Diphtheria also served as the springboard for the first mass use of bacteriological screening in New York City in 1893. Hermann Biggs pointed out that testing to identify actual cases (half of those tested in the diphtheria hospital had not in fact had the disease) was cheaper than disinfecting and quarantining the homes of all suspected cases. Spearheaded in New York, bacteriological testing went on to become an important new tool in the arsenal of public health.[49] The Americans strictly isolated the contagiously ill, a Frenchman noted early in the twentieth century. Physicians reported cases at once by telephone, and patients could be isolated for up to five weeks. This observer concluded that such methods, though accepted in the New World, would be regarded as intolerable in France.[50]

Once Robert Koch had discovered the tubercle bacillus in 1882, tuberculosis became seen not just as a contagious disease but also as one that struck the poor and immigrants in particular.[51] Koch, whom contemporaries and historians often portray as incarnating the Prussian tradition of bacteriological public health, strictly intervening in the lives of individuals to safeguard the community, was astonished to discover that New York City, where tuberculosis sufferers were compulsorily reported to the authorities, had taken a harder line than Prussia.[52] Indeed, Koch wrote to Biggs in 1901 that, to persuade his fellow Prussians to make tuberculosis notifiable, he wished to cite the example of the Americans who, though freedom loving, nonetheless accepted such limitations on their liberties for a higher good.[53] Conversely, reporting of the tubercular was resisted in Britain, as leading to ostracization and concealment of disease. The Medical Office of Health of Birkenhead warned that Britons would not tolerate being overruled as were the people of New York (not a metropolis accustomed to playing the foil to liberty, a role more customarily assumed by Berlin).[54]

Americans combated smallpox with compulsory vaccination, a tactic that in Europe had often been resisted and overturned.[55] During the eighteenth century, many municipalities shunned travelers from infected places. As of 1850, the New York City health officer could order general vaccination of all passengers on ships arriving from infected ports. In 1824, New York City hired physicians to canvass Manhattan and vaccinate anyone not already protected.[56] In the 1890s, schoolchildren in Milwaukee were vaccinated, infected residences were placarded, and the ill were isolated in the city hospital. Though eventually overturned after riots, such measures were adopted largely because of established residents' fears of recent immigrants, above all Germans and Poles, who arrived without immunization and who resisted vaccination, undermining the municipal herd immunity.[57] During the nineteenth century, the National Board of Health maintained an elaborate system of interstate notification as immigrants moved from the East Coast to the Midwest. Sometimes border quarantines against Canada were imposed.[58] Indeed, up until the 1960s, some two hundred thousand border crossers from Mexico were vaccinated annually.

Syphilis and other venereal diseases, in turn, were a slightly peculiar problem. Like the British, the Americans did not regulate prostitution on the Continental model (excepting a brief period in Saint Louis, and continued legalization in parts of Nevada). Instead they outlawed it. Like Britain, American states provided educational campaigns and free medical treatment for victims of venereal diseases. In addition there were more drastic interventions: isolation or quarantine of patients, criminal liability for continued sex while infected, reporting of the disease (introduced in California as of 1911), and compulsory premarital and prenatal tests (used in many states as of the 1930s). As of 1943, Alabama required syphilis tests of all adults between fourteen and fifty.[59]

Nowhere, however, was the quarantinist impulse in American public health clearer than with yellow fever in the South. Starting in the 1870s, the disease gradually became understood as transmissible, and quarantinist techniques were applied. In 1879, when a case was reported in Memphis, orders were issued to inspect all trains leaving infected places, to cleanse and fumigate them, to transfer all passengers and baggage to new trains after five miles and all freight at a distance of fifty, and to heat all mail bags to 250 degrees. During an epidemic in 1888 in Jacksonville, other cities quarantined against that municipality and often each other. Suspected trains were not allowed to pass through uninfected places, much less discharge passengers. The Texas health officer detained and disinfected every person and train coming from east of the Mississippi. Health attests were demanded of travelers. Every house in Jacksonville was fumigated, all infected bedding and clothing was boiled, and other objects were bought and burned by the federal authorities. During the 1890s, railway passengers were forcibly taken to fever camps. In so-called "shotgun" quarantines, trains from infected areas were not allowed to stop in healthy ones. Federal regulations required detention of passengers and fumigation of freight on trains from infected zones headed to points in the South, defined in this case as below Maryland.[60] In 1888, detention camps were first established (between Georgia and Florida) where those traveling north were held for a period sufficient to show that they were not infected—a system, it was hoped, that would end the informal and spontaneous practice of shotgun quarantines. At the end of the Spanish-American War in 1899, with yellow fever threatening to return with the troops, massive feats of quarantinism were performed. More than thirty thousand soldiers were inspected, and some ten thousand detained at a quarantine station at one time. Eighteen thousand tons of baggage were disinfected.[61]

This thoroughly quarantinist impulse in American public health continued during the modern era. Well into the twentieth century, those afflicted with polio, diphtheria, meningitis, influenza, scarlet fever, measles, chicken pox, pneumonia, typhoid, dysentery, encephalitis, septic sore throat, and rubella were forbidden to travel between states. Those with tuberculosis, leprosy, syphilis, or gonorrhea could travel, but only with permission from the public health authorities for their departure and destination points and only if properly treated and isolated during the journey, including disinfection of their traveling quarters upon arrival. Indeed, lepers had to have permission from the surgeon general as well.[62] However superannuated such rules may be in practice, victims of communicable diseases are still in principle forbidden to travel between states without permission from the health officer at their destination. Those suffering from the classic contagious diseases are required to apply for a federal permit for interstate travel.[63]

When the Foreign Quarantine Service was transferred to the Centers for Disease Control in 1967, it was one of the oldest and most prestigious units of the Public Health Service. Its personnel and esprit de corps (including its uniforms, designed and often redesigned by a man in Washington whose full-time job this was) added much to the now-enhanced prowess of the institution in Atlanta. At this time, the Quarantine Service still fulfilled such structurally venerable, though technologically updated, functions as checking x rays and vaccination certificates of arriving ship passengers, passing through the aisles of airplanes inspecting passengers' eyes for signs of jaundice, administering close to two hundred thousand smallpox vaccinations annually to crossers at the Mexican border, and screening and treating Mexican migrant workers for syphilis. Indeed, so traditional did the approach to preventive activities at the border remain that in 1966, the Weir committee, set up to report on such matters, recommended opening the Mexican border, like the Canadian, by dryly noting that smallpox vaccination at the point of entry was too late to be effective. Its logic was much the same as had been pursued a century earlier. One could not both allow international traffic and throw up a palisade impenetrable to communicable disease. Quarantinist attempts at excluding illness disregarded the basic ecological facts of transmissible illness in the jet age.

The nation's foreign wars spurred a concern for imported illnesses—malaria during Korea, venereal diseases in Vietnam. The space program caused NASA to worry about exporting earth microorganisms into the solar system and bringing celestial organisms back. The lunar astronauts were quarantined for twenty-one days upon arrival back home.[64] As recently as the spring of 2000, a panel of leading public health experts from the National Academy of Science's Institute of Medicine recommended tuberculosis screenings of would-be immigrants from Mexico, the Philippines, Vietnam, and other high-incidence countries, not just to discover active tuberculosis but also to determine whether individuals were latent carriers. Victims were not to be denied entry but would hold special visas requiring them to undergo treatment before becoming permanent residents.[65] With the outbreak of the SARS epidemic in the spring of 2003, public health officials were granted powers to isolate suspected arrivals with symptoms, by force if necessary. A traveler from Asia was detained against his will in New York City in April 2003—the first nontubercular person to be quarantined, with one exception, in a quarter century.[66]

The quarantinist impulse was applied not only to foreigners but also to epidemiological outsiders—transients, the homeless, and other marginals—whose numbers swelled in the economic polarization of the century's last decades. Prompted not just by fears of immigrant Others but also by the localization of disease in such marginal groups, American policies against tuberculosis were notably harsh and interventionist. Most drastically, they entailed compulsory incarceration, a procedure that otherwise, in the antibiotic era, was regarded as long outmoded.[67] Directly Observed Therapy, the requirement that the ill take antibiotics in the authorities' presence to ensure a complete course of treatment and thus prevent the emergence of resistant tuberculosis strains, was increasingly imposed on transient and homeless patients. The informal assumption that you take your medicine as the doctor instructs no longer held, it appeared, with certain marginal groups. From 1993, as multi-drug-resistant tuberculosis spread among outcast social groups, noncompliant patients in New York could be detained throughout their treatment and not only, as earlier, for the first few weeks.[68]

Similarly, lepers were isolated in a national institution in Louisiana until well into the twentieth century, and outpatient treatment centers were late in being developed.[69]

Such quarantinist traditions help explain the course of American AIDS policy. Despite common misconceptions, the United States was in fact quite interventionist compared to other developed nations. The fragmented and intermittent public health powers of the national government meant that it took action where it could. It screened immigrants, some public servants, and the army for HIV, much as in the nineteenth century, when border quarantines had been one of the few weapons available in the federal preventive armory.[70] When Congress debated the policy of excluding seropositives from permanent residence—continued despite protests from abroad and at home—Congressman Tom Bliley of Virginia appealed to native traditions: "We have never before permitted immigration of those who were infected in the middle of an epidemic. We should not start now."[71] One might have expected that the legacy of immigration would have sown sympathy for the plight of infected applicants for residence. But instead, many Americans felt it was only fair to use the same rules for current immigrants that had been applied to their ancestors or, on occasion, to themselves.[72]

As with the other nations under the glass here, the American approach to communicable disease during the AIDS era thus continued traditions established—at the latest—during the first cholera epidemics a century and a half earlier. In fact, the only country that veered away from the dominant assumptions of the nineteenth century was Germany. Like the French during their formative experience of cholera in the 1830s, the Germans found that their geoepidemiological position made them straddle significant territorial differences.[73] The easternmost states applied strict quarantinist precautions at first. Those farther to the west were more sanitationist. Hamburg, culturally a Continental outpost of Anglophilic tendencies, was positively liberal.[74] The battle between Robert Koch and Max von Pettenkofer, the public health reformer, embodied the clash of bacteriology and sanitationism. It was made a matter of high politics during the founding years of the empire, as Berlin and Munich battled for supremacy. Despite Pettenkofer's and Rudolf Virchow's socially reformist strategies, the sanitationist approach remained weaker than in Britain. The dramatic bacteriological breakthroughs of the late nineteenth century—the discoveries of Koch, Paul Ehrlich, and others—fostered an individualized curative biomedicine.[75]

Later, public health was stigmatized by the Nazis. Their emphasis on eugenics undermined the field's democratic and reformist credentials, exposing its cruelly interventionist potential. Though the Germans were not alone in their passion for eugenics during the interwar years (Sweden and the United States also passed sterilization laws, for example), they alone pursued the most extreme consequences of racialism, the murder of millions.[76] The Nazis presented their extermination of the Jewish people as an act of public hygiene, similar—in Heinrich Himmler's analogy—to delousing. They managed thus to depict continuities from public health to genocide.[77]

The Nazi tainting of public health left the Germans in a different position than other developed nations during the AIDS era. The drastic subordination of individual liberties to the commonweal possible under the 1900 Contagious Disease Law was not reformed, however, until long after the end of the Second World War. The 1961 law on contagious disease contained little fundamental change. A standard legal textbook testified to the strength of this continuity by blithely noting that the immediate predecessor of the new law was the 1938 Verordnung zur Bekämpfung übertragbarer Krankheiten. This Nazi decree had expanded the list of diseases covered, regulated the details of reporting, unified measures throughout the country, and thus "proved its worth under increasingly difficult external conditions."[78] As a matter of statutory reform, 1945 did not ring in the "zero hour" of German public health. Rather, it was not until the AIDS epidemic provoked a new approach that change was put on the agenda. The decision, though passive, had wide-ranging implications: HIV was not subsumed in the strictures on other transmissible ailments.

The Bavarians and the Swedes relied on much the same prophylactic armamentarium of techniques. And yet their respective political contexts were starkly different. The Swedes remained confident in the rightness of their approach (as always, evil tongues might say), however much they were the odd man out in international comparison. What little criticism they attracted was softened by puzzlement. Why would a country lauded for its civil rights and humanitarianism choose the most drastically communal approach?

Only in the context of the broader Swedish debate of the 1990s, over the unpleasantly exclusionary and functionalistically Benthamite aspects of the Social Democratic welfare state, did this Swedish public health *Sonderweg* make sense.[79] Much of this debate, which is not restricted to Sweden, was exaggerated, and it dealt with sacrificing the well-being of minorities to the dictates of the majority, cementing a scientifically legitimated statutory intrusion into even the most intimate realms. Inspired by Foucault and his followers, debaters denounced much social policy as a form of social control, subordinating individual interests to technocratic social workers and their bureaucracy. Criticism was often anachronistic in its inability to imagine the benefits of the welfare state.[80] And yet there remains a point to be made here. The recent discovery that the Swedish Social Democrats carried out compulsory sterilizations on a scale rivaled only in the Third Reich has shaken beliefs in the exclusively benign nature of their welfare state.[81] In a similar way during the AIDS epidemic, seropositives in Sweden were subjected to one of the most draconian regimes of surveillance and control in the Western world. Few Swedes seem to have suffered twinges of guilt because of it, and the world at large hardly noticed.

The Bavarians, in contrast, were lambasted from all sides for having taken much the same approach as the Swedes. They, too, subjected HIV to the existing strictures of contagious disease control. But in the Bavarian case, the outside world was convinced that, at worst, some inherently evil trait in the German character was resurfacing, or more benignly, that this was what one could expect from conservative Catholics. The difference lay, of course, not in the actions taken but in the ideological context from which they emerged. What Swedish Social Democrats could get away with, German Christian Democratic Catholics took up at their peril. Ironically, the moral conservatism, with its condemnation of prostitution, drug use, and foreigners, that Swedes used to explain the Bavarian *Sonderweg* was the same factor that critical observers used to account for the equally anomalous course of events to the north.[82] It was precisely to avoid the opprobrium heaped on Bavaria that the rest of Germany instead favored one of the most consistently consensual and voluntarist approaches to the epidemic adopted anywhere.

Similarly, it was in the (vain) hope of avoiding pariah status that the Bavarians insisted that, in international comparison, their approach was quite unexceptional. While their opponents found the Bavarian position embarrassing, bringing unwelcome attention to Germany's dark side, the Bavarians and their allies claimed that their strategy in fact was not unusual: they were implementing existing and traditional public health techniques long used against other diseases and widely accepted by the populace at large. Other nations whose ruling parties could not be castigated as reactionary had put through analogous measures.[83] Social Democrats in Sweden had closed down gay saunas, they noted. The Austrian Social Democrats inspected prostitutes and forbade them to work if infected. The Italians, and indeed a host of other nations, had made AIDS a notifiable disease.[84] The Americans had moved away from merely information-based strategies and back toward traditional methods of epidemic disease control, and no one was stricter with foreigners.[85]

The past thus played a larger role than might have been realized by the public health authorities who faced the epidemic and took decisions in the trenches. Each nation reacted in surprisingly different ways to the illness. And each followed a style of prevention largely similar to that adopted during the nineteenth century against the classic contagious diseases. The one exception was non-Bavarian Germany, which carefully sought to avoid measures that resonated with the Nazi past. Such precautions, which were feared by the Germans as inherently tainted, were in fact rooted not in the interwar years but deeper in the nineteenth century. Moreover, they were put in force during the AIDS epidemic not only by the Bavarians but equally by the Swedes, the Austrians and, in some measure, by the Americans.

11. Liberty, Authority, and the State in the AIDS Era

In the age of globalization, HIV is among the most cosmopolitan of life-forms, at home the world over. Despite attempts by even the most isolated of polities to exclude it, it has wrought devastation with grim uniformity everywhere. And yet this ecumenical aggressor has been met and dealt with very differently across the world. Why?

To understand why different nations, even ones with similar cultures and political systems, have pursued various strategies against the epidemic, we need to appraise many factors: the balance of political forces within each nation, the importance attached to privacy, approaches to sexuality, the relative commitment to personal liberty, historical and political traditions, governmental and administrative structures, interactions with already existing legislation, and the value placed on voluntarism. Nevertheless, despite the importance of such contemporary factors, each nation tailored its preventive strategies largely to fit domestic traditions of public health. Basic decisions on dealing with contagious disease were taken, at the latest, during the nineteenth-century cholera epidemics, from the 1830s on. Some nations (the United States, Sweden, and to a lesser extent, France and Germany) adopted quarantinist measures, seeking to keep contagion out and, when it breached the frontiers, isolating and rendering harmless its victims. Others, above all Britain, aimed instead to sanitize the urban environment, giving disease no toehold and undercutting epidemics to avoid the need for quarantinist impositions. Such basic prophylactic stances strongly influenced the response to AIDS a century later.

The effect of past decisions indicates not only that the influence of history and tradition on contemporary public health is stronger than decision makers faced with a current crisis may realize. It also suggests that such choices were, and perhaps still are, made in response to the basic topographical, geographical, and demographic characteristics of each nation—a pro-phylactic deep structure—that has continued to affect public health even over centuries. To illustrate this point, let us survey the sources of the diversity in responses to the epidemic.

THE NATURE OF THE EPIDEMIC

In the age of scientific standardization and globalization, one would hardly expect much variation in the biomedical understanding of AIDS or significant repercussions from such differences. And yet, at the margins such influences were felt. A multidetermined etiology of AIDS—with not just contagion responsible for illness but also environmental, social, immunological, and more broadly health-related factors—might have undermined old-fashioned tactics, with their aim of neutralizing the seed of disease and its carriers. Correlations between national styles of etiology and the preventive strategies adopted were, however, haphazard at best. The Americans, followed by the French, took a primarily biomedical approach, throwing resources at finding a cure, rather than at the socioepidemiological management of the epidemic, which figured more prominently in Germany and Scandinavia. But this dichotomy did not align with the one commonly drawn in terms of treatment between the English-speaking world and the Continent. American and British physicians were believed to be more interested in the microbiological causes of disease, while French and German medical opinion, concerned with illness's terrain, paid more attention to the response of the attacked body, the patient's immune system.[1]

The AIDS denialists and their peculiarly pervasive influence also remain something of a conundrum. Do we add more than grist to trivial stereotypes by pointing out that many of them were residents—though not necessarily natives—of California? More telling is the observation that most were Americans and thus members of the polity that otherwise put its money on biomedicine. And yet what does it say that the denialists found their most receptive audience elsewhere, especially in Britain? Or that they were given a renewed lease on intellectual life by the sympathetic ear lent in Africa to their insistence on the epidemic's social causes?

Nor was the problem posed equivalently in each nation. Africa's heterosexual scourge presented issues different from those of the Mediterranean epidemic, with its focus on intravenous drug users. Within the developed world, the epidemics that struck mainly gays or drug users or hemophiliacs threw up different dilemmas. Drug-related epidemics could spread much more rapidly and suddenly than those driven by sexual behavior—a mercifully less efficient mode of dissemination. They often remained geographically localized, following the contours of the addict population. But their transmission was also more variegated, afflicting women and children and threatening easier access to the heterosexual population.[2] Gay-related epidemics, though inherently limited to one subgroup (except as bisexuals provided a bridge to the general population), spread differently depending on sexual interactions among homosexuals. They proliferated more rapidly where egalitarian sex roles and bathhouse promiscuity were common than where role differentiation and closeted behavior prevailed.

The nature of the epidemic affected the response. If it was seen as limited largely to certain risk groups, then it was logical to aim measures at them—both positively in making resources available and negatively in restricting liberties. In contrast, if seen as threatening all, then broad programs encouraging behavioral change among even average citizens made more sense.[3] Changing patterns of dissemination also had an effect. Traditional public health tactics were vigorously contested at first by gay organizations, which were willing and able to stand up for civil rights. Later, as the epidemic spread to poorer and ill-organized groups, such concerns weakened. As medicine grew better able to treat the disease, inherited techniques, above all testing and contact tracing, regained popularity. When the epidemic began to affect more women during the 1990s, new ethical and political issues arose: should the infected pregnant woman be counseled to abort; could newborns be tested without parental consent; should the HIV status of parents affect their guardianship of children?[4]

And yet, whatever the differences among national experiences of the epidemic, one conclusion is clear: in a simple functionalist sense, sheer numbers did not provoke a quicker or more thorough response. The French, with the highest infection rates in Europe, were slow to react. Germany and Britain, with lower incidences, moved earlier against the epidemic. The first legislative instruments were passed in 1983 by British Columbia, followed shortly by Sweden, Austria, and then California—only the latter of which could plausibly be described as hard-hit.[5] American states that took the most drastic approach often had little direct experience of the disease.[6] Among the fifty or so nations that restricted the access of infected foreigners, incidence rates spanned the gamut. The United States was the Western nation that most sought to prevent the ingress of HIV through testing and excluding foreigners. Yet it also had the highest incidence, and, if anything, it was a net exporter of infection.[7]

IS THERE A POLITICS OF PUBLIC HEALTH?

What, then, explains differences in approach to the epidemic? The most obvious tack is to examine the politics of prevention. Attempts to curtail contagious disease raise—in the guise of public health—the most enduring political dilemma: how to reconcile the individual's claim to autonomy and liberty with the community's concern with safety. When differences in preventive approaches were recognized by observers, they were often attributed to the influence of political variables. Yet what were the political valences of the policies adopted? At a rarified altitude, some differences are simple to explain. Restrictions on the liberties of infected citizens were easier to implement in countries not as beholden as the West to the ideology of civil rights: China, Iran, and Cuba.[8] And yet as we have seen, not just authoritarian governments were tempted by traditional public health solutions.

Conservative critics, who saw no reason why AIDS victims should be exempted from traditional measures, were right on one point. The distinction was not between authoritarian systems that required the ill to knuckle under to strict precautions, and liberal systems that treated all as fellow citizens. The choice was a more interesting one than merely whether to use precautions or not. Was AIDS to be subject to restrictions of the sort imposed against other diseases, and if not, why not?

The belief that AIDS had somehow overcome the classic dilemma of whether to impose communal strictures or observe individual rights was naive, though it was repeated like a mantra by public health professionals.[9] True, the disease's technical peculiarities—its long incubation period, its transmission primarily through irregular and stigmatized habits in sex and recreation—encouraged a virtuous circle where a consensual strategy was both politically palatable and epidemiologically appropriate. Nonetheless, many nations defied this would-be universal logic in order to take quite different approaches. Moreover, starting in the 1990s, all countries were encouraged by the development of treatments to employ traditional tactics once again.[10] Indeed, the very argument that HIV's specific nature encouraged liberal tactics implied that, had it been otherwise, traditional strictures would have remained in order. This suggests that the overall prophylactic fronts had not shifted.[11] The question was not whether to reform public health strategies in general but a smaller one: whether to make an exception for AIDS. Thus, with no end of ideology in public health, the question remains: What were the politics of prevention?

Conservatives were commonly seen as favoring harsh interventions against the infected, giving priority to protecting the community.[12] The governments of Reagan, Bush, Thatcher, and the Bavarian Christian Socialists were blamed both for responding inadequately—taking too little action too late—and for overreacting in a moralizing, punitive fashion against sexual and ethnic outsiders once the initiative was finally seized.[13] Clearly, at this level, politics played a role in the response. Neither Reagan, nor Thatcher, nor the German Christian Democrats were much concerned with the epidemic's initial victims.[14] The French Socialists, coming to power at the dawn of the epidemic in 1981, may have had a friendlier attitude to gays, but the National Front's polarization of AIDS also frightened off the left. At the same time, Social Democrats in Sweden and Austria presided over some of the most drastically interventionist measures in the developed world. Early in the epidemic, the United States and Britain were both governed by conservative parties. Yet they varied significantly in their approach. Indeed, it would be hard to spot common political denominators among the four states that, arguably, took the harshest line: liberalist America, swinging from a Republican to a Democratic president in midepidemic; Social Democratic Austria and Sweden (after the party's return to power in 1982 and except for the bourgeois interlude from 1991 to 1994) and Christian Socialist Bavaria.[15] Conversely, the most consistently consensual approach was taken in an equally polymorphous array of countries: Britain, shifting from Tory to Labour halfway through the epidemic; France under the peculiarities of left-right cohabitation as of the mid-1980s; and Holland, moving from government by a center-right coalition to the Social Democrats in 1989.

Nor did variations in approaches to AIDS correlate well with the usual ideological lineups. American liberals, happy to have the state intervene in other respects, nonetheless found HIV screening a violation of individual liberties. Conservatives, resistant to alleged infractions of civil rights like seat belt or motorcycle helmet laws, saw no contradiction in widespread mandatory testing.[16] Reagan uttered the word *AIDS* for the first time in September 1985 and not again until a speech in April 1987.[17] Thatcher said almost nothing about the epidemic in public and did not mention it in her memoirs. But Mitterrand, the (quasi-) socialist president of France, also had next to nothing to say about it in public. He used the word for the first time only in December 1993 and was duly attacked by the French ACT UP for his tardiness.[18]

That conservatives saw AIDS as an opportunity to argue for reintroducing conventional morality, thrown overboard by the sexual revolution, is true, but unsurprising. Predictably, the right lambasted the immorality and dissolution of modern society as the epidemic's ultimate cause. Such opinion could be heard not just in the United States, where Senator Jesse Helms and other troglodyte populists gave Europeans another chance to smirk at the simple ways of rural Americans. In Europe, above all in France, the skeletons of anti-Semitism and racism rattled in their closets once again. The left also played politics with the epidemic. The traditional left—in France especially—struck a pose of proletarian puritanism. Venereal disease was a symptom of bourgeois decadence. Leftists were able to believe simultaneously that AIDS was the product both of American biological warfare labs and American (here code for gay) sexual profligacy, and that the inadequacies of the American response were symptomatic of a hypercapitalist and puritan society.[19] The frequent French attacks on Anglo-Saxon puritanism and American moralizing (apparently the flip side of American gay hedonism) may also best be understood as elements of a persistent subterranean socioreligious dispute, the attempted revenge of the Catholic Mediterranean on the Protestant North.[20] Certainly, the truly weird, but possibly telling, comments of French Prime Minister Edith Cresson in 1991, during her brief and thoroughly undistinguished reign, on the alleged homosexual proclivities of Englishmen, standing in contrast to the healthy heterosexuality of the French, make whatever sense they possess in these terms.[21]

Elsewhere, leftist opinion also sought to use the epidemic to achieve a revitalization of society. Gays who criticized the promiscuity of homosexual lifestyles, seeking to normalize or heterosexualize their brethren, agreed implicitly with conservatives that gay hedonism was partly to blame.[22] Radicals from what nominally appeared to be the left rejected the pursuit of a biomedical solution. Since AIDS had social causes, or at least cofactors, the epidemic should not end without major changes in society.[23] The AIDS dissidents argued that a microbiological approach diverted efforts to needless precautions (testing, quarantining, and prosecuting transmissive behavior), when in fact the epidemic was caused by personal preference, lifestyle, and social circumstances.[24] They championed an environmental view that denied the need for harsh, contagionist, statutory interventions. Yet just as often their ideas reflected a moralizing approach to personal behavior that condemned gays and drug addicts for noxious habits. They berated Elizabeth Taylor for advising the young to use condoms and not to share needles rather than condemning outright drug use and sleeping around. They sought to saddle gays with their own problems and lambasted the moral neutrality of the view that HIV caused AIDS.[25] As the Berkeley microbiologist Peter Duesberg, the high priest of AIDS dissidents, charitably put it, the

HIV or germ theory lightened the onus on AIDS victims "who were relieved that a God-given, egalitarian virus rather than behavioral factors were to blame for their diseases."[26] Two lunatic fringes here agreed on the cause of the epidemic, whether calling it "the wild lifestyle characteristic of the gay liberation years," as did the denialists, or simply "sodomy," the word of choice for Senator Helms.[27]

Such unholy alliances could also be found between gays, who sought streamlined ways to bring new medicines quickly to the market, and conservatives who opposed on ideological grounds the entire regulatory process.[28] More generally, this curious coincidence of extreme right and left sprang from an agreement across the political divide that AIDS was a symbol of liberal bourgeois capitalist democracy, with its individualism and fixation on pleasures of the flesh. Much as the anti-Semitism of the nineteenth century and the anti-Americanism of the inter- and postwar eras were shared by both left and right in Europe as a formulation of their nostalgic antimodernisms, so too AIDS fit comfortably into this Manichaean teleology.[29]

Environmentalist and social approaches to health were defined from divergent stances. Disease was seen as an outcome of ecological imbalance, with critics attacking industrialization, technology, and capitalism. Or it was seen as the result of social mores, both individual and societal, with the enemy now the laxity, individualism, and hedonism of modern behavior.[30] The lifestyle hypothesis—that something about gay behavior explained the disease—was at first entertained by the CDC, perhaps precisely in reaction to criticism for its having pursued too single-mindedly a microbial explanation of Legionnaires' disease in the mid-1970s. Yet a focus on gays' conduct could all too easily encourage prejudices. The same held doubly for drug addicts. Had the disease first struck straights, one observer speculated, habit and custom would have figured less prominently in the working hypotheses of researchers.[31] Conversely, a biomedical approach was interpreted equally ambiguously. It was considered the position of medical mandarins, insistent on understanding transmissible disease through rigorous application of Koch's Postulates. As so often in the past, germ theory was thought of as reductionist and conservative. And yet biomedicine promised to free AIDS from the moral overtones of a concern with lifestyle.[32] Rather than resulting from practices commonly considered unsavory, illness was seen as the outcome of an unfortunate encounter with malevolent microbes—something that might happen to anyone and that afflicted certain groups for reasons that were neutrally epidemiological rather than condemnably ethical.

IS THERE, THEN, A POLITICAL CULTURE
OF PUBLIC HEALTH?

If politics in a narrow sense does not explain why different nations followed different prophylactic paths, then perhaps the broader political culture does. The line between individual rights and community prerogatives was drawn variously in different nations, though vague generalities are hard to avoid. The French entrusted significant powers to their centralized state, yet reacted allergically to many of its impositions. The Swedes were much more comfortable accepting broad and drastic interventions. The Americans were Janus-faced, tolerating strict measures in certain respects while protecting individual rights in others, and so forth. Did a particular political culture focus on the lives saved by traditional interventions or on the liberties violated, on the rights of patients or of the still uninfected? That Swedes regarded their state as fundamentally benign helps explain why drastic measures—unacceptable elsewhere—were adopted there, supported even by gays and others likely to be their primary objects.[33] Discussing the draft bill of the 1988 Contagious Disease Law, the Swedish Ministry of Social Affairs argued that it was not for the contagiously ill to decide how to live and behave themselves.[34] Could their German colleagues have gotten away with saying something similar? Would it even have occurred to their British peers?

The insistence of the French on the ideology of republican universalism (which they contrasted in caricature to the balkanized multicultural fragmentation of Anglo-American citizenship) focused attention on certain interventions—ones that affected all and were not aimed at high-risk groups.[35] The emphasis on medical confidentiality here hampered techniques in use elsewhere—especially reporting the infected. Instead, emphasis shifted to a form of self-reporting, which unrealistically expected the sick to do the physicians' work for them, or to the polite fiction that a sense of civic duty would encourage infected citizens voluntarily to warn their intimates or at least to avoid transmissive behavior.[36] The balance between state action and voluntarism differed starkly across polities and was much more tilted toward the latter in the Anglo-American realm than on the Continent.[37] Indeed, the very benchmark that observers applied slanted their conclusions. When the French and Germans remarked on the unprecedented activity of voluntary organizations in the epidemic, was it not in comparison with the modesty of such actions in other respects? When the British lamented the slight role accorded the Terence Higgins Trust and other voluntary agencies, was it not on the basis of grander assumptions?[38]

A telling example of the persistence of political culture even beneath vacillations of formal, institutionalized politics came from eastern Europe. The transformation of Communist regimes into democracies and quasi democracies during the 1990s had little effect on their public health strategies. These countries acted consistently across the rupture with Communism. Soviet measures imposed in 1987 required testing of certain foreigners and citizens, including drug addicts, prostitutes, gays, and the contacts of the ill or infected. Knowing exposure of others could result in jail. In 1990, and again in 1994, in what had in the meantime become Russia, precautions were passed that were as strict as earlier ones, or more so. Those suspected of infection were (no longer merely could be) screened and isolated if necessary, including now also vagrants, pregnant women, victims of other STDs, and medical personnel in contact with AIDS. On the other hand, the law also held out carrots: promises of confidentiality and free health care, guarantees against discrimination in employment, education, or housing.[39] Elsewhere in eastern Europe, too, measures remained similar despite the political sea change and were very strict: isolation of the infectious, firm instructions on behavior, criminalization of endangerment and transmission, reporting of seropositives, and screening of foreigners and a broad range of high-risk groups, including sexual contacts and (in Turkmenistan) promiscuous persons in general. The Poles and Bulgarians made treatment compulsory. The Czechs imposed the most detailed behavioral rules on seropositives, requiring them to report changes of residence and marital status; prohibiting their use of public facilities; restricting them to a single sexual partner, with a signed declaration of faithfulness to this person; obliging them to use condoms; outlawing sexually aggressive practices; and forbidding pregnancy.[40]

But political culture could change. Altered political circumstances—the experience of totalitarianism and the civil rights revolution of the postwar years—meant that measures once acceptable, indeed regarded as progressive, democratic, and egalitarian in the interwar period, came to be dismissed as intolerant, restrictive, and dangerous. Where the Scandinavian system in place against venereal disease had been seen as especially egalitarian because it treated all citizens alike, *hart aber gerecht*, the shift in political culture now left such measures to be reviled for their harshness rather than appreciated for their impartiality. The Scots, who had favored a much more compulsory approach to VD early in the century, now swung around to join the voluntarist consensus of the English.[41] Equality had become less important than liberty; individual rights took precedence over the community's needs. The hedonistic individualism of postwar political culture was given concrete legislative expression in public health.

The German prophylactic volte-face exemplified this sea change most dramatically. Though a preventive armamentarium of regulations allowing Swedish-style precautions was at their disposal, it was in fact never deployed outside of Bavaria. Instead, Germany adopted one of the most carefully voluntarist approaches—to the point where (in not making the disease reportable, for example) liberal had become simply lax. In Sweden, anonymous screening was illegal, and all seropositives had to be reported. In West Germany, the opposite extreme held true, with almost no epidemiologically useful reporting at all. After the Nazi experience, the Germans were suspicious of even the state's information-gathering function. Reporting seropositivity was rejected at the same time that public opinion also reacted allergically to plans for a national census. The continuities between the 1953 VD and the 1961 Contagious Disease Laws, on the one hand, and the earlier ones, of 1927 and 1900 respectively, indicated that the break in German public health history came neither after 1933 nor in 1945, but sometime in the 1980s. It was forced into conscious legal formulation at the latest during the AIDS era.

The Bavarians were, in this case, the odd state out, insisting on applying inherited precautions. The irony of such continuities was that, historically, Bavaria had been among the most prophylactically liberal of German states. During the cholera epidemics of the early 1830s, it had pioneered an environmentalist approach. Rather than isolating carriers, the Bavarians had deliberately shunned the strict quarantinism of the Prussians. Instead, they had sought to improve the circumstances of the poorest and most vulnerable. Later in the century, the renowned epidemiologist and reformer Max von Pettenkofer had spoken for a particular Bavarian preventive style that rejected the bacteriological approach of Robert Koch and the powers in Berlin. Instead, Pettenkofer had emphasized sanitationist ideals, however misguided his understanding of cholera etiology proved to be.[42] Now, however, it was Bavaria that upheld the traditionally Prussian approach, while the rest of Germany took a more liberal line—except, of course, those parts of Prussia that had in the meantime become East Germany. The Bavarians, their opponents sneered, sought to preserve the traditions of Prussian bureaucratic statism.[43]

This also put the Bavarians in curious company. Christian Socialists were not only in prophylactic cahoots with Swedish Social Democrats but also, before 1990, with East German Communists. In East Germany, where little need to atone for Fascism was felt, and where the state—now in its new, improved, and ideologically correct version—was still seen as benevolent and trustworthy, the old system was imposed without much soul searching.[44]

East Germany continued the imperial traditions, preserved—by the fiction that it embodied the anti-Fascist current in German history—from doubts that it was doing more than applying common horse sense and valuable experience to epidemics. The 1982 Contagious Disease Law in East Germany continued most aspects of the imperial law of 1900, invoking traditional measures without compunction.[45] AIDS patients were reportable by name, as for any other contagious disease—a precaution that, as observers blithely claimed, not only enjoyed popular approval but also benefited the infected themselves.[46] Victims had to follow physicians' behavioral prescriptions, always use condoms during intercourse, abstain from practices causing lesions, and warn sex partners and medical personnel of their condition. All partners from the previous five years were to be traced and invited for testing. A central registry of seropositives was compiled.[47] While West German political culture had changed, even though the legislative consequences for public health were not drawn until the AIDS era, Bavaria and the German Democratic Republic—Catholic and conservative in one case, secular and socialist in the other—pursued similar approaches to the point of explicit cooperation.[48]

Political culture and traditions thus helped determine public health strategies. Yet there was no simple correspondence between the two. Localities with similar political traditions and cultures adopted different approaches. Blinded seroprevalence studies (anonymous reporting of test results to track disease incidence) were accepted without fuss in the United States but were controversial in Britain, where they were rejected.[49] American states diverged significantly in their techniques—New York and California, for example.[50] Denmark and Sweden, though fellow Nordics, adopted quite different tactics—the former far more liberal.[51] The Teutonic troika—Germany, Switzerland, and Austria—followed different paths. The German government specifically rejected Austrian policies of making AIDS reportable and of medically examining prostitutes.[52] Indeed, within Germany there were stark federal variations. Conversely, much united the tactics of nations with quite different political cultures. Bavaria and Sweden were the epidemic's prophylactic odd couple, joined occasionally by Austria. They combined Social Democracy and Catholicism in a very mixed marriage. Sweden and the United States were also unexpected bedfellows in prevention—the two developed nations that perhaps most consistently imposed traditional measures.

Take the issue of reporting. In Britain and Germany, reporting AIDS or seropositivity was thought to discourage voluntary compliance, driving victims underground. This, of course, could be concluded only on the assumption that citizens distrusted the state and feared its preventive actions. Americans and Swedes appear to have thought differently. In the United States, reporting was widely accepted and instituted. In Colorado, which implemented an early and aggressive reporting program, levels of voluntary testing did not drop appreciably. A study by the CDC suggested that reporting by name would not affect people's willingness to be tested.[53] Similarly, the fear that voluntary testing would decline in Sweden as compulsory measures were implemented proved unfounded.[54] Sweden remained among the most highly tested nations anywhere.

AIDS prevention—indeed public health more generally—was not an issue where clear lines could be drawn from political theory to the practices accepted as palatable. The tilt of the balance between society's claims and individual rights was not a zero-sum distribution. Strong personal rights did not necessarily imply weak social interventions. A resilient sense of communal responsibility and solidarity sometimes permitted impositions on the individual that in weaker and more fragmented societies seemed intolerable. One of the leitmotifs of nineteenth-century debates over such matters had been Continental amazement at the willingness of the English, despite their concern for individual rights, to countenance drastic restrictions of civil liberties in favor of public health—whether isolation of the infectious or forced inspection of private dwellings.[55] Similar puzzlement continued into this epidemic. Why was it that Britain, committed under Thatcher to neoliberalism, nonetheless quickly and decisively intervened against AIDS? Why did nations with otherwise impeccable liberal political instincts, like the United Kingdom and United States, support testing?[56]

The ideological ambiguities of prevention often allowed extremes of left and right to meet. Conservatives and Social Democrats of a certain stripe agreed that the community took precedence over the individual. Both lamented an overemphasis on the rights of the infected and a neglect of society's interests.[57] Both thought that subjecting all to possibly harsh, but equal and effective, measures was the democratic approach. In the nineteenth century, quarantinist precautions were considered democratic because they affected all travelers, whether humble journeymen in third class or leisured tourists. Compulsory vaccination was seen as democratic because thus no one avoided contributing to herd immunity—not even the rich, otherwise able to pay fines for having defaulted on their epidemiological responsibilities. Reporting the names of all syphilitics, not just health insurance members, was democratic, because otherwise the wealthy with their private physicians escaped.[58] A consistent egalitarianism had been the philosophy underlying the Swedish approach to VD prophylaxis. All citizens—not just prostitutes—were subject to the same precautions.

This was now the tradition taken up by supporters of old-fashioned measures for AIDS. While the rich and clever would be protected even if matters were left to private and individual initiative, they claimed, it was the common person who suffered from the state's failure to take action.[59] Social Democrats had earlier been able to argue that—with death the ultimate violator of civil rights—the state should quell infection even at the cost of temporarily suspending individual liberties.[60] This was now the position of conservatives in many countries and of leftists in nations like Sweden, where traditions of subordinating the individual to the community had not yet lost out to postwar individualism. In defending the decision to deny anonymity to those who tested positive, a Swedish Social Democrat argued that the contrary position, taken by Liberals and Communists, would represent a victory for the interests of the individual. At stake, he thought, were the more important and justified concerns of the community.[61]

The individualization of modern public health also made ideological divides less clear. In the choice between individual rights and community prerogatives, which was the position of the left, which of the right? Take the issue of contributory negligence, the degree of culpability that victims of transmissive encounters should bear if they engaged in unprotected sex or shared needles. Was it the liberal position to argue that everyone was his own best quarantine officer, that the condom was the price for sexual pleasure, and that drastic measures were no longer necessary since security was each citizen's responsibility? Or was this a conservative individualization of risk, part of the breakdown of the communal solidarities prized in traditional leftist rhetoric? What, then, about situations where the infecting partner had failed to inform or lied outright about his situation? Was it liberal to argue that, even here, self-protection should be the norm? Or were there circumstances where trust (and therefore liability of the partner who violated it) could be expected?[62] Was a man having gay sex in a bathhouse in a different situation than the long-married faithful woman infected by her husband after his affair? Could the gay lover not expect his partner to divulge his serostatus, and should he therefore share responsibility for his infection if he failed to protect himself? Was it reactionary to prosecute both infecting persons for transmission? To prosecute the husband, but not the gay swinger? Was any attempt to distinguish the two situations an inherent privileging of heterosexual marriage while condemning all other relationships to erotic pariahdom? If a wife was not held to some standard of contributory negligence, would it imply she was paternalistically regarded as a helpless victim? Or would this view of her be a vindication of the trust implicit in the marriage vow?

THE POLITICS OF THE TECHNICAL FIX

Just as individuals differ in their tolerance of risk, so too cultures approach uncertainty differently. Americans are often thought to inhabit a laissez-faire culture of individual responsibility. In fact, they have defined as social risks—requiring statutory action—large swaths of behavior that in other, allegedly more tightly supervised polities like France or Germany, are regarded as individual dangers for which each person assumes responsibility. Sweden and the United States, perhaps surprisingly, are closer in such respects. Nations have quite different ideological neuralgic points. Drugs and medicines are more closely tested before marketing in America than Europe and more strictly regulated in their advertising thereafter. Seat belt laws are enforced with wide variations in stringency—laxly in America and southern Europe, much more strictly in northern Europe. Being required to wear a motorcycle helmet has been redefined in parts of the United States as a symbol of impingement on larger and more important freedoms. It is resisted on principle, and not just as a safety issue. Similarly, speed limits assume for the Germans an ideological aura that they lack elsewhere—outside perhaps of North Dakota. Freie Fahrt für mündige Bürger (freely translatable as "Pedal to the metal: Every citizen's right!) is a slogan inconceivable outside Germany and as incomprehensible to Americans as the insistence on bearing arms as a democratic freedom is to other nations—other than perhaps Switzerland and Israel. Speed limits in general are more tightly regulated in the United States than in Europe, at least south of the river Eider. Smoking and alcohol consumption are regarded as social ills in America. Massive education campaigns and stringent attempts to intervene have been aimed at such habits here more than anywhere in Europe, except for alcohol in Scandinavia. On drug abuse, the Scandinavians take a much harder line than the British and the Dutch.

Defining risk is itself, of course, a social issue. Perhaps we can all agree that Chernobyl was a risk, putting millions in potential harm without their knowledge or ability to take precautions. But whether nuclear power is generally regarded as a problem has varied enormously among cultures. The French are happy to live in the shadow of the cooling towers that produce some 60 percent of their electricity.[63] Their neighbors across the Rhine fret, seeing nuclear power as both a technical danger and a violation of the basic harmony between humans and nature. Gene-altered foodstuffs are regarded with trepidation by Europeans, while happily munched in ignorance by Americans. AIDS, too, raised such broader variances in the culture of risk. Some nations framed it as a social risk justifying massive statutory intervention. Others regarded it as an individual risk, something not requiring strenuous communal action because it could be avoided by acting prudently and sidestepping danger.[64] German Greens scoffed at those who, though willing to tolerate the externalities of industrial society as the price of progress, wanted complete security when it came to AIDS, accepting control, surveillance, and repression to avoid this risk with its comparatively modest lethality.[65]

Posed in terms of public health, the dilemma was whether to treat AIDS as a communal or an individual risk. If a communal risk, the solution was to restrict the infected to render them harmless. If an individual risk, the strategy was to encourage all to take precautions rendering them resistant to infection, and to modify their behaviors to reduce danger. As we have seen, states diverged in their tactics. Some, like Sweden, Bavaria, Austria, and the United States, tended to take a more communal approach than others, like France, Germany, and Britain. Why this was so has been the central concern of this book.

Take the question of seeking to cure AIDS. Though extreme opinion worried lest this would encourage the habits that had helped spread HIV in the first place—whether promiscuity or drug injection—by reducing their consequences, curing the disease was obviously the best solution. And yet not every nation sought with equal energy to achieve this global public good. While the United States and—at a large remove—France poured resources into biomedical research, other nations preferred to coast as free riders. A cure would be the classic Enlightenment achievement, showing that nature could be tamed and providing a public good of universal benefit. The French claimed that they conducted medical research because, reaffirming Enlightenment traditions, they sought a cure for all mankind.[66] Whatever one may think of such rhetoric, it separated them from, say, the Swedes and the Germans, who were apparently not prepared to do the work of humanity. Beyond such universalist posturing, a biomedical solution particularly interested France and the United States because it might allow them to avoid certain problems. Both nations had political and ideological motives for emphasizing a biomedical resolution, for adopting a technical rather than a social approach to the problem.

Most obviously, both were among the hardest-hit industrialized nations.

But beyond pure functionalism, emphasizing biomedical research for all humanity (rather than social science investigations to allow more effective targeting within the nation) enabled the French to gloss over persistent weaknesses in their public health system.[67] Also influential for the French choice was the cultural inclination to see sexuality as an individual, personal, and private choice. The intermediary social groups based on sexual identity—gays above all—that played important roles in the Anglo-Saxon, Dutch, and Scandinavian realms were seen here as politically illegitimate. Biomedicine and its technical fix promised to sidestep such issues.[68]

The Americans, in turn, staked much on biomedicine in hopes of bridging expanding gaps in their health insurance systems. Pouring greater resources into medical research than other nations had been an American tradition since the 1930s. Besides the universalist goal of pursuing public goods, there were political payoffs. Voting for research funding allowed American politicians to demonstrate their support for health, since other avenues of largesse—health insurance for all—were blocked. "Medical research," as Congressman Melvin Laird put it in 1960, "is the best kind of health insurance" the American people could have.[69] For countries with universal and effective health care systems, the epidemic posed less of a political problem. So long as citizens were entitled to reasonable standards of care and the problem did not explode, a new illness was just another blip on the political radar. For these nations, there was less *political* advantage to funding biomedical research than to, say, building hospices for the stricken. (Even in France, the annual budget for indemnifying infected hemophiliacs was many times that for research; in America the proportions were reversed.)[70] For the United States, in contrast, a new epidemic was much less digestible. It suffered the perennial problem of insurance coverage, as the disease struck precisely the groups that were least cared for (as well as articulate sexual minorities with surprisingly adroit political skills).

More generally, the Americans found a biomedical approach consistent with the values of pluralistic democracy. It appealed especially to a multicultural polity—socially, culturally, and sexually balkanized and unable to rely on the cohesion of ethnic and cultural homogeneity or even the classic assimilationist ethos.[71] In a heterogeneous nation, with multiple moral and religious standards, even providing consistent information was fraught with the delicate issue of what could be said to whom. Informal behavioral control could be relied on even less.[72] Seeking biomedically to cure or avoid a stigmatized disease—one spread via behaviors and lifestyles widely regarded as immoral—was the socially and politically most liberal approach. It involved the least tinkering with civil society and its mutually antagonistic proclivities. A biomedical approach promised to spare the United States vexing political choices. By intervening in nature, one could sidestep social interventions. The behavioral change that was unlikely to arise through informal social influence, and whose strict enforcement via rules and laws was difficult, could thus be avoided altogether.[73]

Though promoting condom use, and safe sex in general, also appeared to be a purely technical issue, it too emerged from specific, though often unarticulated, political considerations. First, convincing sexually active citizens that latex offered epidemiological salvation was easier in nations where condoms already robustly served the cause of contraception, as in Japan or Britain, than in France and other Catholic countries, where contraception in general was disputed and condoms were shunned. Beyond this, interposing latex in almost every sexual encounter was a victory for the interests of high-risk groups against those of the average citizen with conventional sexual habits. Condoms were the technical fix that rendered unnecessary the usual means of prevention: testing, reporting, behavioral strictures, and isolation of recalcitrants. Latex also, of course, allowed bypassing the unpopular alternative of monogamy or fidelity, not to mention abstinence.

At stake was either restricting the liberties of high-risk groups or curbing the dangerous—if pleasurable—behavior that put most of the initial victims at risk. Of course, not only gays, or even many gays, were promiscuous. Nor was anal sodomy necessarily the defining feature of gay intercourse. But gay sexual behavior and its remove from mainstream habits became factors in public health decisions. The epidemiologically risky conduct of a subgroup confronted the claims of citizenship. For gays and their allies, the universal law of safe sex sidestepped a negative Hobson's choice. A technical solution was proposed for all, with the goal of sparing certain especially endangered groups even further impositions. Due to the specific nature of AIDS, with the attendant difficulties of deploying traditional measures, this choice was partly preordained. Yet that was not the whole story. In the interests of a customarily despised minority, all citizens were asked to forgo their customary pleasures.

The choice was between imposing legal strictures to discourage and control dangerous behavior, thereby sparing most people the need for individual precautions, and requiring all to throw up their own palisades against infection. As the German Society for Internal Medicine put it, why should one ask legions of uninfected citizens to change their behavior, rather than first and foremost seeking to change seropositives' conduct?[74] Where disease prevention had earlier been a public good, democratization and modern citizenship increasingly privatized it. Citizens were held responsible for their bad habits. Public health came about from the interaction of countless private decisions—a kind of preventive Brownian motion—rather than the imposition of communal norms. Safe sex required latex use by all to ensure that no one was ostracized. Rather than relying on publicly enforceable strictures that permitted a private unencumbrance of behavior, all individuals were expected to curtail and adjust their conduct.

This may well have been a price worth paying. But the costs and benefits were rarely, if ever, discussed in these terms. In the nineteenth century, when victims of contagious disease were forbidden to appear in public, legal strictures sought to preserve citizens' right to walk abroad without fear of infection. It would, in theory, have been possible for all to take personal protective measures, thus avoiding disease, just as requiring all to prepare their own meals would have eliminated the need specifically to forbid typhoid victims from cooking. During the SARS epidemic, face masks became de rigueur in Asian cities. The wife of Tung Chee-Hwa, Hong Kong's chief executive, had protective gear named after her (Betty Suits) when she appeared all but mummified in preventive attire on a visit to a housing project.[75] The choice between individual and communal precautions was not limited to AIDS.

For AIDS, safe sex was considered a small price to pay for avoiding measures to discourage promiscuity, widespread testing, and criminalization of transmission. The logic mimicked that of American gun buffs who argue that, if all were armed, crime would diminish.[76] Just as in Texas each citizen was to be his own police officer, so the condomed were to be their own quarantine officers. As Britain's chief rabbi, Immanuel Jakobovits, put it, it was like sending people into a contaminated atmosphere but providing them with gas masks and protective clothing.[77] All citizens, the German minister of health announced, whether infected or not, must avoid behavior that might infect others.[78] Rather than testing and requiring nontransmissive conduct of the infectious, all citizens were to curtail their behavior as though they too were dangerous. To avoid impositions on the infected, restrictions were instead required of everyone.

THE POLITICS OF PRIVATIZATION

By the AIDS era, public health had become ever more individualized and privatized. With basic sanitary infrastructure in place throughout the developed world, and chronic disease the main enemy, prevention now focused on individual behavior—cultivation of the habits of moderation, prudence, abstemiousness, and risk avoidance, habits that maintained health while sparing citizens intrusive statutory supervision. Economic modernization encouraged this trend. With long life spans the norm, citizens responded to the carrot of possible longevity by shunning avoidable danger. The Struldbruggs, whom Gulliver meets on Luggnagg, exemplify this logic—ancient, risk averse to the extreme, and tedious beyond compare. As life spans lengthen, and preventable accidents become a growing cause of death, we will all become more timid. Public health's individualization also sprang from democratization. Citizens were entrusted with more responsibility, and authorities were reluctant to dictate behavior that was, in any case, unlikely to come about via threats. A taste for low-fat food and plenty of roughage was hard to encourage at gunpoint.

Emphasizing individual rights meant holding citizens, assumed able to control their impulses, responsible for their conduct. Formal controls that governed sexual and other behavior in premodern society loosened, whether the religious and legal injunctions against adultery and fornication, or the close ties between property ownership and reproduction characteristic of peasant societies. Regulation of residence, marriage, dress, and the like was replaced by legal codes that dealt with behavior only at the margins. Rather than using the informal prescriptions of gemeinschaft, together with the strictures of old regime law, modern society governed from within rather than without.

In terms of public health, citizens of democracies were expected to restrain themselves, not have limitations imposed on them. Control shifted, in the sense suggested in the work of Max Weber, Norbert Elias, and Michel Foucault, from external to internal constraints. Emancipation meant less a decrease in control than a displacement of its locus. External control became self-control. Observers of the twentieth-century civil rights revolution often noted the expansion of personal liberty—the emphasis on individual fulfillment rather than communal dictates, the focus on self-expression over self-control.[79] While there was truth to this Whiggish belief in the advance of personal liberty at the expense of group conformity, external freedoms were based on internal strictures. Freedom was not the opposite of control or regulation. Indeed, freedom became the primary program of governance. We were governed, as it were, through our freedom.[80] Self-control and restraint were the preconditions of democracy, of a system that did not enforce behavior with a cudgel.

As part of this shift, health became the morality of modern bourgeois society.[81] Earlier, the imperative had been to act in accord with the precepts of religion. Now the requirements of health and clean living became the codex, the bowels having replaced the soul as the source of the most potent anxieties. In Sinclair Lewis's *Arrowsmith,* Dr. Pickerbaugh, health officer of Zenith, Ohio, advocated a modern social ethos consisting of "good health, good roads, good business, and the single standard of morality." In Foucault's terminology, governmentality replaced external regulation with a quasi-informal system of self-accepted and self-imposed control. Internal strictures now restrained behavior in epidemic circumstances. The modern democratic state, based on informal controls practiced by equal citizens, no longer compelled and coerced, but informed, educated, and hectored. Rather than issuing decrees, it sought to persuade through the techniques of advertising, the social marketing not of products but of behavioral change.[82]

Modern democratic societies could not control citizens' behavior through prescribing conduct, as was possible earlier, and as it perhaps remained the case in dictatorships and autocracies. Instead, they sought to rear, educate, and persuade inhabitants to act as members of a civilized polity. As one observer concluded, while an effective autocracy can mandate public health, democratic regimes can do little more than educate their citizens.[83] The optimistic approach to the AIDS epidemic, which claimed to recognize an overcoming of the eternal conflict between individual rights and community prerogatives, thus rested not just on an ever-expanding realm of individual freedom but equally on a shift in the nature and location of control. We were freer externally only because we exercised more self-control. Yet the individualization of control, the emphasis on voluntary behavioral strictures, meant that society became dependent on individuals' choices. Were the consensus model of AIDS prevention true, then we were, as one commentator put it, "dependent on the emergence of a culture of restraint and responsibility" that would end transmissive behavior.[84] The solution, in another's words, was to decrease formal control and increase informal control over AIDS victims.[85]

In modern polities, the formal rules that still existed to sanction transgressive behavior were no longer assumed to apply to everyone, but only to the small minority of deviants and recalcitrants who actually violated implicit community norms. Laws against bank robbery did not curtail the freedoms of law-abiding citizens.[86] As a Swedish liberal (Folkpartiet) argued, legal restrictions on behavior were compulsory only for the small minority who refused to follow procedures, not for honest citizens.[87] Just as the cow grazing in the center of the field never felt the twitch of the electrified fence, so the freest among us were those who suffered no urge to violate the laws. As nudists can undress only on the assurance that sexual urges have been suppressed, so the modern citizen is free only by conforming.

On the other hand, the growth of sex tourism (*prostiturismo*, in Italian) revealed the dark side of internalizing control. Satisfaction of illicit desires was now outsourced globally.[88] Self-control, combined with the increasing formal prohibition of sexual relations with children, pushed marginalized forms of sexuality abroad, much as Hannah Arendt saw the racism of European society exported to the colonies in the baggage of its adventurers.[89] A chance to abandon the mastery and control expected of citizens at home became one of the attractions of going abroad. Prostitution, as well as a dramatic relaxation of informal controls on drinking, increasingly characterized mass tourism—not only in its exotic locales but also in the sodden excesses of English football hooligans on the Continent.

Holding individuals accountable for their actions and thus their health had two sides: the individual responsibility of democratic citizenship but also the blaming of victims for their own misfortunes. Both were starkly revealed during the AIDS era. Contributory negligence, the responsibility for risk that everyone assumed whenever they had unprotected sex, or shared needles, increasingly erased the distinction between perpetrators and victims—even when seropositives had sex without informing their partners. As one observer phrased it, individuals should always maintain control over their own well-being and never depend on third parties.[90] Guilt and fault were old-fashioned concepts, autonomy and individual action the modern ones. However, when precautions were individualized, making all responsible for themselves, the implication was that, if infection nonetheless ensued, no one was to blame but oneself. Having apparently been thrown out the front door, fault and blame were escorted in again through the back one.[91]

The "civilized" and polite behavior—the restraint imposed on Dionysian instincts, the contact avoidance, and separation of humans from their bodily fluids—that governed everyday conduct in the modern world had obvious effects in curtailing disease. Turn-of-the-century campaigns against tuberculosis transformed spitting—once regarded as an irrepressible instinct, with expectoration akin to excretion—into behavior that has all but vanished (except for that of the occasional baseball pitcher). Even into the twentieth century, syphilis was considered a disease passed along through normal, everyday, but by modern standards primitive, practices. Only with the development of personal hygiene and the sanitization of our everyday interactions did syphilis become a disease transmitted largely via sex. The nonsexual dissemination of VD has long been considered a sign of primitive customs and low cultural development. It indicated that the basic hygienic habits of urban middle-class life (the sanitized interface we present to each other, except in sex—although increasingly even there, depilated, deodorized, belatexed) had not yet been achieved. Sexually transmitted diseases were thus created as a separate and stigmatized class of illness not only because sex was felt to be a sin. Equally, this heralded the triumph of personal hygiene, which left venereal contact as these diseases' predominant mode of transmission.

Conversely, a growing awareness that some diseases passed directly between humans, and did not simply arise from unpropitious environmental circumstances, contributed to the development of polite conduct.[92] Lepers were, in this sense, among the first to bear the brunt of modern civilized and hygienic behavior. Setting them beyond the community's pale, as was once customary, strikes us as brutal only because it was unilateral. But we are all lepers now. Civilized behavior in the sense defined by Norbert Elias is the mutual treatment of all as potentially diseased outcasts. Only in its mutuality is the violence we do to each other obscured. By our natures we are seals, seeking epidermal contact across every square inch. But we have learned to become birds, spacing ourselves equidistantly on the wires.

Syphilis laid bare this process. Since it was evidently spread between individuals, attention focused on the carrier rather than the locality or the environment, as with fevers. Because syphilis was transmitted by voluntary behavior, it was argued, all could protect themselves. The state did not have to take precautions that could best be left to the individual.[93] At the same time, the sexual instinct was regarded in the early modern world as uncontainable. Could individuals mount their own precautions? Not until the sixteenth century did observers, like Fallopius, begin recommending preventive measures—washing the penis after coitus and the like.[94] Slowly, sex came to be regarded as something that could be subordinated to hygienic and epidemiological considerations. Contagion could be fought even in the throes of passion. Self-control and concupiscence were not mutually exclusive. Syphilis also provided an early impetus to behavioral restraint in other ways. In 1529, Erasmus recommended that every man cut his own hair and beard to avoid infection by his barber, that common drinking cups be abolished, and that greetings with a kiss be discouraged.[95]

The system of regulating prostitutes was based on the logic that, by focusing on the most obvious carriers of disease—the purveyors of commercial copulation—the sexual behavior of their clients could be left unhampered. When, late in the nineteenth century, abolitionists sought alternative means of limiting VD, they proposed solutions like criminalizing disease transmission—whether by prostitutes or paterfamilias. Their idea was that all citizens should take responsibility for their actions. By coupling freedom and liberty with individual responsibility for even the most instinctually overdetermined actions, the old system (based on indenturing a caste of sexual untouchables) could be rendered superfluous.[96] The Scandinavian system of sanitary statism (eventually adopted in much of the Western world) assumed that the average citizen, not just prostitutes, should be the target of precautions. This expansion of hygienic behavior to regulate not just the conduct associated with hunger and tactility (table manners, personal hygiene, constraints on contact with others, etc.) but also sex proceeded apace into our own era.[97] Children were taught at the turn of the century to limit their contact with the external world, to shun fixtures and towels in public lavatories; to avoid garbage; not to pick their noses; and to shake hands, rather than kiss, strangers or, ideally, not to touch them at all. Ultimately, it was hoped, male children would internalize the instinct of contact avoidance so firmly that the thought of sex with a public woman would become thoroughly unappetizing.[98]

The voluntary, consensual approach to AIDS instituted a shift from an older use of state power, dictating behavior through law and regulation, to a public health based on individual compliance, conduct, and self-control.[99] AIDS befell a society likely to embrace the ethos of personal restraint, and behavioral change. In the early modern era, lives were nasty, brutish, and short and salvation in the next world beckoned. But modern humans, fixated on the pleasures of the corporeal present, responded to a doctrine dictating abstinence and delayed pleasure in favor of a longer and healthier life.[100]

Respecting civil rights despite the epidemic was thus possible if citizens, suppressing their instincts, acted so as not to harm others. The consensual approach to AIDS shifted the focus from disease carriers to the individual's own defenses, from collective action and control of others to reliance on what we can do for ourselves.[101] The state, unable to relieve individuals of responsibility for their sexual conduct—or so the ministers of health of the German federal states concluded—could not protect them.[102] The Greens agreed: only those, like hemophiliacs, unable to defend themselves, should be protected by the state. Others, who were threatened by consensual acts, had to rely on their own defenses.[103] The Danish Parliament, representative of a nation where this philosophy was not otherwise central to public policy, followed suit: individuals were responsible for their own actions.[104] Such ideas were taken farthest perhaps in the Netherlands. Here, official policy discouraged even voluntary testing of high-risk groups, reasoning that the best way to avoid transmission was behavioral change by all, regardless of serostatus.[105] From one vantage, this was the democratic ethos of individual responsibility. From another, it was a *sauve qui peut* mentality, representing the bankruptcy of public health in its socially reformist, collectivist mode. Life in the latex bunker had become the new ideal for all.

The obvious example of this approach was the condom code. This meant that sex—unless between two people certain of their epidemiological reliability—could occur only with the protection of latex. As a French observer formulated it: unless they were absolutely certain, all men and women, as responsible citizens and subjects of law, should behave sexually as though their partner were infected.[106] The days of sex without responsibility were over, announced the well-known medical historian Roy Porter, drawing the curtain over the 1960s once and for all. Gays could never go back to the heedless promiscuity of the 1970s, Gabriel Rotello warned just as apocalyptically.[107]

But not only did the penis, or the vagina, require sheathing. Society was ever more belatexed, to the point where no contact between strangers took place without precautions. The next step, as a German Green scoffed, was a whole-body condom.[108] A dentist's appointment—an almost informal procedure just a few years earlier—now required sartorial precautions worthy of Bethesda's Level 4 labs.[109] Who today knows the color of his dentist's eyes? Instead of screening patients to determine who needed special precautions, hospitals treated all as potentially infective and applied top-level measures in each instance. The worst-case scenario became the lowest common denominator. Rather than testing prisoners or the arrested, authorities treated each as though a risk and approached them with gloves and masks.[110] The communal chalice now required an epidemiological, as well as theological, leap of faith. The emergency automotive kits issued by the Allgemeine Deutsche Automobil-Club (the German version of the American Automobile Association) now included polyvinyl chloride gloves, in case of accident and the need for first aid. The demand for natural latex went up with the use of condoms; the market for protective gloves, dental dams, and syringe collectors expanded dramatically.[111] Autologous blood banking allowed candidates for surgery to avoid foreign serum and its dangers. Resources that had earlier been collective were individualized as each citizen became a serological monad.[112] The avoidance of others' bodily fluids, so crucial to the Eliasian civilizing process, became almost absolute. Seen in terms of our secretions, we have sealed ourselves off all but hermetically. Making everyone a potential patient, and requiring behavioral change of all, was perhaps the ultimate form of victimology. It created a "society of suspicion," where all had to assume the potential infectedness of everyone else and act accordingly.[113]

Along with latex, abstinence—or at least fidelity and monogamy—now also assumed epidemiological significance. Almost all governments joined in the remoralization of public health by instructing citizens that sexual faithfulness was the best means of avoiding infection.[114] Condoms are good, as a German liberal put it, but fidelity is better—a reversal of Lenin's famous dictum: trust is good, control is better.[115] In the United States, federally funded AIDS education programs encouraged responsible sexual behavior based on fidelity within marriage. The British Education Act of 1986 required that sex education encourage morality and the value of family life. The Czechs forbade seropositives more than one sexual partner.[116]

RIGHT THINKING

Such remoralization also underlined how modern public health relied not just on individuals behaving circumspectly but also on their believing that this was the best way. Physicians in Sweden instructed high-risk patients on the virtues of having a single sexual partner and on safe erotic techniques. Those who rebuffed this advice could be compulsorily isolated. The isolated were to be given psychosocial care to change their attitude, as a condition of eventually freeing them.[117] Nor did the law set clear limits to the duration of isolation: recalcitrants were to be evaluated for changes in attitude. The length of incarceration thus depended on the individual knuckling under to the authorities' expectations. The social minister sought to implement a plan to examine the isolated and release them only provisionally to see whether they had adopted safe habits before allowing them out unconditionally. Encouraging condom use and clean needles was worthwhile, a Social Democrat agreed. More important, however, was penetrating the mindset of dangerous subgroups, like addicts and prostitutes, to learn their codes and make them receptive to changes in attitude.[118]

The Deutsche Gesellschaft zur Bekämpfung der Geschlechtskrankheiten had been the mouthpiece of reform during the great battles over syphilis and prostitution at the turn of the nineteenth century. Now, in the AIDS era, it favored behavioral change, arguing that not compulsory measures but changes in conduct were required. That, in turn, required a change of consciousness.[119] Public health experts thought that certain social groups adopted unhealthy habits and lifestyles. A more contextually oriented approach to prevention should seek to understand why, and to change not just individual behavior but also the very community.[120] The German Greens formulated some of the few objections to such an approach. They argued that the Social Democrats' hopes of instilling change in conduct threatened unwarranted intrusions into citizens' bedrooms. Behavioral modification should not mean a return to the morality of the 1950s.[121]

Here, they touched the nub of the matter. Though the informal, voluntarily adopted behavioral norms were perhaps less harsh than regulations prescribing certain conduct on pain of legal punishment, they still remained a form of control. Self-imposed strictures meant adopting a code of conduct that claimed purely epidemiological justification, yet into which moral, ethical, and other normative evaluations easily crept. There is no educational measure without a repressive element, as one observer put it.[122] Breaking chains of transmission was key, but did this mean monogamy? Or sexual parsimony? Or would sporting a condom at the orgy suffice? Physicians should not prescribe abstinence or monogamy to infected gays, the main Swedish homosexual organization complained, when the goal was not preventing sex as such, but only that involving an exchange of bodily fluids.[123] Was oral sex verboten, or okay so long as it did not include ejaculation in the mouth? Oral sex if it substituted for more dangerous anal practices? Anal sex, but not fisting? French kissing, but not rimming? Monogamy and condoms were ways of avoiding risky sex, but so were encouraging voyeurism, masturbation (mutual, group, or solitary), exhibitionism, telephone and Internet sex, and other unconventional, but epidemiologically unobjectionable, relations.

The solution to the safe sex problem, some brave souls ventured, was perhaps not to fixate on penetrative lovemaking and how to make it innocuous, but to expand the repertoire of erotic practices. For others, the problem with safe sex for gays was that it sought to sanitize and make acceptable homosexual practices that were regarded as distasteful.[124] With anal penetration now frowned on, were gay jerk-off circles a return to schoolboy dalliance, or a brave new venture into sexual terra nova? Was heavy petting a return to the bobbysex fifties or the cutting edge of noncoital innovation?[125] Thanks to the epidemic, fringe sex joined the mainstream. A Nairobi man defended his erotic relationship with a cow, invoking his fear of AIDS. The British minister of public health remarked that there was nothing safe left in sex except bondage and flagellation.[126] In the curious belief that gays would prefer to forego sodomy rather than use condoms, the Dutch government discouraged penetrative anal sex altogether. Before they again criminalized commercial sex in toto, Swedes used educational campaigns to stigmatize and demonize prostitutes.[127]

Voluntary behavioral change, in other words, could mean many things. Who decided what conduct was within the pale? Gays, not surprisingly, feared arguments for sexual parsimony were but veiled attempts to roll back hard-won erotic freedoms. HIV screening was suspect as a new ritual of heterosexuality, designed to stigmatize gays.[128] Whatever their virtues, safe sex campaigns were attacked as cementing the distinction between "normal" heterosexual behavior and "deviant" gay practices. These campaigns were criticized as nailing fast a fixed conception of gay sexual identity. With their focus on anal sex and its implicitly patriarchal primacy of penetration, they encouraged a heterosexualization of homosexual copulative conduct.[129] And what about the recommendations of safe sex—fidelity and/or condoms—in cultures that valued neither? In those, for example, where a transfer of sperm was crucial in lovemaking? Or where, as in New Guinea, regular infusions of seed were considered necessary during pregnancy to construct the fetus? Or where ingestion of semen was thought healthy and beneficial?[130] Among Latin males, penetration was considered paramount, and condoms were feared as counter-erectionary.[131] Safe sex campaigns were attacked for seeking both to control the gay communities of the First World and to limit Africa's population growth by insisting on condoms. Indeed, some believed that such campaigns demonically spread the virus through tainted condoms distributed gratis in the Third World. Others claimed that prosecuting seropositive prostitutes for endangering their clients, far from being a public health measure, covertly sought to control female sexuality.[132]

The inherent contradictions of the problem shone through when the German Green Party warned against moralization and social control if counseling on behavior modification for high-risk groups was provided by advisors from very different backgrounds.[133] Their solution was for self-help groups to offer such services—rather than having, say, Catholic clergy give gays advice on the problematics of anonymous sex. But, of course, the dilemma was that either anonymous promiscuity was dangerous or it was not. If having fellow gays tell you not to go to the bathhouses was preferable to hearing it from Monsignor, it was only because you were likelier to follow their advice. The end effect remained the same: you were supposed to forego the pleasures of the baths. If anything, gay counselors were imposing greater social control—however well-intentioned—than the Church. Similar were the contradictions of the arguments for community-based voluntarist approaches to the epidemic. These assumed that behavioral norms characteristic of a specific subgroup might at one and the same time be epidemiologically safe, yet also differ from the standards of the general population.[134] Removing the doors from the bathhouse cubicles—creating a panoptican of promiscuity—was emblematic of the dilemma: the intent was self-policing of gays in the inner sanctum of their most daring transgression, enlisting homosexuals' own shame to defeat practices that broke the fetters of heterosexual sex but left them vulnerable to infection. At heart, the problem was that, however gussied up in the rhetoric of (multi)cultural sensitivity, certain behaviors were toxic and in need of change.[135]

Gays were particularly affected by this shift of control from the external impositions of an authoritarian state to the internal consensual behavior characteristic of what Foucault called governmentality. Contemporary sexual freedom, such as it is, rests on assumptions of internalized restraint. For gays, the implications were twofold. Resistance to self-restraint meant more than just risky behavior. It was not equivalent to the motorcycle rider who left his helmet at home or the driver who kept his seat belt unfastened. Rejecting safe sex, resisting closure of the bathhouses, or remaining promiscuous indicated a more fundamental refusal to enter into the web of mutually inflecting self-control on which modern democratic polities rested. Foucault's sexual escapades in Toronto and San Francisco early in the epidemic, the presumed occasion of his infection, have been interpreted by his biographer, James Miller, as an ontological *va banque* game with death itself. Knowing that his life was at risk, he still chose to partake of polymorphous pleasures in the baths.[136] One tragic aspect of the epidemic was that it throttled in the crib the most remarkable features of gay sexual behavior. The Dionysian joy of anonymous, multiple, promiscuous sex—bathhouse or not—recaptured a tactility that had been eliminated from civilization in Elias's sense—an infant's pleasure in total corporeal eroticism that bourgeois society had banished, a refound delight in the voluptuousness of bodily fluids before civilization enclosed and separated us behind sanitized interfaces: with shorn hair, banished odors, dried sweat and saliva, sexual fluids neatly shrink-wrapped in latex, in our Vulcan-like disembodiedness.

From this vantage, the efforts of the most "advanced" and liberal governments to include gays in implementing behavioral change made them police themselves. Whereas the old-fashioned approach sought to impose social norms on homosexuals from without, governmentality made gays responsible for their own conduct. Gays could either cooperate with safer sex strategies or face a crackdown: so ran the implicit bargain.[137] The voluntary strategy required not less statutory imposition on the individual than the coercive approach but a different and arguably more thoroughgoing kind. Most obviously, determining whether it was having any effect required extensive information about its subjects. The strategy may not have locked the potentially diseased in lazarettos, but it required the details of their most intimate habits: did you fuck another man up the ass during the last several weeks and, if so, how often and with or without a condom? Do you swallow when someone comes in your mouth? Do you felch? If uncircumcised, are you careful to wash away the smegma *(Vorhautbutter!)*—and so forth in all its epidemiologically relevant detail. While it was laissez-faire in not threatening punishments for certain conduct, the consensual approach was drastically interventionist in wanting to uncover every last detail of behavior said to be voluntarily adopted.[138]

The old-fashioned approach to public health subordinated risky groups to the community. It also defined a clear arena of acceptable behavior, fencing it around with laws and regulations. Those who violated it knew what to expect, but other than the fear of punishment, little control was exerted over their behavior. In contrast, public health in the governmentalist mode may not have punished transgressions. But it sought to ensure compliance and healthy behavior not only by requiring all to conduct themselves in much the same way but also by making them agree that this was for the best. Condoms and sterile needles were technical fixes that might sidestep the problem for the moment, but at the price of continuing behaviors widely regarded as noxious. Better yet, governmentalist public health sought to eliminate the conduct seen as causing the problem: not just sharing, but using needles altogether; not just anal sex, but promiscuity *tout court*. Transgressive behavior was not punished. By changing people's attitudes, it was to be pulled out by its roots. The bourgeois habits of moderation, abstention, and prudence were expected of all citizens. Self-restraint became the basic requirement of modern polities. One of the fundamental issues posed by the epidemic was whether behavior like promiscuity or intravenous drug use—rendered fatal by AIDS—was compatible with democratic citizenship. Gays may have entered the AIDS era seeing themselves as sexual outlaws, in John Rechy's phrase.[139] But the new style of public health, and gays' own interests in not being subject to old-fashioned strictures, meant that they had to adopt the norms of bourgeois, heterosexual society: they had to become sexual insiders.

THE VARIETY OF RESPONSE

It is time to return to the question of why nations varied in their approaches to the epidemic. As we have seen, there was a divergence between those relying on an old-fashioned approach and others willing to try a consensualist or governmentalist mode. Since public health had such apparent political consequences, it might seem intuitive that nations chose strategies according to their political ideologies and traditions. While in part they did, we have also seen that simple correlations were hard to find. Nations reputed to be laissez-faire (the United States) and concerned with civil rights (Sweden) used the most traditional strategy. Others with longer traditions (France) and sometimes quite drastic traditions (Germany) of statutory initiative were markedly hands-off. We have also looked at a series of factors that help explain the divergences: the power of the pertinent interest groups, the nature of the administrative machinery, the role of law and the courts, and the influence of other legislation and public opinion.

That the epidemic first struck ethnic and sexual Others had negative repercussions for prevention. Prejudice and discrimination limited the resources initially devoted to the problem and encouraged more draconian tactics than might otherwise have been the case. Who those "others" were varied by nation: gays at first in the United States, then Haitians, and eventually Afro-Americans and other ethnic minorities; Danes in anxious Sweden; Congolese students in Belgium; Africans throughout Europe; Americans in large parts of the world; Westerners in the East.

But prejudice alone cannot explain the outcomes. Although it entirely missed the tectonic shift in political values that now hampered the application of traditional measures, there was an undeniably rough equity to the conservative query, Why should the victims of this epidemic be exempt from strictures applied to others? Moreover, some of the most extreme proposals (those of the French National Front and the Bavarian government) targeted not only unfavored minorities—gays, prostitutes, foreigners—but also mainstream social groups: military personnel, pregnant and married women, recipients of blood transfusions, and civil servants. In Bavaria, the government threatened to close not only gay saunas but also straight brothels. In San Francisco, the director of public health admitted that only a concern for gay sensibilities had prevented bathhouses from being shut immediately. Had the baths catered to heterosexual exuberance, such establishments would have been closed at once.[140] While prejudice may have been part of it, the story cannot end there.

Seen from another vantage, the epidemic's predation on gays served to mobilize unprecedented political action by high-risk groups. Research and treatment were eventually funded generously. Care was taken to avoid impinging on the civil rights of the sick. The influence of gay movements was crucial, especially in northern Europe and the United States. The stark differences between the gay-focused epidemic here in the early phases, and the high incidence among intravenous drug users in southern Europe (and Scotland), meant that political mobilization would have differed in any case.

Gays were not well organized precisely where drug users were the main victims. Where gays suffered especially, their role was important. And yet, even here, other factors also played a role. While gay organizational clout encouraged a liberal approach in central Europe and the United States, in Scandinavia (especially Sweden and Finland) even a strong homosexual movement did not counteract long traditions of firm state authority over its citizens. Moreover, the later spread of the epidemic among disadvantaged minorities diluted gay influence over the response. Though American gays were well mobilized, they also faced vociferous and powerful right-wing and conservative religious movements without compare in Europe.[141]

Administrative differences were also important. Centralized systems could, in theory, have been early to respond, and some (as in Sweden) were. But others (as in France) tarried. Federalized ones had the chance to tailor their response to local peculiarities, though also the disadvantage of being unable to tame excessive measures that found regional favor. The nature of the social policy machinery was crucial. American seropositives, bereft of a national health system and often lost in the cracks of private insurance, were relegated to the last resort of Medicaid. A consensual approach rested on an implicit promise of treatment or, at least, care. What incentive did the stricken have to cooperate if they were not offered medical attention once the news proved bad? This was the lesson drawn in the nineteenth century by the Swedish system of VD prevention—that you had to promise treatment to impose surveillance—and the conclusion of the British interwar experience: that voluntary arrangements were effective if care was readily available. In nations with universal health insurance, this was no problem. In the United States it was. Indeed, advocates of voluntary testing here proposed offering health care for seropositives as a carrot.[142]

In being protected against discrimination, however, American seropositives enjoyed the advantage of existing legislation for the handicapped. American legal guarantees for the disabled were extensive, largely thanks to affirmative action and other attempts to ensure a fair chance for formerly outcast ethnic minorities. In the United States, with health care largely contingent on employment, protections against discrimination in hiring and firing were more important than in Europe, where people were often covered as citizens, not employees. Conversely, in Europe, where firing, if not hiring, was subject to broad legal regulation, employers were permitted greater latitude in investigating, questioning, and screening applicants than in the United States. Such frontline hurdles were less crucial in America, given the employer's ability to terminate jobs later on. In this case, too, the individual's privacy was inversely related to the benefits that citizens expected from the state.

The epidemic sparked brushfires of extreme public opinion in much the same way across all nations. Grassroots opinion among those outside the high-risk core was often panicky. Many were willing to impose drastic measures on epidemiological outsiders. The experts of the policy-making pantheon, in contrast, generally took a considered view, downplaying the risks and the need for harsh statutory incursions. But the respective influence of these two voices varied among nations. The more populistically democratic a polity was, and the more permeable to public opinion, the more influence extreme opinions had. If anything, this reversed a notable idea in the history of public health, Erwin Ackerknecht's claim that authoritarian governments tended to intervene harshly with little concern for individual rights, while liberal ones sought to avoid violating liberties.[143] At the heart of this dilemma lay the classic tension between democracy and liberty, the vox populi and enlightened moderation. Was it good or bad to incorporate grassroots opinion in formulating policy? If it meant listening to the epidemic's victims, probably good. If it meant responding to the vox populi, not necessarily so. Putting decision making into the hands of professionals and experts kept the rabble at arm's length. Yet it also meant stilling victims' voices. In the United States, the extremists of gay activism and fundamentalist moralism did public battle. In France, both ends of the spectrum were muzzled after initial politicization from the right. Sweden, in contrast, though attentive to civil rights, allowed a professional caste of decision makers free rein in ways that victims elsewhere would have found intolerable.

SOCIAL HETEROGENEITY

We have explored such particular factors behind the divergent approaches taken. It remains to consider some of the most general issues at stake. The choice between traditionalist and governmentalist public health approaches to AIDS posed the question of how control was exerted in different polities—formally or informally. That, in turn, broached the assumptions that any society could make without comment or discussion. The intuitive rule of thumb would seem to be that the more homogeneous a polity—ethnically, religiously, socially—the more it can rely on unspoken, informal norms of correct behavior. A balkanized, heterogeneous society, in contrast, must count on formal criteria imposed by law and authority.[144] In heterogeneous societies, it was tempting to assign moral valuation to diseases, seeing them as the outcome of unfortunate lifestyle choices. Such condemnation might be less common in homogeneous polities, where the difference between those struck and those spared could more plausibly be regarded as an unfortunate encounter with malevolent microorganisms. In Norway, for example, leprosy had been easily medicalized and treated with scientific impartiality as the outcome of a bacillus, not of the victim's morality, lifestyle, or choice. Elsewhere, where the disease's victims overlapped with racial minorities, other prejudices colored its popular etiology.[145] AIDS presented a similar situation.

In societies where most people enjoyed broadly comparable socioeconomic standards, common behavioral norms could more easily be assumed. Poverty and its circumstances were important factors in facilitating the spread of AIDS in both First and Third Worlds. Male promiscuity and polygamy, widespread commercial sex, and the rejection of condoms—all of which helped spread HIV in Africa—were the outcome of women's economic disadvantages. In the developed world, prostitution and drug use were the epidemiologically pertinent behaviors closely tied to poverty. In nations with a wide divergence in affluence, the epidemic's nature and the response to it differed from those where most citizens had access to health care, disability pensions, and other forms of social security. Such differences not only separated the Third from the First World but also distinguished between the United States, at one extreme among developed nations, and northern Europe, at the other. The presence of an underclass, reinforced by ethnic markers and afflicted by poverty's consequences, was one of the most important factors. The more an underclass existed apart from the mainstream, the greater the dilemmas concerning a disease that attacked it especially.[146]

Societies have adopted the norms of modern personal hygiene at different times. Traveling in Italy in the 1780s, Goethe marveled that the natives still defecated in the streets. Even today, the sense of shame attached to excretion varies among cultures—as anyone can attest who has compared the privacy assured even men at Swedish urinals to the all-but-public micturation still common in the French countryside. Sanitary reformers in southern Europe at the turn of the century often complained that they could not make the same assumptions as their colleagues to the north. Abolishing the regulation of prostitution, one argued, worked only in civilized nations that respected personal and public hygiene.[147] The Mediterranean countries, they calculated, imposed theoretically strict laws, honoring them in the breach. The North took a more laissez-faire approach, which rested in its liberality on common habits of propriety, a respect for the law, and well-developed sanitary and medical infrastructure.[148] The shift to informal control took place early in Britain. By nineteenth-century Continental standards, the English were clean, their cities hygienic. Hence, they could be the first to dispense with quarantine. The British were moral, sexually circumspect, and willing to conduct themselves so as not to spread venereal disease. Hence, they could do without officially regulated prostitution.

Immigration complicated things, undermining shared behavioral assumptions and informal control. That was especially America's problem. Since it could not rely on commonly accepted standards of conduct among its rainbow-hued citizenry, the United States instituted often stringent precautions. America's social heterogeneity—especially the presence of an ever more permanent underclass, distinguished both racially and socioeconomically, and comparatively neglected by social policy—influenced public health. Tuberculosis prevention, for example, focused on transients and the marginal. Considered likely to act transmissively, the infected were often incarcerated. Such measures continued in the United States even into the postwar era, when tuberculosis became treatable with drugs, and traditional techniques, including isolation, slipped into anachronism elsewhere.[149] Directly Observed Therapy—administering antibiotics under supervision to ensure a complete course of treatment—was required of transient and homeless patients during the AIDS epidemic. Prominent public health scholars had once argued in the 1950s that precautions against tuberculosis did not require legal compulsion because they had "acquired the compelling strength of common sense."[150] It should come as no surprise that common sense had become much less common during the AIDS era.

Social pathologies and the weaknesses of American welfare policy meant that certain issues, especially health care, were debated more urgently than in Europe during the AIDS era. Homelessness, which worsened at this time, was linked to AIDS by the likelihood that those without housing were drug injectors and suffered from STDs or tuberculosis. The nation faced tandem epidemics—one among gays, the other among ghettoized ethnic minorities.[151] The first of these received much attention, the second much less. In 1993, the National Research Council argued provocatively that, with AIDS increasingly affecting ethnic minorities, the epidemic would soon disappear—not by ending, but because its victims were socially invisible. In Cuba, by way of contrast, high-risk groups were an elite, favored by travel abroad and in contact with infected foreigners.[152] Hence the oft-remarked good conditions of the quarantine camps.

Minorities, in turn, reacted in tandem to their marginalized status. Blacks distrusted government interventions and often saw the epidemic as an excuse for persecution. Nonetheless, they were also more willing than whites to endorse coercive policies.[153] Blacks were stratified both by their ethnicity and by class divisions among themselves. What from the outside was seen as black sexual behavior or drug use was black lower-class, or otherwise marginal, conduct. Black gays and intravenous drug users were doubly stigmatized, not only as blacks by others but also as minorities of the minority.[154] Partly because black leaders regarded harm minimization as neglect (or genocide in the most heated rhetoric) in the effort to prevent and treat drug abuse, needle exchanges were controversial in the United States. Black gays' concerns, in turn, tended to get short shrift, given the prevalence of traditional attitudes toward homosexuality in this culture.[155]

American ethnic heterogeneity also made perinatal transmission an issue fraught with tension. The political delicacy of abortion made it tactically difficult to counsel infected expectant mothers to terminate pregnancies (an issue that the United States shared with European nations outside Scandinavia). Abortion, indeed any limits on the reproductive freedom of seropositive women, was out of bounds. Sterilization and eugenic policies had harmed black females especially and other ethnic minorities in the past. Combined with a tradition of protecting women's reproductive rights, including that of bearing forseeably handicapped offspring, this meant that even counseling the pregnant on the virtues of voluntary HIV testing caused an outcry in New York City during the mid-1980s. Opponents charged that advising such women to terminate their pregnancies was tantamount to genocide.[156] The experience of sickle-cell anemia had set a precedent. Though public health officials had initially proposed mandatory testing, they quickly abandoned all but voluntary tactics as racist (since the disease strikes mainly blacks) and useless (since there was as yet no cure).[157]

American social heterogeneity was also reflected in other aspects of policy. Social stratification meant that making decisions locally and including members of affected minority communities was more important than in Europe, the Continent especially. Programs and organizations developed for minorities were more common in the United States and more common in— by European standards—self-consciously multicultural Britain than on the Continent. (Similar programs were also instituted in explicitly multicultural Australia.) In other European nations, AIDS organizations specific to migrants were either late creations or nonexistent.[158] Cultural heterogeneity also forced American education campaigns to be variegated, taking linguistic, religious, and cultural differences into account—though in Europe, too, the increasing presence of Muslims with distinct views of sexuality raised similar problems.[159] The American Public Health Service quickly discovered that its message had to be tailored to specific communities, not addressed to all citizens. Not just American puritanism but also the variety of sensibilities to take into account (many of them neither Protestant nor puritan) help explain why education campaigns here were less sexually explicit, indeed why advertising generally remains erotically more timid than in northern Europe.[160] Hispanics, heavily Catholic, resisted frank sexuality in information campaigns, as did equally prudish Native Americans.[161] Cultural heterogeneity alone, however, did not determine the variety of the informational response. National attitudes toward assimilation and the nature of citizenship also played a role.[162] The French, who also had large ethnic and religious minorities, took an explicitly assimilationist approach. On the assumption that minorities would become mainstreamed into the dominant culture, they saw no need to tailor campaigns to subgroups.

And yet such obvious examples of cultural heterogeneity did not determine everything. Why did Sweden—arguably the most economically, socially, culturally, ethnically, and religiously homogenous nation in the Western World—not trust informal social control and the voluntary behavioral change thus, in theory, made possible? The Swedes worried especially about recalcitrants, the behavioral outsiders who—impervious to informal control—threatened to wreak havoc by persisting in risky behavior. On them, drastic sanctions were imposed. Legal action was needed against those who rejected physicians' behavioral prescriptions, the authorities insisted in 1985, rebutting the argument that only voluntary measures would prevent victims from disappearing underground. With AIDS threatening to spread out of high-risk groups, more drastic restrictions were required, they continued, as they closed gay bathhouses.[163] The Swedish approach was heavily colored by its concern about outsiders who threatened the general population. A fixation on foreigners, whether resident Somalians, visiting Poles, or neighboring Danes, was a leitmotif here. Strict measures, especially isolation of recalcitrant seropositives, were aimed at prostitutes and drug addicts.[164]

Disease transmission via drug users preoccupied the Swedes. It was a short step from the compulsory treatment of addicts that had long been policy here (most recently in the Law on the Treatment of Addicts of 1981) to the draconian strategy broached in 1986, when the government sought to establish more institutions for the isolation and treatment of infected addicts. Strict treatment was also aimed at addicts in attempts to circumscribe medical confidentiality, allowing authorities to share information about the infected. Addicts were seen as unpredictable and dangerous. Young girls risked infection by having sex with them, one conservative cautioned.[165] The dangers they posed, especially the double whammy of addicted prostitutes, were a preoccupation of the Swedish discussion, with little sympathy spared for the victims. As one local authority put it, these were groups that disregarded others in their addictive and mercenary pursuits, without a care for transmission. Such subcultures lacked normal concepts of honor and solidarity. Unreachable by education and unlikely to follow physicians' prescriptions, they required stronger means of control, like isolation. Even the Communists sometimes defenders of civil rights, were satisfied with modifications in proposed measures to direct them no longer at gays but at drug addicts and prostitutes, who were not among their primary voting base.[166]

Other nations, too, had analogous concerns. There was a similar demonization in the German terms for those who transmitted disease by not curbing their behavior. The government threatened harsh measures against people who endangered others through *uneinsichtiges* or malicious conduct, those who were reckless and *unbelehrbar*.[167] The Bavarian authorities justified their *Sonderweg,* much on the Swedish model, with a similar concern for the "hard kernel" of recalcitrants—prostitutes, psychotics, illiterates, and especially drug addicts and desperados—who refused to change their behavior regardless of education campaigns. For them, the heavy hand of traditional measures should be kept ready. The Scots worried about "revenge sex." In the United States, Congressman William Dannemeyer anticipated the actions of "AIDS terrorists." Senator Helms apparently fretted that AIDS terrorists employed as food handlers might spit in the salad.[168] And yet, with respect to drug addicts, such fears were ventilated in substitution and harm minimization policies elsewhere. The makers of these policies agreed, in effect, to sacrifice addicts on the altar of public health. This logic of accepting the evil of chemical dependency while limiting the danger to others was rejected in Sweden, where long traditions of temperance and abstinence still held sway. Given Sweden's equal fear of addicts, the conclusion drawn here was that it was better to level strict measures at them, rendering them harmless by isolating them, than to tamper with their habits.

THE HAND OF THE PAST

One of the themes explored here has been the influence of past decisions on present public health policies. Historians live, of course, to argue that the past matters. In this case, the past did have more of an influence than most of the practitioners and decision makers, faced with the urgency of a major crisis, perhaps realized. A Swedish local health officer might have argued that, naturally, the infectious who refused to curb potentially transmissive behavior should be isolated. Her English colleague would have claimed that, to the contrary, doing so would drive the infected underground, defeating public health's larger purpose. Both of them would have thought that they were expressing the rudest common sense, self-evident to all persons of goodwill. Neither might have realized that, in fact, they were giving voice to long-standing, broadly held yet largely unformulated assumptions of their respective public health establishments, indeed of their political cultures.

These basic, unarticulated, yet influential public health presuppositions had originated at the latest a century and a half before the current crisis. During the cholera epidemics of the early nineteenth century, Western nations began assuming the basic preventive stances they would continue. The Mediterranean nations adopted strict quarantinist precautions, fearing the import of contagion via the transport of goods from the Orient, especially with the opening of the Suez Canal in 1869. Britain, conversely, blessed by a position more remote from the immediate avenues of contagious peregrination, and impelled by the imperative logic of its trading prowess, refused to submit to strictures on the flows of traffic across its borders. Instead, it adopted sanitationist methods of cleansing the urban environment, rendering it resistant to contagion. Free trade and public health were not incompatible in its view. For its part, France straddled an epidemiological fault line, contagionist along its Mediterranean shores yet favoring the English approach on the Atlantic. The result was preventive indecision and tergiversation. Germany too vacillated, initially contagionist as the cholera epidemic of 1832 struck its eastern flank, first to be affected among the western European nations. Later, however, it joined the British in resisting French and Mediterranean demands for across-the-board contagionist precautions. The Swedes, in turn, followed a curiously Mediterranean approach—not of course because of any geographic proximity, but because their peripheral location allowed them to close off access at crucial nodal points, and because no compelling commercial interests demanded—as in Britain—more openness. The United States, too, imposed contagionist precautions, fearing the ingress of contagion carried along by successive waves of immigrants.

Such nineteenth-century decisions on the basic orientation of public health reflected fundamental differences among countries in terms of their geographic placement in the flows of contagion, in terms of their topography (could they close off access or were their borders inherently porous), and in terms of the demographic streams that lapped at their shores or left them untouched. Geography, topography, and demography (or what I have elsewhere called geoepidemiology) helped determine each nation's preventive response when faced with onslaughts of epidemic disease in the nineteenth century.[169] Were they among the first struck by cholera in the 1830s, and therefore obliged to respond with no precedence other than the plague and the precautions marshaled against it, as in the case of the German states, especially Prussia? Or did they, like the French and British, enjoy the advantages of a favorable placement along the learning curve, permitting them to observe that drastic quarantinist precautions taken elsewhere proved fruitless and, therefore, to chose more lenient alternatives? Topographic and demographic characteristics encouraged certain responses: the Americans' emphasis on quarantinist strictures at the nodal points through which immigrants arrived, or the Swedes' decision for similar precautions because of their epidemiologically favorable peripheral placement in both geography and the networks of commercial intercourse.

Geoepidemiological factors had played a role a century earlier; it would be unsurprising if they continued to do so. The heavy hand of the past is, of course, not necessarily a dead one. That certain traditions exist does not automatically ensure their continued success. Having failed in the past, policies were sometimes changed. The poor results of locking up thousands of prostitutes, and of the strict controls on the venereally diseased imposed by the Americans early in the century, were taken as good reasons to try a different approach now. The (non-Bavarian) Germans were prompted by the Nazi experience to change preventive tactics during the epidemic, even though they were legislatively well equipped to impose traditional solutions. Nonetheless, the continuity of geoepidemiology's influence remained strong. Nations do not often change their geography or topography, and even basic demographic factors continued to have a similar influence across the decades.

During the AIDS era, one geoepidemiological factor was the colonial connections still, or at least recently, maintained by some nations. In France in 1986, 11 percent of AIDS patients came from Equatorial Africa. Although this diminished thereafter, the African connection remained an issue. The National Front whipped up anxiety over the exposure of soldiers in former French colonies.[170] The Belgian case was clearer. HIV here was spread with striking frequency through heterosexual contact with persons from former African colonies. Almost a quarter of early non-African Belgian AIDS patients had contracted it heterosexually from former residents of central Africa. During the early 1980s, almost three-quarters of Belgian AIDS cases came from Africa. In the Brussels subway, graffiti announced "Black = AIDS" in a way that would have been much less plausible elsewhere.[171] The Belgians and Germans screened African students. The British too, with their continued African military connections, worried about this source of infection, though without drawing any practical conclusions.[172]

In a more general sense, many nations worried about the import of disease from abroad, some with more justification than others. Over one-third of early AIDS patients in Greece had resided in epidemic areas. The overwhelming majority of eastern European cases came at first from abroad. Close to half of Bulgarian AIDS patients were international seafarers.[173] Even more than sex with another male, the main risk factor of those voluntarily tested in Britain during the mid-1990s was having lived in or visited Africa. Of French patients infected heterosexually during the 1980s and early 1990s, three-quarters were from or had partners from Africa or the Caribbean.[174] Of infected Danes, some 14 percent had caught it abroad. Fully half of all heterosexually acquired cases here were suffered by Danes having visited foreign, mostly sub-Saharan, countries. Of Swedes, over half of those infected heterosexually had been so via intercourse abroad. Of nonimmigrant Norwegians, over a quarter were infected outside the nation's borders.[175]

Swedes were among those who most consistently redeployed arguments of the sort they had marshaled in the nineteenth century to justify their prophylactic *Sonderweg*. As then, they considered themselves epidemiologically beleaguered from all sides—not just by the barbarian hordes from Russia and the East. Even the Danes, who during the earlier cholera epidemics had been regarded as epidemiological Continentals and therefore suspect, were now seen as loose living and decadent. Copenhagen exerted a powerful attraction for Swedish gays. As then, the Swedes nonetheless also saw their own geoepidemiological situation as favorable. Thanks to their peripheral position in this, as in so many epidemics (winter may be the single greatest public health intervention in the world, as the economist Jeffrey Sachs once remarked),[176] the Swedes also now enjoyed a favorable placement along the learning curve. In 1985, when deciding to treat seropositivity like other contagious diseases, the government analyzed Sweden's situation hopefully: HIV had not yet reached beyond limited high-risk groups. Decisive intervention promised to restrict its percolation into the general population. Sweden's sparse population density, its extensive countryside with few large cities, offered unfavorable conditions for spread. Its well-developed health system stood readier than most to meet the challenges. Sweden had the advantage of epidemiological backwardness (a three-year delay compared to the United States) in learning from the others' experiences. It was the Swedish authorities' hope that their "small, well-organized country" could act more effectively than sprawling and chaotic nations.[177] Sweden's situation was thus—so ran the implicit argument—like the nations (Iran, Cuba, and countries in eastern Europe) that had not yet been hard hit or indeed hit at all. Slamming the barn door shut was not yet useless. Drastic and quarantinist measures remained more persuasive here than in already infected nations. It was for such reasons that Sweden remained a nation where the headline of the largest daily—filling the entire front page tabloid-style—could announce the death by transmissible disease of a Swedish tourist in the epidemiological morass that is the great abroad, in this case meningitis in Greece.[178] In short, the anxieties and measures prompted by epidemiological Otherness that in the United States were attached also to ethnic minorities at home were focused more exclusively in Sweden on foreigners and Swedish contacts abroad.

Geoepidemiology's influence was felt elsewhere as well. Much as in the days of cholera, the French were hamstrung between different approaches partly determined by geopolitical realities. In the nineteenth century, they had straddled a preventive dilemma that pitted the Mediterranean ports (more fearful of disease import than concerned to preserve trade profits, and therefore quarantinist) against the Atlantic (with reversed priorities). Much as France straddled the butter/oil line, so epidemiologically it was poised astride divergent prophylactic worldviews. During the AIDS era, France experienced at least three different varieties of epidemic: the northern European pattern of transmission primarily among gay men in Paris; the Mediterranean drug-related variety along the southeastern coast, in Marseilles, Cannes, and Nice; and the Third World pattern of spread among heterosexuals in the Antilles and Guiana. French public health officials attributed their unusually high case load to such coincidences.[179] The question remains whether their lackluster response did not also reflect, as it had a century and a half earlier, this peculiar geoepidemiological position. Similar in its juxtaposition of different epidemics within one polity (though different in the lack of a clear north-south divide) was the American case (along with the South African, Chinese, and Brazilian cases), which combined elements of both the gay epidemic and Third World transmission patterns in the ghettos.[180]

Geoepidemiology also played a role in more specific circumstances. Collecting information on the infected, and requiring that the authorities be notified about seropositives, was undermined in nations either so small or subdivided into sufficiently intimate administrative districts that, even with anonymity preserved, it would be easy to guess the identity of the reported. In both Sweden and Switzerland, even anonymous screening was questioned because of the informal knowledge available in small societies.[181] The irregularity of the epidemic's spread—it was regionally bunched in urban areas, sparing the rural hinterlands—influenced the response in all nations, aggravating the perennial tensions between rustic and metropolitan. The approaches taken varied regionally, and local resistance sprang up against directives issued from national centers: between Bonn and Munich, between Paris and the southeast, Rome and Lombardy, London and Edinburgh. But beyond conclusions at this level, geography was not destiny. Different urban areas had different sorts of epidemics: Paris's was gay-focused, while in Marseilles it shared the Mediterranean orbit's focus on drugs; San Francisco's epidemic struck middle-class white gay males, New York's was as much concerned with ethnic minorities and addicts.[182] And urban fears could be displaced abroad. Though the Swedish epidemic was concentrated in the local metropolises of Stockholm, Gothenburg, and Malmö, the education campaigns focused on the dangers emanating from Copenhagen.[183]

Obviously, neither geoepidemiology nor history determined everything. We have looked in detail at the mosaic of factors that help explain why Western nations took such surprisingly divergent approaches to a largely common public health problem. And yet it is also clear that, with the exception of Germany, each of the nations under the microscope here approached AIDS in much the same way that it had dealt with cholera 150 years earlier. One can debate whether similar geoepidemiological factors continued to exert an influence late in the 1900s as they had a century before, or whether the decisions arrived at then acquired a kind of path determinacy that gave past choices purchase on the present, even with the decline of the initial causes. Either way, it is striking both how nations' responses to the epidemic diverged among them and how continuous public health strategies remained over a long duration in a given country.

The choice among strategies was between a communal and an individualistic one. Was society and its protection reason to subordinate individual rights? Or was there a solution that relied on voluntary changes in citizens' behavior without needing to compel them? Despite a general tendency toward individualistic, voluntary, and consensual solutions, nations varied in their political and prophylactic instincts—some more willing to exalt the group and its needs over the individual. The ultimate dilemma raised by the AIDS epidemic is whether—in an age of democratic polities ever more characterized by individualization, an ethos of personal hedonism, and the dissolution of collective solidarities—public goods and communal responses are still possible. Just as we are losing confidence that postpolitical democracies can fight wars any longer—perhaps even in self-defense—so too we find it ever harder to require of the particular citizen any sacrifice for the group. In an era of individuals, are we capable of protecting ourselves against collective threats?

POSTSCRIPT: AIDS IN THE NEW MILLENNIUM

This is a volume of contemporary history. It has to end somewhere. The epidemic, however, has not. In the Third World, it is the most horrendous public health disaster of many centuries. The cause of twenty-five million deaths and forty million infections so far, it strikes the young and economically active, crippling already undeveloped economies and slashing life expectancies. Alas, the metaphors of the Black Death, so overextended in the developed world early in the epidemic, seem only too apt when applied to Africa and possibly parts of Asia. Infection rates among precisely those citizens most crucial for economic progress are skyrocketing. AIDS orphans are raised, if lucky, by their grandparents. Administrations, devastated as cohorts of civil servants fall ill and perish, find it hard to act. In some nations, more teachers die than retire.[184]

In the developed world, in contrast, the disease is becoming manageable—a chronic, though still ultimately fatal, disease. Here, the seropositive has become almost emblematic of the human condition in the era of ever more glaring knowledge of our own mortality. Given accurate information about our genetic foibles, we will soon all know the date of our likely death and its specific cause, and we will pass what remains of our lives in the shadow of that insight—much as seropositives do now.[185] AIDS has become almost routinized and treatable, if not yet curable. AZT was the first major breakthrough, followed in the mid-1990s by protease and entry inhibitors. Highly active antiretroviral therapy has now made AIDS a disease more like cancer than the plague.

In the meantime, public health has moved from the margins to the center of politics. AIDS put it on the front pages along with resurgences of classic epidemic diseases. New, viciously infectious diseases grabbed the headlines. Anthrax became a weapon of terrorism, and, after 9/11, Western military leaders feared the possibility of suicide smallpox spreaders. Did AIDS bring a new orientation in the balance between individual rights and the community's hopes to protect itself? This claim would have been undermined by the repoliticization of public health even had there been no independent reasons for questioning it. As we have seen, some have argued that the AIDS epidemic was treated in an exceptionalist manner. Rather than imposing traditional strictures on its victims, modern public health realized that AIDS victims' civil rights had to be respected.[186] And yet we have also seen that this view of AIDS exceptionalism is doubtful. A consensual approach was pursued only for a short period in certain nations. Some countries, like Sweden and parts of Germany, were happy to continue old-fashioned tactics. Even where a more voluntarist approach was followed, it was gradually weakened by other developments. Once gays were no longer the primary victims, patients' civil rights were emphasized less. Once treatments were available, inherited measures had logic, and not just precedence, on their side.[187]

Reactions to other epidemic diseases also demonstrated that, even if AIDS was treated unusually, this was more an exception than the harbinger of a sea change in public health. Victims of tuberculosis who were considered unable to follow a protracted regimen of treatment on their own were medicated while under official custody to prevent drug-resistant strains from developing. With the SARS epidemic of 2003, the traditional artillery of public health was wheeled out once again. In China, tens of thousands were quarantined, and the authorities threatened to execute any who deliberately spread the disease. Visitors to Singapore were passed through thermal scanners to detect the feverish. American authorities were granted powers to detain suspected victims against their will. In New York City, an arrival from Asia with symptoms was compulsorily quarantined.[188]

In retrospect and seen comparatively, the exceptional approach to AIDS taken by public health may have been just that, an exception. Some nations may have adopted a consensual strategy for a certain phase of the epidemic's development. But will exceptionalism characterize approaches to the epidemic in the future? In more than a sampling of nations? Does it foreshadow any more thoroughgoing change in public health strategies? For such questions the answers seem uncertain. More broadly, are there lessons to be drawn from the experience of the West by other parts of the world? There is no lockstep between democracy and a certain style of disease prevention. Obviously, a system that pays attention to individual rights and the claims of minorities, however defined, will be more inclined than an authoritarian one to tread lightly in disease prevention. And yet, even here, the Swedish and—to a lesser extent—the American experience shows that the classic dilemma of liberal politics raises its head in disease prevention. The claims of the majority to security have here ridden more roughly over individuals' rights than in other developed nations.

Democracy has expanded with heartening inexorability during the post–cold war period. Yet any direct translation into a consensual approach to epidemic disease control is hard to detect. The nations of the former East Bloc have seen little cause to modify quarantinist public health precautions inherited from a totalitarian past, when, in turn, they had been taken over from authoritarian predecessors. In the Third World, the problem is less preexisting legislation than a lack of effective measures. Only 17 percent of the world's nations, with about 5 percent of global AIDS cases, enjoy specific legislation protecting the epidemic's victims against social discrimination. Only 11 percent have measures to promote condom use. Few of these countries are in the developing world. In contrast, a quarter of the world's population lives under legal regimes that allow victims of the epidemic to be quarantined.[189]

Many developing nations began democratizing around the same time as the epidemic, and many will start and continue to do so in years to come. What influence, if any, will such political changes have on public health? And vice versa? Government authority must be transparent and accountable to be legitimate; it must be effective and efficient to be enforceable. Complaints of the sort heard in Kenya, that the National AIDS Control Council kept to itself, refusing to speak to the press and failing to win the public's confidence, threaten to undermine preventive efforts.[190] If education and persuasion are to be central to prevention, a free, independent, and trustworthy mass media are required. Moreover, because illicit behavior remains a significant avenue of transmission, even in the Third World, taboos must be broken. In India, for example, after *Jasoos Vijay*, a TV detective series, dealt with the issue, 40 percent of its audience of 150 million discussed AIDS.[191] If consensual efforts require an unstigmatizing approach, can this be reconciled with customs prevalent in parts of the developing world that treat sexual minorities, not to mention women, appallingly? If potential victims are to be persuaded to change their behavior, how does one deal with traditional, prescientific forms of medicine that claim, and convince their clients, that they are able to cure the disease?[192]

More broadly, if modern public health depends on citizens' self-policing and their adherence to the standards of risk avoidance, how uniform does this require conduct to be throughout the world? Must other cultures now adopt behavioral norms determined in, and possibly dictated by, the industrialized world? If so, is this a form of cultural imperialism or merely a part of the benign globalization that is proceeding apace anyhow? Do American-style civil liberties make sense in developing nations? Or will leaders there argue that they are unaffordable or culturally untransplantable?[193] Even observers from the English-speaking professorate, lucky enough not to have to chose in the trade-off they themselves suggest, see an emphasis on civil rights in epidemics as a lesser substitution for more thorough social and economic reform.[194] If rigorous protection of individual liberties is no longer the centerpiece of AIDS policies in the First World, what is the likelihood of it being repeated in the Third? Will the exceptionalism of the response to AIDS, partial as it was, be skipped entirely in developing nations?

Being optimistic, may we hope for new relations between First and Third Worlds, partly prompted by AIDS? Certainly the increasing recognition that the epidemic has international security implications, that it threatens to destabilize a large part of the globe, encourages the industrialized West not to ignore its developing cousins. The movement to override market principles in the pricing of new medicines in the Third World bespeaks an unprecedented—however limited—sense of international solidarity. To be sure, public health issues, broadly speaking, are being recognized as unsolvable within national borders. When Chernobyl made vegetables radioactive throughout central Europe, nuclear energy became everyone's problem. When Australians breathe the smoke of Indonesian farmers' fires, air pollution is no longer a matter to be solved within any one region. In the age of mass tourism, contagious disease inherently becomes a global issue. Epidemiologically, the world is more interconnected than ever. The fear of disease is the dark side of globalization.[195] High-speed trains, jet airplanes, hotel rooms, and fold-out sofas were the main facilitators in recent epidemics, whether cholera arriving in California from Latin America, Marburg fever in Marburg from Africa, SARS in Toronto from China, AIDS in San Francisco from Haiti and the Dominican Republic, or syphilis in Tokyo or Düsseldorf from Bangkok.

In the nineteenth century, the ever denser interconnections among social classes in rapidly growing cities helped prompt the better-off to realize that they could not ignore the plight of the dispossessed except at their own peril.[196] Not altruism, in other words, but mutual dependence and self-protection were the motor forces of the early welfare state—and much stronger motives for solidaristic reform than mere charitable instinct.[197] If there is any lining in this epidemic with even a glint of silver, it may be that, finally, the First World is coming to realize that it cannot ignore the Third without harming itself. Let us not, however, think about the price that has been paid for this insight, if insight it proves to be. Down that road lies madness.

Notes

INTRODUCTION: SLAVES TO THE PAST

1. Lars Magnusson, "The Role of Path Dependence in the History of Regulation," in Magnusson and Jan Ottosson, eds., *The State, Regulation, and the Economy: A Historical Perspective* (Cheltenham, U.K., 2001), p. 111.

2. Some of the classics of the field are Douglass C. North, *Institutions, Institutional Change, and Economic Performance* (Cambridge, 1990); W. Brian Arthur, *Increasing Returns and Path Dependence in the Economy* (Ann Arbor, 1994); Jack A. Goldstone, "Initial Conditions, General Laws, Path Dependence, and Explanation in Historical Sociology," *American Journal of Sociology* 104, 3 (1998); Stanley Liebowitz and Steven Margolis, "Path Dependence, Lock In, and History," *Journal of Law, Economics, and Organization* 11, 1 (1995).

3. Paul A. David, "Understanding the Economics of QWERTY: The Necessity of History," in William N. Parker, ed., *Economic History and the Modern Economist* (Oxford, 1986); Stanley Liebowitz and Stephen Margolis, "The Fable of the Keys," *Journal of Law and Economics* 33, 1 (April 1990).

4. Jacob S. Hacker, *The Divided Welfare State: The Battle over Public and Private Social Benefits in the United States* (Cambridge, 2002), p. 55.

5. James F. Tent, *Mission on the Rhine* (Chicago, 1983); Jerzy Hausner, Bob Jessop, and Klaus Nielsen, eds., *Strategic Choice and Path Dependency in Post-Socialism: Institutional Dynamics in the Transformation Process* (Brookfield, VT, 1995).

1. BODILY FLUIDS AND CITIZENSHIP

1. Nancy Tomes, "The Making of a Germ Panic, Then and Now," *American Journal of Public Health* 90, 2 (February 2000), p. 192.

2. Dorothy Nelkin, "Cultural Perspectives on Blood," in Eric A. Feldman and Ronald Bayer, eds., *Blood Feuds: AIDS, Blood, and the Politics of Medical Disaster* (New York, 1999), pp. 284–87.

3. Bernadette Pratt Sadler, "When Rape Victims' Rights Meet Privacy Rights: Mandatory HIV Testing, Striking the Fourth Amendment Balance," *Washington Law Review* 67 (1992), pp. 203–4.

4. Arthur and Marilouise Kroker, "Panic Sex in America," in Arthur and Marilouise Kroker, eds., *Body Invaders: Sexuality and the Postmodern Condition* (London, 1988), p. 10; William G. Staples, *The Culture of Surveillance: Discipline and Social Control in the United States* (New York, 1997), pp. 95–96; John Gilliom, *Surveillance, Privacy, and the Law: Employee Drug Testing and the Politics of Social Control* (Ann Arbor, 1997), p. 6; F. Allan Hanson, *Testing Testing: Social Consequences of the Examined Life* (Berkeley, 1993), pp. 131–32.

5. Jean-François Fogel and Bertrand Rosenthal, *Fin de siècle à la Havane: Les secrets du pouvoir cubain* (Paris, 1993), p. 364.

6. Henry E. Sigerist, "Kultur und Krankheit," *Kyklos* 1 (1928), p. 62. Similarly: Hans Halter, ed., *Todesseuchen AIDS* (Reinbek, 1985), p. 22.

7. Jean Baudrillard, *The Transparency of Evil: Essays on Extreme Phenomena* (London, 1993), pp. 63–67; Ian Young, *The AIDS Dissidents: An Annotated Bibliography* (Metuchen, NJ, 1993), p. 130 and passim; Susan J. Palmer, "AIDS as Metaphor," *Society* 26 (1989), p. 48; Kathleen Kete, "*La rage* and the Bourgeoisie: The Cultural Context of Rabies in the French Nineteenth Century," *Representations* 22 (1988), pp. 93–94; Boris Velimirovic, "NATC: A Delusive Approach," *AIDS-Forschung* 5 (1993), pp. 261–62.

8. Susan Sontag, *AIDS and Its Metaphors* (New York, 1989), p. 10.

9. Elaine Showalter, *Sexual Anarchy: Gender and Culture at the Fin de Siècle* (New York, 1990), pp. 188–90; Werner Thönnessen, *The Emancipation of Women: The Rise and Decline of the Women's Movement in German Social Democracy 1863–1933* (London, 1973), pp. 22, 37; *Sitzungsberichte der verfassunggebenden Preussischen Landesversammlung*, 1919–21, 25 February 1920, col. 9946–47; Fernand Mignot, *Le péril vénérien et la prophylaxie des maladies vénériennes* (Paris, 1905), p. 145; Norman Naimark, *The Russians in Germany: A History of the Soviet Zone of Occupation, 1945–1949* (Cambridge, MA, 1995), p. 97.

10. André Glucksmann, *La fêlure du monde: Éthique et sida* (n.p., 1994), p. 120; Marita Sturken, *Tangled Memories: The Vietnam War, the AIDS Epidemic, and the Politics of Remembering* (Berkeley, 1997), p. 167; Michael Pollak, "Attitudes, Beliefs, and Opinions," in Michael Pollak, ed., *AIDS: A Problem for Sociological Research* (London, 1992), p. 24; Johannes Gründel, "AIDS—eine ethische Herausforderung an die Christen," in Bistum Essen, ed., *AIDS—eine medizinische und eine moralische Herausforderung* (Nettetal, n.d.), pp. 39–40.

11. Baudrillard, *Transparency of Evil*, pp. 8–9.

12. Peter Baldwin, *Contagion and the State in Europe, 1830–1930* (Cambridge, 1999), pp. 284–86; Stephanie C. Kane, *AIDS Alibis: Sex, Drugs, and Crime in the Americas* (Philadelphia, 1998), pp. 55–56; Gayle S. Rubin, "Elegy for the Valley of the Kings: AIDS and the Leather Community in San Francisco, 1981–1996," in Martin P. Levine et al., eds., *In Changing Times: Gay Men and Lesbians Encounter HIV/AIDS* (Chicago, 1997), p. 111; Jenny Kitzinger and

David Miller, " 'African AIDS': The Media and Audience Beliefs," in Peter Aggleton et al., eds., *AIDS: Rights, Risk, and Reason* (London, 1992), p. 40.

13. Stuart Close, "Vaccine Virus and Degeneration," *Anti-Vaccinator: Illustrated Annual of the International Antivaccination-League*, ed. H. Molenaar, 1 (1911), p. 30; Nils Thyresson, *Från Fransoser till AIDS: Kapitel ur de veneriska sjukdomarnas historia i Sverige* (n.p., 1991), pp. 32–33.

14. Nicolas Mauriac, *Le mal entendu: Le sida et les médias* (Paris, 1990), pp. 141–43; Renée Sabatier, *Blaming Others* (Philadelphia, 1988), p. 43.

15. Manuel Carballo, "Le rôle des facteurs sociaux et comportementaux dans l'infection par le HIV et dans le SIDA," in Jean Martin, ed., *Faire face au SIDA* (Lausanne, 1988), p. 70; Memo by David Miller, House of Commons, 1986–87, Social Services Committee, *Problems Associated with AIDS*, 13 May 1987, vol. 2, p. 157; Paula A. Treichler, "AIDS, HIV, and the Cultural Construction of Reality," in Gilbert Herdt and Shirley Lindenbaum, eds., *The Time of AIDS* (Newbury Park, 1992); Elizabeth Fee and Nancy Krieger, "Understanding AIDS: Historical Interpretations and the Limits of Biomedical Individualism," *American Journal of Public Health* 83, 10 (October 1993), pp. 1482–83; Tim Rhodes, "Risk, Injecting Drug Use, and the Myth of an Objective Social Science," in Joshua Oppenheimer and Helena Reckitt, eds., *Acting on AIDS: Sex, Drugs, and Politics* (London, 1997), p. 60; Casper G. Schmidt, "The Group-Fantasy Origin of AIDS," *Journal of Psychohistory* 12, 1 (1984); David Caron, *AIDS in French Culture: Social Ills, Literary Cures* (Madison, 2001), pp. 96–87.

16. Daniel Borrillo, "AIDS and Human Rights: A Societal Choice," in Daniel Borrillo and Anne Masseran, eds., *Sida et droits de l'homme: L'épidémie dans un Etat de droit* (Strasbourg, 1991), pp. 222, 238, 248; François Bachelot and Pierre Lorane, *Une société au risque du sida* (Paris, 1988), p. 22; BT *Verhandlungen* 11/8, 2 April 1987, p. 427B; Eric Fuchs, "Le SIDA, réflexions éthiques," in Jean Martin, ed., *Faire face au SIDA* (Lausanne, 1988), p. 60; RD *Prot*, 1986/87:50 (16 December 1986), p. 7.

17. *Congressional Record* (House), 30 June 1987, 133, p. 18379.

18. Simon Watney, *Practices of Freedom: Selected Writings on HIV/AIDS* (Durham, NC, 1994), pp. 26, 49–52, 58–59, 118–19.

19. Christopher Hamlin, *Public Health and Social Justice in the Age of Chadwick: Britain, 1800–1854* (Cambridge, 1998).

20. Christopher Hamlin, "State Medicine in Great Britain," in Dorothy Porter, ed., *The History of Public Health and the Modern State* (Amsterdam, 1994), pp. 135–36.

21. Lion Murard and Patrick Zylberman, *L'hygiène dans la république: La santé publique en France, ou l'utopie contrariée (1870–1918)* (Paris, 1996); Anthony S. Wohl, *Endangered Lives: Public Health in Victorian Britain* (London, 1983).

22. Elizabeth Fee and Dorothy Porter, "Public Health, Preventive Medicine, and Professionalization: Britain and the United States in the Nineteenth Century," in Elizabeth Fee and Roy M. Acheson, eds., *A History of Education in*

Public Health (Oxford, 1991), pp. 33–35; John Duffy, *The Sanitarians: A History of American Public Health* (Urbana, 1990), p. 206.

23. Elizabeth Fee, *Disease and Discovery: A History of the Johns Hopkins School of Hygiene and Public Health, 1916–1939* (Baltimore, 1987), pp. 20–21; Barron H. Lerner, *Contagion and Confinement: Controlling Tuberculosis along the Skid Road* (Baltimore, 1998), p. 170; Judith Walzer Leavitt, *Typhoid Mary: Captive to the Public's Health* (Boston, 1996), pp. 23–25.

24. Dorothy Porter, ed., *The History of Public Health and the Modern State* (Amsterdam, 1994), pp. 124, 237–39.

25. Margaret Humphreys, *Yellow Fever and the South* (New Brunswick, 1992), p. 122.

26. Paul Starr, *The Social Transformation of American Medicine* (New York, 1982), pp. 189–94.

27. From the now massive literature spawned by this approach, begun by Norbert Elias and elaborated most prominently by Foucault: Colin Jones and Roy Porter, eds., *Reassessing Foucault: Power, Medicine, and the Body* (London, 1994); Graham Burchell et al., eds., *The Foucault Effect: Studies in Governmentality* (Chicago, 1991); Johan Goudsblom, "Zivilisation, Ansteckungsangst und Hygiene: Betrachtungen über ein Aspekt des europäischen Zivilisationsprozesses," in Peter Gleichmann et al., eds., *Materialen zu Norbert Elias' Zivilisationstheorie* (Frankfurt, 1977); Nikolas Rose, *Governing the Soul: The Shaping of the Private Self,* 2d ed. (London, 1999).

28. Françoise Hildesheimer, *La terreur et la pitié: L'ancien régime à l'épreuve de la peste* (Paris, 1990), p. 24.

29. Jane Lewis, *What Price Community Medicine? The Philosophy, Practice, and Politics of Public Health since 1919* (Brighton, 1986), pp. 5–6, 19–20.

30. David S. Barnes, *The Making of a Social Disease: Tuberculosis in Nineteenth-Century France* (Berkeley, 1995), pp. 14–15; Nancy Tomes, *The Gospel of Germs: Men, Women, and the Microbe in American Life* (Cambridge, MA, 1998), p. 105.

31. Dora B. Weiner, *The Citizen-Patient in Revolutionary and Imperial Paris* (Baltimore, 1993).

32. Gunnar Broberg and Mattias Tydén, *Oönskade i folkhemmet: Rashygien och sterilisering i Sverige* (Stockholm, 1991); Maija Runcis, *Steriliseringar i folkhemmet* (Stockholm, 1998); Maciej Zaremba, *De rena och de andra: Om tvångssteriliseringar, rashygien och arvsynd* (n.p., 1999); Gunnar Broberg and Nils Roll-Hansen, eds., *Eugenics and the Welfare State* (East Lansing, 1996); Stefan Kuhl, *The Nazi Connection: Eugenics, American Racism, and German National Socialism* (Oxford, 1994); Patrick Zylberman, "Les damnés de la démocratie puritaine: Stérilisations en Scandinavie, 1929–1977," *Le Mouvement Social* 187 (1999), pp. 99–125.

33. Michael Burleigh and Wolfgang Wippermann, *The Racial State: Germany, 1933–1945* (Cambridge, 1991), p. 290; Mark Mazower, *Dark Continent: Europe's Twentieth Century* (New York, 1999), ch. 3; Robert N. Proctor, *The Nazi War on Cancer* (Princeton, 1999), pp. 124–25.

34. Jane Lewis, "The Public's Health: Philosophy and Practice in Britain in the Twentieth Century," in Elizabeth Fee and Roy M. Acheson, eds., *A History of Education in Public Health* (Oxford, 1991), pp. 198, 204.

35. Rüdiger Jacob, *Krankheitsbilder und Deutungsmuster: Wissen über Krankheit und dessen Bedeutung für die Praxis* (Opladen, 1995), p. 278; Daniel M. Fox, "AIDS and the American Health Polity: The History and Prospects of a Crisis of Authority," *Milbank Quarterly* 64, suppl. 1 (1986), pp. 8–12; Charles Rosenberg, "Banishing Risk: Continuity and Change in the Moral Management of Disease," in Allan M. Brandt and Paul Rozin, eds., *Morality and Health* (New York, 1997), p. 37; Barbara Gutmann Rosenkrantz, *Public Health and the State: Changing Views in Massachusetts, 1842–1936* (Cambridge, MA, 1972), p. 145.

36. Peter N. Stearns, *Battleground of Desire: The Struggle for Self-Control in Modern America* (New York, 1999).

37. Bryan S. Turner, *The Body and Society: Explorations in Social Theory,* 2d ed. (London, 1996), p. 210; Stephen Davies, *The Historical Origins of Health Fascism* (London, 1991); Proctor, *Nazi War on Cancer,* p. 12.

38. Allan M. Brandt, "Behavior, Disease, and Health in the Twentieth-Century United States," in Allan M. Brandt and Paul Rozin, eds., *Morality and Health* (New York, 1997), pp. 68–69; Jonathan Mann et al., "Toward a New Health Strategy to Control the HIV/AIDS Pandemic," *Journal of Law, Medicine, and Ethics* 22, 1 (1994), p. 49; Richard G. Parker, "Empowerment, Community Mobilization, and Social Change in the Face of HIV/AIDS," *AIDS,* 10, suppl. 3 (1996), pp. S28–29; Tim Rhodes, "Individual and Community Action in HIV Prevention," in Tim Rhodes and Richard Hartnoll, eds., *AIDS, Drugs, and Prevention* (London, 1996), pp. 1–2; Paul Farmer, "Women, Poverty, and AIDS," in Farmer et al., eds., *Women, Poverty, and AIDS: Sex, Drugs, and Structural Violence* (Monroe, ME, 1996), pp. 28–29.

39. Admittedly an exaggeration. While smokers appear to pay for the external costs imposed by their habits via taxes on tobacco, the same does not hold for drinkers of alcohol. William G. Manning et al., "The Taxes of Sin: Do Smokers and Drinkers Pay Their Way?" *JAMA* 261, 11 (1989), p. 1608.

40. Chris Bennett and Ewan Ferlie, *Managing Crisis and Change in Health Care: The Organizational Response to HIV/AIDS* (Buckingham, 1994), pp. 37–39.

41. Dorothy Porter, *Health, Civilization, and the State: A History of Public Health from Ancient to Modern Times* (London, 1999), pp. 291–96; Barnes, *Making of a Social Disease,* p. 220; David McBride, *From TB to AIDS: Epidemics among Urban Blacks since 1900* (Albany, 1991), pp. 32, 48.

42. Elizabeth W. Etheride, "Pellagra: An Unappreciated Reminder of Southern Distinctiveness," in Todd L. Savitt and James Harvey Young, eds., *Disease and Distinctiveness in the American South* (Knoxville, 1988); Milton Terris, "The Changing Relationships of Epidemiology and Society: The Robert Cruikshank Lecture," *Journal of Public Health Policy* 6 (1985), pp. 19–23.

43. For lessons drawn for AIDS from this example: Joan Shenton, *Positively False: Exposing the Myths around HIV and AIDS* (London, 1998), p. xxix.

44. Baldwin, *Contagion and the State*, pp. 21–23; Dennis Altman, *Power and Community: Organizational and Cultural Responses to AIDS* (London, 1994), pp. 16–17; Neil Small, "The Changing Context of Health Care in the UK: Implications for HIV/AIDS," in Peter Aggleton et al., eds., *AIDS: Foundations for the Future* (London, 1994), p. 27.

45. Richard Wilkinson, *Unhealthy Societies: The Afflictions of Inequality* (London, 1996); Nancy Adler et al., "Socioeconomic Status and Health: The Challenge of the Gradient," in Jonathan M. Mann et al., eds., *Health and Human Rights* (New York, 1999), p. 182; Klaus Hurrelmann, *Sozialisation und Gesundheit: Somatische, psychische und soziale Risikofaktoren im Lebenslauf* (Weinheim, 1988); Richard Smith, *Unemployment and Health* (Oxford, 1987); Mel Bartley, *Authorities and Partisans: The Debate on Unemployment and Health* (Edinburgh, 1992); Andreas Mielck, ed., *Krankheit und soziale Ungleichheit* (Opladen, 1994); Finn Diderichsen et al., eds., *Klass och ohälsa* (n.p., 1991); Ralf Schwarzer and Anja Leppin, *Sozialer Rückhalt und Gesundheit* (Göttingen, 1989).

46. Martin J. Walker, *Dirty Medicine: Science, Big Business, and the Assault on Health Care*, rev. ed. (London, 1994), ch. 7.

47. Ulrich Beck, *Risk Society: Towards a New Modernity* (Newbury Park, CA, 1992).

48. Tim Rhodes, "Outreach, Community Change, and Community Empowerment: Contradictions for Public Health and Health Promotion," in Peter Aggleton et al., eds., *AIDS: Foundations for the Future* (London, 1994), pp. 49, 58–60.

49. John J. Hanlon and George E. Pickett, *Public Health: Administration and Practice*, 8th ed. (St. Louis, 1984), p. 4. Similarly: International Federation of Red Cross and Red Crescent Societies, *AIDS, Health, and Human Rights: An Explanatory Manual* (n.p., 1995), p. 31.

50. Jonathan M. Mann et al., "Health and Human Rights," *Health and Human Rights* 1, 1 (1994), p. 20.

51. R. S. Downie et al., *Health Promotion: Models and Values*, 2d ed. (Oxford, 1996), pp. 1–4, 19–20, 34–37.

52. Steve Kroll-Smith and H. Hugh Floyd, *Bodies in Protest: Environmental Illness and the Struggle over Medical Illness* (New York, 1997), pp. 1–2; Deborah Lupton, *The Imperative of Health: Public Health and the Regulated Body* (London, 1995), p. 50; Meredith Minkler, "Health Education, Health Promotion, and the Open Society: An Historical Perspective," *Health Education Quarterly* 16, 1 (1989), pp. 24–25; Bryan S. Turner, *Regulating Bodies* (London, 1992), pp. 130–31.

53. Erwin H. Ackerknecht, "Anticontagionism between 1821 and 1867," *Bulletin of the History of Medicine* 22, 5 (September–October 1948); Erwin H. Ackerknecht, *Medicine at the Paris Hospital, 1794–1848* (Baltimore, 1967), pp. 156–57; Henry E. Sigerist, *Civilization and Disease* (Ithaca, 1944), p. 91.

54. Saul Friedländer, *Nazi Germany and the Jews* (New York, 1997), 1:100; Burleigh and Wippermann, *Racial State*, p. 107; Marcel Reich-Ranicki, *Mein*

Leben (Stuttgart, 1999), pp. 205–7; Paul Weindling, *Epidemics and Genocide in Eastern Europe, 1890–1945* (Oxford, 2000), pp. 273–74; Proctor, *Nazi War on Cancer,* p. 46.

55. James C. Scott, *Seeing Like a State: How Certain Schemes to Improve the Human Condition Have Failed* (New Haven, 1998), p. 155.

56. Baldwin, *Contagion and the State,* ch. 5.

57. Fee and Krieger, "Understanding AIDS," pp. 1481–83; Cindy Patton, *Inventing AIDS* (New York, 1990), p. 18; Tony Barnett and Alan Whiteside, *AIDS in the Twenty-first Century: Disease and Globalization* (Houndmills, U.K., 2002), ch. 3.

58. Jon Cohen, "The Duesberg Phenomenon," *Science* 266 (1994), pp. 1642–49; Steven B. Harris, "The AIDS Heresies: A Case Study in Skepticism Taken Too Far," *Skeptic* 3, 2 (1995).

59. Nancy F. McKenzie, ed., *The AIDS Reader: Social Political and Ethical Issues* (New York, 1991), sect. 1; Barry D. Adam, "The State, Public Policy, and AIDS Discourse," *Contemporary Crises* 13 (1989), p. 8; *Newsweek* 28 August 2000, pp. 54–56; James Monroe Smith, *AIDS and Society* (Upper Saddle River, NJ, 1996), pp. 26–28.

60. *New York Times,* 19 March 2000, p. 9; 23 April 2000, p. 10; 7 May 2000, p. 15; 14 May 2000, sect. 4, p. 4; *Economist,* 3 November 2001, p. 82; Chris McGreal, "Thabo Mbeki's Catastrophe," *Prospect* (March 2002), pp. 42–47; Catherine Campbell, *"Letting Them Die": Why HIV/AIDS Intervention Programmes Fail* (Oxford, 2003), p. 158.

61. *Los Angeles Times,* 10 July 2000, p. A11; *New York Times,* 9 July 2000, p. A15.

62. Meredeth Turshen, "Is AIDS Primarily a Sexually Transmitted Disease?" in Nadine Job-Spira et al., eds., *Santé publique et maladies à transmission sexuelle* (Montrouge, 1990), p. 347; Michel Jossay and Yves Donadieu, *Le SIDA* (Paris, 1987), pp. 167–79; Mauriac, *Le mal entendu,* pp. 76–77; Rolf Rosenbrock, "The Role of Policy in Effective Prevention and Education," in Dorothee Friedrich and Wolfgang Heckmann, eds., *Aids in Europe: The Behavioural Aspect* (Berlin, 1995), 5:25–26; Rolf Rosenbrock, "Aids-Prävention und die Aufgaben der Sozialwissenschaften," in Rolf Rosenbrock and Andreas Salmen, eds., *Aids-Prävention* (Berlin, 1990), p. 18; Gene M. Shearer and Ursula Hurtenbach, "Is Sperm Immunosuppressive in Male Homosexuals and Vasectomized Men?" *Immunology Today* 3, 6 (1982), pp. 153–54; G. M. Shearer and A. S. Rabson, "Semen and AIDS," *Nature* 308, 5956 (15 March 1984), p. 230; Henri H. Mollaret, "The Socio-Ecological Interpretation of the Appearance of Really New Infections," in Charles Mérieux, ed., *SIDA: Épidémies et sociétés* (n.p., 1987), p. 112; Paula A. Treichler, "AIDS, Homophobia, and Biomedical Discourse: An Epidemic of Signification," in Douglas Crimp, ed., *AIDS: Cultural Analysis, Cultural Activism* (Cambridge, 1988), pp. 53–54; J. A. Sonnabend, "The Etiology of AIDS," *AIDS Research* 1, 1 (1983), p. 9; Peter H. Duesberg, *Infectious AIDS: Have We Been Misled?* (Berkeley, 1995), pp. 328–33, 539; Peter Duesberg, ed., *AIDS: Virus- or Drug Induced?* (Dordrecht, 1996), pp. 71, 78, 179; Peter Dues-

berg, *Inventing the AIDS Virus* (Washington, DC, 1996), chs. 7, 8, pp. 595–96; Robert S. Root-Bernstein, *Rethinking AIDS: The Tragic Cost of Premature Consensus* (New York, 1993), pp. 26–30, ch. 10; Jad Adams, *AIDS: The HIV Myth* (New York, 1989), ch. 4; Walker, *Dirty Medicine*, ch. 16.

63. *Nature* 406 (2000), pp. 15–16.

64. Young, *AIDS Dissidents*, p. 2; Bernard Paillard, *Notes on the Plague Years: AIDS in Marseilles* (New York, 1998), ch. 7.

65. Raymond A. Smith, *Encyclopedia of AIDS* (Chicago, 1998), p. 5; John Nguyet Erni, *Unstable Frontiers: Technomedicine and the Cultural Politics of "Curing" AIDS* (Minneapolis, 1994), pp. 8–12.

66. Duesberg, *Infectious AIDS*, pp. 333, 336–38, 539; Paul E. Pezza, "The Viral Model for AIDS: Paradigmatic Dominance, Politics, or Best Approximation of Reality?" in David Buchanan and George Cernada, eds., *Progress in Preventing AIDS? Dogma, Dissent, and Innovation* (Amityville, NY, 1998), pp. 123–27; Steven Epstein, *Impure Science: AIDS, Activism, and the Politics of Knowledge* (Berkeley, 1996), chs. 2–4.

67. John Hardie, *AIDS, Dentistry, and the Illusion of Infection Control: Questioning the HIV Hypothesis* (Lewiston, NY, 1995); John Lauritsen, *The AIDS War: Propaganda, Profiteering, and Genocide from the Medical-Industrial Complex* (New York, 1993); Harris, "AIDS Heresies," p. 48.

68. Elinor Burkett, *The Gravest Show on Earth: America in the Age of AIDS* (Boston, 1995), ch. 2; Epstein, *Impure Science*, p. 129; Joan H. Fujimura and Danny Y. Chou, "Dissent in Science: Styles of Scientific Practice and the Controversy over the Cause of AIDS," *Social Science and Medicine* 38, 8 (1994), p. 1020.

69. Harris, "AIDS Heresies," p. 58; Jonathan M. Mann and Daniel J. M. Tarantola, eds., *AIDS in the World II* (New York, 1996), p. 430.

70. Mirko D. Grmek, *History of AIDS* (Princeton, 1990), pp. 157–58; William A. Rushing, *The AIDS Epidemic: Social Dimensions of an Infectious Disease* (Boulder, 1995), p. 39.

71. Marie A. Muir, *The Environmental Contexts of AIDS* (New York, 1991); Ute Canaris, "Gesundheitspolitische Aspekte im Zusammenhang mit AIDS," in Johannes Korporal and Hubert Malouschek, eds., *Leben mit AIDS — Mit AIDS leben* (Hamburg, 1987), p. 279; Rolf Rosenbrock, "AIDS and Preventive Health Policy," *Veröffentlichungsreihe des Internationalen Instituts für vergleichende Gesellschaftsforschung/Arbeitspolitik des Wissenschaftszentrums Berlin*, IIVG/pre87–208 (Berlin, May 1987), p. 22; Scott Burris, "Public Health, 'AIDS Exceptionalism' and the Law," *John Marshall Law Review* 27 (1994), p. 272.

72. Jean-Paul Lévy, preface to Jacques Foyer and Lucette Khaïat, *Droit et Sida: Comparaison internationale* (Paris, 1994), p. 5; Gerald M. Oppenheimer, "In the Eye of the Storm: The Epidemiological Construction of AIDS," in Elizabeth Fee and Daniel M. Fox, eds., *AIDS: The Burdens of History* (Berkeley, 1988), p. 291.

73. Fee and Krieger, "Understanding AIDS," pp. 1477–78, 1481–83; Jonathan M. Mann et al., "Health and Human Rights," in Mann et al., eds.,

Health and Human Rights (New York, 1999), p. 17; Paul Farmer, *Infections and Inequalities: The Modern Plagues* (Berkeley, 1999), p. 52.

74. Tamsin Wilton, *EnGendering AIDS: Deconstructing Sex, Text, and Epidemic* (London, 1997), pp. 51–52.

75. *Los Angeles Times*, 23 May 2000, p. A6; 10 July 2000, p. A11. However, antiretrovirals were allowed in state hospitals as of the spring of 2002. *Economist*, 27 April 2002, p. 78.

76. Mann et al., "Toward a New Health Strategy to Control the HIV/AIDS Pandemic," pp. 49–50; Jonathan Mann, "Global AIDS: Revolution, Paradigm, and Solidarity," *AIDS* 4, suppl. 1 (1990), p. S249. On Mann, see Peter Söderholm, *Global Governance of AIDS: Partnerships with Civil Society* (Lund, 1997), ch. 9; Scott Burris and Lawrence O. Gostin, "The Impact of HIV/AIDS on the Development of Public Health Law," in Ronald O. Valdiserri, ed., *Dawning Answers: How the HIV/AIDS Epidemic Has Helped to Strengthen Public Health* (Oxford, 2003), pp. 108–9.

77. P. Gillies et al., "Is AIDS a Disease of Poverty?" *AIDS Care* 8, 3 (1996), p. 353; Margaret Connors, "Sex, Drugs, and Structural Violence: Unraveling the Epidemic among Poor Women in the United States," in Farmer, *Women, Poverty, and AIDS*, pp. 92–93; Lawrence Gostin and Lane Porter, eds., *International Law and AIDS* (n.p., 1992), p. 263; Kane, *AIDS Alibis*, pp. 5, 33; Rolf Rosenbrock, "Strategie und Politik für wirksame AIDS-Prävention," *AIDS-Forschung* 2 (1994), p. 90.

78. Richard G. Parker, "Empowerment, Community Mobilization, and Social Change in the Face of HIV/AIDS," *AIDS* 10, suppl. 3 (1996), pp. S28–30.

79. Frank Becker and Klaus-Dieter Beisswenger, eds., *Solidarität der Uneinsichtigen: Aktionstag 9. Juli 1988 Frankfurt a.M.* (Berlin, 1988), p. 14.

80. S. R. Friedman and D. C. Des Jarlais, "HIV among Drug Injectors: The Epidemic and the Response," *AIDS Care* 3, 3 (1991), p. 242; Samuel R. Friedman et al., "Multiple Racial/Ethnic Subordination and HIV among Drug Injectors," in Merrill Singer, ed., *The Political Economy of AIDS* (Amityville, NY, 1998), p. 120.

81. Nicholas Freudenberg, quoted in Scott Burris, "Education to Reduce the Spread of HIV," in Burris et al., eds., *AIDS Law Today* (New Haven, 1993), p. 87.

82. William Muraskin, "Hepatitis B as a Model (and Anti-Model) for AIDS," in Virginia Berridge and Philip Strong, eds., *AIDS and Contemporary History* (Cambridge, 1993), pp. 126–27.

83. J. Mann, "Worldwide Epidemiology of AIDS," and J. Mann, "AIDS Prevention and Control," in Alan F. Fleming et al., *The Global Impact of AIDS* (New York, 1988), pp. 5–6, 203; Söderholm, *Global Governance*, pp. 10–11, 23, 28.

84. Norman Howard-Jones, *The Scientific Background of the International Sanitary Conferences, 1851–1938* (Geneva, 1975); W. F. Bynum, "Policing Hearts of Darkness: Aspects of the International Sanitary Conferences," *History and Philosophy of the Life Sciences* 15 (1993); Baldwin, *Contagion and the State*, ch. 3.

85. Simon Watney, "The Spectacle of AIDS," in Douglas Crimp, ed., *AIDS: Cultural Analysis, Cultural Activism* (Cambridge, 1988), p. 83; Turshen, "Is AIDS Primarily a Sexually Transmitted Disease?" p. 347.

86. Baldwin, *Contagion and the State*, pp. 411–13.

87. Ibid., ch. 4.

88. Friedr. Alexander Simon jun., *Die indische·Brechruhr oder Cholera morbus* (Hamburg, 1831), p. vii; Leviseur, *Praktische Mittheilungen zur Diagnose, Prognose u. Cur der epidemischen Cholera* (Bromberg, 1832), p. iii; *Hansard Parliamentary Debates*, vol. 88 (1846), col. 227.

89. Mann, "Worldwide Epidemiology," pp. 5–6.

90. Except, as in this case, perhaps to the French, among whom traditional boundaries between private and public are still more staidly maintained: Mauriac, *Le mal entendu*, p. 10.

91. In Britain, for example, the details of gay sex broached during policy discussion among ministers led to scenes described as "surrealist." This was an issue, after all, that prompted parliamentary questions to the secretary of state for social services for advice on the dangers of "the practice known as French kissing" (answer: a theoretical possibility of transmission, but no known cases). *Hansard*, vol. 107 (19 December 1986), col. 780; Patricia Day and Rudolf Klein, "Interpreting the Unexpected: The Case of AIDS Policy Making in Britain," *Journal of Public Policy* 9, 3 (1989), p. 346.

92. *Los Angeles Times*, 11 July 2000, p. A1, A18; World Bank, *Confronting AIDS: Public Priorities in a Global Epidemic* (Oxford, 1997), p. 25; *International Herald Tribune*, 8 July 2002, p. 7.

93. Center for Strategic and International Studies, *Global HIV/AIDS: A Strategy for U.S. Leadership* (Washington, DC, 1994), pp. 3–4, 26–28.

94. Jean de Savigny, *Le Sida et les fragilités françaises: Nos réactions face à l'épidémie* (Paris, 1995), p. 342.

95. Aquilino Morelle, *La défaite de la santé publique* (Paris, 1996), p. 88.

96. Gerry Kearns, "Zivilis or Hygaeia: Urban Public Health and the Epidemiological Transition," in Richard Lawton, ed., *The Rise and Fall of Great Cities* (London, 1989), p. 100.

97. Howard M. Leichter, *Free to Be Foolish: Politics and Health Promotion in the United States and Great Britain* (Princeton, 1991), p. 29, ch. 3.

98. Laurie Garrett, *The Coming Plague: Newly Emerging Diseases in a World Out of Balance* (New York, 1994); Arno Karlen, *Plague's Progress: A Social History of Man and Disease* (London, 1995), ch. 1; Madeleine Drexler, *Secret Agents: The Menace of Emerging Infections* (Washington, DC, 2002); Jonathan B. Tucker, *Scourge: The Once and Future Threat of Smallpox* (New York, 2001).

99. *Public Health in England: The Report of the Committee of Inquiry into the Future Development of the Public Health Function* (Cm 289; London, 1988), p. 1; Peter A. Selwyn, "Tuberculosis and AIDS: Epidemiologic, Clinical, and Social Dimensions," *Journal of Law, Medicine, and Ethics* 21, 3–4 (1993), pp. 280–86; Lerner, *Contagion and Confinement*, ch. 8; S. C. McCombie, "AIDS in

Cultural, Historic ,and Epidemiologic Context," in Douglas A. Feldman, ed., *Culture and AIDS* (New York, 1990), p. 10.

100. Virginia Berridge, "AIDS, Drugs, and History," *British Journal of Addiction* 87, 3 (1992), p. 365.

101. Ronald O. Valdiserri, *Preventing AIDS: The Design of Effective Programs* (New Brunswick, 1989), pp. 24–25.

102. Jeffrey Weeks, "AIDS and the Regulation of Sexuality," in Virginia Berridge and Philip Strong, eds., *AIDS and Contemporary History* (Cambridge, 1993), p. 24.

103. Michael Pollak quoted in Emmanuel Hirsch, *Le SIDA: Rumeurs et faits* (Paris, 1987), p. 39; Michael Bartos, "Community vs. Population: The Case of Men Who Have Sex with Men," in Peter Aggleton et al., eds., *AIDS: Foundations for the Future* (London, 1994), p. 83; Baldwin, *Contagion and the State*, pp. 411–13.

104. Daniel M. Fox, "Chronic Disease and Disadvantage: The New Politics of HIV Infection," *Journal of Health Politics, Policy, and Law* 15, 2 (summer 1990), pp. 343–44; Virginia Berridge, "AIDS and Contemporary History," in Virginia Berridge and Philip Strong, eds., *AIDS and Contemporary History* (Cambridge, 1993), p. 3; Elizabeth Fee and Daniel M. Fox, "The Contemporary Historiography of AIDS," *Journal of Social History* 23, 2 (winter 1989), pp. 303–6; Virginia Berridge, *AIDS in the UK: The Making of Policy, 1981–1994* (Oxford, 1996), pp. 182–83; Daniel M. Fox, "The Politics of HIV Infection: 1989–1990 as Years of Change," in Elizabeth Fee and Daniel M. Fox, eds., *AIDS: The Making of a Chronic Disease* (Berkeley, 1992), pp. 125–28; Elizabeth Fee and Nancy Krieger, "Thinking and Rethinking AIDS: Implications for Health Policy," *International Journal of Health Sciences* 23, 2 (1993), pp. 330–31.

105. Lucette Khaïat, "Nouveau virus et vieux démons: Le droit face au sida, une approache comparative," in Eric Heilmann, ed., *Sida et libertés: La régulation d'une épidemie dans un état de droit* (n.p., 1991), p. 73; Paul Farmer, *AIDS and Accusation: Haiti and the Geography of Blame* (Berkeley, 1992), p. 122; Alan M. Kraut, *Silent Travelers: Germs, Genes, and the "Immigrant Menace"* (New York, 1994), pp. 260–61.

106. J. Arras, "The Fragile Web of Responsibility: AIDS and the Duty to Treat," *Hastings Center Report* 18, 2 (1988), pp. 10–20; Shirley Lindenbaum, "Knowledge and Action in the Shadow of AIDS," in Gilbert Herdt and Shirley Lindenbaum, eds., *The Time of AIDS* (Newbury Park, 1992), p. 323; Mann, "AIDS Prevention and Control," p. 205; Shirley Lindenbaum, "Imagines of Catastrophe: The Making of an Epidemic," in Merrill Singer, ed., *The Political Economy of AIDS* (Amityville, NY, 1998), p. 50.

107. *Le Monde*, 29 November 1986, p. 11a.

108. F. Grémy and A. Bouckaert, "Santé publique et sida: Contribution du sida à la critique de la raison médicale," *Ethique* 12, 2 (1994), p. 20.

109. Dudley Clendinen and Adam Nagourney, *Out for Good: The Struggle to Build a Gay Rights Movement in America* (New York, 1999), pp. 484–85.

110. *Le Monde*, 1 July 1987, p. 15e; Michael Pollak, *Les homosexuels et le*

sida: Sociologie d'une épidémie (Paris, 1988), p. 164; Pierre Mathiot, "Le sida dans la stratégie et la rhétorique du Front National," in Pierre Favre, ed., *Sida et politique: Les premiers affrontements (1981–1987)* (Paris, 1992), p. 192.

111. *Congressional Record* (House), 14 July 1983, 129, p. 19360.

112. Not until the early 1990s did the German federal health ministers note that a massive expansion from the original risk groups had not taken place. "Entschliessung der 63. Konferenz der für das Gesundheitswesen zuständigen Minister und Senatoren der Länder vom 22. bis 23. November 1990 in Berlin," *AIDS-Forschung* 6, 1 (January 1991), pp. 28–29. Similarly in France: Monika Steffen, "Les modèles nationaux d'adaptation aux défis d'une épidémie," *Revue française de sociologie* 41, 1 (2000), p. 23.

113. William H. Masters, Virginia E. Johnson, Robert C. Kolodny, *Crisis: Heterosexual Behavior in the Age of AIDS* (New York, 1988); William B. Johnston and Kevin R. Hopkins, *The Catastrophe Ahead: AIDS and the Case for a New Public Policy* (New York, 1990); Michael Fumento, *The Myth of Heterosexual AIDS* (New York, 1990); Gertrud Lenzer, "Aids in Amerika," in Ernst Burkel, ed., *Der AIDS-Komplex: Dimensionen einer Bedrohung* (Frankfurt, 1988), pp. 204–6.

114. Monika Steffen, "AIDS and Political Systems," in Dorothee Friedrich and Wolfgang Heckmann, eds., *Aids in Europe: The Behavioural Aspect* (Berlin, 1995), 5:38; Mann and Tarantola, *AIDS in the World II*, p. 58.

115. Aran Ron and David E. Rogers, "AIDS in the United States: Patient Care and Politics," *Dædalus* 118, 2 (spring 1989), pp. 46, 48; David C. Colby and David G. Baker, "State Policy Responses to the AIDS Epidemic," *Publius* 18, 3 (summer 1988), p. 115; Sandra Panem, *The AIDS Bureaucracy* (Cambridge, MA, 1988), p. 17; Omar L. Hendrix, "New York City Health and Hospitals Corporation," in John Griggs, ed., *AIDS: Public Policy Dimensions* (New York, 1987), p. 141; Ira Cohen and Ann Elder, "Major Cities and Disease Crises: A Comparative Perspective," *Social Science History* 13, 1 (1989), pp. 45–46.

116. Philippe Pedrot, "La protection sociale du malade atteint du SIDA," in Brigitte Feuillet-Le Mintier, ed., *Le SIDA: Aspects juridiques* (Paris, 1995), p. 176; Lutz Horn, "Die Behandlung von AIDS in ausgewählten Mitgliedstaaten des Europarates—ein rechtsvergleichender Überblick," in Hans-Ullrich Gallwas et al., eds., *Aids und Recht* (Stuttgart, 1992), pp. 198, 200; Ronald Bayer and David L. Kirp, "An Epidemic in Political and Policy Perspective," in Kirp and Bayer, eds., *AIDS in the Industrialized Democracies* (New Brunswick, 1992), p. 2.

117. Françoise F. Hamers and Jean-Baptiste Brunet, "Différences géographiques et tendances récentes de l'épidémie de VIH/sida en Europe," in Nathalie Bajos et al., *Le sida en Europe: Nouveaux enjeux pour les sciences sociales* (Paris, 1998), p. 14; Jean Dhommeaux, "Les dimensions internationales de la pandémie de VIH/SIDA," in Brigitte Feuillet-Le Mintier, ed., *Le SIDA: Aspects juridiques* (Paris, 1995), p. 220.

118. Susan Kippax et al., *Sustaining Safe Sex: Gay Communities Respond to AIDS* (London, 1993), pp. 11–12; Barbara A. Misztal, "AIDS in Australia: Dif-

fusion of Power and Making of Policy," in Barbara A. Misztal and David Moss, eds., *Action on AIDS: National Policies in Comparative Perspective* (New York, 1990), p. 190; Deborah J. Terry et al., eds., *The Theory of Reasoned Action: Its Application to Aids-Preventive Behaviour* (Oxford, 1993), p. ix.

119. Françoise F. Hamers et al., "The HIV Epidemic Associated with Injecting Drug Use in Europe: Geographic and Time Trends," *AIDS* 11 (1997), pp. 1365–66; J. B. Brunet et al., "La surveillance du SIDA en Europe," *Revue d'epidemiologie et de santé publique* 34 (1986), p. 132.

120. Vittorio Agnoletto et al., "AIDS and Legislation in Italy," in Martin Breum and Aart Hendriks, eds., *AIDS and Human Rights* (Copenhagen, 1988), p. 88; James W. Dearing, "Foreign Blood and Domestic Politics: The Issue of AIDS in Japan," in Elizabeth Fee and Daniel M. Fox, eds., *AIDS: The Making of a Chronic Disease* (Berkeley, 1992), pp. 327–28; Erik Albæk, "Denmark: AIDS and the Political 'Pink Triangle,'" in David L. Kirp and Ronald Bayer, eds., *AIDS in the Industrialized Democracies* (New Brunswick, 1992), p. 295.

121. *Hansard*, vol. 108 (20 January 1987), col. 536.

122. Berridge, *AIDS in the UK*, pp. 246–49; *Hansard*, vol. 110 (9 February 1987), col. 129; vol. 111 (26 February 1987), col. 408.

123. *Public Health Reports*, 103, suppl. 1 (1988), pp. 23, 91, 94; Fox, "Chronic Disease and Disadvantage," p. 345; Sabatier, *Blaming Others*, p. 7.

124. Meinrad A. Koch, "Surveys on AIDS in Europe (What Do They Tell Us?)," in M. A. Koch and F. Deinhardt, eds., *AIDS Diagnosis and Control: Current Situation* (Munich, 1988), p. 72.

125. A. Hiersche and M. Schrappe, "Clinical Course of HIV-Infected Adults in Europe," in Matthias Schrappe, ed., *AIDS-SIDA: A Comparison between Europe and Africa* (Stuttgart, 1993), p. 49; Farmer, *AIDS and Accusation*, p. 127; Samuel V. Duh, *Blacks and Aids: Causes and Origins* (Newbury Park, 1991), pp. 59–60.

126. Kathleen M. Sullivan and Martha A. Field, "AIDS and the Coercive Power of the State," *Harvard Civil Rights–Civil Liberties Law Review* 23 (1988), p. 150.

127. Albert R. Jonsen and Jeff Stryker, eds., *The Social Impact of AIDS in the United States* (Washington, DC, 1993), pp. 10, 25. But see also Burris, "Public Health, 'AIDS Exceptionalism' and the Law."

128. Edward King, "HIV Prevention and the New Virology," in Joshua Oppenheimer and Helena Reckitt, eds., *Acting on AIDS: Sex, Drugs, and Politics* (London, 1997), pp. 19–20; Fox, "Chronic Disease and Disadvantage," pp. 343–44; Ronald Bayer, "AIDS, Public Health, and Civil Liberties: Consensus and Conflict in Policy," in Frederick G. Reamer, ed., *AIDS and Ethics* (New York, 1991), pp. 43–44; Jonsen and Stryker, *Social Impact*, pp. 25–42; D. P. Francis, "Targeting Clinical and Preventive Care to and around HIV-Infected Persons: The Concept of Early Intervention," in F. Paccaud et al., eds., *Assessing AIDS Prevention* (Basel, 1992), pp. 257–62; Carol Levine and Ronald Bayer, "The Ethics of Screening for Early Intervention in HIV Disease," *American Journal of Public Health* 79, 12 (1989), p. 1661; BT *Verhandlungen* 12/12, 28 February

1991, p. 597A; M. A. Schiltz and Th. G. M. Sandfort, "HIV-Positive People, Risk, and Sexual Behaviour," *Social Science and Medicine* 50 (2000), pp. 1571–88.

129. Ronald Bayer et al., "The American, British, and Dutch Responses to Unlinked Anonymous HIV Seroprevalence Studies: An International Comparison," *AIDS* 4 (1990), p. 285; Swiss Institute of Comparative Law, *Comparative Study on Discrimination against Persons with HIV or AIDS* (Strasbourg, 1993), p. 139.

130. *LA Weekly*, 5 April–11 April 1996, pp. 13–14; Mann and Tarantola, *AIDS in the World II*, p. 335; Peter A. Selwyn, "Tuberculosis and AIDS: Epidemiologic, Clinical, and Social Dimensions," *Journal of Law, Medicine, and Ethics* 21, 3–4 (1993), pp. 280–86; Lerner, *Contagion and Confinement*, ch. 8.

131. Ronald Bayer, "AIDS, Public Health, and Civil Liberties," pp. 26–28; David L. Kirp and Ronald Bayer, "The Second Decade of AIDS: The End of Exceptionalism?" in Kirp and Bayer, eds., *AIDS in the Industrialized Democracies* (New Brunswick, 1992), p. 369; Fox, "Chronic Disease and Disadvantage," p. 349.

132. David Moss, "A Republican Framework for Comparing Policy Responses to HIV/AIDS: Two Roads from Machiavelli" (paper presented at a conference of the Council for European Studies Research Planning Group "Responding to HIV/AIDS," University of New Orleans, 3–5 October 1991), p. 3; Rolf Rosenbrock et al., "The Aids Policy Cycle in Western Europe: From Exceptionalism to Normalization," Wissenschaftszentrum Berlin für Sozialforschung, *Veröffentlichungsreihe der Arbeitsgruppe Public Health*, P99–202 (Berlin, 1999); Rolf Rosenbrock et al., "The Normalization of AIDS in Western European Countries," *Social Science and Medicine* 50 (2000), pp. 1607–29.

133. John C. Cutler and R. C. Arnold, "Venereal Disease Control by Health Departments in the Past: Lessons for the Present," *American Journal of Public Health* 78, 4 (April 1988), p. 375.

134. BT *Drucksache* 10/4071, 23 October 1985.

135. "Let us assume we can develop medicines able to do in an AIDS virus before it does any harm, indeed halt its emergence altogether" Andrew Hacker stated in the *Wall Street Journal* (21 May 1987), clearly worried at the prospect. "Will that mean we will go back to multiple partners and sharing bloodied needles?" *Congressional Record* (House), 9 June 1987, 133, p. 15113.

136. Norman E. Himes, *Medical History of Contraception* (New York, 1970), ch. 8; A.-J.-B. Parent-Duchatelet, *De la prostitution dans la ville de Paris*, 2d ed. (Paris, 1837), 2:534–37; Erica-Marie Benabou, *La prostitution et la police des mœurs au XVIIIe siècle* (Paris, 1987), p. 426; Jacques Donzelot, *The Policing of Families* (New York, 1979), p. 172.

137. Ed Jeanselme, *Traité de la syphilis* (Paris, 1931), 1:378.

138. Gordon T. Stewart, "The Epidemiology and Transmission of AIDS: A Hypothesis Linking Behavioural and Biological Determinants to Time, Person and Place," in Peter Duesberg, *AIDS: Virus- or Drug Induced?* (Dordrecht, 1996), p. 180; House of Commons, *Problems Associated with AIDS*, vol. 3, pp. 180–81; Jonsen and Stryker, *Social Impact*, p. 131; BT *Verhandlungen* 10/184,

10 December 1985, pp. 14068B-14069D; Charles Perrow and Mauro F. Guillén, *The AIDS Disaster: The Failure of Organizations in New York and the Nation* (New Haven, 1990), p. 7.

139. House of Commons, *Problems Associated with AIDS*, vol. 3, p. 35.

140. Michael L. Closen et al., *AIDS: Cases and Materials* (Houston, 1989), p. 182; *Congressional Record* (House), 1 October 1985, 131, p. 25521.

141. BT *Verhandlungen* 11/71, 14 April 1988, p. 4810C; Virginie Linhart, "Le silence de l'église," in Pierre Favre, ed., *Sida et politique: Les premiers affrontements (1981–1987)* (Paris, 1992), p. 128; Deborah Lupton, *Moral Threats and Dangerous Desires: AIDS in the News Media* (London, 1994), pp. 74–75; Gabriel Rotello, *Sexual Ecology: AIDS and the Destiny of Gay Men* (New York, 1997), pp. 10–13.

142. *Congressional Record* (House), 9 June 1987, 133, p. 15113.

143. Edmund Stoiber, "Kontinuität bayerischer AIDS-Politik," *AIDS-Forschung* 11 (1989), p. 573.

144. Philip M. Kayal, *Bearing Witness: Gay Men's Health Crisis and the Politics of AIDS* (Boulder, 1993), pp. 53–54, 92–95; Rotello, *Sexual Ecology*, pp. 109, 188–90, ch. 8; Patricia Illingworth, *AIDS and the Good Society* (London, 1990), p. 15; Lauritsen, *The AIDS War*, pp. 188–90.

145. Kane, *AIDS Alibis*, p. 33; Nancy Krieger, introduction to Krieger and Glen Margo, eds., *AIDS: The Politics of Survival* (Amityville, NY, 1994,), p. ix.

146. Edmund White, "AIDS Awareness and Gay Culture in France," in Joshua Oppenheimer and Helena Reckitt, eds., *Acting on AIDS: Sex, Drugs, and Politics* (London, 1997), p. 340; Claude Évin and Bruno Durieux, *La lutte contre le sida en France* (Paris, 1992), p. 36.

147. Stephen P. Strickland, *Politics, Science, and Dread Disease: A Short History of United States Research Policy* (Cambridge, MA, 1972); Victoria A. Harden, *Inventing the NIH: Federal Biomedical Research Policy, 1887–1937* (Baltimore, 1986), p. 25.

148. Philip R. Lee and Peter S. Arno, "AIDS and Health Policy," in John Griggs, ed., *AIDS: Public Policy Dimensions* (New York, 1987), p. 10; William Winkenwerder et al., "Federal Spending for Illness Caused by the Human Immunodeficiency Virus," *New England Journal of Medicine* 320, 24 (1989), pp. 1599, 1603.

149. John Street, "British Government Policy on AIDS: Learning Not to Die of Ignorance," *Parliamentary Affairs* 41 (October 1988), p. 495; House of Commons, *Problems Associated with AIDS*, vol. 2, p. 153; Misztal, "AIDS in Australia," p. 190.

150. *Hansard*, vol. 144 (13 January 1989), col. 1147; *RD Prot*, 1985/86, Bihang, Socialutskottets betänkande 1985/86:15, p. 10.

151. Mann and Tarantola, *AIDS in the World II*, p. 203; Michael Balter, "Europe: AIDS Research on a Budget," *Science*, 280 (19 June 1998), p. 1856.

152. Christophe Martet, *Les combattants du sida* (Paris, 1993), p. 223.

153. *RD Prot*, 1985/86, Bihang, Prop. 171, pp. 19–20; 1987/88, Bihang, Prop. 79, p. 42; 1986/87:109 (23 April 1987), p. 140. This, of course, implied that the

quality of Swedish research was up to snuff, but that the Swedish government simply saw no reason to be doing it.

154. Bundesrat, *Verhandlungen* 580, 25 September 1987, p. 305A; BT *Drucksache* 11/7200, 31 May 1990, pp. 292–93; Bernhard Fleckenstein and Volker ter Meulen, "Memorandum der Gesellschaft für Virologie zur Finanzkrise der AIDS-Forschung in der Bundesrepublik Deutschland," *AIDS-Forschung* 2 (1992), pp. 59–60; P. Brown, "Has the AIDS Research Epidemic Spread Too Far?" *New Scientist* 5, 1993, pp. 12–15; Sonja Kiessling and Wolfgang Vettermann, "Effektivität staatlich geförderter Forschung: Eine Analyse für den Bereich AIDS," *AIDS-Forschung* 5 (1995), pp. 245–49.

155. *Hansard*, Lords (10 December 1986), col. 1204; *New York Times*, 23 January 1998, p. B2.

156. *IDHL* 38, 3 (1987), p. 489; 39, 2 (1988), pp. 369–70; 39, 1 (1988), p. 39; 39, 3 (1988), pp. 623–26; Vincent E. Gil, "Behind the Wall of China: AIDS Profile, AIDS Policy," in Douglas A. Feldman, ed., *Global AIDS Policy* (Westport, 1994), pp. 12–13.

157. *IDHL* 42, 1 (1991), pp. 16–17; 44, 1 (1993), p. 28.

158. Ronald Bayer and Cheryl Healton, "Controlling AIDS in Cuba," *New England Journal of Medicine* 320, 15 (1989), pp. 1022–23; Olga Mesa Castillo et al., "La legislation cubaine face au SIDA," in Jacques Foyer and Lucette Khaïat, *Droit et Sida: Comparaison internationale* (Paris, 1994), pp. 133–35; Jennifer L. Manlowe, "Gender, Freedom and Safety: Does the US Have Anything to Learn from Cuban AIDS Policy?" in Nancy Goldstein and Jennifer L. Manlowe, eds., *The Gender Politics of HIV/AIDS in Women* (New York, 1997), pp. 385–99; Paul Farmer, *The Uses of Haiti* (Monroe, ME, 1994), pp. 264–66, 286–87; Marvin Leiner, *Sexual Politics in Cuba: Machismo, Homosexuality, and AIDS* (Boulder, CO, 1994), ch. 5.

159. *IDHL* 40, 4 (1989), p. 830; 46, 3 (1995), pp. 316–17.

160. Rolf Rosenbrock, "AIDS: Fragen und Lehren für Public Health," Wissenschaftszentrum Berlin für Sozialforschung, *Veröffentlichungsreihe der Forschungsgruppe Gesundheitsrisiken und Präventionspolitik*, P92–206 (Berlin, April 1992), p. 9; Kaye Wellings, "HIV/AIDS Prevention: The European Approach," in Dorothee Friedrich and Wolfgang Heckmann, eds., *Aids in Europe: The Behavioural Aspect* (Berlin, 1995), 1:52; Kirp and Bayer, "The Second Decade," p. 365; BT *Drucksache* 11/2495, 16 June 1988, p. 76; Georges Vigarello, *Le sain et le malsain* (Paris, 1993), p. 296; S. Fluss and J. Lau Hansen, "La réponse du législateur face au Vih/Sida: Aperçu international," in Jacques Foyer and Lucette Khaïat, *Droit et Sida: Comparaison internationale* (Paris, 1994), p. 470; John Harris and Søren Holm, "If Only AIDS Were Different!" *Hastings Center Report* 23, 6 (1993), p. 6.

161. Michael Pollak, "Introduction à la discussion: Systèmes de lutte contre les MST et sciences sociales," in Nadine Job-Spira et al., eds., *Santé publique et maladies à transmission sexuelle* (Montrouge, 1990), pp. 107–8; Daniel Defert, "Police sanitaire ou droit commun?" in Emmanuel Hirsch, *Aides: Solidaires* (Paris, 1991), p. 539; Françoise Héritier-Augé, preface to Eric Heilmann, ed., *Sida*

et libertés: La régulation d'une épidemie dans un état de droit (n.p., 1991), p. 12; Berridge, *AIDS in the UK*, p. 55; Jonathan M. Mann, "AIDS: Discrimination and Public Health," in WHO, *Legislative Responses to AIDS* (Dordrecht, 1989), p. 292; Lawrence O. Gostin and Zita Lazzarini, *Human Rights and Public Health in the AIDS Pandemic* (New York, 1997), pp. xv, 2, 51–52.

162. One of the leitmotifs of Baldwin, *Contagion and the State.*

163. And in fact many observers point out such divergences: Vera Boltho-Massarelli and Michael O'Boyle, "Droits de l'homme et santé publique, une nouvelle alliance," in Heilmann, *Sida et libertés*, p. 46; N. J. Mazen, "VIH et SIDA: Pour une réelle prévention," in Nadine Job-Spira et al., eds., *Santé publique et maladies à transmission sexuelle* (Montrouge, 1990), pp. 326–27; Jean-Paul Lévy, preface to Jacques Foyer and Lucette Khaïat, *Droit et Sida: Comparaison internationale* (Paris, 1994), p. 6; Mary Catherine Bateson and Richard Goldsby, *Thinking AIDS* (Reading, MA, 1988), p. 122; Monika Steffen, *The Fight against AIDS: An International Public Policy Comparison between Four European Countries: France, Great Britain, Germany, and Italy* (Grenoble, 1996), p. 11; Hans Moerkerk with Peter Aggleton, "AIDS Prevention Strategies in Europe: A Comparison and Critical Analysis," in Peter Aggleton et al., eds., *AIDS: Individual, Cultural, and Policy Dimensions* (London, 1990), p. 182; Sev S. Fluss, "National AIDS Legislation: An Overview of Some Global Developments," in Lawrence Gostin and Lane Porter, eds., *International Law and AIDS* (n.p., 1992), p. 8; Mildred Blaxter, *AIDS: Worldwide Policies and Problems* (London, 1991), p. 24; John A. Harrington, "AIDS, Public Health and the Law: A Case of Structural Coupling?" *European Journal of Health Law* 6 (1999).

164. Michael Pollak, *The Second Plague of Europe: AIDS Prevention and Sexual Transmission among Men in Western Europe* (Binghamton NY, 1994), pp. 7–8.

165. William Rubenstein, "Law and Empowerment: The Idea of Order in the Time of AIDS," *Yale Law Journal* 98 (1989), p. 986.

166. Bernd Schünemann, "Die Rechtsprobleme der AIDS-Eindämmung," in Bernd Schünemann and Gerd Pfeiffer, eds., *Die Rechtsprobleme von AIDS* (Baden-Baden, 1988), p. 378; Petra Wilson, "Colleague or Viral Vector? The Legal Construction of the HIV-Positive Worker," *Law and Policy* 16, 3 (1994), pp. 300–301.

167. Luc Montagnier, *Vaincre le SIDA: Entretiens avec Pierre Bourget* (Paris, 1986), p. 148; *Congressional Record* (House), 11 March 1993, pp. 1204, 1208; (Senate) 18 February 1993, p. 1763.

168. Bayer and Kirp, "An Epidemic in Political and Policy Perspective," pp. 4–5; David L. Kirp et al., *Learning by Heart: AIDS and Schoolchildren in America's Communities* (New Brunswick, 1989), p. 289; Markus Müller, *Zwangsmassnahmen als Instrument der Krankheitsbekämpfung: Das Epidemiengesetz und die Persönliche Freiheit* (Basel, 1992), p. 90; Vera Boltho-Massarelli, "Incidences ethiques du Sida dans le cadre sanitaire et social," in Daniel Borrillo and Anne Masseran, eds., *Sida et droits de l'homme: L'épidémie dans un Etat de droit* (Strasbourg, 1991), p. 23; Birgit Westphal Christensen et al., *AIDS:*

Prævention og kontrol i Norden (Stockholm, 1988), p. 66; Wellings, "HIV/AIDS Prevention, 1:52; Lucette Khaïat, "Nouveau virus et vieux démons: Le droit face au sida, une approache comparative," in Eric Heilmann, ed., *Sida et libertés: La régulation d'une épidemie dans un état de droit* (n.p., 1991), pp. 64–65; Barry D. Adam, "The State, Public Policy, and AIDS Discourse," *Contemporary Crises* 13, 1 (March 1989), p. 11; Colby and Baker, "State Policy Responses to the AIDS Epidemic," pp. 116–17; David Hirsch, "SIDA et droit en Australie," in Jacques Foyer and Lucette Khaïat, *Droit et Sida: Comparaison internationale* (Paris, 1994), p. 69; Jonathan Glasson, "Public Health and Human Rights: Finding a Balance in HIV Prevention," in David FitzSimons et al., eds., *The Economic and Social Impact of AIDS in Europe* (London, 1995), p. 234; Volker Koch, *Zu einer sozialen Ätiologie von AIDS: Der soziologische Beitrag zur Krankheitserklärung* (Bremen, 1989), pp. 17–18; Tonny Dina Maria Zeegers Paget, *AIDS and Public Health Measures: A Global Survey of the Activities of Legislatures, 1983–1993* (Groningen, 1996), p. 23; B. D. Bytchenko, "A Search for Effective Strategies against AIDS: Points for Discussion," in M. A. Koch and F. Deinhardt, eds., *AIDS Diagnosis and Control: Current Situation* (Munich, 1988), pp. 59–60; Michael T. Isbell, "AIDS and Public Health: The Enduring Relevance of a Communitarian Approach to Disease Prevention," *AIDS and Public Policy Journal* 8, 4 (1993); Günter Frankenberg, "Aids und Grundgesetz—eine Zwischenbilanz," in Cornelius Prittwitz, ed., *Aids, Recht und Gesundheitspolitik* (Berlin, 1990), p. 94; Richard Freeman, "The Politics of AIDS in Britain and Germany," in Peter Aggleton et al., eds., *AIDS: Rights, Risk, and Reason* (London, 1992), p. 54; Pierre Darbeda, "Les prisons face au Sida: Vers des normes européennes," *Revue de science criminelle et de droit pénal comparé* 4 (1990), p. 825; Wolfgang Riekenbrauck, "Toxicomanie et S.I.D.A. dans les prisons allemandes: L'exemple de la Nord Rhénanie-Westphalie," in Jean-Marie Guffens, ed., *Toxicomanie, Hépatites, S.I.D.A.* (n.p., 1994), pp. 451–52; Howard H. Hiatt, "The AIDS Epidemic: Social, Cultural, and Political Issues in Industrialized Countries," in J. M. Dupuy et al., eds., *SIDA 2001: AIDS 2001* (Paris, 1989), p. 69; Borrillo, "AIDS and Human Rights," p. 238; Werner Reutter, "Aids, Politik und Demokratie: Ein Vergleich aids-politischer Massnahmen in Deutschland und Frankreich," Wissenschaftszentrum Berlin für Sozialforschung, *Veröffentlichungsreihe der Forschungsgruppe Gesundheitsrisiken und Präventionspolitik*, P92–205 (Berlin, April 1992), p. 2; Rosenbrock, "AIDS: Fragen und Lehren für Public Health," p. 9; *AIDS: Fakten und Konsequenzen: Endbericht der Enquête-Kommission des 11. Deutschen Bundestages "Gefahren von AIDS und wirksame Wege zu ihrer Eindämmung"* (Bonn, 1990), p. 327; BT Drucksache 11/7200, 31 May 1990, p. 175; Daniel Fox et al., "AIDS and Economics: An International Perspective," in Robert F. Hummel et al., eds., *AIDS: Impact on Public Policy* (New York, 1986), p. 142; Matthias Weikert, "AIDS Prevention: Cooperation of NGOs and GOs," in Dorothee Friedrich and Wolfgang Heckmann, eds., *Aids in Europe: The Behavioural Aspect* (Berlin, 1995), 4:58; *Congressional Record* (House), 13 June 1990, p. 3522; Spiros Simitis, "Gesundheitsrechtliche Aspekte der Bekämpfung von AIDS," *AIDS-Forschung* 1, 4 (April

1986), p. 212; Suzanne Sangree, "Control of Childbearing by HIV-Positive Women," *Buffalo Law Review* 41, 2 (spring 1993), p. 313; BT *Verhandlungen* 12/12, 28 February 1991, p. 590C; Prosper Schücking, "Recht und AIDS: Verfassungsrechtliche Schutzpflichten für die Gesunden und Freiheitsrechte der Menschen mit HIV," in Behörde für Arbeit, Gesundheit und Soziales der Freien und Hansestadt Hamburg, *Dokumentation des Internationalen Symposiums "HIV/AIDS-Homosexualität/Bisexualität" 6. Oktober 1991 bis 9. Oktober 1991 in Hamburg* (Hamburg, 1991), p. 234.

169. Patrick Wachsmann, "Le Sida ou la gestion de la peur par l'état de droit," in Daniel Borrillo and Anne Masseran, eds., *Sida et droits de l'homme: L'épidémie dans un Etat de droit* (Strasbourg, 1991), p. 14; Michael G. Koch, *AIDS: Vom Molekül zur Pandemie* (Heidelberg, 1987), p. 236; Hans D. Pohle and Dieter Eichenlaub, "Kann die weitere Ausbreitung von AIDS verhindert werden?" *AIDS-Forschung* 2, 3 (March 1987), p. 121; Jean Martin, "Le SIDA et les pouvoirs publics: Potential et limites de leur action," in Jean Martin, ed., *Faire face au SIDA* (Lausanne, 1988), p. 111; Günter Frankenberg, *AIDS-Bekämpfung im Rechtsstaat* (Baden-Baden, 1988), pp. 14, 26; Canaris, "Gesundheitspolitische Aspekte," p. 299; Bayer, "AIDS, Public Health, and Civil Liberties: Consensus and Conflict in Policy," p. 27; Felix Herzog, "Das Strafrecht im Kampf gegen 'Aids-Desperados,'" in Ernst Burkel, ed., *Der AIDS-Komplex: Dimensionen einer Bedrohung* (Frankfurt, 1988), p. 343; Rebecca Bennett and Charles A. Erin, eds., *HIV and AIDS: Testing, Screening, and Confidentiality* (Oxford, 1999), pp. 69, 229; Richard D. Mohr, *Gays/Justice: A Study of Ethics, Society, and Law* (New York, 1988), pp. 217, 242; Richard A. Mohr, "AIDS, Gays, and State Coercion," *Bioethics* 1, 1 (1987), p. 49.

170. See references in chapter 7. Similar arguments were heard in France too: Michael Pollak, "AIDS Policy in France: Biomedical Leadership and Preventive Impotence," in Barbara A. Misztal and David Moss, eds., *Action on AIDS: National Policies in Comparative Perspective* (New York, 1990), p. 87.

171. Wolfgang Spann, "Überlegungen zur Bekämpfung der weiteren Ausbreitung der Erkrankung AIDS," *AIDS-Forschung* 2, 5 (May 1987), p. 242.

172. Memo by Dr. Ronald Bolton, House of Commons, *Problems Associated with AIDS*, vol. 3, pp. 206–11. Similar arguments from the National Front in France: *Le Monde*, 3 December 1986, p. 36.

173. Müller, *Zwangsmassnahmen als Instrument der Krankheitsbekämpfung*, p. 88; Hans-Ulrich Gallwas, "AIDS und Recht aus verfassungsrechtlicher Sicht," in Gallwas et al., eds., *Aids und Recht* (Stuttgart, 1992), pp. 28–29; Michael G. Koch, "Stellungnahme zur AIDS-Problematik: Antworten auf Fragen der Presse," *AIDS-Forschung* 3, 10 (October 1988), p. 545; Peter Gauweiler, "Zur Notwendigkeit eines geschlossenen Gesamtkonzepts staatlicher Massnahmen zur Bekämpfung der Weltseuche AIDS," in Bernd Schünemann and Gerd Pfeiffer, eds., *Die Rechtsprobleme von AIDS* (Baden-Baden, 1988), pp. 50–51; Bachelot and Lorane, *Une société au risque du sida*, pp. 52, 85, 92–94, 103; Bayer, "AIDS, Public Health, and Civil Liberties," pp. 34–35.

174. Wolfgang Spann, "Überlegungen zur Bekämpfung der weiteren Aus-

breitung der Erkrankung AIDS," *AIDS-Forschung* 2, 5 (May 1987), p. 242; Bachelot and Lorane, *Une société au risque du sida*, pp. 85, 92–93; Memo from the Conservative Family Campaign, House of Commons, *Problems Associated with AIDS*, vol. 3, p. 36; Vagn Greve and Annika Snare, *AIDS: Nogle retspolitiske spørgsmål*, 5th ed. (Copenhagen, 1987), p. 18; *RD Prot*, 1985/86, Bihang, Prop. 13, p. 10; *Congressional Record* (Senate), 25 January 1989, 135, p. 397; (House) 12 June 1990, p. 3484.

175. Koch, "Stellungnahme," p. 603; T. Krech, "Syphilis und AIDS: Eine historische Parallele," *Fortschritte der Medizin* 106, 21 (1988), p. 441; Mark Scherzer, "Private Insurance," in Scott Burris et al., eds., *AIDS Law Today* (New Haven, 1993), p. 419; D. C. Jayasuriya, *AIDS: Public Health and Legal Dimensions* (Dordrecht, 1988), p. 43.

176. BT *Drucksache* 10/6299, 4 November 1986, p. 7; 11/7200, 31 May 1990, p. 174; *Congressional Record* (House), 13 June 1990, p. 3522; (Senate) 14 January 1991, p. 879; Bundesrat, *Verhandlungen* 580, 25 September 1987, p. 299B; Gert G. Frösner, "Wie kann die weitere Ausbreitung von AIDS verlangsamt werden?" *AIDS-Forschung* 2, 2 (1987), p. 65.

177. Kirp, *Learning by Heart*, p. 35; Peter Gauweiler, *Was tun gegen AIDS?* (Percha am Starnberger See, 1989), pp. 11, 76; Ronald Bayer, *Private Acts, Social Consequences: AIDS and the Politics of Public Health* (New York, 1989), p. 53; *Congressional Record* (House), 30 June 1987, 133, p. 18379.

178. Annika Snare, "The Legal Treatment of AIDS in Denmark," in Martin Breum and Aart Hendriks, eds., *AIDS and Human Rights* (Copenhagen, 1988), p. 41; H. Jäger, ed., *AIDS und HIV-Infektionen* (n.p., n.d.), ix–2.3.3, pp. 1–5.

179. Koch, "Stellungnahme," p. 545.

180. For examples of such correlations, see Ernst Drucker, "Communities at Risk: The Social Epidemiology of AIDS in New York City," in Richard Ulack and William F. Skinner, eds., *AIDS and the Social Sciences* (Lexington, KY, 1991), p. 63; Nora Kizer Bell, "Ethical Issues in AIDS Education," in Frederick G. Reamer, ed., *AIDS and Ethics* (New York, 1991), p. 137; Bachelot and Lorane, *Une société au risque du sida*, p. 52; *Hansard*, vol. 144 (13 January 1989), col. 1126; Olli Stålström and Outi Lithén, "AIDS in Finland," in Martin Breum and Aart Hendriks, eds., *AIDS and Human Rights* (Copenhagen, 1988), p. 48; Gert G. Frösner, "AIDS-Bekämpfung: Die unterschiedliche Seuchenbekämpfung in verschiedenen Ländern," *AIDS-Forschung* 11 (1989), p. 606; Wilton, *EnGendering AIDS*, p. 36; Kirp and Bayer, "The Second Decade," p. 368; BT *Verhandlungen* 12/12, 28 February 1991, p. 593B-C; Tomas J. Philipson and Richard A. Posner, *Private Choices and Public Health: The AIDS Epidemic in an Economic Perspective* (Cambridge, MA, 1993), p. 205; Gauweiler, *Was tun gegen AIDS?*, p. 133; Bayer, "AIDS, Public Health, and Civil Liberties," p. 27; Gerry V. Stimson and Martin C. Donoghoe, "Health Promotion and the Facilitation of Individual Change," in Tim Rhodes and Richard Hartnoll, eds., *AIDS, Drugs and Prevention* (London, 1996), p. 16; Barry D. Adam, "Sociology and People Living with AIDS," in Joan Huber and Beth E. Schneider, eds., *The Social Context of AIDS* (Newbury Park, CA, 1992), p. 12; Nadine Marie, "Le Sida dans l'ex-URSS," in Jacques Foyer and

Lucette Khaïat, *Droit et Sida: Comparaison internationale* (Paris, 1994), p. 439; Jean-Paul Jean, "Les problèmes juridiques soulevés par le développement des MST et leur prévention," in Nadine Job-Spira et al., eds., *Santé publique et maladies à transmission sexuelle* (Montrouge, 1990), p. 125; Dan E. Beauchamp, *The Health of the Republic: Epidemics, Medicine, and Moralism as Challenges to Democracy* (Philadelphia, 1988), p. 206; Madeleine Leijonhufvud, *HIV-smitta: Straff- och skadeståndsansvar* (Stockholm, 1993), p. 49; Jacques Foyer and Lucette Khaïat, introduction to Foyer and Khaïat, *Droit et Sida: Comparaison internationale* (Paris, 1994), pp. 18–19; Bayer, *Private Acts, Social Consequences*, pp. 170–71; Lucette Khaïat, "The Law and AIDS: Issues and Objectives," *Medicine and Law* 12 (1993), p. 6.

2. WHAT CAME FIRST

1. Herbert Tröndle, *Strafgesetzbuch*, 48th ed. (Munich, 1997), p. 1168.

2. Barbara Breitbach et al., "AIDS-Bekämpfung und Bundes-Seuchengesetz," *Kritische Justiz* 21, 1 (1988), p. 64.

3. Peter Baldwin, *Contagion and the State in Europe, 1830–1930* (Cambridge, 1999), ch. 5.

4. Owsei Temkin, "On the History of 'Morality and Syphilis,'" in Temkin, *The Double Face of Janus* (Baltimore, 1977), pp. 472–84.

5. Larry Gostin, "The Future of Communicable Disease Control: Toward a New Concept in Public Health Law," *Milbank Quarterly* 64, suppl. 1 (1986), p. 83.

6. John C. Cutler and R. C. Arnold, "Venereal Disease Control by Health Departments in the Past: Lessons for the Present," *American Journal of Public Health* 78, 4 (April 1988), pp. 372–74; Allan M. Brandt, *No Magic Bullet: A Social History of Venereal Disease in the United States since 1880*, exp. ed. (New York, 1987), pp. 147–54.

7. Michael Mills et al., "The Acquired Immunodeficiency Syndrome: Infection Control and Public Health Law," *New England Journal of Medicine* 314, 14 (3 April 1986), p. 935; William Curran et al., *AIDS: Legal and Regulatory Policy* (Frederick, MD, 1988), pp. 21, 42, 85, 108; Frank P. Grad, *Public Health Law Manual: A Handbook on the Legal Aspects of Public Health Administration and Enforcement* (n.p., 1970), p. 43.

8. William J. Novak, *The People's Welfare: Law and Regulation in Nineteenth-Century America* (Chapel Hill, 1996), ch. 6 and passim; William R. Brock, *Investigation and Responsibility: Public Responsibility in the United States, 1865–1900* (Cambridge, 1984); Daniel T. Rodgers, *Atlantic Crossings: Social Politics in a Progressive Age* (Cambridge, MA, 1998), pp. 80–81.

9. Barron H. Lerner, *Contagion and Confinement: Controlling Tuberculosis along the Skid Road* (Baltimore, 1998).

10. Curran, *AIDS*, pp. 10–23, 102–3.

11. Norbert Schmacke, "Aids und Seuchengesetze," in Cornelius Prittwitz, ed., *Aids, Recht und Gesundheitspolitik* (Berlin, 1990), p. 22.

12. *Reichsgesetzblatt* 1940, pt. 1, pp. 456, 1459, 1514; 1941, pt. 1, p. 128.

13. *Reichsgesetzblatt* 1934, pt. 1, p. 532, §12; 1938, pt. 1, p. 1721; BT *Drucksache*, 3/1888, p. 18.

14. Paul Weindling, *Epidemics and Genocide in Eastern Europe, 1890–1945* (Oxford, 2000).

15. BT *Drucksache* 1/3232, p. 10; BT *Verhandlungen*, 23 April 1952, pp. 8859D-60A, 8863A-B. Though for an example of Nazi measures against syphilis regarded as useless and setting harmful precedent, see BT *Drucksache* 11/7200, 31 May 1990, pp. 167.

16. Stefan Kirchberger, "Public-Health Policy in Germany, 1945–1949," in Donald W. Light and Alexander Schuller, eds., *Political Values and Health Care: The German Experience* (Cambridge, 1986), p. 207.

17. BT *Drucksache* 1/104; 1/529; 1/3232; *Bundesgesetzblatt*, 1953, p. 700.

18. BT *Verhandlungen*, 1 March 1950, p. 1461A-B; 23 April 1952, pp. 8859D, 8862A, 8863A-64A; 12 June 1953, pp. 13419D-20D.

19. BT *Drucksache*, 3/1888; 3/2662. For a detailed account of the law, see Wolfgang Schumacher and Egon Meyn, *Bundes-Seuchengesetz*, 4th ed. (Cologne, 1992).

20. *RD Prot*, 1968, Bihang, Prop. 36; *SFS* 1968:231.

21. *RD Prot*, 1968, Bihang, Prop. 36, p. 27.

22. Ibid., pp. 27, 69.

23. Ibid., p. 26.

24. 26 Geo. 5 & 1 Edw. 8, c. 49.

25. François Burdeau, "Propriété privée et santé publique: Étude sur la loi du 15 février 1902," in Jean-Louis Harouel, ed., *Histoire du droit social: Mélanges en hommage à Jean Imbert* (Paris, 1989); Ann-Louise Shapiro, "Private Rights, Public Interest, and Professional Jurisdiction: The French Public Health Law of 1902," *Bulletin of the History of Medicine* 54, 1 (spring 1980); Paul Strauss and Alfred Fillassier, *Loi sur la protection de la santé publique (Loi du 15 Février 1902)*, 2d ed. (Paris, 1905); Baldwin, *Contagion and the State*, ch. 3.

26. Baldwin, *Contagion and the State*, ch. 5.

27. Hans Halter, " 'Sterben, bevor der Morgen graut': Aids und die grossen Seuchen," in Hans Halter, ed., *Todesseuche AIDS* (Reinbek, 1985), p. 28.

28. D. P. Francis, "Targeting Clinical and Preventive Care to and around HIV-Infected Persons: The Concept of Early Intervention," in F. Paccaud et al., eds., *Assessing AIDS Prevention* (Basel, 1992), p. 257.

29. Scott Burris, "Public Health, 'AIDS Exceptionalism,' and the Law," *John Marshall Law Review* 27 (1994), p. 260.

30. BT *Verhandlungen* 10/246, 13 November 1986, p. 19095A-B.

31. *RD Prot*, 1986/87, Bihang, Prop. 2, pp. 22–23, 26.

32. Manfred Steinbach, "Zur Strategie der staatlichen AIDS-Bekämpfung," in Bernd Schünemann and Gerd Pfeiffer, eds., *Die Rechtsprobleme von AIDS* (Baden-Baden, 1988), p. 63.

33. Peter Gauweiler, "Zur Notwendigkeit eines geschlossenen Gesamtkonzepts staatlicher Massnahmen zur Bekämpfung der Weltseuche AIDS," in

Bernd Schünemann and Gerd Pfeiffer, eds., *Die Rechtsprobleme von AIDS* (Baden-Baden, 1988), p. 54.

3. FIGHTING THE PREVIOUS WAR:
TRADITIONAL PUBLIC HEALTH STRATEGIES AND AIDS

1. Nancy E. Allin, "The AIDS Pandemic: International Travel and Immigration Restrictions and the World Health Organization's Response," *Virginia Journal of International Law* 28 (1988), p. 1043; Ronald Bayer et al., "Public Health and Private Rights: Health, Social and Ethical Perspectives," in Robert F. Hummel et al., eds., *AIDS: Impact on Public Policy* (New York, 1986), p. 23.

2. *Congressional Record* (Senate), 9 April 1987, 133, p. 8773; (House) 5 May 1987 (133), pp. 11270–71.

3. Peter Baldwin, *Contagion and the State in Europe, 1830–1930* (Cambridge, 1999), pp. 411–15; Nayan Shah, *Contagious Divides: Epidemics and Race in San Francisco's Chinatown* (Berkeley, 2001), pp. 89, 95.

4. James Harvey Young, "AIDS and Deceptive Therapies," in *American Health Quackery* (Princeton, 1992); Bernard Paillard, *Notes on the Plague Years: AIDS in Marseilles* (New York, 1998), pp. 43–44.

5. Paul Farmer, *AIDS and Accusation: Haiti and the Geography of Blame* (Berkeley, 1992), p. 221.

6. D. C. Jayasuriya, *AIDS: Public Health and Legal Dimensions* (Dordrecht, 1988), p. 23; Larry Gostin, "The Future of Communicable Disease Control: Toward a New Concept in Public Health Law," *Milbank Quarterly* 64, suppl. 1 (1986), pp. 83–84; Arnold J. Rosoff, "The AIDS Crisis: Constitutional Turning Point?" *Law, Medicine, and Health Care* 15, 1–2 (summer 1987), p. 81.

7. Lotta Westerhäll and Ake Saldeen, "Réflexions sur le Sida et le droit suédois," in Jacques Foyer and Lucette Khaïat, *Droit et Sida: Comparaison internationale* (Paris, 1994), pp. 405–6.

8. Annika Snare, "The Legal Treatment of AIDS in Denmark," in Martin Breum and Aart Hendriks, eds., *AIDS and Human Rights* (Copenhagen, 1988), p. 35; Vagn Greve and Annika Snare, *AIDS: Nogle retspolitiske spørgsmål*, 5th ed. (Copenhagen, 1987), p. 18.

9. H. D. C. Roscam Abbing, "AIDS, Human Rights, and Legislation in the Netherlands," in Martin Breum and Aart Hendriks, eds., *AIDS and Human Rights* (Copenhagen, 1988), pp. 97, 99.

10. Larry O. Gostin, "Public Health Strategies for Confronting AIDS: Legislative and Regulatory Policy in the United States," *JAMA* 261, 11 (17 March 1989), p. 1626; Arthur S. Leonard, "Discrimination," in Scott Burris et al., eds., *AIDS Law Today* (New Haven, 1993), p. 306; Ronald Bayer and David L. Kirp, "The United States: At the Center of the Storm," in Kirp and Bayer, eds., *AIDS in the Industrialized Democracies* (New Brunswick, 1992), p. 27; Albert R. Jonsen and Jeff Stryker, eds., *The Social Impact of AIDS in the United States* (Washington, DC, 1993), pp. 30–31; William Curran et al., *AIDS: Legal and Regulatory Policy* (Frederick, MD, 1988), pp. 23, 109; IDHL 37, 3 (1986), pp.

544–45; Martha A. Field and Kathleen M. Sullivan, "AIDS and the Criminal Law," *Law, Medicine, and Health Care* 15, 1–2 (summer 1987), p. 58.

11. AIDES, *Droit et S.I.D.A.: Guide juridique*, 3d. ed. (Paris, 1996), p. 62; Michel Danti-Juan, "Quelques reflexions en droit penal français sur les problemes posés par le sida," *Revue de droit penal et de criminologie* 68 (1988), p. 634; Frédéric Ocqueteau, "La répression pénale dans la lutte contre le sida: Solution ou alibi?" in Eric Heilmann, ed., *Sida et libertés: La régulation d'une épidemie dans un état de droit* (n.p., 1991), p. 245; Daniel Borrillo and Anne Masseran, eds., *Sida et droits de l'homme: L'épidémie dans un Etat de droit* (Strasbourg, 1991), p. 223.

12. Vittorio Agnoletto et al., "AIDS and Legislation in Italy," in Martin Breum and Aart Hendriks, eds., *AIDS and Human Rights* (Copenhagen, 1988), p. 90; Lutz Horn, "Die Behandlung von AIDS in ausgewählten Mitgliedstaaten des Europarates—ein rechtsvergleichender Überblick," in Hans-Ullrich Gallwas et al., eds., *Aids und Recht* (Stuttgart, 1992), pp. 206–7.

13. Margaret Duckett, ed., *Australia's Response to AIDS* (Canberra, 1986), p. 19; Barbara A. Misztal, "AIDS in Australia: Diffusion of Power and Making of Policy," in Barbara A. Misztal and David Moss, eds., *Action on AIDS: National Policies in Comparative Perspective* (New York, 1990), p. 195. Similar variations in Guatemala, Hungary, and Poland: WHO, *Legislative Responses to AIDS* (Dordrecht, 1989), pp. 89–93, 130; S. S. Fluss and D. K. Latto, "The Coercive Element in Legislation for the Control of AIDS and HIV Infection: Some Recent Developments," *AIDS and Public Policy Journal* 2, 3 (summer–fall 1987), p. 14; *IDHL* 37, 1 (1986), pp. 21–23.

14. *SFS* 1985:742.

15. Smittskyddskommittén, *Om smittskydd*, Statens offentliga utredningar 1985:37, pp. 32–38, 66–68, 90–93, 104–6, 155.

16. Seropositivity and AIDS tended to be kept conceptually and legally separate for a longer period in other nations: BT *Drucksache* 10/2473, 26 November 1984; BT *Verhandlungen* 11/71, 14 April 1988, p. 4809A-B.

17. In the 1985 legislation, seropositives could, in principle, be isolated for a lifetime, with no automatic process of appealing or reconsidering the length of their hospitalization: *RD Prot*, 1986/87, Bihang, Socialutskottets betänkande 9, pp. 16–17; Benny Henriksson, "Swedish AIDS Policy from a Human Rights Perspective," in Martin Breum and Aart Hendriks, eds., *AIDS and Human Rights* (Copenhagen, 1988), pp. 128, 131.

18. S. A. Månsson, "Psycho-Social Aspects of HIV Testing: The Swedish Case," *AIDS Care* 2, 1 (1990), p. 8; Benny Henriksson and Hasse Ytterberg, "Sweden: The Power of the Moral(istic) Left," in David L. Kirp and Ronald Bayer, eds., *AIDS in the Industrialized Democracies* (New Brunswick, 1992), p. 325; Benny Henriksson, *Social Democracy or Societal Control? A Critical Analysis of Swedish AIDS Policy* (Stockholm, 1988), p. 28; Swiss Institute of Comparative Law, *Comparative Study on Discrimination against Persons with HIV or AIDS* (Strasbourg, 1993), p. 21.

19. *RD Prot*, 1986/87, Bihang, Socialutskottets betänkande 9, pp. 16–17, 22;

RD Prot, 1987/88, Bihang, Socialutskottets betänkande 10, p. 25; *RD Prot*, 1985/86, Bihang, Prop. 13, pp. 1, 9, 12–13, 15; *SFS* 1985:786; *RD Prot*, 1988/89, Bihang, Prop. 5, pp. 1–3, 81; *SFS* 1988:1472.

20. *IDHL* 40, 4 (1989), pp. 833–35.

21. Greve and Snare, *AIDS: Nogle retspolitiske spørgsmål*, p. 18; BT *Druck-sache* 11/2495, 16 June 1988, p. 89; Madeleine Leijonhufvud, *HIV-smitta: Straff- och skadeståndsansvar* (Stockholm, 1993), p. 31; Raymond A. Smith, *Encyclopedia of AIDS* (Chicago, 1998), p. 209; Timothy Harding and Marinette Ummel, "Consensus on Non-Discrimination in HIV Policy," *Lancet* 341, 8836 (1993), pp. 24–25; Renée Danziger, "HIV Testing and HIV Prevention in Sweden," *British Medical Journal* 7127 (24 January 1994), pp. 293–96.

22. Wolf-Rüdiger Schenke, "AIDS aus verwaltungsrechtlicher Perspektive," and Hans-Ulrich Gallwas, "AIDS und Recht aus verfassungsrechtlicher Sicht," in Gallwas, *Aids und Recht* (Stuttgart, 1992), pp. 28–29, 36; "Entschliessung der 59. Konferenz der für das Gesundheitswesen zuständigen Minister und Senatoren der Länder (GMK) am 17./18. November 1988 in Berlin," in Bundesministerium für Jugend, Familie, Frauen und Gesundheit, *Aidsbekämpfung in der Bundesrepublik Deutschland* (n.p., n.d.), p. 94; Otfried Seewald, "Aids als Herausforderung an den Verfassungsstaat des Grundgesetzes," in Ernst Burkel, ed., *Der AIDS-Komplex: Dimensionen einer Bedrohung* (Frankfurt, 1988), p. 303; Heino Mönnich and Marius Fiedler, *Das Handeln der Berliner Gesundheitsverwaltung am Beginn der AIDS-Epoche* (Berlin, 1988), p. 56.

23. "Die rechtliche Beurteilung von Eingriffsmassnahmen und ihre Gewichtung im Rahmen der Gesamtstrategie der AIDS-Bekämpfung," *AIDS-Forschung* 4 (1989), p. 209.

24. Otfried Seewald, "Zur Verantwortlichkeit des Bürgers nach dem Bundes-Seuchengesetz," *Neue Juristische Wochenschrift* 40 (9 September 1987), p. 2269; Wolfgang Schumacher and Egon Meyn, *Bundes-Seuchengesetz*, 4th ed. (Cologne, 1992), pp. 35, 104–5; W. H. Eberbach, "Rechtliche Rahmenbedingungen für die Krankheit AIDS in der Bundesrepublik Deutschland 1988," *Das öffentliche Gesundheitswesen* 50 (1988), p. 459; Wilfried Bottke," SIDA et droit en République fédérale d'Allemagne," in Jacques Foyer and Lucette Khaïat, *Droit et Sida: Comparaison internationale* (Paris, 1994), pp. 28–29; Walter Bachmann, "Seuchenrechtliche Aspekte der HIV-Infektion," *AIDS-Forschung* 2, 2 (1987), pp. 100–103; "Rechtsgutachten des Ministeriums für Arbeit, Gesundheit und Soziales des Landes Nordrhein-Westfalen, Stand 15. 3. 1988," *AIDS-Forschung* 9 (1988), pp. 528–29; Wilfried Bottke, "AIDS und Recht," *AIDS-Forschung* 8 (1993), pp. 419–28.

25. Schenke, "AIDS aus verwaltungsrechtlicher Perspektive," pp. 49–51.

26. "Bekanntmachung des Bayerischen Staatsministeriums des Innern vom 19. 5. 1987 zum Vollzug des Seuchenrechts, des Ausländerrechts und des Polizeirechts," *AIDS-Forschung* 2, 6 (1987), p. 346; "Bayerischer Verwaltungsgerichtshof: Beschluss vom 24. November 1987," *AIDS-Forschung* 5 (1988), pp. 283–84.

27. *AIDS: Fakten und Konsequenzen: Endbericht der Enquête-Kommission*

des 11. Deutschen Bundestages "Gefahren von AIDS und wirksame Wege zu ihrer Eindämmung" (Bonn, 1990), pp. 337–38; BT *Drucksache* 11/7200, 31 May 1990, pp. 176–77; Martina Rübsaamen, "Der Ansteckungsverdacht im Sinne des Bundes-Seuchengesetzes insbesondere im Zusammenhang mit AIDS," *AIDS-Forschung* 2, 3 (1987), pp. 166–67; 2, 4 (1987), p. 212.

28. Jochen Hofmann, "Verfassungs- und verwaltungsrechtliche Probleme der Virus-Erkrankung Aids unter besonderer Berücksichtigung des bayerischen Massnahmenkatalogs," *Neue Juristische Wochenschrift* 41 (1988), p. 1490; Andreas Costard, *Öffentlich-rechtliche Probleme beim Auftreten einer neuen übertragbaren Krankheit am Beispiel AIDS* (Berlin, 1989), p. 89; Hans-Ullrich Gallwas, "Gesundheitsrechtliche Aspekte der Bekämpfung von AIDS," *AIDS-Forschung* 1 (1986), p. 36.

29. Bayerisches Staatsministerium des Innern, *Strategie gegen AIDS* (Munich [1989]), pp. 25–26; Bottke," SIDA et droit en République fédérale d'Allemagne," pp. 23–24; BT *Drucksache* 10/3829, No. 74, 13 September 1985; "Entschliessung der Sondersitzung der Konferenz der für das Gesundheitswesen zuständigen Minister und Senatoren der Länder (GMK) vom 27.3.1987 in Bonn," in Bundesministerium für Jugend, Familie, Frauen und Gesundheit, *Aidsbekämpfung in der Bundesrepublik Deutschland* (n.p., n.d.), pp. 87, 94.

30. BT *Drucksache* 11/1548, 17 December 1987, p. 3; 11/680, 7 August 1987; BT *Verhandlungen* 11/43, 26 November 1987, p. 2965B; BT *Drucksache* 11/54, No. 36, 13 March 1987; BT *Verhandlungen* 11/5, 19 March 1987, pp. 230D–31A; "Entschliessung der 63. Konferenz der für das Gesundheitswesen zuständigen Minister und Senatoren der Länder vom 22. bis 23. November 1990 in Berlin," *AIDS-Forschung* 6, 1 (1991), pp. 28–29; Bundesrat, *Verhandlungen* 580, 25 September 1987, p. 307A.

31. BT *Drucksache* 11/54, No. 36, 13 March 1987.

32. BT *Drucksache* 10/6746, No. 93, 12 December 1986; Ute Canaris, "Gesundheitspolitische Aspekte im Zusammenhang mit AIDS," in Johannes Korporal and Hubert Malouschek, eds., *Leben mit AIDS—Mit AIDS leben* (Hamburg, 1987), pp. 271–74, 300.

33. BT *Drucksache* 11/1548, 17 December 1987, pp. 1–3; BT *Verhandlungen* 11/8, 2 April 1987, p. 427C; "Koalitionsvereinbarung: Massnahmen zur Bekämpfung von AIDS," 9 March 1987, in Günter Frankenberg, *AIDS-Bekämpfung im Rechtsstaat* (Baden-Baden, 1988), p. 159.

34. BT *Drucksache* 11/2495, 16 June 1988, pp. 73, 76; BT *Verhandlungen* 11/103, 27 October 1988, pp. 7051D-7053A.

35. BT *Drucksache* 11/7200, 31 May 1990, pp. 13–14, 174–75, 187, 206–7. On internal battles within the commission, see Johannes Frhr. v. Gayl, *Das Parlamentarische Institut der Enquête-Kommission am Beispiel der Enquête-Kommission "AIDS" des Deutschen Bundestages* (Frankfurt, 1993).

36. Canaris, "Gesundheitspolitische Aspekte," pp. 276–77; Werner Reutter, "Aids, Politik und Demokratie: Ein Vergleich aids-politischer Massnahmen in Deutschland und Frankreich," Wissenschaftszentrum Berlin für Sozialforschung, *Veröffentlichungsreihe der Forschungsgruppe Gesundheitsrisiken*

und Präventionspolitik, P92–205 (Berlin, April 1992), pp. 19–20; Roland Czada and Heidi Friedrich-Czada, "Aids als politisches Konfliktfeld und Verwaltungsproblem," in Rolf Rosenbrock and Andreas Salmen, eds., *Aids-Prävention* (Berlin, 1990), p. 263.

37. Spiros Simitis, "Gesundheitsrechtliche Aspekte der Bekämpfung von AIDS," *AIDS-Forschung* 1, 4 (April 1986), pp. 211–12; BT *Verhandlungen* 10/152, 4 September 1985, p. 11415B; 11/71, 14 April 1988, p. 4804B; 11/103, 27 October 1988, p. 7052C-D; 11/71, 14 April 1988, pp. 4810A, 4812C.

38. BT *Drucksache* 11/274, 14 May 1987; BT *Verhandlungen* 11/71, 14 April 1988, p. 4803B; 11/92, 9 September 1988, p. 6299C; 11/43, 26 November 1987, p. 2958B; Rita Süssmuth, *AIDS: Wege aus der Angst* (Hamburg, 1987), pp. 26–29.

39. BT *Drucksache* 11/54, No. 36, 13 March 1987; 11/934, Nos. 52–53, 9 October 1987; BT *Verhandlungen* 11/185, 14 December 1989, p. 14357A-C.

40. BT *Verhandlungen* 11/71, 14 April 1988, p. 4809D; Hofmann, "Verfassungs- und verwaltungsrechtliche Probleme," p. 1489; Bayerisches Staatsministerium des Innern, *Strategie gegen AIDS,* pp. 25–26; Bayerisches Staatsministerium für Arbeit und Sozialordnung, Familie, Frauen und Gesundheit, *Die Krankheit AIDS: Ansteckungswege, Schutzmöglichkeiten, Konsequenzen,* 3d ed. (Munich, 1993), pp. 35–36.

41. BT *Drucksache* 11/7200, 31 May 1990, p. 178.

42. Staatssekretärsausschuss "AIDS" der Bayerischen Staatsregierung, *Konzept der Bayerischen Staatsregierung zur Bekämpfung der Immunschwächekrankheit AIDS* (Munich, n.d.), pp. 6–7, 12 ff; H. Jäger, ed., *AIDS und HIV-Infektionen* (n.p., n.d.), xv–1.3.1; Frankenberg, *AIDS-Bekämpfung,* pp. 179 ff; WHO, *Legislative Responses,* pp. 52–59; *IDHL* 38, 3 (1987), pp. 478–86; Bundesrat, *Verhandlungen* 580, 25 September 1987, p. 300B.

43. "Verwaltungsgericht München, Beschluss vom 13. September 1988," *AIDS-Forschung* 12 (1988), pp. 694–96.

44. Wolfgang Lippstreu, "AIDS und Gewerberecht," *AIDS-Forschung* 8 (1987), pp. 469–75.

45. Douglas Webb, *HIV and AIDS in Africa* (London, 1997), p. 173.

46. Tonny Dina Maria Zeegers Paget, *AIDS and Public Health Measures: A Global Survey of the Activities of Legislatures, 1983–1993* (Groningen, 1996), p. 127; Dineke Zeegers, "AIDS and the Law: A Comparative Overview," *Comparative Law Yearbook* 11 (1992), p. 217.

47. *IDHL* 38, 3 (1987), pp. 504–7; D. E. Woodhouse et al., "Restricting Personal Behaviour: Case Studies on Legal Measures to Prevent the Spread of HIV," *International Journal of STD and AIDS* 4, 1 (1993), pp. 115–16.

48. Ronald Bayer and Amy Fairchild-Carrino, "AIDS and the Limits of Control: Public Health Orders, Quarantine, and Recalcitrant Behavior," *American Journal of Public Health* 83, 10 (1993), pp. 1471–76; Donald H. J. Hermann, "AIDS and the Law," in Frederick G. Reamer, ed., *AIDS and Ethics* (New York, 1991), pp. 294–95; Ronald Elsberry, "AIDS Quarantine in England and the United States," *Hastings International and Comparative Law Review* 10

(1986), pp. 132–33, 145; Nancy Ford and Michael D. Quam, "AIDS Quarantine: The Legal and Practical Implications," *Journal of Legal Medicine* 8, 3 (1987), pp. 378–80; Larry Gostin, "The Politics of AIDS: Compulsory State Powers, Public Health, and Civil Liberties," *Ohio State Law Journal* 49 (1989), p. 1029; Institute of Medicine, *Confronting AIDS: Directions for Public Health, Health Care, and Research* (Washington, DC, 1986), p. 127.

49. Lorne E. Rozovsky and Fay A. Rozovsky, *AIDS and Canadian Law* (Toronto, 1992), pp. 32–33.

50. Public Health (Infectious Diseases) Regulations 1985, S.I. 1985/434; David Goss and Derek Adam-Smith, *Organizing AIDS: Workplace and Organizational Responses to the HIV/AIDS Epidemic* (London, 1995), p. 120; House of Commons, 1986–87, Social Services Committee, *Problems Associated with AIDS*, 13 May 1987, vol. 2, p. 73; Paul Sieghart, *AIDS and Human Rights: A UK Perspective* (London, 1989), pp. 45–46.

51. *Hansard Parliamentary Debates*, vol. 71 (21 January 1985), col. 347; vol. 71 (23 January 1985), col. 464; vol. 75 (21 March 1985), col. 591; vol. 73 (20 February 1985), col. 499; Simon Garfield, *The End of Innocence: Britain in the Time of AIDS* (London, 1994), p. 72; Elsberry, "AIDS Quarantine," p. 141.

52. Marlene C. McGuirl and Robert N. Gee, "AIDS: An Overview of the British, Australian, and American Responses," *Hofstra Law Review* 14, 107 (1985), pp. 112–13; Margaret Brazier and Maureen Mulholland, "Droit et Sida: Le Royaume-uni," in Jacques Foyer and Lucette Khaïat, *Droit et Sida: Comparaison internationale* (Paris, 1994), p. 372; Chris Bennett and Ewan Ferlie, *Managing Crisis and Change in Health Care: The Organizational Response to HIV/AIDS* (Buckingham, 1994), p. 68; House of Commons, *Problems Associated with AIDS*, vol. 1, p. lix.

53. Paillard, *Notes*, pp. 237–38.

54. Memo by Dr. Ronald Bolton, House of Commons, *Problems Associated with AIDS*, vol. 3, pp. 206–11.

55. House of Commons, *Problems Associated with AIDS*, vol. 2, pp. 70–71; BT *Drucksache* 11/2495, 16 June 1988, pp. 84, 116; Catherine Hankins, "Recognizing and Countering the Psychosocial and Economic Impact of HIV on Women in Developing Countries," in José Catalán et al., eds., *The Impact of AIDS: Psychological and Social Aspects of HIV Infection* (Amsterdam, 1997), p. 129.

56. William B. Rubenstein et al., *The Rights of People Who Are HIV Positive* (Carbondale, IL. 1996), p. 27; Colin A. M. E. d'Eça, "Medico-Legal Aspects of HIV Infection and Disease," in Richard Haigh and Dai Harris, eds., *AIDS: A Guide to the Law*, 2d ed. (London, 1995), pp. 114–15; Margaret Brazier and Mary Lobjoit, "Fiduciary Relationship: An Ethical Approach and a Legal Concept," in Rebecca Bennett and Charles A. Erin, eds., *HIV and AIDS: Testing, Screening, and Confidentiality* (Oxford, 1999), pp. 181–86; Andrew Grubb and David S. Pearl, *Blood Testing, AIDS, and DNA Profiling: Law and Policy* (Bristol, 1990), ch. 1. Although there was dispute on this issue in the United Kingdom: Gregor Heemann, *AIDS und Arbeitsrecht: Rechtliche Fragen bei der Begrün-*

dung und Beendigung von Arbeitsverhältnissen in der Bundesrepublik Deutschland und in England (Baden-Baden, 1992), pp. 153–54.

57. Bayer and Kirp, "The United States," p. 27.

58. Klaus Geppert, "AIDS und Strafvollzug," in Andrzej J. Szwarc, ed., *AIDS und Strafrecht* (Berlin, 1996), pp. 238–39; BT *Drucksache* 11/2495, 16 June 1988, pp. 86–87; Herbert Tröndle, *Strafgesetzbuch*, 48th ed. (Munich, 1997), pp. 1166–67; Günter Hirsch, "AIDS-Test bei Krankenhauspatienten," *AIDS-Forschung* 3 (1988), pp. 159–60; Friedrich Baumhauer, "Legal Measures Employed in Germany for Coping with AIDS," in AIDS-Forum D.A.H., *Aspects of AIDS and AIDS-Hilfe in Germany* (Berlin, 1993), p. 110.

59. RD *Prot*, 1985/86, Bihang, Socialutskottets betänkande 4, p. 10; RD *Prot*, 1985/86:33 (21 November 1985), p. 19.

60. Brazier and Mulholland, "Droit et Sida: Le Royaume-uni," p. 368; Margaret Brazier, "Common Law Chaos: Screening for HIV," in Wayland Kennet, ed., *Parliaments and Screening: A Conference on the Ethical and Social Problems Arising from Testing and Screening for HIV and AIDS* (Paris, 1995), p. 36.

61. Birgit Westphal Christensen et al., *AIDS: Prævention og kontrol i Norden* (Stockholm, 1988), pp. 120–22.

62. Frank Höpfel, "Strafrechtliche Probleme des HIV-Tests," in Andrzej J. Szwarc, ed., *AIDS und Strafrecht* (Berlin, 1996), p. 103.

63. Patrick Wachsmann, "Le Sida ou la gestion de la peur par l'état de droit," in Daniel Borrillo and Anne Masseran, eds., *Sida et droits de l'homme: L'épidémie dans un Etat de droit* (Strasbourg, 1991), p. 16; *Congressional Record* (House), 13 June 1990, pp. 3542–43; Gayl, *Parlamentarische Institut der Enquête-Kommission*, p. 54; Gert G. Frösner, "Wie kann die weitere Ausbreitung von AIDS verlangsamt werden?" *AIDS-Forschung*, 2, 2 (1987), p. 64.

64. Hans D. Pohle and Dieter Eichenlaub, "Kann die weitere Ausbreitung von AIDS verhindert werden?" *AIDS-Forschung*, 2, 3 (March 1987), p. 120; Jörg Lücke, *Aids im amerikanischen und deutschen Recht* (Berlin, 1989), pp. 120–21; *IDHL*, 39, 1 (1988), pp. 31–32.

65. House of Commons, *Problems Associated with AIDS*, vol. 2, pp. 70–71.

66. Gerd Paul and Loretta Walz, eds., *Eine Stadt Lebt mit AIDS: Hilfe und Selbsthilfe in San Francisco* (Berlin, 1986), pp. 46–47; Frank Rühmann, *AIDS: Eine Krankheit und ihre Folgen*, 2d ed. (Frankfurt, 1985), p. 145; John Street and Albert Weale, "Britain: Policy-making in a Hermetically Sealed System," in David L. Kirp and Ronald Bayer, eds., *AIDS in the Industrialized Democracies* (New Brunswick, 1992), p. 207.

67. Höpfel, "Strafrechtliche Probleme," pp. 113–14, 126.

68. RD *Prot*, 1987/88, Bihang, Socialutskottets betänkande 10, p. 25; 1988/89, Bihang, Prop. 5, pp. 104–6.

69. RD *Prot*, 1987/88:94 (6 April 1988), pp. 23, 27; 1988/89, Bihang, Prop. 5, p. 3; *SFS* 1988:1473, 1988:1474; RD *Prot*, 1986/87:110 (24 April 1987), pp. 45–46; Höpfel, "Strafrechtliche Probleme," pp. 114–15; Henriksson and Ytterberg, "Sweden," p. 323.

70. P. O. Träskman, "Att döda genom kärlek: Straffrättsdogmatik och rättspolitik i slagskuggan av HIV," *Retfærd* 16, 1 (1993), p. 42.

71. Rubenstein et al., *Rights of People*, p. 35; Mark H. Jackson, "The Criminalization of HIV," in Nan D. Hunter and William B. Rubenstein, eds., *AIDS Agenda: Emerging Issues in Civil Rights* (New York, 1992), pp. 252–53; Michael Fumento, *The Myth of Heterosexual AIDS* (New York, 1990), p. 99; Gene W. Matthews and Verla S. Neslund, "The Initial Impact of AIDS on Public Health Law in the United States—1986," *JAMA* 257, 3 (1987), p. 345; Nancy Lee Jones, "Les différents aspects juridiques des problèmes posés par le SIDA aux États-unis," in Jacques Foyer and Lucette Khaïat, *Droit et Sida: Comparaison internationale* (Paris, 1994), p. 207; Theodore J. Stein, *The Social Welfare of Women and Children with HIV and AIDS: Legal Protections, Policy, and Programs* (New York, 1998), p. 100.

72. Lücke, *Aids*, p. 81; AIDES, *Droit et S.I.D.A*, pp. 26–27.

73. Westerhäll and Saldeen, "Réflexions sur le Sida," pp. 389–92; *RD Prot*, 1988/89, Bihang, Prop. 5, p. 261.

74. *IDHL* 38, 2 (1987), pp. 253–54; 42, 2 (1991), pp. 245–54.

75. Allan M. Brandt, *No Magic Bullet: A Social History of Venereal Disease in the United States since 1880*, exp. ed. (New York, 1987), pp. 148–49; Allan M. Brandt, "AIDS in Historical Perspective: Four Lessons from the History of Sexually Transmitted Diseases," *American Journal of Public Health* 78, 4 (April 1988), p. 369.

76. *IDHL* 38, 3 (1987), p. 508; 39, 3 (1988), p. 633; Institute of Medicine, *Confronting AIDS: Update 1988* (Washington, DC, 1988), p. 77; WHO, *Legislative Responses*, p. 229.

77. James F. Childress, "Mandatory HIV Screening and Testing," in Frederick G. Reamer, ed., *AIDS and Ethics* (New York, 1991), p. 63; June E. Osborn, "Public Health and the Politics of AIDS," *Dædalus* 118, 3 (summer 1989), p. 135; Donald H. J. Hermann and William P. Schurgin, *Legal Aspects of AIDS* (Deerfield, IL, 1991), §4:04.

78. Lücke, *Aids*, p. 70; *Le Monde*, 17 December 1988, p. 1; 13 December 1991, p. 13.

79. Raffaele d'Amelio et al., "A Global Review of Legislation on HIV/AIDS: The Issue of HIV Testing," *Journal of Acquired Immune Deficiency Syndromes* 28, 2 (2001), pp. 175; Monika Steffen, "Crisis Governance in France: The End of Sectoral Corporatism?" in Mark Bovens et al., eds., *Success and Failure in Public Governance: A Comparative Analysis* (Cheltenham, U.K., 2001), pp. 477–78.

80. *Public Health Reports* 103, suppl. 1 (1988), pp. 60–61; Michael Tanner and the ALEC National Working Group on State AIDS Policy, *The Politics of Health: A State Response to the AIDS Crisis* (n.p., 1989), p. 103.

81. Swiss Institute of Comparative Law, *Comparative Study*, p. 15; *RD Prot*, 1987/88, Bihang, Socialutskottets betänkande 10, p. 26; WHO, *Legislative Responses*, p. 166; *RD Prot*, 1986/87, Bihang, Socialutskottets betänkande 9, p. 22; Virginie Linhart, "L'intervention tardive et dispersée des partis et des syndi-

cats," in Pierre Favre, ed., *Sida et politique: Les premiers affrontements (1981–1987)* (Paris, 1992), p. 139.

82. Nadine Marie, "Le Sida dans l'ex-URSS," in Jacques Foyer and Lucette Khaïat, *Droit et Sida: Comparaison internationale* (Paris, 1994), pp. 434–37; Christopher Williams, *AIDS in Post-Communist Russia and Its Successor States* (Aldershot, U.K., 1995), p. 59; Barbara A. Misztal, "AIDS in Poland: The Fear of Unmasking Intolerance," in Barbara A. Misztal and David Moss, eds., *Action on AIDS: National Policies in Comparative Perspective* (New York, 1990), p. 169.

83. *RD Prot*, 1986/87:109 (23 April 1987), p. 143; 1986/87:110 (24 April 1987), pp. 45–46; 1987/88, Bihang, Socialutskottets betänkande 10, p. 23; 1987/88, Bihang, Prop. 79, pp. 15–16.

84. M. Lagergren et al., "Anonymous Inquiries in Sweden Regarding the Individual's Motives for HIV-Antibody Testing Autumn 1987 and 1988," *AIDS Education and Prevention* 2, 3 (1990), p. 171; Månsson, "Psycho-Social Aspects," p. 5; *RD Prot*, 1987/88, Bihang, Prop. 79, p. 15; BT *Drucksache* 11/2495, 16 June 1988, p. 89; Jonathan M. Mann and Daniel J. M. Tarantola, eds., *AIDS in the World II* (New York, 1996), p. 6; Julie Margot Feinsilver, *Healing the Masses: Cuban Health Politics at Home and Abroad* (Berkeley, 1993), p. 83; Ronald Bayer and Cheryl Healton, "Controlling AIDS in Cuba," *New England Journal of Medicine* 320, 15 (1989), p. 1022; Marvin Leiner, *Sexual Politics in Cuba: Machismo, Homosexuality, and AIDS* (Boulder, CO, 1994), p. 117.

85. *RD Prot*, 1987/88, Bihang, Prop. 79, pp. 6–7.

86. Anders Blaxhult et al., "Evaluation of HIV Testing in Sweden, 1985–1991," *AIDS* 7 (1993), p. 1629; Anders Foldspang and Else Smith, *Overvågning af HIV og AIDS i Danmark* (Copenhagen, 1992), p. 13; Bundeszentrale für gesundheitliche Aufklärung, *Aids im öffentlichen Bewusstsein der Bundesrepublik 1996* (Cologne, 1997), p. 74.

87. Horn, "Die Behandlung von AIDS," p. 198; *RD Prot*, 1985/86, Bihang, Socialutskottets betänkande 4, p. 12.

88. *SFS* 1985:562; *RD Prot*, 1985/86, Bihang, Socialutskottets betänkande 4, p. 13; Benny Henriksson, "Aids—föreställningar om en verklighet," in Henriksson, ed., *Aids: Föreställningar om en verklighet* (Stockholm, 1987), p. 56.

89. *RD Prot*, 1985/86:33 (21 November 1985), pp. 7, 11–14; 1985/86, Bihang, Socialutskottets betänkande 15, pp. 10, 22–23; *SFS* 1986:197, 1986:198; *RD Prot*, 1985/86, Socialutskottets betänkande 25, pp. 4–5, 9; 1985/86:109 (4 April 1986), p. 9; 1985/86:157 (30 May 1986), pp. 5, 9; 1986/87, Bihang, Socialutskottets betänkande 9, p. 1; 1986/87, Bihang, Socialutskottets betänkande 19, p. 2; 1986/87:50 (16 December 1986), p. 5.

90. BT *Drucksache* 11/2495, 16 June 1988, p. 90.

91. *RD Prot*, 1988/89, Bihang, Socialutskottets betänkande 9, p. 1.

92. *RD Prot*, 1988/89:44 (13 December 1988), p. 12.

93. Christensen et al., *AIDS*, p. 65.

94. WHO, *Legislative Responses*, p. 81; AIDES, *Droit et S.I.D.A*, pp. 26–27;

Monika Steffen, *The Fight against AIDS: An International Public Policy Comparison between Four European Countries: France, Great Britain, Germany, and Italy* (Grenoble, 1996), p. 59; Michel Setbon, *Pouvoirs contre SIDA: De la transfusion sanguine au dépistage: Decisions et pratiques en France, Grande-Bretagne et Suède* (Paris, 1993), p. 198; Lucette Khaïat, "Nouveau virus et vieux démons: Le droit face au sida, une approache comparative," in Eric Heilmann, ed., *Sida et libertés: La régulation d'une épidemie dans un état de droit* (n.p., 1991), p. 76.

95. *Le Monde*, 17 December 1988, p. 1; 13 December 1991, p. 13; Annie Serfaty and Norma Oliveira, "Dispositif des consultations de dépistage anonyme et gratuit du VIH," in Agence nationale de recherches sur le sida, *Le dépistage du VIH: Politiques et pratiques* (Paris, 1996), p. 23.

96. *Le Monde*, 13 December 1991, p. 13; 12 December 1991, p. 13; 18 December 1991, p. 9; 21 December 1991, p. 11; 19 March 1992, p. 12; 25 March 1992, p. 19; 26 March 1992, p. 10; 3 April 1992, p. 13; 28 October 1993, p. 8; 29 November 1993, p. 7; 1 December 1993, p. 10; 15 December 1993, p. 7; 19 November 1994, p. 11; *Journal Officiel, Débats*, Assemblée Nationale, 29 November 1993, p. 6532.

97. Ronald Bayer, "AIDS, Public Health, and Civil Liberties: Consensus and Conflict in Policy," in Frederick G. Reamer, ed., *AIDS and Ethics* (New York, 1991), pp. 37–38, 41; Bayer and Kirp, "The United States," pp. 25–27.

98. BT *Verhandlungen* 11/103, 27 October 1988, pp. 7054C-55C; 12/12, 28 February 1991, p. 586B-C; BT *Drucksache* 11/7200, 31 May 1990, p. 187, 189–90.

99. Patricia Day and Rudolf Klein, "Interpreting the Unexpected: The Case of AIDS Policy Making in Britain," *Journal of Public Policy* 9, 3 (1989), pp. 345–46; Street and Weale, "Britain" p. 207; Setbon, *Pouvoirs contre SIDA*, pp. 261–62, 265.

100. *Hansard*, vol. 113 (23 March 1987), col. 72; vol. 114 (7 April 1987), col. 153; vol. 131 (12 April 1988), col. 101; vol. 133 (10 May 1988), col. 143.

101. Martin Sieber, *Die Bedeutung des HIV-Tests für die Aids-Prävention* (Bern, 1995), p. 20.

102. Michel Setbon, "La normalisation paradoxale du sida," *Revue française de sociologie* 41, 1 (2000), p. 70; Michel Setbon, "Approche comparative internationale du dépistage de l'infection par le VIH comme politique publique," in Agence nationale de recherches sur le sida, *Le dépistage du VIH: Politiques et pratiques* (Paris, 1996), pp. 15–16.

103. BT *Drucksache* 11/2495, 16 June 1988, p. 88; Jan K. van Wijngaarden, "The Netherlands: AIDS in a Consensual Society," in David L. Kirp and Ronald Bayer, eds., *AIDS in the Industrialized Democracies* (New Brunswick, 1992), p. 264.

104. Marie-Ange Schiltz and Philippe Adam, "Le test de dépistage au VIH: Diffusion parmi les homo et bisexuels français," in Agence nationale de recherches sur le sida, *Le dépistage du VIH: Politiques et pratiques* (Paris, 1996), p. 41.

105. BT *Drucksache* 11/7200, 31 May 1990, p. 374; BT *Verhandlungen* 11/103, 27 October 1988, p. 7057A; Wolfram H. Eberbach, "Anonymisierte Prävalenz- und Inzidenzstudie zu HIV: Rechtliche und politische Aspekte," *AIDS-Forschung* 6 (1989), pp. 283–87.

106. House of Commons, *Problems Associated with AIDS*, vol. 1, pp. x–xii; vol. 2, p. 298.

107. Ronald Bayer et al., "The American, British, and Dutch Responses to Unlinked Anonymous HIV Seroprevalence Studies: An International Comparison," *AIDS* 4 (1990), pp. 284–86; Bayer and Kirp, "The United States," p. 26; Lücke, *Aids*, pp. 54 ff; Harold Edgar and Hazel Sandomire, "Medical Privacy Issues in the Age of AIDS: Legislative Options," *American Journal of Law and Medicine* 16, 1–2 (1990), pp. 171–72.

108. Mildred Blaxter, *AIDS: Worldwide Policies and Problems* (London, 1991), p. 21; John Street, "A Fall in Interest? British AIDS Policy, 1986–1990," in Virginia Berridge and Philip Strong, eds., *AIDS and Contemporary History* (Cambridge, 1993), p. 230; Alistair Orr, "The Legal Implications of AIDS and HIV Infection in Britain and the United States," in Brenda Almond, ed., *AIDS: A Moral Issue* (London, 1990), p. 123; Virginia Berridge, *AIDS in the UK: The Making of Policy, 1981–1994* (Oxford, 1996), pp. 150–51, 212–13; Andrew Grubb and David S. Pearl, *Blood Testing, AIDS, and DNA Profiling: Law and Policy* (Bristol, 1990), p. 24; *Hansard*, vol. 144 (13 January 1989), col. 1103–4, 1121–22, 1124, 1144, 1146.

109. Van Wijngaarden, "The Netherlands," p. 273; Bayer et al., "American, British, and Dutch Responses," p. 288; Theo Sandfort, "Pragmatism and Consensus: The Dutch Response to HIV," in Sandfort, ed., *The Dutch Response to HIV: Pragmatism and Consensus* (London, 1998), p. 6.

110. Erik Albæk, "Denmark: AIDS and the Political 'Pink Triangle,'" in David L. Kirp and Ronald Bayer, eds., *AIDS in the Industrialized Democracies* (New Brunswick, 1992), p. 295; Erik Albæk, "AIDS: The Evolution of a Non-Controversial Issue in Denmark" (paper presented at the American Political Science Association meeting, 1990), p. 11; Viggo Hagstrøm, *AIDS som juridisk problem* (n.p., 1988), p. 30; Christensen et al., *AIDS*, pp. 26, 120–22.

111. RD *Prot*, 1987/88, Bihang, Prop. 79, p. 15; 1986/87, Bihang, Socialutskottets betänkande 19, pp. 26–27; 1987/88, Bihang, Prop. 79, p. 30; Henriksson and Ytterberg, "Sweden," p. 331.

112. Gallwas, "AIDS und Recht," pp. 30–31; Lücke, *Aids*, pp. 59–60.

113. Robert N. Proctor, *The Nazi War on Cancer* (Princeton, 1999), pp. 44–45.

114. BT *Drucksache* 11/122, 1 April 1987; Colin J. Bennett, *Regulating Privacy: Data Protection and Public Policy in Europe and the United States* (Ithaca, 1992), p. 41.

115. BT *Drucksache* 11/7200, 31 May 1990, pp. 271–72; 12/4080, 8 January 1993, no. 81; BT *Verhandlungen* 12/147, 12 March 1993, p. 12630B-C; Bayerisches Staatsministerium für Arbeit und Sozialordnung, Familie, Frauen und Gesundheit, *Die Krankheit AIDS*, p. 37,

116. Wolf Kirschner, *HIV-Surveillance: Inhaltliche und methodische Prob-*

leme bei der Bestimmung der Ausbreitung von HIV-Infektionen (Berlin, 1993), pp. 7–8, 46, 95; BT Drucksache 11/7200, 31 May 1990, pp. 293–94, 317; Gert G. Frösner, "AIDS-Bekämpfung: Die unterschiedliche Seuchenbekämpfung in verschiedenen Ländern," AIDS-Forschung 11 (1989), p. 605.

117. Sev S. Fluss and Dineke Zeegers, "Reporting of AIDS and Human Immunodeficiency Virus (HIV) Infection: A Worldwide Review of Legislative and Regulatory Patterns and Issues," AIDS and Public Policy Journal 5, 1 (1990), pp. 32–36.

118. House of Commons, Problems Associated with AIDS, vol. 1, p. lviii.

119. Michael Mills et al., "The Acquired Immunodeficiency Syndrome: Infection Control and Public Health Law," New England Journal of Medicine 314 (1986), p. 931; IDHL 37, 4 (1986), pp. 780–85; 38, 1 (1987), pp. 51–52; Mann and Tarantola, AIDS in the World II, p. 7.

120. Congressional Record (Senate), 14 January 1991, p. 879; Bayer, "AIDS, Public Health, and Civil Liberties," p. 42; Institute of Medicine, Confronting AIDS, pp. 118–19; Jonsen and Stryker, Social Impact, pp. 30–31; Ronald Bayer, "The Dependent Center: The First Decade of the AIDS Epidemic in New York City," in David Rosner, ed., Hives of Sickness: Public Health and Epidemics in New York City (New Brunswick, 1995), pp. 142–43; IDHL 38, 1 (1987), pp. 42–43.

121. Congressional Record (House), 13 June 1990, p. 3532; Bayer and Kirp, "The United States," pp. 28–29; Donald H. J. Hermann, "AIDS and the Law," in Frederick G. Reamer, ed., AIDS and Ethics (New York, 1991), pp. 286–88; Tanner and the ALEC National Working Group on State AIDS Policy, Politics of Health, pp. 25–26; Lawrence O. Gostin, "The AIDS Litigation Project: A National Review of Court and Human Rights Commission Decisions," JAMA 263, 14 (11 April 1990), p. 1962.

122. Rubenstein et al., Rights of People, pp. 44, 58–59; Los Angeles Times, 10 December 1998, p. A32; New York Times, 29 July 1999, p. A19; James W. Buehler, "HIV and AIDS Surveillance: Public Health Lessons Learned," in Ronald O. Valdiserri, ed., Dawning Answers: How the HIV/AIDS Epidemic Has Helped to Strengthen Public Health (New York, 2003), p. 34.

123. IDHL 34, 4 (1983), p. 748; Charles Mérieux, ed., SIDA: Épidémies et sociétés (n.p., 1987), p. 174; Horn, "Die Behandlung von AIDS," p. 198.

124. Christensen et al., AIDS, p. 28; Hagstrøm, AIDS, p. 26; IDHL 35, 1 (1984), p. 54; 37, 4 (1986), p. 770; 39, 3 (1988), p. 630; 46, 1 (1995), pp. 26–28; Snare, "Legal Treatment of AIDS," p. 35; Olli Stålström and Outi Lithén, "AIDS in Finland," in Martin Breum and Aart Hendriks, eds., AIDS and Human Rights (Copenhagen, 1988), p. 49; Beatrice Irene Tschumi Sangvik, Dänemark, Norwegen, Schweden und die Schweiz in Auseinandersetzung mit HIV und Aids (Zürich, 1994), ch. 2.

125. Henriksson, "Aids—föreställningar om en verklighet," p. 56.

126. Hans Ytterberg and Bo Widegren, "Strid om lagstiftningen kring AIDS i Sverige," Retfærd 9, 34 (1986), p. 20.

127. Månsson, "Psycho-Social Aspects," pp. 8–9; Benny Henriksson,

"Swedish AIDS Policy from a Human Rights Perspective," p. 126; David H. Flaherty, *Protecting Privacy in Surveillance Societies* (Chapel Hill, 1989), pp. 4–5.

128. Westerhäll and Saldeen, "Réflexions sur le Sida," pp. 395–96; Christensen et al., *AIDS*, p. 59; Henriksson, "Swedish AIDS Policy from a Human Rights Perspective," p. 130; *SFS* 1985:786; 1987:271.

129. Christensen et al., *AIDS*, p. 25; WHO, *Legislative Responses*, p. 181; *IDHL* 39, 1 (1988), pp. 60–69; BT *Drucksache* 12/6700, 31 January 1994, p. 108.

130. Agnoletto et al., "AIDS and Legislation in Italy," p. 90; David Moss, "AIDS in Italy: Emergency in Slow Motion," in Barbara A. Misztal and David Moss, eds., *Action on AIDS: National Policies in Comparative Perspective* (New York, 1990), p. 144; *IDHL* 38, 4 (1987), pp. 767–68; 42, 1 (1991), pp. 17–18; Jayasuriya, *AIDS*, p. 77.

131. *IDHL* 39, 3 (1988), pp. 628–29; 40, 1 (1989), p. 56; Jacques Foyer and Lucette Khaïat "Droit et SIDA: La situation française," in Foyer and Khaïat, *Droit et Sida: Comparaison internationale* (Paris, 1994), p. 254; Claude Évin and Bruno Durieux, *La lutte contre le sida en France* (Paris, 1992), p. 19; Françoise Barré-Sinoussi et al., *Le SIDA en questions* (Paris, 1987), p. 60.

132. *IDHL* 39, 1 (1988), pp. 33–34; WHO, *Legislative Responses*, p. 83.

133. House of Commons, *Problems Associated with AIDS*, vol. 1, p. lix; David Feldman, *Civil Liberties and Human Rights in England and Wales* (Oxford, 1993), pp. 299–300.

134. *Hansard*, vol. 103 (28 October 1986), col. 123; vol. 111 (27 February 1987), col. 449; vol. 113 (27 March 1987), col. 678; House of Commons, *Problems Associated with AIDS*, vol. 3, pp. 111–12.

135. BT *Drucksache* 12/6700, 31 January 1994, p. 108; Michael G. Koch, "Stellungnahme zur AIDS-Problematik: Antworten auf Fragen der Presse," *AIDS-Forschung* 3, 10 (October 1988), p. 541.

136. BT *Drucksache* 10/3749, No. 46; Hofmann, "Verfassungs- und verwaltungsrechtliche Probleme," p. 1489.

137. BT *Drucksache* 10/4071, 23 October 1985; 10/4516, 10 December 1985; BT *Verhandlungen* 10/152, 4 September 1985, p. 11415B.

138. BT *Drucksache* 11/7200, 31 May 1990, pp. 187, 338.

139. BT *Drucksache* 10/6299, 4 November 1986, pp. 5–7; BT *Verhandlungen* 10/246, 13 November 1986, pp. 19093A-94A; BT *Drucksache* 11/1548, 17 December 1987, p. 4; Rita Süssmuth, "Massnahmen der Bundesregierung zur AIDS-Bekämpfung," *AIDS-Forschung* 1, 1 (January 1986), p. 4.

140. Wolfgang Spann, "Überlegungen zur Bekämpfung der weiteren Ausbreitung der Erkrankung AIDS," *AIDS-Forschung* 2, 5 (May 1987), p. 242; Staatssekretärsausschuss "AIDS" der Bayerischen Staatsregierung, *Konzept der Bayerischen Staatsregierung*, p. 7; Bundesrat, *Drucksache* 294/87, 16 July 1987, p. 2.

141. Bundesrat, *Drucksache* 456/87, 3 November 1987; Bundesrat, *Verhandlungen* 580, 25 September 1987, p. 306C; Meinrad A. Koch et al., *AIDS und HIV in der Bundesrepublik Deutschland: Bericht zum 31. Dezember 1989* (Munich, 1990), pp. 17, 117; Kirschner, *HIV-Surveillance*, pp. 10, 64–67.

142. Günther Beckstein, "Die Anonyme Unverknüpfbare HIV-Test— machbar und notwendig," *AIDS-Forschung* 8 (1992), pp. 395–98.

143. "Entschliessung der 57. Konferenz der für das Gesundheitswesen zuständigen Minister und Senatoren der Länder am 19./20. November 1987 in Osnabrück," in Bundesministerium für Jugend, Familie, Frauen und Gesundheit, *Aidsbekämpfung in der Bundesrepublik Deutschland* (n.p., n.d.), p. 90; Koch et al., *AIDS und HIV*, p. 76.

144. Ronald Bayer and Kathleen E. Toomey, "HIV Prevention and the Two Faces of Partner Notification," *American Journal of Public Health* 82, 8 (1992), p. 1159; James T. Dimas and Jordan H. Richland, "Partner Notification and HIV Infection: Misconceptions and Recommendations," *AIDS and Public Policy Journal* 4, 4 (1989), p. 207; D. E. Woodhouse et al., "Restricting Personal Behaviour: Case Studies on Legal Measures to Prevent the Spread of HIV," *International Journal of STD and AIDS* 4, 1 (1993), pp. 116–17.

145. This was the subterfuge with which the French, for example, sought to preserve their rigid interpretation of medical secrecy with an acknowledgment that sometimes it made sense to warn unsuspecting third parties. Barré-Sinoussi et al., *Le SIDA en questions*, p. 59.

146. Chandler Burr, "The AIDS Exception: Privacy vs. Public Health," *Atlantic Monthly* 279 (June 1997), pp. 60–61.

147. Cornelius Prittwitz, "Strafrechtliche Aspekte von HIV-Infektion und Aids," in Prittwitz, ed., *Aids, Recht und Gesundheitspolitik* (Berlin, 1990), pp. 137–39; Alain Bergdoll, "L'approche juridique: Sida, droits et libertés," in Emmanuel Hirsch, *Aides: Solidaires* (Paris, 1991), p. 542; Jaqueline Bouton, "Le secret médical et le sida," in Eric Heilmann, ed., *Sida et libertés: La régulation d'une épidemie dans un état de droit* (n.p., 1991), p. 139.

148. Larry Gostin and William J. Curran, "Legal Control Measures for AIDS: Reporting Requirements, Surveillance, Quarantine, and Regulation of Public Meeting Places," *American Journal of Public Health* 77, 2 (February 1987), pp. 215–16; William J. Curran et al., "AIDS: Legal and Policy Implications of the Application of Traditional Disease Control Measures," *Law, Medicine, and Health Care* 15, 1–2 (summer 1987), p. 31; RD Prot, 1988/89, Bihang, Prop. 5, p. 206.

149. *Congressional Record* (Senate), 15 May 1990, p. 6225.

150. Elinor Burkett, *The Gravest Show on Earth: America in the Age of AIDS* (Boston, 1995), p. 208; *Congressional Record* (Senate), 15 May 1990, p. 6224.

151. Christensen et al., *AIDS*, p. 117.

152. Hagstrøm, *AIDS*, p. 44. Just as the Japanese thought that their gays were not as promiscuous as the Western variety. John Whittier Treat, *Great Mirrors Shattered: Homosexuality, Orientalism, and Japan* (New York, 1999), p. 29.

153. Bayer, "AIDS, Public Health, and Civil Liberties," p. 43.

154. American Bar Association, AIDS Coordinating Committee, *AIDS: The Legal Issues* (Washington, DC, 1988), pp. 49–51; Donald H. J. Hermann, "Liability Related to Diagnosis and Transmission of AIDS," *Law, Medicine and Health Care* 15, 1–2 (summer 1987), p. 38; Hermann and Schurgin, *Legal Aspects*, §2:18.

155. Edgar and Sandomire, "Medical Privacy Issues," p. 159.

156. Joni N. Gray et al., *Ethical and Legal Issues in AIDS Research* (Baltimore, 1995), p. 118; Institute of Medicine, *Confronting AIDS: Update 1988*, pp. 80–81; Mark Blumberg, *AIDS: The Impact On the Criminal Justice System* (Columbus, 1990), p. 6; Michael L. Closen et al., *AIDS: Cases and Materials* (Houston, 1989), p. 651; *Report of the Presidential Commission on the Human Immunodeficiency Virus Epidemic* (Washington, DC, 1988), pp. 75–76, 128–29.

157. Tanner and the ALEC National Working Group on State AIDS Policy, *Politics of Health*, p. 28; Rubenstein et al., *Rights of People*, pp. 61–62; S. Eric Lamboi and Francisco S. Sy, "The Impact of AIDS on State Public Health Legislation in the United States: A Critical Review," *AIDS Education and Prevention* 1, 4 (1989), p. 333.

158. Jonsen and Stryker, *Social Impact of AIDS*, pp. 32–33; IDHL 42, 2 (1991), pp. 245–54; Burr, "The AIDS Exception," p. 64.

159. Hermann and Schurgin, *Legal Aspects*, §4:06; Donald H. J. Hermann, "Liability Related to Diagnosis and Transmission of AIDS," *Law, Medicine, and Health Care* 15, 1–2 (1987), p. 40; Edgar and Sandomire, "Medical Privacy Issues," p. 161.

160. Rubenstein et al., *Rights of People*, p. 86.

161. IDHL 38, 3 (1987), pp. 504–7; Joyner Sims, "AIDS-Related Crime in Florida," in Clark C. Abt and Kathleen M. Hardy, eds., *AIDS and the Courts* (Cambridge, MA, 1990), p. 243; Suzanne Sangree, "Control of Childbearing by HIV-Positive Women," *Buffalo Law Review* 41, 2 (spring 1993), pp. 351–52.

162. Christensen et al., *AIDS*, pp. 26, 117–18.

163. Foyer and Khaïat, "Droit et SIDA," p. 255.

164. Olivier Guillod et al., *Drei Gutachten über rechtliche Fragen im Zusammenhang mit AIDS* (Bern, 1991), pp. 206–7, 276–77.

165. Frans van den Boom and Paul Schnabel, "The Impact of AIDS on the Dutch Health Care System," in Theo Sandfort, ed., *The Dutch Response to HIV: Pragmatism and Consensus* (London, 1998), p. 158.

166. House of Commons, *Problems Associated with AIDS*, vol. 1, p. lx; vol. 2, p. 10.

167. R. G. S. Aitken, "AIDS: Some Myths and Realities," *Law Society's Gazette* 84 (1987), p. 240; *Hansard*, vol. 72 (7 February 1985), col. 682: Berridge, *AIDS in the UK*, pp. 255–56; Street and Weale, "Britain," p. 191.

168. Sheila M. Rothman, *Living in the Shadow of Death: Tuberculosis and the Social Experience of Illness in American History* (New York, 1994), p. 189; Baldwin, *Contagion and the State*, pp. 442–46; Judith Walzer Leavitt, *The Healthiest City: Milwaukee and the Politics of Health Reform* (Princeton, 1982), p. 246.

169. Dorothy Porter and Roy Porter, "The Enforcement of Health: The British Debate," in Elizabeth Fee and Daniel M. Fox, eds., *AIDS: The Burdens of History* (Berkeley, 1988), p. 107; Bridget Towers, "Politics and Policy: Historical Perspectives on Screening," in Virginia Berridge and Philip Strong, eds., *AIDS and Contemporary History* (Cambridge, 1993), p. 67; Setbon, *Pouvoirs contre SIDA*, pp. 342–44.

170. BT *Drucksache* 11/3483, 24 November 1988; 11/7200, 31 May 1990, pp. 199–201; 12/2344, 25 March 1992, p. 23; 11/2495, 16 June 1988, p. 108. This was rejected by the government: BT *Drucksache* 12/2344, 25 March 1992, p. 23.

171. *Congressional Record* (Senate), 25 January 1989, 135, pp. 397–98; 135, 21 September 1989, p. 11606.

172. *RD Prot*, 1985/86:33 (21 November 1985), p. 17.

173. *Le Monde*, 10 October 1987, p. 18e.

174. David L. Kirp and Ronald Bayer, "The Second Decade of AIDS: The End of Exceptionalism?" in Kirp and Bayer, *AIDS in the Industrialized Democracies* (New Brunswick, 1992), p. 367; Albæk, "AIDS: The Evolution," p. 11; *Journal Officiel, Débats*, Assemblée Nationale, 31 May 1994, p. 2411; Stephan Ruppen, *AIDS: Ein Ratgeber für Rechtsfragen rund um AIDS* (Zurich, 1989), p. 79; Signild Vallgårda, *Folkesundhed som Politik: Danmark og Sverige fra 1930 til i Dag* (Århus, 2003), p. 249.

175. James C. Mohr, *Doctors and the Law: Medical Jurisprudence in Nineteenth-Century America* (New York, 1993), pp. 115–16.

176. Stein, *Social Welfare*, pp. 99–100; Rubenstein et al., *Rights of People*, pp. 41, 50; Jayasuriya, *AIDS*, p. 36; Lücke, *Aids*, p. 49; Tanner and the ALEC National Working Group on State AIDS Policy, *Politics of Health*, p. 68.

177. Chai R. Feldblum, "Workplace Issues: HIV and Discrimination," in Nan D. Hunter and William B. Rubenstein, eds., *AIDS Agenda: Emerging Issues in Civil Rights* (New York, 1992), p. 285.

178. John Duffy, *A History of Public Health in New York City, 1625–1866* (New York, 1968), p. 129.

179. Hermann, "AIDS and the Law," p. 288.

180. Bernard M. Dickens, "Legal Rights and Duties in the AIDS Epidemic," *Science* 239, 4840 (5 February 1988), p. 581.

181. Bayer and Toomey, "HIV Prevention," p. 1162; Joseph D. Piorkowski Jr., "Between a Rock and a Hard Place: AIDS and the Conflicting Physician's Duties of Preventing Disease Transmission and Safeguarding Confidentiality," *Georgetown Law Journal* 76 (1987), p. 197.

182. Robert B. Gainor, "To Have and to Hold: The Tort Liability for the Interspousal Transmission of AIDS," *New England Law Review* 23 (1988–89), p. 895.

183. Andrew Grubb and David S. Pearl, *Blood Testing, AIDS, and DNA Profiling: Law and Policy* (Bristol, 1990), ch. 2; Feldman, *Civil Liberties and Human Rights*, pp. 392–98.

184. *Hansard*, vol. 106 (2 December 1986), col. 611.

185. Orr, "Legal Implications of AIDS and HIV Infection," pp. 117, 136; d'Eça, "Medico-Legal Aspects," pp. 118–20; Swiss Institute of Comparative Law, *Comparative Study*, p. 31; Kenneth M. Boyd, "HIV Infection and AIDS: The Ethics of Medical Confidentiality," *Journal of Medical Ethics* 18 (1992), pp. 173–79.

186. Jonathan Grimshaw, "AIDS and Human Rights in the United Kingdom," in Martin Breum and Aart Hendriks, eds., *AIDS and Human Rights* (Copenhagen, 1988), p. 142; Alistair Orr, "Legal AIDS: Implications of AIDS and

HIV for British and American Law," *Journal of Medical Ethics* 15 (1989), p. 63; *Hansard*, vol. 90 (20 January 1986), col. 64–65.

187. Ulrich Amelung, *Der Schutz der Privatheit im Zivilrecht: Schadenersatz und Gewinnabschöpfung bei Verletzung des Rechts auf Selbstbestimmung über personenbezogene Informationen im deutschen, englischen und US-amerikanischen Recht* (Tübingen, 2002), pp. 129–57.

188. *Hansard* (12 February 1988), col. 657–58; vol. 147 (21 February 1989), col. 608.

189. Peter Roth, "AIDS and Insurance: Some Very British Questions," in David FitzSimons et al., eds., *The Economic and Social Impact of AIDS in Europe* (London, 1995), p. 288; Elsberry, "AIDS Quarantine," p. 129.

190. Benny Henriksson, ed., *Aids: Föreställningar om en verklighet* (Stockholm, 1987), pp. 56–57, 107; Westerhäll and Saldeen, "Réflexions sur le Sida," pp. 400–401; *RD Prot*, 1986/87, Bihang, Prop. 2, pp. 1, 20–21.

191. Andreas Costard, *Öffentlich-rechtliche Probleme beim Auftreten einer neuen übertragbaren Krankheit am Beispiel AIDS* (Berlin, 1989), p. 71; Dieter Meurer, "AIDS und strafrechtliche Probleme der Schweigepflicht," in Andrzej J. Szwarc, ed., *AIDS und Strafrecht* (Berlin, 1996), p. 137; *Der Spiegel* 28 (1987), p. 45.

192. *AIDS: Fakten und Konsequenzen*, pp. 386, 404; W. Eberbach, *Rechtsprobleme der HTLV-III-Infektion (AIDS)* (Berlin, 1986), pp. 32–33; Meurer, "AIDS und strafrechtliche Probleme," pp. 144–48; Bernd Schünemann, "AIDS und Strafrecht," in Andrzej J. Szwarc, ed., *AIDS und Strafrecht* (Berlin, 1996), pp. 41–42; Erwin Deutsch, *Rechtsprobleme von AIDS* (Bergisch Gladbach, 1988), p. 13; Wolfgang Spann and Randolph Penning, "Neue Problemstellungen in der Rechtsmedizin durch AIDS," *AIDS-Forschung* 1, 12 (1986), p. 639; Gerhard H. Schlund, "Zur Berufsverschwiegenheit bei AIDS," *AIDS-Forschung* 2, 7 (1987), p. 405; BT *Drucksache* 11/7200, 31 May 1990, p. 212.

193. Catherine Manuel, "HIV Screening: Benefits and Harms for the Individual and the Community," in Rebecca Bennett and Charles A. Erin, eds., *HIV and AIDS: Testing, Screening, and Confidentiality* (Oxford, 1999), pp. 70–71; Baldwin, *Contagion and the State*, pp. 442–46.

194. Ana Paula Fialho Lopes, "Du silence à 'l'aveu': Les intellectuels et le sida de la mort de Foucault (1984) à la mort de J. P. Aron (1988)," in Pierre Favre, ed., *Sida et politique: Les premiers affrontements (1981–1987)* (Paris, 1992), pp. 151–52; Thomaïs Douraki, "La protection juridique des malades atteints du SIDA," *Revue internationale de criminologie et de police technique* 2 (1990), p. 241; Emily Apter, "Fantom Images: Hervé Guibert and the Writing of 'sida' in France," in Timothy F. Murphy and Suzanne Poirier, eds., *Writing AIDS: Gay Literature, Language, and Analysis* (New York, 1993), p. 86.

195. Aquilino Morelle, *La défaite de la santé publique* (Paris, 1996), p. 295; Anne-Marie Casteret, *L'affaire du sang* (Paris, 1992), p. 100; Daniel Defert, "Une expérience collective," in Emmanuel Hirsch, *Aides: Solidaires* (Paris, 1991), pp. 63–64; Bouton, "Le secret médical et le sida," p. 130 and Françoise Degott-Kieffer, "Maladies nouvelles et droit du travail, le cas de l'infection par

le VIH," in Eric Heilmann, ed., *Sida et libertés: La régulation d'une épidemie dans un état de droit* (n.p., 1991), p. 218. The Swiss too recognized a limited right for physicians not to inform patients of their own diagnosis. Guillod, *Drei Gutachten*, pp. 99–100.

196. François-Régis Cerruti, *Medilex: Guide juridique médical* (Levallois-Perret, 1996), ch. 1, pt. 3; Sabine Michalowski, "Medical Confidentiality and Medical Privilege: A Comparison of French and German Law," *European Journal of Health Law* 5 (1998), pp. 95–96.

197. Jean de Savigny, *Le Sida et les fragilités françaises: Nos réactions face à l'épidémie* (Paris, 1995), p. 277; *Le Monde*, 3–4 July 1988, p. 8.

198. AIDES, *Droit et S.I.D.A*, p. 35; Barré-Sinoussi, *Le SIDA en questions*, p. 59; Khaïat, "Nouveau virus et vieux démons," p. 92; Philippe Auvergnon, ed., *Le droit social à l'epreuve du SIDA* (n.p., n.d.), pp. 46–47; Pierre Kayser, *La protection de la vie privée: Protection du secret de la vie privée* (Paris, 1984), p. 245.

199. *Le Monde*, 7 April 1994, p. 11; 12 April 1994; 25 May 1994, p. 10; 31 May 1994, p. 14; 1 June 1994, p. 26; *Journal Officiel, Débats*, Assemblée Nationale, 31 May 1994, p. 2404; Alain Sobel, "Policy Making under Changing Political Situations: The French National AIDS Council and AIDS Control Policies," in Dorothee Friedrich and Wolfgang Heckmann, eds., *Aids in Europe: The Behavioural Aspect* (Berlin, 1995), 4:92; Vèronique Barabe-Bouchard, "La famille et le SIDA," in Brigitte Feuillet-Le Mintier, ed., *Le SIDA: Aspects juridiques* (Paris, 1995), pp. 33–36.

200. Nancy Tomes, "The Making of a Germ Panic, Then and Now," *American Journal of Public Health* 90, 2 (February 2000), p. 195.

201. Leonard J. Nelson III, "International Travel Restrictions and the AIDS Epidemic," *American Journal of International Law* 81 (1987), p. 231; Allin, "AIDS Pandemic," p. 1056.

202. WHO, *Legislative Responses*, pp. 38, 97, 103, 191, 194; Jean-Pierre Cabestan, "SIDA et droit en Chine populaire," in Jacques Foyer and Lucette Khaïat, *Droit et Sida: Comparaison internationale* (Paris, 1994), p. 100; S. S. Fluss and D. K. Latto, "The Coercive Element in Legislation for the Control of AIDS and HIV Infection: Some Recent Developments," *AIDS and Public Policy Journal* 2, 3 (summer–fall 1987), p. 15; Marie, "Le Sida dans l'ex-URSS," pp. 433–37; Williams, *AIDS in Post-Communist Russia*, p. 59, 73–74, 160–61; *IDHL* 38, 4 (1987), p. 769–71; 41, 3 (1990), pp. 431–32; 42, 1 (1991), pp. 21–25.

203. Tomas J. Philipson and Richard A. Posner, *Private Choices and Public Health: The AIDS Epidemic in an Economic Perspective* (Cambridge, MA, 1993), p. 152; Sarah Santana et al., "Human Immunodeficiency Virus in Cuba: The Public Health Response of a Third World Country," in Nancy Krieger and Glen Margo, eds., *AIDS: The Politics of Survival* (Amityville, NY, 1994), p. 168; Julie Margot Feinsilver, *Healing the Masses: Cuban Health Politics at Home and Abroad* (Berkeley, 1993), pp. 82–84.

204. Aart Hendriks, *AIDS and Mobility: The Impact of International Mobility on the Spread of HIV and the Need and Possibility for AIDS/HIV Prevention Programmes* (Copenhagen, 1991), p. 20.

205. Brenda Almond, "Introduction: War of the World," in Almond, ed., *AIDS: A Moral Issue* (London, 1990), p. 20; B. D. Bytchenko, "A Search for Effective Strategies against AIDS: Points for Discussion," in M. A. Koch and F. Deinhardt, eds., *AIDS Diagnosis and Control: Current Situation* (Munich, 1988), p. 55; Jürgen Kölzsch, "HIV-/Aids-Beratungs- und Betreuungsmodell an der Charité-Hautklinik Berlin," in Doris Schaeffer et al., eds., *Aids-Krankenversorgung* (Berlin, 1992), p. 190; Williams, *AIDS in Post-Communist Russia*, p. 163; "Russia Enacts Travel Restrictions, Mandates Testing of Some Workers," *AIDS Policy and Law* 21 April 1995, p. 7.

206. Left-wing critics of the Reagan Strategic Defense Initiative drew parallels between the Star Wars missile shield and safer sex, both seeking security behind a thin and improbable veil of protection. Michael Bochow, "Reactions of the Gay Community to AIDS in East and West Berlin," in AIDS-Forum D.A.H., *Aspects of AIDS and AIDS-Hilfe in Germany* (Berlin, 1993), p. 27.

207. Kölzsch, "HIV-/Aids-Beratungs- und Betreuungsmodell an der Charité-Hautklinik Berlin," p. 190; Niels Sönnichsen, "Überlegungen und Erfahrungen zur Verhütung und Bekämpfung des Syndroms des erworbenen Immundefektes (AIDS) in der DDR," *AIDS-Forschung* 2, 10 (October 1987), pp. 549–50; Günter Grau, *AIDS: Krankheit oder Katastrophe?* (Berlin, 1990), p. 80; Stephan Dressler, "Blood 'Scandal' and AIDS in Germany," in Eric A. Feldman and Ronald Bayer, eds., *Blood Feuds: AIDS, Blood, and the Politics of Medical Disaster* (New York, 1999), p. 195.

208. Anders Foldspang and Else Smith, *Overvågning af HIV og AIDS i Danmark* (Copenhagen, 1992), pp. 18, 45–47; Sarah N. Qureshi, "Global Ostracism of HIV-Positive Aliens: International Restrictions Barring HIV-Positive Aliens," *Maryland Journal of International Law and Trade* 19 (1995), pp. 117–18; Sangvik, *Dänemark, Norwegen, Schweden und die Schweiz*, p. 106; Danziger, "HIV Testing and HIV Prevention," pp. 293–96; Matti Hayry and Heta Hayry, "AIDS and a Small North European Country: A Study in Applied Ethics," *International Journal of Applied Philosophy* 3, 3 (1987), p. 52.

209. *Congressional Record* (Senate), 17 February 1993, p. 1719; (Senate) 7 May 1990, p. 5738.

210. Guy S. Goodwin-Gill, "AIDS and HIV, Migrants, and Refugees," in Mary Haour-Knipe and Richard Rector, eds., *Crossing Borders: Migration, Ethnicity, and AIDS* (London, 1996), p. 56; Margaret Duckett and Andrew J. Orkin, "AIDS-Related Migration and Travel Policies and Restrictions: A Global Survey," *AIDS* 3, suppl. 1 (1989), p. S251; Éric Seizelet, "Le droit face au SIDA en Corée du sud," in Jacques Foyer and Lucette Khaïat, *Droit et Sida: Comparaison internationale* (Paris, 1994), p. 113.

211. Swiss Institute of Comparative Law, *Comparative Study*, p. 103; *IDHL* 40, 1 (1989), p. 59; Virginia van der Vliet, "Apartheid and the Politics of AIDS," in Douglas A. Feldman, ed., *Global AIDS Policy* (Westport, 1994), p. 109.

212. Chetan Bhatt and Robert Lee, "Official Knowledges: The Free Market, Identity Formation, Sexuality, and Race in the HIV/AIDS Sector," in Joshua

Oppenheimer and Helena Reckitt, eds., *Acting on AIDS: Sex, Drugs, and Politics* (London, 1997), p. 204.

213. WHO, *Legislative Responses*, p. 191; Jean-Pierre Legrand, "Les personnes de nationalité étrangère et le Sida," in Michel Vincineau, ed., *Le Sida: Un défi aux droits* (Brussels, 1991), pp. 764–65; Swiss Institute of Comparative Law, *Comparative Study*, pp. 107–8; Bernard M. Dickens et al., "HIV Screening: The International Implications," in Lawrence Gostin and Lane Porter, eds., *International Law and AIDS* (n.p., 1992), pp. 111–12; Michel Hubert, "AIDS in Belgium: Africa in Microcosm," in Barbara A. Misztal and David Moss, eds., *Action on AIDS: National Policies in Comparative Perspective* (New York, 1990), p. 106; Terry Morehead Dworkin and Elies Steyger, "AIDS Victims in the European Community and the United States: Are They Protected from Unjustified Discrimination?" *Texas International Law Journal* 24 (1989), p. 314; Jean-François Revel, "AIDS and Political Manipulation," in Charles Mérieux, ed., *SIDA: Épidémies et sociétés* (n.p., 1987), p. 36; Renée Sabatier, *Blaming Others: Prejudice, Race, and Worldwide AIDS* (London, 1988), pp. 110–13.

214. *AIDS: Fakten und Konsequenzen*, p. 610; BT *Drucksache* 11/4043, 21 February 1989; BT *Verhandlungen* 10/184, 12 December 1985, p. 14086B-C; Canaris, "Gesundheitspolitische Aspekte," p. 300; BT *Drucksache* 11/218; 11/295, 19 May 1987; 11/647, 28 July 1987; BT *Verhandlungen* 12/12, 28 February 1991, p. 588D; Mönnich and Fiedler, *Handeln der Berliner Gesundheitsverwaltung*, pp. 93–94.

215. *IDHL* 38, 4 (1987), pp. 762–63; 41, 1 (1990), p. 39; David Hirsch, "SIDA et droit en Australie," in Jacques Foyer and Lucette Khaïat, *Droit et Sida: Comparaison internationale* (Paris, 1994), pp. 94–95; David T. Evans, *Sexual Citizenship: The Material Construction of Sexualities* (London, 1993), p. 125; Deutsche AIDS-Hilfe, Berlin, *Restrictions of Entry and Residence for People with HIV/AIDS: A Global Survey* (Frankfurt, November 1991), p. 30; Frösner, "AIDS-Bekämpfung," p. 599; Rozovsky and Rozovsky, *AIDS and Canadian Law*, p. 72.

216. BT *Verhandlungen* 11/13, 21 May 1987, pp. 795D-796C, 798A-B, 801A; 11/60, 24 February 1988, pp. 4149D-50A; BT *Drucksache* 11/6485, 15 February 1990.

217. Lücke, *Aids*, pp. 64–65; Deutsche AIDS-Hilfe, *Restrictions of Entry and Residence*, p. 32.

218. Ian A. Macdonald, *Immigration Law and Practice* (London, 1983), p. 115; BT *Drucksache* 11/7200, 31 May 1990, pp. 252–55; Schenke, "AIDS aus verwaltungsrechtlicher Perspektive," in p. 60; *AIDS: Fakten und Konsequenzen*, pp. 482–88; Walter Zitzelsberger, "Ausländerrechtliche Aspekte der AIDS-Problematik," *AIDS-Forschung* 1 (1988), pp. 49–53; "Rechtliche Aspekte der HIV-Infektion und der AIDS-Erkrankung," *AIDS-Forschung* 7 (1988), p. 411.

219. Bundesrat, *Drucksache* 295/87, 16 July 1987; Jäger, *AIDS und HIV-Infektionen*, ix-2.1.1, p. 1; *AIDS-Forschung* 2, 10 (October 1987), p. 582; Guenter Frankenberg, "Germany: The Uneasy Triumph of Pragmatism," David

L. Kirp and Ronald Bayer, eds., *AIDS in the Industrialized Democracies* (New Brunswick, 1992), p. 128.

220. Deutsche AIDS-Hilfe, *Restrictions of Entry and Residence*, p. 15; Michael Kirby, "Inefficient Laws Will Not Protect Countries against AIDS," *Washington Post*, 2 February 1988.

221. WHO, *Legislative Responses*, p. 79; *IDHL* 39, 2 (1988), pp. 363–64; Claude Got, *Rapport sur le SIDA* (Paris, 1989), p. 42; Swiss Institute of Comparative Law, *Comparative Study*, p. 239.

222. *RD Prot*, 1986/87:109 (23 April 1987), p. 140; Westerhäll and Saldeen, "Réflexions sur le Sida," p. 393; Henriksson and Ytterberg, "Sweden," p. 331; Leijonhufvud, *HIV-smitta*, p. 16. This was also true in Germany: Friedrich Baumhauer, "Legal Measures Employed in Germany for Coping with AIDS," in AIDS-Forum D.A.H., *Aspects of AIDS and AIDS-Hilfe in Germany* (Berlin, 1993), p. 107.

223. *Hansard*, vol. 108 (16 January 1987), col. 342; Berridge, *AIDS in the UK*, p. 116; Swiss Institute of Comparative Law, *Comparative Study*, pp. 103–4; House of Commons, *Problems Associated with AIDS*, vol. 3, p. 78; Allin, "AIDS Pandemic," p. 1054; Eibe Riedel, "Internationale und europarechtliche Aspekte von AIDS," in Hans-Ullrich Gallwas et al., eds., *Aids und Recht* (Stuttgart, 1992), p. 220.

224. *Hansard*, vol. 111 (2 March 1987), col. 466; vol. 146 (10 February 1989), col. 820; Wesley Gryk, "AIDS and Immigration," in Richard Haigh and Dai Harris, eds., *AIDS: A Guide to the Law*, 2d ed. (London, 1995), pp. 82–83; Qureshi, "Global Ostracism," p. 91.

225. Gryk, "AIDS and Immigration," p. 79; Horn, "Die Behandlung von AIDS," p. 204.

226. Setbon, *Pouvoirs contre SIDA*, pp. 366–67; Faith G. Pendleton, "The United States Exclusion of HIV-Positive Aliens: Realities and Illusions," *Suffolk Transnational Law Review* 18 (1995), pp. 298–99; Lia Macko, "Acquiring a Better Global Vision: An Argument against the United States' Current Exclusion of HIV-Infected Immigrants," *Georgetown Immigration Law Journal* 9 (1995), p. 546; Juan P. Osuna, "The Exclusion from the United States of Aliens Infected with the AIDS Virus," *Houston Journal of International Law* 16, 1 (1993), p. 14.

227. Robert M. Wachter, *The Fragile Coalition: Scientists, Activists, and AIDS* (New York, 1991), pp. 113–15, 124–25, 134; *Congressional Record* (Senate), 5 April 1990, pp. 4069–70.

228. Claude Évin and Bruno Durieux, *La lutte contre le sida en France* (Paris, 1992), p. 103.

229. *IDHL* 38, 3 (1987), p. 502.

230. Carol Leslie Wolchok, "AIDS at the Frontier: United States Immigration Policy," *Journal of Legal Medicine* 10, 1 (1989), pp. 127–29; Wachter, *Fragile Coalition*, pp. 28–31; Lücke, *Aids*, p. 61; Jayasuriya, *AIDS*, p. 42.

231. Rubenstein et al., *Rights of People*, p. 315; Goodwin-Gill, "AIDS and HIV, Migrants, and Refugees," pp. 62–63; Christopher H. Foreman Jr., *Plagues*,

Products, and Politics: Emergent Public Health Hazards and National Policy-making (Washington, DC, 1994), p. 64; Larry O. Gostin et al., "Screening Immigrants and International Travelers for the Human Immunodeficiency Virus," *New England Journal of Medicine* 322, 24 (14 June 1990), p. 1743; Allin, "AIDS Pandemic," p. 1055.

232. Timothy F. Murphy, *Ethics in an Epidemic: AIDS, Morality, and Culture* (Berkeley, 1994), pp. 129–33; *Report of the Presidential Commission*, p. 156; *AIDS-Nachrichten aus Forschung und Wissenschaft* 3 (1991), pp. 1–2; Donna I. Dennis, "HIV Screening and Discrimination: The Federal Example," in Scott Burris et al., eds., *AIDS Law Today* (New Haven, 1993), pp. 203–5; Edward J. Lynch, "Medical Exclusion and Admissions Policy: Statutes and Strictures," *New York University Journal of International Law and Politics* 23 (1991), pp. 1004–8; Dickens, "HIV Screening," p. 110.

233. Pendleton, "The United States Exclusion of HIV-Positive Aliens," pp. 277, 295; *Congressional Record* (House), 11 March 1993, p. 1205.

234. *Congressional Record*, Extensions of Remarks, 22 March 1994, pp. 506–7; Qureshi, "Global Ostracism," p. 96.

235. House of Commons, *Problems Associated with AIDS*, vol. 3, p. 134; van Wijngaarden, "The Netherlands," p. 260. During the 1994 Fourth International Gay Games, New York City earned some four hundred million dollars. Gary W. Dowsett, "Governing Queens: Gay Communities and the State in Contemporary Australia," in Mitchell Dean and Barry Hindess, eds., *Governing Australia: Studies in Contemporary Rationalities of Government* (Cambridge, 1998), p. 139.

236. Legrand, "Les personnes de nationalité étrangère," p. 766; Dickens, "HIV Screening," pp. 111–12; Hubert, "AIDS in Belgium," p. 106.

237. Adrian Favell and Randall Hansen, "Markets against Politics: Migration, EU Enlargement, and the Idea of Europe," *Journal of Ethnic and Migration Studies* 28, 4 (2002); Christian Joppke, "Asylum and State Sovereignty: A Comparison of the United States, Germany, and Britain," in Joppke, ed., *Challenge to the Nation-State: Immigration in Western Europe and the United States* (Oxford, 1998), pp. 112–13.

4. PATIENTS INTO PRISONERS: RESPONSIBILITY, CRIME, AND HEALTH

1. Larry O. Gostin, "Public Health Strategies for Confronting AIDS: Legislative and Regulatory Policy in the United States," *JAMA* 261, 11 (17 March 1989), p. 1626; Ronald Bayer, "AIDS, Public Health, and Civil Liberties: Consensus and Conflict in Policy," in Frederick G. Reamer, ed., *AIDS and Ethics* (New York, 1991), p. 45; Donald H. J. Hermann and William P. Schurgin, *Legal Aspects of AIDS* (Deerfield, IL, 1991), §9:03; Larry Gostin, "The Politics of AIDS: Compulsory State Powers, Public Health, and Civil Liberties," *Ohio State Law Journal* 49 (1989), p. 1038.

2. William J. Novak, *The People's Welfare: Law and Regulation in Nineteenth-Century America* (Chapel Hill, 1996), ch. 5.

3. Nikolas Rose, *Governing the Soul: The Shaping of the Private Self*, 2d ed. (London, 1999); Nikolas Rose, *Powers of Freedom: Reframing Political Thought* (Cambridge, 1999); Peter N. Stearns, *Battleground of Desire: The Struggle for Self-Control in Modern America* (New York, 1999).

4. Peter Baldwin, "The Return of the Coercive State? Behavioral Control in Multicultural Society," in John A. Hall et al., eds., *The Nation-State under Challenge: Autonomy and Capacity in a Changing World* (Princeton, 2003).

5. Ingemar Folke, "Anteckningar om prostitutionen och lagen," in Gunilla Fredelius, ed., *Ett onödigt ont: En antologi mot porr och prostitution* (Stockholm, 1978), p. 45; Tomas Söderblom, *Horan och batongen: Prostitution och repression i folkhemmet* (Stockholm, 1992), p. 176; Margaret Davis, *Lovers, Doctors, and the Law* (New York, 1988), p. 82; Bernard M. Dickens, "Legal Rights and Duties in the AIDS Epidemic," *Science* 239, 4840 (5 February 1988), p. 580; David Feldman, *Civil Liberties and Human Rights in England and Wales* (Oxford, 1993), pp. 513–14.

6. Peter Baldwin, *Contagion and the State in Europe, 1830–1930* (Cambridge, 1999), pp. 429–34.

7. Scott Burris, "Fear Itself: AIDS, Herpes, and Public Health Decisions," *Yale Law and Policy Review* 3, 479 (1985), pp. 496–504; Mark Blumberg, *AIDS: The Impact on the Criminal Justice System* (Columbus, 1990), p. 53; Harold Edgar and Hazel Sandomire, "Medical Privacy Issues in the Age of AIDS: Legislative Options," *American Journal of Law and Medicine* 16, 1–2 (1990), p. 161; Andrew Grubb and David S. Pearl, *Blood Testing, AIDS and DNA Profiling: Law and Policy* (Bristol, 1990), p. 8.

8. BT *Verhandlungen* 11/71, 14 April 1988, pp. 4806D–07A.

9. Wilfried Bottke, "Strafrechtliche Probleme von AIDS und der AIDS-Bekämpfung," in Bernd Schünemann and Gerd Pfeiffer, eds., *Die Rechtsprobleme von AIDS* (Baden-Baden, 1988), p. 180; Madeleine Leijonhufvud, *HIV-smitta: Straff- och skadeståndsansvar* (Stockholm, 1993), pp. 60–61, 73–74, 102–9; Frédéric Ocqueteau, "La répression pénale dans la lutte contre le sida: Solution ou alibi?" in Eric Heilmann, ed., *Sida et libertés: La régulation d'une épidemie dans un état de droit* (n.p., 1991), p. 235; Felix Herzog, "Das Strafrecht im Kampf gegen 'Aids-Desperados,'" in Ernst Burkel, ed., *Der AIDS-Komplex: Dimensionen einer Bedrohung* (Frankfurt, 1988), p. 343; Michael Tanner and the ALEC National Working Group on State AIDS Policy, *The Politics of Health: A State Response to the AIDS Crisis* (n.p., 1989), p. 87; Mark H. Jackson, "The Criminalization of HIV," in Nan D. Hunter and William B. Rubenstein, eds., *AIDS Agenda: Emerging Issues in Civil Rights* (New York, 1992), pp. 242–52.

10. Jacob A. Heth, "Dangerous Liaisons: Criminalizing Conduct Related to HIV Transmission," *Willamette Law Review* 29 (1993), p. 851.

11. Kathleen M. Sullivan and Martha A. Field, "AIDS and the Coercive Power of the State," *Harvard Civil Rights–Civil Liberties Law Review* 23

(1988), pp. 163–65; Larry Gostin, "The Politics of AIDS: Compulsory State Powers, Public Health, and Civil Liberties," *Ohio State Law Journal* 49 (1989), p. 1053; Donald H. J. Hermann, "AIDS and the Law," in Frederick G. Reamer, ed., *AIDS and Ethics* (New York, 1991), p. 297; William B. Rubenstein et al., *The Rights of People Who Are HIV Positive* (Carbondale, IL, 1996), p. 76; Otfried Seewald, "Aids als Herausforderung an den Verfassungsstaat des Grundgesetzes," in Ernst Burkel, ed., *Der AIDS-Komplex: Dimensionen einer Bedrohung* (Frankfurt, 1988), p. 302; Herbert Tröndle, *Strafgesetzbuch*, 48th ed. (Munich, 1997), p. 1191; Bernd Schünemann, "AIDS und Strafrecht," in Andrzej J. Szwarc, ed., *AIDS und Strafrecht* (Berlin, 1996), pp. 19–22, 37, 63; Klaus Scherf, *AIDS und Strafrecht* (Baden-Baden, 1992), pp. 61–68; Monika Steffen, *The Fight against AIDS: An International Public Policy Comparison between Four European Countries: France, Great Britain, Germany, and Italy* (Grenoble, 1996), p. 53.

12. In *Bowers v. Hardwick* 1986, where the Supreme Court refused to extend privacy protections to consensual homosexual relations. William N. Eskridge Jr., *Gaylaw: Challenging the Apartheid of the Closet* (Cambridge, MA, 1999), p. 171; Michael L. Closen et al., *AIDS: Cases and Materials* (Houston, 1989), p. 679.

13. Cornelius Nester, "AIDS: Strafzumessung und Sicherungsmassnahmen," in Andrzej J. Szwarc, ed., *AIDS und Strafrecht* (Berlin, 1996), p. 214; Michael Kirby, "AIDS and the Law," *Dædalus* 118, 3 (summer 1989), p. 108; Rubenstein et al., *Rights of People*, p. 75; Dieter Meurer, "AIDS und Strafrecht," in Hans-Ullrich Gallwas et al., eds., *Aids und Recht* (Stuttgart, 1992), p. 117.

14. Jean-Paul Jean, "Les problèmes juridiques soulevés par le développement des MST et leur prévention," in Nadine Job-Spira et al., eds., *Santé publique et maladies à transmission sexuelle* (Montrouge, 1990), p. 125; BT Drucksache 11/7200, 31 May 1990, pp. 164–68, 171–72; *Report of the Presidential Commission on the Human Immunodeficiency Virus Epidemic* (Washington, DC, 1988), p. 130; Andreas Salmen, "Aktuelle Erfordernisse der Aidsprävention," in Rolf Rosenbrock and Andreas Salmen, eds., *Aids-Prävention* (Berlin, 1990), p. 94; H. Jäger, ed., *AIDS und HIV-Infektionen* (n.p., n.d.), ix–2.3.3, pp. 1–5; American Bar Association, *Policy on AIDS and the Criminal Justice System* (Chicago, 1989), pp. 5–6.

15. Leijonhufvud, *HIV-smitta*, p. 80; Martha A. Field and Kathleen M. Sullivan, "AIDS and the Criminal Law," *Law, Medicine, and Health Care* 15, 1–2 (summer 1987), p. 46.

16. Nester, "AIDS," p. 215; Hubert Rottleuthner, "Probleme der rechtlichen Regulierung von Aids," in Rolf Rosenbrock and Andreas Salmen, eds., *Aids-Prävention* (Berlin, 1990), p. 123; Andrzej J. Szwarc, *AIDS und Strafrecht* (Berlin, 1996), pp. 231, 234.

17. *Congressional Record* (Senate), 11 July 1991, p. 9796; (Senate) 18 July 1991, p. 10342.

18. Arthur Kreuzer, "Sozialwissenschaftlich-kriminologische Vorbehalte gegenüber der strafrechtsdogmatisch-kriminalpolitischen Aids-Diskussion," in

Cornelius Prittwitz, ed., *Aids, Recht und Gesundheitspolitik* (Berlin, 1990), p. 118; *AIDS: Fakten und Konsequenzen: Endbericht der Enquête-Kommission des 11. Deutschen Bundestages "Gefahren von AIDS und wirksame Wege zu ihrer Eindämmung"* (Bonn, 1990), p. 316; BT *Verhandlungen* 11/110, 24 November 1988, p. 7748B; 11/103, 27 October 1988, p. 7055 B-C; BT *Drucksache* 11/7200, 31 May 1990, p. 165.

19. Vagn Greve and Annika Snare, "Retssystemet v. Aids?" *Retfærd* 9, 34 (1986), p. 11.

20. Hermann and Schurgin, *Legal Aspects,* §3:17.

21. Ibid., §4:16; §9:26.50.

22. Herzog, "Das Strafrecht im Kampf gegen 'Aids-Desperados,'" pp. 331 ff; Peter H. Stephenson, "Le SIDA, la syphilis et la stigmatisation: La genèse des politiques et des préjugés," *Anthropologie et sociétés* 15, 2–3 (1991), p. 91; André Glucksmann, *La fêlure du monde: Éthique et sida* (n.p., 1994), p. 155; Stephanie C. Kane, *AIDS Alibis: Sex, Drugs, and Crime in the Americas* (Philadelphia, 1998), pp. 170–71; Michael Fumento, *The Myth of Heterosexual AIDS* (New York, 1990), p. 61; Nicolas Mauriac, *Le mal entendu: Le sida et les médias* (Paris, 1990), p. 113; Bernard Paillard, *Notes on the Plague Years: AIDS in Marseilles* (New York, 1998), p. 11; Dennis Altman, *Global Sex* (Chicago, 2001), p. 144; *Journal Officiel, Débats,* Assemblée Nationale, 20 June 1991, p. 3433.

23. *Los Angeles Times,* 6 December 1998; 24 October 1998, p. A18; Rolf Dietrich Herzberg, "Die strafrechtliche Haftung für die Infizierung oder Gefährdung durch HIV," in Andrzej J. Szwarc, ed., *AIDS und Strafrecht* (Berlin, 1996), p. 61; *New York Times,* 29 July 1999, p. A19.

24. Schünemann, "AIDS und Strafrecht," pp. 19–22, 37; Scherf, *AIDS und Strafrecht,* pp. 46–50, 55–56; Roland Christiani, *AIDS und Zufallsbekanntschaften: Die Haftung der Virusträgers für die Infektion seines Partners* (Regensburg, 1993), pp. 18, 34–37; Maren Sedelies, *Arbeitsrechtliche Probleme im Umgang mit der Immunschwächekrankheit Aids* (Aachen, 1992), pp. 156–57, 179; Arnulf F. Günther, "Die Strafbarkeit des AIDS-Infizierten beim sexueller Verkehr," (Ph.D. diss., University of Kiel, 1988), passim.

25. Szwarc, *AIDS und Strafrecht,* pp. 63, 124, 231–34; Wilfried Bottke, "Die Immission infektiösen Ejakulats bei ungeschütztem Geschlechtsverkehr zwischen HIV-Infizierten und minderjährigen Jugendlichen," *AIDS-Forschung* 11 (1988), pp. 628–39.

26. "Amtsgericht Kempten (Allgäu), Urteil vom 1. Juli 1988," *AIDS-Forschung* 11 (1988), pp. 640–44; "Landgericht Kempten (Allgäu), Urteil vom 20. Januar 1989," *AIDS-Forschung* 5 (1989), pp. 256–60; Scherf, *AIDS und Strafrecht,* pp. 35–36; Walter Scheuerl, *Aids und Strafrecht: Die Strafbarkeit HIV-infizierter Personen beim Vollziehen sexueller Kontakte* (Münster, 1992), pp. 57–58; Daniel Borrillo and Anne Masseran, eds., *Sida et droits de l'homme: L'épidémie dans un Etat de droit* (Strasbourg, 1991), pp. 225–26; Anne Le Gallou, "SIDA et droit pénal," in Brigitte Feuillet-Le Mintier, ed., *Le SIDA: Aspects juridiques* (Paris, 1995), pp. 146–47; Ronald Turner, "AIDS and Employment:

Asymptomatic Human Immunodeficiency Virus Carriers and Section 504 of the Rehabilitation Act," *AIDS and Public Policy Journal* 5, 4 (1990), pp. 168–69.

27. David L. Kirp and Ronald Bayer, "The Second Decade of AIDS: The End of Exceptionalism?" in Kirp and Bayer, eds., *AIDS in the Industrialized Democracies* (New Brunswick, 1992), p. 368; Dickens, "Legal Rights and Duties," p. 583.

28. Baldwin, *Contagion and the State,* pp. 429–36; Leijonhufvud, *HIV-smitta,* p. 94; W. Spann, "Gerichtsmedizinische Aspekte der HIV-Infektion," *AIDS-Forschung* 12 (1987), p. 701.

29. Lotta Westerhäll and Ake Saldeen, "Réflexions sur le Sida et le droit suédois," in Jacques Foyer and Lucette Khaïat, eds., *Droit et Sida: Comparaison internationale* (Paris, 1994), p. 410; Swiss Institute of Comparative Law, *Comparative Study on Discrimination against Persons with HIV or AIDS* (Strasbourg, 1993), p. 62; Leijonhufvud, *HIV-smitta,* pp. 15, 35–37.

30. Borrillo and Masseran, *Sida et droits de l'homme,* p. 223–26; Claude Got, *Rapport sur le SIDA* (Paris, 1989), p. 82; Michel Danti-Juan, "Quelques reflexions en droit penal français sur les problemes posés par le sida," *Revue de droit penal et de criminologie* 68 (1988), pp. 636–39; Monika Steffen, "AIDS and Political Systems," in Dorothee Friedrich and Wolfgang Heckmann, eds., *Aids in Europe: The Behavioural Aspect* (Berlin, 1995), 5:37–38; AIDES, *Droit et S.I.D.A.: Guide juridique,* 3d ed. (Paris, 1996), pp. 153–54; Brigitte Feuillet-Le Mintier, ed., *Le SIDA: Aspects juridiques* (Paris, 1995), pp. 69, 146; Ocqueteau, "La répression pénale," pp. 241–44.

31. Alistair Orr, "Legal AIDS: Implications of AIDS and HIV for British and American Law," *Journal of Medical Ethics* 15 (1989), p. 65; Gerald Forlin and Piers Wauchope, "AIDS and the Criminal Law," *Law Society's Gazette* 84, 12 (25 March 1987), pp. 884–85; Margaret Brazier and Maureen Mulholland, "Droit et Sida: Le Royaume-uni," in Jacques Foyer and Lucette Khaïat, eds., *Droit et Sida: Comparaison internationale* (Paris, 1994), pp. 374, 380; *Hansard Parliamentary Debates,* vol. 119 (16 July 1987), col. 604.

32. Angus Hamilton, "The Criminal Law and HIV Infection," in Richard Haigh and Dai Harris, eds., *AIDS: A Guide to the Law,* 2d ed. (London, 1995), pp. 27–30; Leslie J. Moran, *The Homosexual(ity) of Law* (London, 1996), pp. 180–91; Anthony P. M. Coxon, *Between the Sheets: Sexual Diaries and Gay Men's Sex in the Era of AIDS* (London, 1996), p. 132.

33. Simon Bronitt, "Spreading Disease and the Criminal Law," *Criminal Law Review* (1994), pp. 21–22, 27.

34. *IDHL* 45, 1 (1994).

35. Harlon L. Dalton, "Criminal Law," in Scott Burris et al., eds., *AIDS Law Today* (New Haven, 1993), pp. 250–51; Monika Steffen, "France: Social Solidarity and Scientific Expertise," in David L. Kirp and Ronald Bayer, eds., *AIDS in the Industrialized Democracies* (New Brunswick, 1992), p. 242.

36. Albert R. Jonsen and Jeff Stryker, eds., *The Social Impact of AIDS in the United States* (Washington, DC, 1993), p. 36; *Congressional Record* (House), 13 June 1990, p. 3532; (House) 31 July 1990, pp. 6031–32, 6046; Rubenstein et al.,

Rights of People, p. 81; Ronald Bayer and David L. Kirp, "The United States: At the Center of the Storm," in Kirp and Bayer, eds., AIDS in the Industrialized Democracies (New Brunswick, 1992), p. 32; IDHL 37, 3 (1986), pp. 544–45; Tanner and the ALEC National Working Group on State AIDS Policy, Politics of Health, p. 87; Los Angeles Times, 27 April 2002, p. A14.

37. D. C. Jayasuriya, AIDS: Public Health and Legal Dimensions (Dordrecht, 1988), p. 29; Kirby, "AIDS and the Law," pp. 102, 107; Margaret Duckett, ed., Australia's Response to AIDS (Canberra, 1986), p. 33.

38. Bundesrat, Drucksache 294/87, 16 July 1987, pp. 31–32; Staatssekretärsausschuss "AIDS" der Bayerischen Staatsregierung, Konzept der Bayerischen Staatsregierung zur Bekämpfung der Immunschwächekrankheit AIDS (Munich, n.d.), pp. 12 ff.

39. "Landgericht Nürnberg-Fürth—13. Strafkammer, Urteil vom 16. November 1987," AIDS-Forschung 5 (1988), pp. 278–82; BT Drucksache 11/7200, 31 May 1990, p. 191; Wolfgang Schumacher and Egon Meyn, Bundes-Seuchengesetz, 4th ed; (Cologne, 1992), pp. 165–67; Meurer, "AIDS und Strafrecht," p. 118; W. Eberbach, Rechtsprobleme der HTLV-III-Infektion (AIDS) (Berlin, 1986), pp. 8–9; Scherf, AIDS und Strafrecht, pp. 29–31; "Landgericht München I, 6. Strafkammer, Urteil vom 20. Juli 1987," AIDS-Forschung 11 (1987), pp. 648–51; "Landgericht München I—Jugendkammer, Urteil vom 12.4.1991," AIDS-Forschung 6, 11 (November 1991), p. 598.

40. Manfred Bruns, "AIDS, Prostitution und das Strafrecht," Neue Juristische Wochenschrift 40, 12 (1987), p. 693; Jäger, ed., AIDS und HIV-Infektionen, ix–2.3.11, pp. 1–2, 4. Similarly in Switzerland: Roger Gaillard, "Virus et médias," in Jean Martin, ed., Faire face au SIDA (Lausanne, 1988), p. 91.

41. Jacques Foyer and Lucette Khaïat "Droit et SIDA: La situation française," in Foyer and Khaïat, eds., Droit et Sida: Comparaison internationale (Paris, 1994), p. 239.

42. Swiss Institute of Comparative Law, Comparative Study, p. 63; Ocqueteau, "La répression pénale," p. 234; Hermann and Schurgin, Legal Aspects, §9:05, supplement; Scherf, AIDS und Strafrecht, p. 41; Foyer and Khaïat "Droit et SIDA," p. 240; Leijonhufvud, HIV-smitta, p. 38; "Amtsgericht München, Urteil vom 24. 11. 1989," AIDS-Forschung 5 (1990), p. 248.

43. Swiss Institute of Comparative Law, Comparative Study, pp. 63–64.

44. Scherf, AIDS und Strafrecht, p. 177; Bottke, "Strafrechtliche Probleme," p. 181.

45. Cornelius Prittwitz, "Strafrechtliche Aspekte von HIV-Infektion und Aids," in Prittwitz, Aids, Recht und Gesundheitspolitik, p. 141; Jäger, AIDS und HIV-Infektionen, ix–2.3.4, pp. 1, 5; Schünemann, "AIDS und Strafrecht," pp. 19–22, 37; Ocqueteau, "La répression pénale," p. 247; Scheuerl, Aids und Strafrecht, pp. 161–262.

46. Leijonhufvud, HIV-smitta, pp. 46–49; Scherf, AIDS und Strafrecht, pp. 35–36.

47. IDHL 39, 3 (1988), pp. 626–27; 44, 1 (1993), pp. 27–28; 44, 2 (1993), p. 229; WHO, Legislative Responses to AIDS (Dordrecht, 1989), p. 193.

48. *IDHL* 39, 3 (1988), p. 633; 42, 2 (1991), pp. 245–54; Jayasuriya, *AIDS*, p. 29; Kirby, "AIDS and the Law," p. 107; WHO, *Legislative Responses*, pp. 224, 228; Hermann and Schurgin, *Legal Aspects*, §9:05.50; Heth, "Dangerous Liaisons," pp. 844–45.

49. Robert B. Gainor, "To Have and to Hold: The Tort Liability for the Interspousal Transmission of AIDS," *New England Law Review* 23 (1988–89), p. 907.

50. Ksenija Savin, "Sex, Culture, Law, and AIDS: Draft for a Research Project," in Dorothee Friedrich and Wolfgang Heckmann, eds., *Aids in Europe: The Behavioural Aspect* (Berlin, 1995), 4:302–3; Swiss Institute of Comparative Law, *Comparative Study*, p. 65; Diana Brahams, "AIDS and the Law," *New Law Journal* 137 (1987), p. 751.

51. Leijonhufvud, *HIV-smitta*, pp. 25, 38–39.

52. Baldwin, *Contagion and the State*, pp. 434–36.

53. Mildred Blaxter, *AIDS: Worldwide Policies and Problems* (London, 1991), p. 6.

54. Got, *Rapport sur le SIDA*, pp. 42, 221–22; WHO, *Legislative Responses*, p. 75; *IDHL* 38, 4 (1987), pp. 766–67; Michel Danti-Juan, "Quelques reflexions en droit penal français sur les problemes posés par le sida," *Revue de droit penal et de criminologie* 68 (1988), p. 636; Staatssekretärsausschuss "AIDS" der Bayerischen Staatsregierung, *Konzept der Bayerischen Staatsregierung*, pp. 12 ff; Günter Frankenberg, *AIDS-Bekämpfung im Rechtsstaat* (Baden-Baden, 1988), pp. 196–97; Hans-Georg Koch, "AIDS und Schwangerschaft: Strafrechtliche Probleme," in Andrzej J. Szwarc, ed., *AIDS und Strafrecht* (Berlin, 1996), pp. 190–91.

55. WHO, *Legislative Responses*, pp. 119, 174; *IDHL* 38, 3 (1987), p. 492; 39, 1 (1988), p. 56; Sundhedsbestyrelsen, *AIDS: Sygdommen AIDS og retningslinier til forebyggelse af HIV-infektion* (n.p. [Copenhagen], 1988), p. 24; Socialstyrelsens författningssamling 1986:1.

56. Hermann and Schurgin, *Legal Aspects*, §4:16, 4:23; Gena Corea, *The Invisible Epidemic: The Story of Women and AIDS* (New York, 1992), p. 48.

57. Michael D. Kirby, "AIDS: Epidemic and Society, Element of Synthesis," in Charles Mérieux, ed., *SIDA: Épidémies et sociétés* (n.p., 1987), pp. 192–93; Robin Gorna, *Vamps, Virgins, and Victims: How Can Women Fight AIDS?* (London, 1996), pp. 240–43; Chloe O'Gara and Anna C. Martin, "HIV and Breast-Feeding: Informed Choice in the Face of Medical Ambiguity," in Lynellyn D. Long and E. Maxine Ankrah, eds., *Women's Experiences with HIV/AIDS* (New York, 1996), p. 221; Thomas C. Quinn et al., "Special Considerations for Developing Nations," in Philip A. Pizzo and Catherine M. Wilfert, eds., *Pediatric AIDS*, 2d ed. (Baltimore, 1994), p. 37.

58. Inger Marie Conradsen, "Hiv, graviditet og hvad så?" *Retfærd* 17, 2 (1994), pp. 36, 39–41.

59. House of Commons, 1986–87, Social Services Committee, *Problems Associated with AIDS*, 13 May 1987, vol. 2, pp. 70–71; *Los Angeles Times*, 10 July 2002, p. A3.

60. Friedrich Nietzsche, *The Birth of Tragedy*, ch. 3, vs. 19–24.

61. George Rosen, *Preventive Medicine in the United States, 1900–1975* (New York, 1975), p. 41.

62. Bayer, "AIDS, Public Health, and Civil Liberties," p. 41; Ronald Bayer, "Perinatal Transmission of HIV Infection: The Ethics of Prevention," in Lawrence O. Gostin, ed., *AIDS and the Health Care System* (New Haven, 1990), pp. 66–68; Nan D. Hunter, "AIDS Prevention and Civil Liberties: The False Security of Mandatory Testing," *Aids and Public Policy Journal* 2, 3 (summer–fall 1987), p. 5.

63. Penelope Ploughman, "Public Policy versus Private Rights: The Medical, Social, Ethical and Legal Implications of the Testing of Newborns for HIV," *AIDS and Public Policy Journal* 10, 4 (1995–96), p. 190; Rubenstein et al., *Rights of People*, p. 205; Nan D. Hunter, "Complications of Gender: Women and HIV Disease," in Hunter and William B. Rubenstein, eds., *AIDS Agenda: Emerging Issues in Civil Rights* (New York, 1992), p. 17.

64. *Los Angeles Times,* 29 February 2000, p. A14; Hermann and Schurgin, *Legal Aspects,* §3:38, §4:23; Suzanne Sangree, "Control of Childbearing by HIV-Positive Women," *Buffalo Law Review* 41, 2 (spring 1993), pp. 327–28; Closen, *AIDS: Cases and Materials,* pp. 463–65.

65. *Congressional Record* (House), 31 July 1990, p. 6046; Nan D. Hunter, "Complications of Gender: Women, AIDS, and the Law," in Beth E. Schneider and Nancy E. Stoller, eds., *Women Resisting AIDS: Feminist Strategies of Empowerment* (Philadelphia, 1995), pp. 37, 44; Sangree, "Control of Childbearing," p. 346.

66. Dickens, "Legal Rights and Duties," p. 583.

67. Eberbach, *Rechtsprobleme,* pp. 19–21, 30–31; Koch, "AIDS und Schwangerschaft," pp. 185–89; Alexander Utz, "Schadensrechtliche Probleme im Zusammenhang mit einer HIV-Infektion," *AIDS-Forschung* 2 (1988), pp. 98–99; Gerhard H. Schlund, "Juristische Aspekte beim erworbenen Immun-Defekt-Syndrom (AIDS)," *AIDS-Forschung* 10 (1986), p. 566.

68. Douglas A. Feldman, "Sacrificing Basic Civil Liberties," *Anthropology Newsletter* (December 1993), p. 2; Lorraine Sherr, *HIV and AIDS in Mothers and Babies* (London, 1991), pp. 91–93. The surveys were done in Scotland and New York.

69. Elinor Burkett, *The Gravest Show on Earth: America in the Age of AIDS* (Boston, 1995), p. 240; Hunter, "Complications of Gender: Women and HIV Disease," p. 19; Rebecca Bennett, "Should We Routinely Test Pregnant Women for HIV?" in Bennett and Charles A. Erin, eds., *HIV and AIDS: Testing, Screening, and Confidentiality* (Oxford, 1999), pp. 235–36; Sangree, "Control of Childbearing," pp. 338–40; Sandra Panem, *The AIDS Bureaucracy* (Cambridge, MA, 1988), p. 128; Cheri Pies, "AIDS, Ethics, Reproductive Rights: No Easy Answers," in Beth E. Schneider and Nancy E. Stoller, eds., *Women Resisting AIDS: Feminist Strategies of Empowerment* (Philadelphia, 1995), pp. 325–26.

70. House of Commons, *Problems Associated with AIDS,* vol. 1, p. xii; Foyer and Khaïat, "Droit et SIDA," p. 231; Westerhäll and Saldeen, "Réflexions sur le Sida," p. 412; Sundhedsbestyrelsen, *AIDS,* p. 24; Szwarc, *AIDS und Strafrecht,* p. 204.

71. Bayer, "Perinatal Transmission of HIV Infection," pp. 62–65, 69–70.

72. Amitai Etzioni, *The Limits of Privacy* (New York, 1999), pp. 22–23; Rubenstein et al., *Rights of People*, p. 205; Theodore J. Stein, *The Social Welfare of Women and Children with HIV and AIDS: Legal Protections, Policy, and Programs* (New York, 1998), pp. 93, 109–11; *Los Angeles Times*, 15 October 1998; 17 October 1998, p. A20.

73. Teresa Cameron, "Mandatory HIV Testing of Newborns in New York State: What Are the Implications?" *Journal of Health and Social Policy* 14, 3 (2002), pp. 59–61; Burkett, *Gravest Show on Earth*, pp. 239–41; Hunter, "Complications of Gender: Women, AIDS, and the Law," p. 46; Sangree, "Control of Childbearing," p. 356; Katherine L. Acuff, "Prenatal and Newborn Screening: State Legislative Approaches and Current Practice Standards," in Ruth R. Faden et al., eds., *AIDS, Women, and the Next Generation* (New York, 1991), p. 133; Chandler Burr, "The AIDS Exception: Privacy vs. Public Health," *Atlantic Monthly* 279 (June 1997), p. 65.

74. RD Prot, 1986/87, Bihang, Socialutskottets betänkande 19, p. 27; *IDHL* 39, 1 (1988), pp. 58–60; Michael Pollak, "AIDS Policy in France: Biomedical Leadership and Preventive Impotence," in Barbara A. Misztal and David Moss, eds., *Action on AIDS: National Policies in Comparative Perspective* (New York, 1990), p. 91; Monika Steffen, "AIDS Policies in France," in Virginia Berridge and Philip Strong, eds., *AIDS and Contemporary History* (Cambridge, 1993), p. 255; Swiss Institute of Comparative Law, *Comparative Study*, p. 16.

75. Viggo Hagstrøm, *AIDS som juridisk problem* (n.p., 1988), p. 51; Alistair Orr, "The Legal Implications of AIDS and HIV Infection in Britain and the United States," in Brenda Almond, ed., *AIDS: A Moral Issue* (London, 1990), p. 125; Donald H. J. Hermann and Scott Burris, "Torts: Private Lawsuits about HIV," in Burris et al., eds., *AIDS Law Today* (New Haven, 1993), pp. 340–42; Arnold J. Rosoff, "The AIDS Crisis: Constitutional Turning Point?" *Law, Medicine, and Health Care* 15, 1–2 (summer 1987), p. 84.

76. Hartmut Schulz, *Haftung für Infektion* (Frankfurt, 1988), pp. 18–20; Foyer and Khaïat, "Droit et SIDA," p. 234; Westerhäll and Saldeen, "Réflexions sur le Sida," pp. 406–9; Leijonhufvud, *HIV-smitta*, pp. 140–41.

77. Eric A. Feldman and Ronald Bayer, eds., *Blood Feuds: AIDS, Blood, and the Politics of Medical Disaster* (New York, 1999); Erwin Deutsch, "AIDS und Hämophilie in Frankreich und Deutschland," *AIDS-Forschung* 3 (1993), pp. 153–60; Monika Steffen, "Crisis Governance in France: The End of Sectoral Corporatism?" in Mark Bovens et al., eds., *Success and Failure in Public Governance: A Comparative Analysis* (Cheltenham, U.K., 2001); Jonathan M. Mann and Daniel J. M. Tarantola, eds., *AIDS in the World II* (New York, 1996), p. 289.

5. DISCRIMINATION AND ITS DISCONTENTS: PROTECTING THE VICTIMS

1. Cornelius Nester, "AIDS: Strafzumessung und Sicherungsmassnahmen," in Andrzej J. Szwarc, ed., *AIDS und Strafrecht* (Berlin, 1996), pp. 227,

232; Cornelius Nestler-Tremel, *AIDS und Strafzumessung* (Frankfurt, 1992); BT *Drucksache* 11/3243, 31 October 1988; Angus Hamilton, "The Criminal Law and HIV Infection," in Richard Haigh and Dai Harris, eds., *AIDS: A Guide to the Law,* 2d ed. (London, 1995), pp. 24–27, 30–31; Mark Blumberg, *AIDS: The Impact on the Criminal Justice System* (Columbus, 1990), pp. 54–55.

2. BT *Verhandlungen* 11/103, 27 October 1988, p. 7050D.

3. C. Everett Koop, "Individual Freedom and the Public Interest," in Alan F. Fleming et al., *The Global Impact of AIDS* (New York, 1988), p. 308; Paul Sieghart, *AIDS and Human Rights: A UK Perspective* (London, 1989), p. 19; Cathy Jean Cohen, "Power, Resistance, and the Construction of Crisis: Marginalized Communities Respond to AIDS" (Ph.D. diss., University of Michigan, 1993), pp. 210–15; Peter Lewis Allen, *The Wages of Sin: Sex and Disease, Past and Present* (Chicago, 2000), pp. 127–34.

4. Jonathan M. Mann, "AIDS: Discrimination and Public Health," in WHO, *Legislative Responses to AIDS* (Dordrecht, 1989), p. 292; House of Commons, 1986–87, Social Services Committee, *Problems Associated with AIDS,* 13 May 1987, vol. 3, pp. 23–25.

5. Ronald Bayer, *Private Acts, Social Consequences: AIDS and the Politics of Public Health* (New York, 1989), ch. 3.

6. Johanna Pindyck, "AIDS and the Blood Service System," in John Griggs, ed., *AIDS: Public Policy Dimensions* (New York, 1987), p. 87; Ronald Bayer, "Blood and AIDS in America," in Eric Feldman and Bayer, eds., *Blood Feuds: AIDS, Blood, and the Politics of Medical Disaster* (New York, 1999), p. 25; William B. Rubenstein et al., *The Rights of People Who Are HIV Positive* (Carbondale, IL, 1996), p. 93; Heather G. Miller et al., eds., *AIDS: The Second Decade* (Washington, DC, 1990), p. 22; Ronald Bayer and David L. Kirp, "The United States: At the Center of the Storm," in Kirp and Bayer, eds., *AIDS in the Industrialized Democracies* (New Brunswick, 1992), p. 22.

7. D. C. Jayasuriya, *AIDS: Public Health and Legal Dimensions* (Dordrecht, 1988), p. 40; IDHL 37, 4 (1986), pp. 764–65; 38, 1 (1987), pp. 33–35.

8. David Moss, "AIDS in Italy: Emergency in Slow Motion," in Barbara A. Misztal and Moss, eds., *Action on AIDS: National Policies in Comparative Perspective* (New York, 1990), p. 146; John Street, "British Government Policy on AIDS: Learning Not to Die of Ignorance," *Parliamentary Affairs* 41 (October 1988), p. 496; Andrew Grubb and David S. Pearl, *Blood Testing, AIDS, and DNA Profiling: Law and Policy* (Bristol, 1990), p. 79; *Hansard Parliamentary Debates,* vol. 69 (4 December 1984), col. 160; vol. 72 (4 February 1985), col. 450; vol. 72 (5 February 1985), col. 498.

9. RD *Prot,* 1984/85, Bihang, Socialutskottets betänkande 24, pp. 5–6; 1987/88, Bihang, Socialutskottets betänkande 10, p. 26; IDHL 37, 1 (1986), p. 27; Béatrice Thomas-Tual, "La fonction publique et le SIDA," in Brigitte Feuillet-Le Mintier, ed., *Le SIDA: Aspects juridiques* (Paris, 1995), p. 191.

10. Swiss Institute of Comparative Law, *Comparative Study on Discrimination against Persons with HIV or AIDS* (Strasbourg, 1993), p. 15; Jayasuriya, *AIDS,* p. 22; IDHL 40, 2 (1989), p. 378; 41, 1 (1990), p. 48; 43, 4 (1992), p. 733.

11. Anne Marie Moulin, "Reversible History: Blood Transfusion and the Spread of AIDS in France," in Caroline Hannaway et al., eds., *AIDS and the Public Debate* (Amsterdam, 1995), p. 177; Pierre Favre, "La gestion administrative du Sida," in Favre, ed., *Sida et politique: Les premiers affrontements (1981–1987)* (Paris, 1992), pp. 84–85; Frédéric Martel, *Le rose et le noir: Les homosexuels en France depuis 1968* (Paris, 1996), p. 226; *IDHL* 37, 3 (1986), pp. 536–37; Sebastian Roché, "Le sida en politique," *Revue politique et parlementaire* (1991), p. 37; *Journal Officiel, Débats*, Assemblée Nationale, 23 October 1991, p. 4926; Erik Albæk, "AIDS: The Evolution of a Non-Controversial Issue in Denmark" (paper presented at the American Political Science Association, 1990), p. 9; Erik Albæk, "The Never-Ending Story? The Political and Legal Controversies over HIV and the Blood Supply in Denmark," in Eric Feldman and Ronald Bayer, eds., *Blood Feuds: AIDS, Blood, and the Politics of Medical Disaster* (New York, 1999), p. 164.

12. *RD Prot*, 1984/85, Bihang, Socialutskottets betänkande 24, p. 6.

13. Edward King, *Safety in Numbers: Safer Sex and Gay Men* (London, 1993), p. 42; Eric A. Feldman, "HIV and Blood in Japan," in Feldman and Ronald Bayer, eds., *Blood Feuds: AIDS, Blood, and the Politics of Medical Disaster* (New York, 1999), p. 65.

14. Paul Farmer, *AIDS and Accusation: Haiti and the Geography of Blame* (Berkeley, 1992), p. 122; James Harvey Young, "AIDS and the FDA," in Caroline Hannaway et al., eds., *AIDS and the Public Debate* (Amsterdam, 1995), p. 48; Alan M. Kraut, "Plagues and Prejudice: Nativism's Construction of Disease in Nineteenth- and Twentieth-Century New York City," in David Rosner, ed., *Hives of Sickness: Public Health and Epidemics in New York City* (New Brunswick, 1995), pp. 65–66; *Congressional Record* (Senate), 14 January 1991, p. 884; Dorothy Nelkin, "Cultural Perspectives on Blood," in Eric Feldman and Ronald Bayer, eds., *Blood Feuds: AIDS, Blood, and the Politics of Medical Disaster* (New York, 1999), p. 280.

15. D. C. Jayasuriya, "AIDS-Related Legislation in the Context of the Third AIDS Pandemic," *Law, Medicine, and Health Care* 18, 1–2 (1990), p. 45; David Goss and Derek Adam-Smith, *Organizing AIDS: Workplace and Organizational Responses to the HIV/AIDS Epidemic* (London, 1995), p. 9; Don Nutbeam and Virginia Blakey, "The Concept of Health Promotion and AIDS Prevention: A Comprehensive and Integrated Basis for Action in the 1990s," *Health Promotion International* 5, 3 (1990), p. 235; Tonny Dina Maria Zeegers Paget, *AIDS and Public Health Measures: A Global Survey of the Activities of Legislatures, 1983–1993* (Groningen, 1996), p. 17; Harold Edgar and Hazel Sandomire, "Medical Privacy Issues in the Age of AIDS: Legislative Options," *American Journal of Law and Medicine* 16, 1–2 (1990), p. 211.

16. Dudley Clendinen and Adam Nagourney, *Out for Good: The Struggle to Build a Gay Rights Movement in America* (New York, 1999), pp. 523, 526–30; David L. Kirp and Ronald Bayer, "The Second Decade of AIDS: The End of Exceptionalism?" in Kirp and Bayer, eds., *AIDS in the Industrialized Democracies*

(New Brunswick, 1992), p. 372; *Hansard*, vol. 144 (13 January 1989), col. 1137; Goss and Adam-Smith, *Organizing AIDS*, p. 150.

17. John Borneman, "AIDS in the Two Berlins," in Douglas Crimp, ed., *AIDS: Cultural Analysis, Cultural Activism* (Cambridge, 1988), p. 225.

18. Wolfgang Heckmann, "AIDS: Soziale Veränderungen und soziale Arbeit," in Max Busch et al., eds., *HIV/AIDS und Straffälligkeit* (Bonn, 1991), p. 5.

19. Karen M. Offen, *European Feminisms, 1700–1950* (Stanford, 2000); Anne Cova, "French Feminism and Maternity: Theories and Policies 1890–1918," in Gisela Bock and Pat Thane, eds., *Maternity and Gender Policies* (London, 1991); Mona Ozouf, *Women's Words: Essay on French Singularity* (Chicago, 1997); Christoph Sachsse, *Mütterlichkeit als Beruf: Sozialarbeit, Sozialreform und Frauenbewegung 1871–1929,* 2d ed. (Opladen, 1994); Ann Taylor Allen, *Feminism and Motherhood in Germany, 1800–1914* (New Brunswick, 1991).

20. Ute Canaris, "Gesundheitspolitische Aspekte im Zusammenhang mit AIDS," in Johannes Korporal and Hubert Malouschek, eds., *Leben mit AIDS — Mit AIDS leben* (Hamburg, 1987), p. 288; Guenter Frankenberg, "Germany: The Uneasy Triumph of Pragmatism," David L. Kirp and Ronald Bayer, eds., *AIDS in the Industrialized Democracies* (New Brunswick, 1992), pp. 123–24.

21. Eileen Boris, " 'The Right to Work Is the Right to Live!' Fair Employment and the Quest for Social Citizenship," in Manfred Berg and Martin H. Geyer, eds., *Two Cultures of Rights: The Quest for Inclusion and Participation in Modern America and Germany* (Cambridge, 2002); Paul Burstein, *Discrimination, Jobs, and Politics: The Struggle for Equal Employment Opportunity in the United States since the New Deal* (Chicago, 1985), pp. 7–8.

22. William B. Rubenstein, ed., *Lesbians, Gay Men, and the Law* (New York, 1993), p. xviii.

23. Goss and Adam-Smith, *Organizing AIDS*, p. 139; Vagn Greve and Annika Snare, "Retssystemet v. Aids?" *Retfærd* 9, 34 (1986), p. 16; Alistair Orr, "The Legal Implications of AIDS and HIV Infection in Britain and the United States," in Brenda Almond, ed., *AIDS: A Moral Issue* (London, 1990), p. 114; Vera Boltho-Massarelli and Michael O'Boyle, "Droits de l'homme et santé publique, une nouvelle alliance," in Eric Heilmann, ed., *Sida et libertés: La régulation d'une épidemie dans un état de droit* (n.p., 1991), pp. 39–40; Olli Stålström and Outi Lithén, "AIDS in Finland," in Martin Breum and Aart Hendriks, eds., *AIDS and Human Rights* (Copenhagen, 1988), p. 51; Swiss Institute of Comparative Law, *Comparative Study*, pp. 256–57, 392, 405, 425.

24. Rob Tielman and Hans Hammelburg, "World Survey on the Social and Legal Position of Gays and Lesbians," in Aart Hendriks et al., eds., *The Third Pink Book: A Global View of Lesbian and Gay Liberation and Oppression* (Buffalo, 1993), pp. 274, 280, 282, 308, 312; Mark Bell, "Sexual Orientation and Antidiscrimination Policy: The European Community," in Terrell Carver and Véronique Mottier, eds., *Politics of Sexuality: Identity, Gender, Citizenship* (London, 1998).

25. David Feldman, *Civil Liberties and Human Rights in England and Wales* (Oxford, 1993), pp. 525–29.

26. Anne-Sophie Rieben Schizas, "Employment, the Law, and HIV: An Overview of European Legislation," in David FitzSimons et al., eds., *The Economic and Social Impact of AIDS in Europe* (London, 1995), p. 308; Brian Doyle, *Disability, Discrimination, and Equal Opportunities: A Comparative Study of the Employment Rights of Disabled Persons* (London, 1995), chs. 2, 3.

27. David Newell, "The Contract of Employment," *New Law Journal* 140 (1990), p. 992; *Hansard* (25 May 1994), col. 354; 26 May 1994, col. 485–542; Goss and Adam-Smith, *Organizing AIDS*, p. 122.

28. Ulrich-Arthur Birk, "AIDS im Sozialrecht," in Max Busch et al., eds., *HIV/AIDS und Straffälligkeit* (Bonn, 1991), p. 41–43; Swiss Institute of Comparative Law, *Comparative Study*, p. 265.

29. AIDES, *Droit et S.I.D.A.: Guide juridique*, 3d ed. (Paris, 1996), p. 41; Gérard Bach-Ignasse, "Le Sida et la vie politique française," in Michael Pollak et al., eds., *Homosexualités et Sida* (n.p., n.d. [1991]), p. 104; Jean-Pierre Laborde, "Quelques observations à propos de la loi du 12 juillet 1990 relative à la protection des personnes contre les discriminations en raison de leur état de santé ou de leur handicap," *Droit social* 7–8 (1991), p. 617.

30. Gregor Heemann, *AIDS und Arbeitsrecht: Rechtliche Fragen bei der Begründung und Beendigung von Arbeitsverhältnissen in der Bundesrepublik Deutschland und in England* (Baden-Baden, 1992), pp. 54–55, 138–39; Gill Green, "Processes of Stigmatization and Their Impact on the Employment of People with HIV," in David FitzSimons et al., eds., *The Economic and Social Impact of AIDS in Europe* (London, 1995), p. 251. For a similar logic in the United States, see Michael L. Closen et al., *AIDS: Cases and Materials* (Houston, 1989), p. 320.

31. Bernard Richmond, "HIV and Employment," in Richard Haigh and Dai Harris, eds., *AIDS: A Guide to the Law,* 2d ed. (London, 1995), pp. 51–52; Petra Wilson, "Discrimination in the Workplace: Protection and the Law in the UK," in David FitzSimons et al., eds., *The Economic and Social Impact of AIDS in Europe* (London, 1995), p. 312; Jeffrey A. Mello, *AIDS and the Law of Workplace Discrimination* (Boulder, 1995), p. 71.

32. *Le Monde*, 29 January 1988, p. 10; American Bar Association, AIDS Coordinating Committee, *AIDS: The Legal Issues* (Washington, DC, 1988), p. 85; Stålström and Lithén, "AIDS in Finland," p. 52; *Hansard*, vol. 144 (13 January 1989), col. 1137; Benny Henriksson and Hasse Ytterberg, "Sweden: The Power of the Moral(istic) Left," in David L. Kirp and Ronald Bayer, eds., *AIDS in the Industrialized Democracies* (New Brunswick, 1992), p. 330; *AIDS: Fakten und Konsequenzen: Endbericht der Enquête-Kommission des 11. Deutschen Bundestages "Gefahren von AIDS und wirksame Wege zu ihrer Eindämmung"* (Bonn, 1990), p. 223; BT *Verhandlungen* 11/71, 14 April 1988, p. 4809A-B; Michel Vincineau, "Les homosexuels face au Sida," in Vincineau, ed., *Le Sida: Un défi aux droits* (Brussels, 1991), p. 467; *Le Monde*, 4 March 1993.

33. Anne M. Trebilcock, "AIDS and the Workplace: Some Policy Pointers

from International Labour Standards," *International Labour Review* 128, 1 (1989), pp. 34–35; *Le Monde*, 29 January 1988, p. 10; Horst Schröder, "Les pratiques de dépistage du Sida aux communautés européennes," in Michel Vincineau, ed., *Le Sida: Un défi aux droits* (Brussels, 1991), pp. 58–60, 65–66; F. Cotti, "SIDA: La panoplie extravagante des mesures légales et policières," *Médicine et hygiène* 46 (10 February 1988), p. 437; Jonathan M. Mann and Daniel J. M. Tarantola, eds., *AIDS in the World II* (New York, 1996), p. 334.

34. Schizas, "Employment, the Law, and HIV," p. 304; Swiss Institute of Comparative Law, *Comparative Study*, p. 111.

35. Margaret Brazier and Maureen Mulholland, "Droit et Sida: Le Royaume-uni," in Jacques Foyer and Lucette Khaïat, eds., *Droit et Sida: Comparaison internationale* (Paris, 1994), p. 383; Wilson, "Discrimination in the Workplace," p. 314; Wilfried Bottke," SIDA et droit en République fédérale d'Allemagne," in Jacques Foyer and Lucette Khaïat, eds., *Droit et Sida: Comparaison internationale* (Paris, 1994), pp. 36–37; Lotta Westerhäll and Ake Saldeen, "Réflexions sur le Sida et le droit suédois," in Jacques Foyer and Lucette Khaïat, eds., *Droit et Sida: Comparaison internationale* (Paris, 1994), p. 414; Swiss Institute of Comparative Law, *Comparative Study*, pp. 113, 119; Françoise Degott-Kieffer, "Maladies nouvelles et droit du travail, le cas de l'infection par le VIH," in Eric Heilmann, ed., *Sida et libertés: La régulation d'une épidemie dans un état de droit* (n.p., 1991), p. 221; *AIDS-Forschung* 2, 10 (October 1987), p. 566.

36. WHO, *Legislative Responses*, pp. 1, 64; *IDHL* 39, 2 (1988), pp. 358–60.

37. Alistair Orr, "Legal AIDS: Implications of AIDS and HIV for British and American Law," *Journal of Medical Ethics* 15 (1989), p. 66; Brazier and Mulholland, "Droit et Sida," p. 383; Green, "Processes of Stigmatization," p. 251; Jonathan Grimshaw, "AIDS and Human Rights in the United Kingdom," in Martin Breum and Aart Hendriks, eds., *AIDS and Human Rights* (Copenhagen, 1988), p. 144; Richmond, "HIV and Employment," p. 45; Orr, " Legal Implications of AIDS," p. 129; Heemann, *AIDS und Arbeitsrecht*, pp. 151–52, 185; Petra Wilson, "Colleague or Viral Vector? The Legal Construction of the HIV-Positive Worker," *Law and Policy* 16, 3 (1994), pp. 302–3; Swiss Institute of Comparative Law, *Comparative Study*, pp. 113, 116; *Hansard*, vol. 190 (1 May 1991), col. 234.

38. Annika Snare, "The Legal Treatment of AIDS in Denmark," in Martin Breum and Aart Hendriks, eds., *AIDS and Human Rights* (Copenhagen, 1988), p. 41; Viggo Hagstrøm, *AIDS som juridisk problem* (n.p., 1988), p. 84; Schizas, "Employment, the Law, and HIV," pp. 305–6; Swiss Institute of Comparative Law, *Comparative Study*, pp. 113, 116; Henriksson and Ytterberg, "Sweden," p. 330; Westerhäll and Saldeen, "Réflexions sur le Sida," p. 414.

39. Heemann, *AIDS und Arbeitsrecht*, pp. 60–69, 86–87; Maren Sedelies, *Arbeitsrechtliche Probleme im Umgang mit der Immunschwächekrankheit Aids* (Aachen, 1992), pp. 17–20; Winfried Mummenhoff, "Arbeitsrechtliche Problemkreise bei HIV-Infektionen," in Hans-Ullrich Gallwas et al., eds., *Aids und Recht* (Stuttgart, 1992), pp. 156–60; Bottke, "SIDA et droit," pp. 35–36; Jörg Lücke, *Aids im amerikanischen und deutschen Recht* (Berlin, 1989), p. 149; BT

Drucksache 11/7200, 31 May 1990, pp. 218–19; Swiss Institute of Comparative Law, *Comparative Study*, pp. 112, 267–68.

40. Degott-Kieffer, "Maladies nouvelles et droit du travail," p. 217; Philippe Auvergnon, ed., *Le droit social à l'epreuve du SIDA* (n.p., n.d.), pp. 140–41; Jacques Foyer and Lucette Khaïat "Droit et SIDA: La situation française," in Foyer and Khaïat, eds., *Droit et Sida: Comparaison internationale* (Paris, 1994), pp. 247–49; Claude Got, *Rapport sur le SIDA* (Paris, 1989), p. 273.

41. Memo from the Department of Employment, House of Commons, *Problems Associated with AIDS*, vol. 3, p. 135; Brazier and Mulholland, "Droit et Sida," p. 383; Wilson, "Discrimination in the Workplace," pp. 312–14; Street, "British Government Policy on AIDS," p. 498; Grimshaw, "AIDS and Human Rights," p. 144; Bottke," SIDA et droit," p. 36; Lücke, *Aids*, pp. 145–47; Mummenhoff, "Arbeitsrechtliche Problemkreise," p. 166; Werner Hinrichs, "AIDS und Arbeitsrecht," in Max Busch et al., eds., *HIV/AIDS und Straffälligkeit* (Bonn, 1991), p. 73.

42. Westerhäll and Saldeen, "Réflexions sur le Sida," pp. 413–14; Hagstrøm, *AIDS som juridisk problem*, pp. 76, 83; Halvor Moxnes, "AIDS and Human Rights in Norway," in Martin Breum and Aart Hendriks, eds., *AIDS and Human Rights* (Copenhagen, 1988), p. 111; Harald Stabell, "Retten til arbeid for HIV/AIDS-smittede," in Turid Eikvam and Arne Grønningsæter, eds., *AIDS og samfunnet* (n.p., 1987), p. 105; Harald Stabell, "Aids og retten til arbeid," *Retfærd* 10, 37 (1987), pp. 101–5.

43. Got, *Rapport*, p. 275; Swiss Institute of Comparative Law, *Comparative Study*, pp. 112–13, 118; Schizas, "Employment, the Law, and HIV," p. 307; Degott-Kieffer, "Maladies nouvelles et droit du travail," p. 219.

44. Gene W. Matthews and Verla S. Neslund, "The Initial Impact of AIDS on Public Health Law in the United States—1986," *JAMA* 257, 3 (1987), p. 345; Closen et al., *AIDS*, pp. 263–64, 271–76; Wendy E. Parmet, "AIDS and the Limits of Discrimination Law," *Law, Medicine, and Health Care* 15, 1–2 (1987), pp. 61–66; Chai R. Feldblum, "Workplace Issues: HIV and Discrimination," in Nan D. Hunter and William B. Rubenstein, eds., *AIDS Agenda: Emerging Issues in Civil Rights* (New York, 1992), pp. 274–75.

45. Ronald Turner, "AIDS and Employment: Asymptomatic Human Immunodeficiency Virus Carriers and Section 504 of the Rehabilitation Act," *AIDS and Public Policy Journal* 5, 4 (1990).

46. Terry Morehead Dworkin and Elies Steyger, "AIDS Victims in the European Community and the United States: Are They Protected from Unjustified Discrimination?" *Texas International Law Journal* 24 (1989), p. 308; Mello, *AIDS and the Law*, pp. 34–35; Lawrence O. Gostin, "The AIDS Litigation Project: A National Review of Court and Human Rights Commission Decisions," *JAMA* 263, 15 (18 April 1990), p. 2086; Rubenstein et al., *Rights of People*, p. 275; Donald H. J. Hermann and William P. Schurgin, *Legal Aspects of AIDS* (Deerfield, IL, 1991), §6:05.

47. Donald H. J. Hermann, "AIDS and the Law," in Frederick G. Reamer, ed., *AIDS and Ethics* (New York, 1991), pp. 280–81; Lücke, *Aids*, p. 128; Larry

Gostin, "Traditional Public Health Strategies," in Scott Burris et al., eds., *AIDS Law Today* (New Haven, 1993), pp. 66–67.

48. Hermann and Schurgin, *Legal Aspects,* §§10:05, 10:16; Wendy E. Parmet, "Discrimination and Disability: The Challenges of the ADA," *Law, Medicine, and Health Care* 18, 4 (1990), pp. 332–38; Feldblum, "Workplace Issues," p. 286; Matthew E. Turowski, "AIDS in the Workplace: Perceptions, Prejudices, and Policy Solutions," *Ohio Northern University Law Review* 20 (1993), pp. 143–45.

49. Goss and Adam-Smith, *Organizing AIDS,* pp. 145–47; Arthur S. Leonard, "Discrimination," in Scott Burris et al., eds., *AIDS Law Today* (New Haven, 1993), p. 301; Simon LeVay and Elisabeth Nonas, *City of Friends: A Portrait of the Gay and Lesbian Community in America* (Cambridge, MA, 1995), p. 277.

50. Thomas B. Stoddard and Walter Rieman, "AIDS and the Rights of the Individual," in Dorothy Nelkin et al., eds., *A Disease of Society: Cultural and Institutional Responses to AIDS* (Cambridge, 1991), pp. 256–57; Theodore J. Stein, "Disability-Based Employment Discrimination against Individuals Perceived to Have AIDS and Individuals Infected with HIV or Diagnosed with AIDS: Federal and New York Statutes and Case Law," *AIDS and Public Policy Journal* 10, 3 (1995), pp. 123–30; Janine M. Dlutowski, "Employment Discrimination," *Harvard Journal of Law and Public Policy* 9, 3 (summer 1986), pp. 739–51; Nancy Ford and Michael D. Quam, "AIDS Quarantine: The Legal and Practical Implications," *Journal of Legal Medicine* 8, 3 (1987), p. 381; Lücke, *Aids,* p. 124; *IDHL* 38, 1 (1987), pp. 42–43; Hermann, "AIDS and the Law," p. 282; Rubenstein et al., *Rights of People,* p. 244.

51. Swiss Institute of Comparative Law, *Comparative Study,* pp. 123, 313, 397; Olivier Corten et al., "Europe des droits de l'homme ou Europe du Sida?" in Michel Vincineau, ed., *Le Sida: Un défi aux droits* (Brussels, 1991), p. 94; Hagstrøm, *AIDS som juridisk problem,* p. 85.

52. Monika Steffen, "AIDS Policies in France," in Virginia Berridge and Philip Strong, eds., *AIDS and Contemporary History* (Cambridge, 1993), p. 25; O. S., "Le sida et la fonction publique," *L'actualité juridique: Droit administratif* (20 April 1988), pp. 270–71; Thomas-Tual, "La fonction publique," p. 194; Michael Pollak, "AIDS Policy in France: Biomedical Leadership and Preventive Impotence," in Barbara A. Misztal and David Moss, eds., *Action on AIDS: National Policies in Comparative Perspective* (New York, 1990), p. 95; Bach-Ignasse, "Le Sida," p. 103; AIDES, *Droit et S.I.D.A.: Guide juridique,* pp. 100–101.

53. *Hansard,* vol. 114 (22 April 1987), col. 627; vol. 114 (23 April 1987), col. 654; vol. 116 (13 May 1987), col. 215.

54. Hans-Ulrich Gallwas, "AIDS und Recht aus verfassungsrechtlicher Sicht," in Gallwas et al., eds., *Aids und Recht* (Stuttgart, 1992), p. 31; Norbert Kathke, "Die Begutachtung von anti-HIV-positiven Personen durch das Gesundheitsamt," *AIDS-Forschung* 12 (1986), p. 666; Wolf-Rüdiger Schenke, "AIDS aus verwaltungsrechtlicher Perspektive," in Hans-Ullrich Gallwas et al.,

eds., *Aids und Recht* (Stuttgart, 1992), p. 54; Ottfried Seewald, "Verfassungs- und verwaltungsrechtliche Aspekte von Aids," in Cornelius Prittwitz, ed., *Aids, Recht und Gesundheitspolitik* (Berlin, 1990), p. 48; "Die rechtliche Beurteilung von Eingriffsmassnahmen und ihre Gewichtung im Rahmen der Gesamtstrategie der AIDS-Bekämpfung," *AIDS-Forschung* 4 (1989), p. 218.

    55. BT *Drucksache* 11/1588, 5 January 1988; BT *Verhandlungen* 11/26, 16 September 1987, p. 1717B; Lücke, *Aids*, p. 109.

    56. H. Jäger, ed., *AIDS und HIV-Infektionen* (n.p., n.d.), xv–1.3.1, p. 4; WHO, *Legislative Responses*, p. 60; Staatssekretärsausschuss "AIDS" der Bayerischen Staatsregierung, *Konzept der Bayerischen Staatsregierung zur Bekämpfung der Immunschwächekrankheit AIDS* (Munich, n.d.), p. 23; Günter Frankenberg, *AIDS-Bekämpfung im Rechtsstaat* (Baden-Baden, 1988), p. 141; BT *Drucksache* 11/7200, 31 May 1990, p. 227; Manfred Seume, "Der HIV-Antikörpertest bei Einstellungsuntersuchungen von Beamtenbewerbern," *AIDS-Forschung* 12 (1987), pp. 703–7.

    57. "Bayerisches Verwaltungsgericht Ansbach: Beschluss vom 21. January 1988," *AIDS-Forschung* 6 (1988), p. 355; "Rechtsgutachten des Ministeriums für Arbeit, Gesundheit und Soziales des Landes Nordrhein-Westfalen, Stand 15. 3. 1988," *AIDS-Forschung* 9 (1988), pp. 525–26; *AIDS: Fakten und Konsequenzen*, pp. 426–27; BT *Drucksache* 11/7200, 31 May 1990, p. 225.

    58. Kelvin Widdows, "AIDS and the Workplace: Some Approaches at the National Level," *International Journal of Comparative Labour Law and Industrial Relations* 4, 3 (1988), p. 148.

    59. Lücke, *Aids*, pp. 104–6; Mello, *AIDS and the Law*, p. 29.

    60. William H. L. Dornette, ed., *AIDS and the Law*, 1991 Cumulative Supplement (New York, 1987), p. 67; Lücke, *Aids*, p. 104.

    61. Raffaele d'Amelio et al., "A Global Review of Legislation on HIV/AIDS: The Issue of HIV Testing," *Journal of Acquired Immune Deficiency Syndromes* 28, 2 (2001), p. 177; Lücke, *Aids*, pp. 95–97; Donna I. Dennis, "HIV Screening and Discrimination: The Federal Example," in Scott Burris et al., eds., *AIDS Law Today* (New Haven, 1993), pp. 189–94; Bernard M. Dickens et al., "HIV Screening: The International Implications," in Lawrence Gostin and Lane Porter, eds., *International Law and AIDS* (n.p., 1992), pp. 102–6; Rubenstein et al., *Rights of People*, pp. 33–34; *IDHL* 38, 4 (1987), pp. 771–72; 42, 3 (1991), p. 445.

    62. Swiss Institute, *Comparative Study* of Comparative Law, p. 165; WHO, *Legislative Responses*, pp. 73–74; *IDHL* 39, 2 (1988), pp. 361–63; *Le Monde*, 13 December 1991, p. 13; Thomas-Tual, "La fonction publique," p. 190.

    63. BT *Drucksache* 10/3829, No. 71, 13 September 1985; 11/909, 7 October 1987; 11/1116, No. 74, 2 November 1987; 11/1116, Nos. 54–55, 3 November 1987; 11/7200, 31 May 1990, pp. 122–25; Lücke, *Aids*, pp. 102–5; Christoph Veit, "AIDS und die Bundeswehr," in Hans-Ullrich Gallwas et al., eds., *Aids und Recht* (Stuttgart, 1992), pp. 111–13.

    64. Benny Henriksson, *Social Democracy or Societal Control? A Critical Analysis of Swedish AIDS Policy* (Stockholm, 1988), p. 19; Lutz Horn, "Die Behandlung von AIDS in ausgewählten Mitgliedstaaten des Europarates—ein

rechtsvergleichender Überblick," in Hans-Ullrich Gallwas et al., eds., *Aids und Recht* (Stuttgart, 1992), p. 198; *RD Prot*, 1986/87, Bihang, Socialutskottets betänkande 19, pp. 1–2, 27; 1987/88, Bihang, Prop. 79, p. 30; *Hansard*, vol. 124 (14 December 1987), col. 415; Swiss Institute of Comparative Law, *Comparative Study*, p. 166.

65. *Hansard*, vol. 127 (9 February 1988), col. 135; vol. 133 (20 May 1988), col. 612.

66. Peter Baldwin, *Contagion and the State in Europe, 1830–1930* (Cambridge, 1999), pp. 510–15.

67. Rolf Rosenbrock, "AIDS and Preventive Health Policy," *Veröffentlichungsreihe des Internationalen Instituts für Vergleichende Gesellschaftsforschung/Arbeitspolitik des Wissenschaftszentrums Berlin*, IIVG/pre87–208 (Berlin, May 1987), p. 26.

68. *Congressional Record*, Extensions of Remarks, 14 June 1994, pp. 1212–13.

69. Bundesrat, *Verhandlungen* 580, 25 September 1987, p. 307B; David Wilson, "Preventing Transmission of HIV in Heterosexual Prostitution," in Lorraine Sherr, ed., *AIDS and the Heterosexual Population* (Chur, 1993), p. 68; Beth E. Schneider and Valerie Jenness, "Social Control, Civil Liberties, and Women's Sexuality," in Schneider and Nancy E. Stoller, eds., *Women Resisting AIDS: Feminist Strategies of Empowerment* (Philadelphia, 1995), p. 81.

70. Michael Bloor, *The Sociology of HIV Transmission* (London, 1995), p. 53; Blumberg, *AIDS*, pp. 91–98; U. Tirelli et al., "HIV Infection in 403 Female Prostitutes in Italy," in N. Loimer et al., eds., *Drug Addiction and AIDS* (Vienna, 1991), pp. 35–36; Françoise F. Hamers and Jean-Baptiste Brunet, "Différences géographiques et tendances récentes de l'épidémie de VIH/sida en Europe," in Nathalie Bajos et al., *Le sida en Europe: Nouveaux enjeux pour les sciences sociales* (Paris, 1998), p. 15.

71. B. Velimirovic, "AIDS as a Social Phenomenon," in M. A. Koch and F. Deinhardt, eds., *AIDS Diagnosis and Control: Current Situation* (Munich, 1988), p. 44; Dennis Altman, forward to Peter Aggleton, ed., *Men Who Sell Sex: International Perspectives on Male Prostitution and HIV/AIDS* (Philadelphia, 1999), p. xiv; Douglas Webb, *HIV and AIDS in Africa* (London, 1997), pp. 126–27; Nancy Romero-Daza and David Himmelgreen, "More Than Money for Your Labor: Migration and the Political Economy of AIDS in Lesotho," in Merrill Singer, ed., *The Political Economy of AIDS* (Amityville, NY, 1998), pp. 193–96.

72. Department of Health and Human Services, Public Health Service, *AIDS: A Public Health Challenge* (Washington, DC, October 1987), 1:2–19.

73. Andrzej J. Szwarc, ed., *AIDS und Strafrecht* (Berlin, 1996), p. 213; Koch, "Stellungnahme zur AIDS-Problematik: Antworten auf Fragen der Presse," p. 673; BT *Verhandlungen* 10/246, 13 November 1986, p. 19095A-B.

74. BT *Drucksache* 11/2495, 16 June 1988, p. 86.; Staatssekretärsausschuss "AIDS" der Bayerischen Staatsregierung, *Konzept der Bayerischen Staatsregierung*, pp. 12 ff. The TÜV is the automobile inspection test.

75. Velimirovic, "AIDS as a Social Phenomenon," p. 44; Frank Höpfel, "Strafrechtliche Probleme des HIV-Tests," in Andrzej J. Szwarc, ed., *AIDS und Strafrecht* (Berlin, 1996), p. 106.

76. Lucette Khaïat, "Et pour etre juriste, on n'en est pas moins homme: Quelques réactions en droit comparé," in Daniel Borrillo and Anne Masseran, eds., *Sida et droits de l'homme: L'épidémie dans un Etat de droit* (Strasbourg, 1991), p. 218; Peter Raschke and Claudia Ritter, *Eine Grossstadt lebt mit Aids: Strategien der Prävention und Hilfe am Beispiel Hamburgs* (Berlin, 1991), p. 162.

77. Memo by the Women and AIDS Working Group, House of Commons, *Problems Associated with AIDS*, vol. 3, pp. 195–96; *Hansard*, vol. 146 (9 February 1989), col. 761; BT *Drucksache* 10/6299, 4 November 1986, pp. 7–8.

78. *Le Monde*, 3 December 1986, p. 36; 12 December 1990, p. 10; 21 March 1991, p. 14; Foyer and Khaïat, "Droit et SIDA," p. 228; Bach-Ignasse, "Le Sida," p. 104; Pierre Favre, ed., *Sida et politique: Les premiers affrontements (1981–1987)* (Paris, 1992), pp. 116, 143.

79. *RD Prot*, 1985/86:33 (21 November 1985), p. 21; 1985/86, Bihang, Justitieutskottets betänkande 20, pp. 1–3; 1985/86:130 (29 April 1986), pp. 116–18; 1987/88, Bihang, Justitieutskottets betänkande 12, pp. 1–4, 15; Britt-Inger Lind and Torsten Fredriksson, *Kärlek för pengar? En bok om prostitutionsprojektet i Malmö 1976–80* (Stockholm, 1980), p. 197.

80. "Violence against Women: Government Bill 1997/98:55," Swedish Government Offices, Fact Sheet, 1999; Judith Kilvington et al., "Prostitution Policy in Europe: A Time of Change?" *Feminist Review* 67 (2001), p. 83.

81. *Le Monde*, 16 April 1987; BT *Drucksache* 11/7200, 31 May 1990, p. 16; Ine Vanwesenbeeck and Ron de Graaf, "Sex Work and HIV in the Netherlands," in Theo Sandfort, ed., *The Dutch Response to HIV: Pragmatism and Consensus* (London, 1998), p. 103.

82. WHO, *Legislative Responses*, p. 17; *IDHL* 37, 3 (1986), pp. 533–35; 44, 4 (1993), pp. 598–601; Horn, "Die Behandlung von AIDS," p. 209; Sev S. Fluss, "National AIDS Legislation: An Overview of Some Global Developments," in Lawrence Gostin and Lane Porter, eds., *International Law and AIDS* (n.p., 1992), p. 22; S. S. Fluss and D. K. Latto, "The Coercive Element in Legislation for the Control of AIDS and HIV Infection: Some Recent Developments," *AIDS and Public Policy Journal* 2, 3 (summer–fall 1987), p. 12; Jayasuriya, *AIDS*, p. 77.

83. Staatssekretärsausschuss "AIDS" der Bayerischen Staatsregierung, *Konzept der Bayerischen Staatsregierung*, pp. 12 ff.

84. *Hansard*, vol. 106 (3 December 1986), col. 634; vol. 146 (9 February 1989), col. 761.

85. Westerhäll and Saldeen, "Réflexions sur le Sida," pp. 394–95; *IDHL* 39, 4 (1988), pp. 832–33; Helena G. Papaevangelou, "AIDS and Human Rights in Greece," in Martin Breum and Aart Hendriks, eds., *AIDS and Human Rights* (Copenhagen, 1988), p. 72.

86. *IDHL* 38, 4 (1987), pp. 770–71; 42, 1 (1991), pp. 21–25; 44, 2 (1993), pp. 223–28; 39, 4 (1988), pp. 830–32.

87. Dornette, ed., *AIDS and the Law,* p. 67; WHO, *Legislative Responses,* p. 230; *IDHL* 39, 3 (1988), p. 634.

88. *IDHL* 38, 2 (1987), pp. 253–54; Heather G. Miller et al., eds., *AIDS: The Second Decade* (Washington, DC, 1990), pp. 277–79; Hermann and Schurgin, *Legal Aspects,* §9:25; Jayasuriya, *AIDS,* p. 85; Lücke, *Aids,* pp. 71, 76; Institute of Medicine, *Confronting AIDS: Update 1988* (Washington, DC, 1988), p. 78.

89. Farmer, *AIDS and Accusation,* ch. 14; E. Antonio de Moya and Rafael Garcia, "Three Decades of Male Sex Work in Santo Domingo," in Peter Aggleton, ed., *Men Who Sell Sex: International Perspectives on Male Prostitution and HIV/AIDS* (Philadelphia, 1999), pp. 132–36; David T. Evans, *Sexual Citizenship: The Material Construction of Sexualities* (London, 1993), pp. 109–13.

90. Aart Hendriks, *AIDS and Mobility: The Impact of International Mobility on the Spread of HIV and the Need and Possibility for AIDS/HIV Prevention Programmes* (Copenhagen, 1991), p. 22; Dennis Altman, *Global Sex* (Chicago, 2001), p. 110.

91. Signe Ettrup Larsen, "International prostitution," *Retfærd* 14, 4 (1991), pp. 33–48; "Entschliessung der 63. Konferenz der für das Gesundheitswesen zuständigen Minister und Senatoren der Länder vom 22. bis 23. November 1990 in Berlin," *AIDS-Forschung* 6, 1 (January 1991), pp. 28–29; BT *Drucksache* 11/7200, 31 May 1990, pp. 156–61; 12/4485, 5 March 1993, pp. 5, 13; 12/4528, 10 March 1993; BT *Verhandlungen* 12/147, 12 March 1993, pp. 12622C, 12635D; *AIDS: Fakten und Konsequenzen,* p. 30; Erik Cohen, "Tourism and AIDS in Thailand," *Annals of Tourism Research* 15 (1988), pp. 467–86; Leonard J. Nelson III, "International Travel Restrictions and the AIDS Epidemic," *American Journal of International Law* 81 (1987), p. 235; Gundo Aurel Weiler, "HIV und Tourismus: Deutsche Freier auf den Philippinen," in Anja Bestmann et al., eds., *Aids—weltweit und dichtdran* (Saarbrücken, 1997); Mario Vargas Llosa, "Crossing the Moral Boundary," *New York Times,* 7 January 2001, sect. 4, p. 17.

92. Stanislav Andreski, *Syphilis, Puritanism, and Witch Hunts* (London, 1989), p. 169; Frank Hausser, "Sida et prison: Quelles politiques, quelles réglementations?" in Eric Heilmann, ed., *Sida et libertés: La régulation d'une épidemie dans un état de droit* (n.p., 1991), p. 259; *Hansard,* vol. 144 (13 January 1989), col. 1115, 1125, 1151.

93. Theodore M. Hammett et al., "AIDS in Prisons in the USA," in Philip A. Thomas and Martin Moerings, eds., *AIDS in Prison* (Aldershot, U.K., 1994), p. 143; Hermann, "AIDS and the Law," p. 283; Edgar and Sandomire, "Medical Privacy Issues," p. 196; Bernadette Pratt Sadler, "When Rape Victims' Rights Meet Privacy Rights: Mandatory HIV Testing, Striking the Fourth Amendment Balance," *Washington Law Review* 67 (1992), pp. 199–200; *IDHL* 39, 4 (1988), p. 836; 42, 2 (1991), pp. 245–54; *Report of the Presidential Commission on the Human Immunodeficiency Virus Epidemic* (Washington, DC, 1988), pp. 134–35; Michael Tanner and the ALEC National Working Group on State AIDS Policy, *The Politics of Health: A State Response to the AIDS Crisis* (n.p., 1989), p. 46; Hermann and Schurgin, *Legal Aspects,* §8:12.

94. Mukesh Kapila and Maryan J. Pye, "The European Response to AIDS," in Jaime Sepulveda et al., eds., *AIDS: Prevention through Education* (New York, 1992), p. 223.

95. Klaus Geppert, "AIDS und Strafvollzug," in Andrzej J. Szwarc, ed., *AIDS und Strafrecht* (Berlin, 1996), pp. 238–39; Johannes Feest and Heino Stöver, "AIDS in Prisons in Germany," in Philip A. Thomas and Martin Moerings, eds., *AIDS in Prison* (Aldershot, U.K., 1994), p. 23; Raschke and Ritter, *Eine Grossstadt*, p. 193; Swiss Institute of Comparative Law, *Comparative Study*, pp. 145–47; Karl-Heinrich Schäfer, "AIDS im Strafvollzug: Eine besondere Aufgabe für die Landesjustizverwaltung," and Angelika Sauer, "AIDS und Recht im Strafvollzug aus medizinischer Sicht," in Hans-Ullrich Gallwas et al., eds., *Aids und Recht* (Stuttgart, 1992), pp. 131, 145; Justizminister des Landes Nordrhein-Westfalen, *Im Gespräch: AIDS im Strafvollzug: Protokoll des Symposiums am 2. Oktober 1985 in Düsseldorf* (Düsseldorf, n.d.), pp. 23, 26–27; Karl-Heinrich Schäfer, "AIDS: Ansätze zu einer Problembewältigung auf der Ebene von Landesjustizverwaltung und Parlament," in Max Busch et al., eds., *HIV/AIDS und Straffälligkeit* (Bonn, 1991), p. 180; *AIDS: Fakten und Konsequenzen*, p. 283; Staatssekretärsausschuss "AIDS" der Bayerischen Staatsregierung, *Konzept der Bayerischen Staatsregierung*, pp. 7–9; Johann Singhartinger, *AIDS als Anlass—Kontrolle als Konzept: Entwicklungen am Beispiel Strafvollzug* (Munich, 1987), pp. 124–25.

96. Birgit Westphal Christensen et al., *AIDS: Prævention og kontrol i Norden* (Stockholm, 1988), pp. 25, 63, 206; Westerhäll and Saldeen, "Réflexions sur le Sida," p. 411; Horn, "Die Behandlung von AIDS," p. 198.

97. *Hansard*, vol. 137 (19 July 1988), col. 569; vol. 93 (6 March 1986), col. 236; vol. 107 (8 December 1986), col. 81; Memo from the Home Office, House of Commons, *Problems Associated with AIDS*, vol. 3, p. 77; Dineke Zeegers, "Droit et Sida: Perspectives aux Pay-Bas," in Jacques Foyer and Lucette Khaïat, eds., *Droit et Sida: Comparaison internationale* (Paris, 1994), p. 333.

98. Swiss Institute of Comparative Law, *Comparative Study*, pp. 145, 148–49; Orr, "The Legal Implications of AIDS," p. 131.

99. Bernard Paillard, *Notes on the Plague Years: AIDS in Marseilles* (New York, 1998), p. 195; Hausser, "Sida et prison," pp. 260–61; *Le Monde*, 24 May 89, p. 10.

100. Raymond A. Smith, *Encyclopedia of AIDS* (Chicago, 1998), p. 213; *IDHL* 37, 3 (1986), p. 542; 45, 1 (1994); Moss, "AIDS in Italy," p. 145.

101. Katja Høegh, "Dansk AIDS-bekæmpelse: Frivillighed—for hvem?" *Retfærd* 11, 1 (1988), pp. 40–41; BT *Drucksache* 11/7200, 31 May 1990, pp. 148–50; Christian Dertinger, "Vom Umgang des Vollzuges mit AIDS," in Max Busch et al., eds., *HIV/AIDS und Straffälligkeit* (Bonn, 1991), p. 170; Karl Peter Rotthaus, "AIDS im Strafvollzug," in Hans-Ullrich Gallwas et al., eds., *Aids und Recht* (Stuttgart, 1992), pp. 139–40; *AIDS: Fakten und Konsequenzen*, p. 286; Rubenstein et al., *Rights of People*, pp. 306–7; *Hansard*, vol. 119 (16 July 1987), col. 603; vol. 147 (22 February 1989), col. 635; Swiss Institute of Comparative Law, *Comparative Study*, p. 51; Una Padel, "HIV, Prisons, and Prisoners'

Rights," in Richard Haigh and Dai Harris, eds., *AIDS: A Guide to the Law*, 2d ed. (London, 1995), pp. 132–33; *RD Prot*, 1986/87, Bihang, Prop. 2, p. 26; Paillard, *Notes*, p. 198.

102. Staatssekretärsausschuss "AIDS" der Bayerischen Staatsregierung, *Konzept der Bayerischen Staatsregierung*, pp. 7–9; Swiss Institute of Comparative Law, *Comparative Study*, p. 52; *AIDS: Fakten und Konsequenzen*, p. 29; Closen et al., *AIDS*, pp. 730–36; Alexa Freeman, "HIV in Prison," in Scott Burris et al., eds., *AIDS Law Today* (New Haven, 1993), p. 271; Blumberg, *AIDS*, p. 231; J. Michael Quinlan, "The Federal Prisons Management Response to AIDS," in Clark C. Abt and Kathleen M. Hardy, eds., *AIDS and the Courts* (Cambridge, MA, 1990), pp. 94–95; *IDHL* 42, 2 (1991), pp. 255–57.

103. Hammett et al., "AIDS in Prisons," p. 145; Albert R. Jonsen and Jeff Stryker, eds., *The Social Impact of AIDS in the United States* (Washington, DC, 1993), p. 187; Rubenstein et al., *Rights of People*, p. 308; Tanner and the ALEC National Working Group on State AIDS Policy, *Politics of Health*, p. 47; Pollak, "AIDS Policy in France," p. 90; Foyer and Khaïat, "Droit et SIDA," pp. 255–56; John de Wit and Gazet van Antwerpen, "AIDS in Prisons in Belgium," in Philip A. Thomas and Martin Moerings, eds., *AIDS in Prison* (Aldershot, U.K., 1994), p. 80.

104. Schäfer, "AIDS im Strafvollzug"; Sauer, "AIDS und Recht im Strafvollzug," pp. 134, 145; Marita P., *AIDS hat mir das Leben gerettet: Meine Jahre zwischen Edelstrich und Drogensumpf* (Berlin, 1993), p. 72; Wolfram H. Eberbach, "AIDS im Strafvollzug," in Bernd Schünemann and Gerd Pfeiffer, eds., *Die Rechtsprobleme von AIDS* (Baden-Baden, 1988), p. 263; *AIDS: Fakten und Konsequenzen*, p. 286.

105. *Hansard*, vol. 93 (3 March 1986), col. 49; vol. 144 (13 January 1989), col. 1142; Orr, "Legal Implications of AIDS," p. 131; Orr, "Legal AIDS" p. 62; John L. Kilgour, "AIDS in Prisons in England and Wales," in Alan F. Fleming et al., *The Global Impact of AIDS* (New York, 1988), p. 324–25; Swiss Institute of Comparative Law, *Comparative Study*, pp. 148–49; Virginia Berridge, *AIDS in the UK: The Making of Policy, 1981–1994* (Oxford, 1996), p. 261; Padel, "HIV, Prisons, and Prisoners' Rights," pp. 132–33.

106. *International Herald Tribune*, 10 June 1999, p. 5; Duckett, *Australia's Response to AIDS*, pp. 21, 29, 39.

107. *Prison and Criminological Aspects of the Control of Transmissible Diseases including AIDS and Related Health Problems in Prisons: Recommendation No. R (93) 6 Adopted by the Committee of Ministers of the Council of Europe on 18 October 1993* (Strasbourg, 1995), pp. 9–10.

108. Hammett et al., "AIDS in Prisons," pp. 146–47; Freeman, "HIV in Prison," p. 285; Theodore M. Hammett, "Correctional Facilities Survey Findings on AIDS," in Clark C. Abt and Kathleen M. Hardy, eds., *AIDS and the Courts* (Cambridge, MA, 1990), p. 100; Jonsen and Stryker, *Social Impact of AIDS*, p. 185; *Los Angeles Times*, 30 November 2001, p. A1.

109. *Hansard*, vol. 143 (6 December 1988), col. 108; vol. 152 (3 May 1989), col. 111; Philip A. Thomas, "AIDS in Prisons in England and Wales," in Thomas

and Martin Moerings, eds., *AIDS in Prison* (Aldershot, U.K., 1994), p. 54; John Street and Albert Weale, "Britain: Policy-Making in a Hermetically Sealed System," in David L. Kirp and Ronald Bayer, eds., *AIDS in the Industrialized Democracies* (New Brunswick, 1992), pp. 207–8; Street, "British Government Policy," p. 497; Bob Watt, "HIV/AIDS and European Human Rights Law," *European Human Rights Law Review* 1 (2000), p. 60.

110. Westerhäll and Saldeen, "Réflexions sur le Sida," p. 412; *Le Monde*, 6 August 1987, p. 8a; Annie Serfaty, "L'infection par le VIH liée à l'usage de drogues en France," *Sida, toxicomanie: Une lecture documentaire* (n.p., November 1993), p. 74; Hausser, "Sida et prison" p. 262; Alain Sobel, "Policy Making under Changing Political Situations: The French National AIDS Council and AIDS Control Policies," in Dorothee Friedrich and Wolfgang Heckmann, eds., *Aids in Europe: The Behavioural Aspect* (Berlin, 1995), 4:91; *Le Monde*, 24 May 1989, p. 10; Foyer and Khaïat, "Droit et SIDA," p. 256.

111. J. Jepsen, "Drug Policies in Denmark," in Hans-Jörg Albrecht and Anton van Kalmthout, eds., *Drug Policies in Western Europe* (Freiburg, 1989), pp. 113–14; Pierre Darbeda, "Les prisons face au Sida: Vers des normes européennes," *Revue de science criminelle et de droit pénal comparé* 4 (1990), p. 826.

112. Feest and Stöver, "AIDS in Prisons in Germany," pp. 27–28; BT *Drucksache* 11/7200, 31 May 1990, pp. 146, 284; Schäfer, "AIDS im Strafvollzug," pp. 134–35; *AIDS: Fakten und Konsequenzen*, pp. 280–81; Vereinigung Berliner Strafverteidiger, *AIDS im Strafvollzug: Strafe wegen AIDS?* (Berlin, n.d. [1987]), pp. 14–15; Deutsche AIDS-Hilfe e.v., *AIDS im Strafvollzug* (Berlin, 1993), p. 8.

113. Wolfram H. Eberbach, "Arztrechtliche Aspekte bei AIDS," *AIDS-Forschung* 2, 5 (1987), pp. 282–83; Gostin, "AIDS Litigation Project," p. 2089; Abigail Zuger and Steven H. Miles, "Physicians, AIDS, and Occupational Risk: Historic Traditions and Ethical Obligations," *JAMA* 258, 14 (1987), pp. 1926–27; "Straf-, zivil-, arbeits- und beamtenrechtliche Aspekte von AIDS," *AIDS-Forschung* 6 (1986), p. 318; Olivier Guillod et al., *Drei Gutachten über rechtliche Fragen im Zusammenhang mit AIDS* (Bern, 1991), p. 354.

114. Blumberg, *AIDS*, p. 5; Sev S. Fluss and Dineke Zeegers, "AIDS, HIV, and Health Care Workers: Some International Legislative Perspectives," *Maryland Law Review* 48 (1989), pp. 87–88; Paget, *AIDS and Public Health Measures*, ch. 10; American Bar Association, AIDS Coordinating Committee, *AIDS: The Legal Issues* (Washington, DC, 1988), p. 86; Diana Brahams, "AIDS and the Law," *New Law Journal* 137 (1987), p. 749; Paget, *AIDS*, p. 60.

115. IDHL 37, 1 (1986), pp. 28–29; 38, 4 (1987), pp. 761–62; 39, 1 (1988), p. 55; 39, 3 (1988), p. 631; RD Prot, 1985/86, Bihang, Socialutskottets betänkande 15, p. 6; Benny Henriksson, "Swedish AIDS Policy from a Human Rights Perspective," in Martin Breum and Aart Hendriks, eds., *AIDS and Human Rights* (Copenhagen, 1988), p. 128; WHO, *Legislative Responses*, p. 167; RD Prot, 1987/88, Bihang, Socialutskottets betänkande 10, pp. 24, 33; Moxnes, "AIDS and Human Rights," p. 110; Christensen et al., *AIDS*, p. 64.

116. Wolfgang Schumacher and Egon Meyn, *Bundes-Seuchengesetz*, 4th ed. (Cologne, 1992), p. 23; "Korrespondenz," *AIDS-Forschung* 2, 5 (1987), pp. 292–93; BT *Drucksache* 11/2495, 16 June 1988, pp. 86–87; 11/7200, 31 May 1990, pp. 206–7.

117. Colin A. M. E. d'Eça, "Medico-Legal Aspects of HIV Infection and Disease," in Richard Haigh and Dai Harris, eds., *AIDS: A Guide to the Law*, 2d ed. (London, 1995), p. 116; Margaret Brazier and Mary Lobjoit, "Fiduciary Relationship: An Ethical Approach and a Legal Concept," in Rebecca Bennett and Charles A. Erin, eds., *HIV and AIDS: Testing, Screening, and Confidentiality* (Oxford, 1999), p. 185.

118. *IDHL* 39, 1 (1988), pp. 31–32; AIDES, *Droit et S.I.D.A*, pp. 28–29; Brigitte Feuillet-Le Mintier, "SIDA, séropositivité et droit des personnes," in Feuillet-Le Mintier, ed., *Le SIDA: Aspects juridiques* (Paris, 1995), p. 7; Monika Steffen, "France: Social Solidarity and Scientific Expertise," in David L. Kirp and Ronald Bayer, eds., *AIDS in the Industrialized Democracies* (New Brunswick, 1992), p. 221.

119. Hermann, "AIDS and the Law," p. 283; Jonsen and Stryker, *Social Impact*, p. 59. Though the presidential commission thought that exposed personnel had the right to know the serostatus of patients. *Report of the Presidential Commission*, pp. 30–34.

120. Hermann and Schurgin, *Legal Aspects*, §2:24; *IDHL* 41, 4 (1990), pp. 609–11; 42, 4 (1991), pp. 649–50; 43, 1 (1992), p. 40.

121. *Congressional Record* (House), 31 July 1990, pp. 6037–38; *IDHL* 38, 1 (1987), p. 45; Hermann, "AIDS and the Law," p. 285; Lücke, *Aids*, p. 113.

122. Ann N. James, "Legal Aspects of AIDS: The Chasm between Public Health Practices and Societal Norms," in Gerald Schochetman and J. Richard George, eds., *AIDS Testing*, 2d ed. (New York, 1994), p. 322; Katharine Park, "Kimberly Bergalis, AIDS, and the Plague Metaphor," in Marjorie Garber et al., eds., *Media Spectacles* (New York, 1993), p. 236.

123. *Congressional Record* (Senate), 10 July 1991, p. 9476; (Senate) 18 July 1991, pp. 10346, 10357; Norman Daniels, *Seeking Fair Treatment: From the AIDS Epidemic to National Health Care Reform* (New York, 1995), p. 53; Elinor Burkett, *The Gravest Show on Earth: America in the Age of AIDS* (Boston, 1995), pp. 230–32; Inge B. Corless, "Much Ado about Something: The Restriction of HIV-Infected Health-Care Providers," *AIDS and Public Policy Journal* 7, 2 (1992), p. 84.

124. David B. Feinberg, *Queer and Loathing: Rants and Raves of a Raging AIDS Clone* (New York, 1994), p. 143.

125. Larry Gostin, "The HIV-Infected Health Care Professional: Public Policy, Discrimination, and Patient Safety," *Law, Medicine, and Health Care* 18, 4 (1990), p. 304; Mark Barnes et al., "The HIV-Infected Health Care Professional: Employment Policies and Public Health," *Law, Medicine, and Health Care* 18, 4 (1990), pp. 319–22.

126. Jonsen and Stryker, *Social Impact*, p. 89; Steven Epstein, *Impure Science: AIDS, Activism, and the Politics of Knowledge* (Berkeley, 1996), pp. 8–14;

Peter S. Arno and Karyn L. Feiden, *Against the Odds: The Story of AIDS Drug Development, Politics, and Profits* (New York, 1992), pp. 243–44; Victoria A. Harden, "The NIH and Biomedical Research on AIDS," in Caroline Hannaway et al., eds., *AIDS and the Public Debate* (Amsterdam, 1995), p. 30; Robert M. Wachter, "AIDS, Activism, and the Politics of Health," *New England Journal of Medicine* 326, 2 (1992), p. 131; Mariana Valverde, *Diseases of the Will: Alcohol and the Dilemmas of Freedom* (Cambridge, 1998), p. 122.

127. William Muraskin, "Hepatitis B as a Model (and Anti-Model) for AIDS," in Virginia Berridge and Philip Strong, eds., *AIDS and Contemporary History* (Cambridge, 1993), p. 126; William Muraskin, "The Silent Epidemic: The Social, Ethical and Medical Problems Surrounding the Fight against Hepatitis B," *Journal of Social History* 22, 2 (1988), pp. 283–84.

128. Mark Barnes et al., "The HIV-Infected Health Care Professional: Employment Policies and Public Health," *Law, Medicine, and Health Care* 18, 4 (1990), pp. 313–14; Daniels, *Seeking Fair Treatment*, p. 41; *Congressional Record* (Senate), 15 July 1991, pp. 9977–79; Bayer and Kirp, "The United States," p. 17; Rubenstein et al., *Rights of People*, pp. 251–52; James, "Legal Aspects of AIDS," p. 322.

129. BT *Drucksache* 12/1336, 18 October 1991, p. 2; Swiss Institute of Comparative Law, *Comparative Study*, p. 31; *AIDS: HIV-Infected Health Care Workers: Report of the Recommendations of the Expert Advisory Group on AIDS* (London, March 1988), p. 6; Berridge, *AIDS in the UK*, p. 257.

130. Widdows, "AIDS and the Workplace," p. 151; *IDHL* 39, 3 (1988), pp. 627–28; RD Prot, 1985/86, Bihang, Socialutskottets betänkande 1985/86:15, p. 6; "Die Bayerische Staatskanzlei teilt mit," *AIDS-Forschung* 2, 3 (March 1987).

131. BT *Drucksache* 11/1620, Nos. 18–20, 23 December 1987; Institute of Medicine, *Confronting AIDS: Update 1988*, p. 10; David M. Bell, "HIV Infection in Health Care Workers: Occupational Risk and Prevention," in Lawrence O. Gostin, ed., *AIDS and the Health Care System* (New Haven, 1990), pp. 121–22; WHO, *Legislative Responses*, p. 77; Christensen et al., *AIDS*, p. 62; Lucette Khaïat, "Nouveau virus et vieux démons: Le droit face au sida, une approache comparative," in Eric Heilmann, ed., *Sida et libertés: La régulation d'une épidemie dans un état de droit* (n.p., 1991), p. 76.

132. Got, *Rapport*, p. 278; Michel Setbon, *Pouvoirs contre SIDA: De la transfusion sanguine au dépistage: Decisions et pratiques en France, Grande-Bretagne et Suède* (Paris, 1993), p. 264; Monika Steffen, *The Fight against AIDS: An International Public Policy Comparison between Four European Countries: France, Great Britain, Germany, and Italy* (Grenoble, 1996), p. 53; Peter Roth, "AIDS and Insurance: Some Very British Questions," in David FitzSimons et al., eds., *The Economic and Social Impact of AIDS in Europe* (London, 1995), p. 284; House of Commons, *Problems Associated with AIDS*, vol. 1, p. lxi.

133. Peter Roth and Wesley Gryk, "AIDS and Insurance," in Richard Haigh and Dai Harris, eds., *AIDS: A Guide to the Law*, 2d ed. (London, 1995), p. 94; Swiss Institute of Comparative Law, *Comparative Study*, p. 97.

134. Pierre Lascoumes, "De la sélection des risques à la discrimination: Les pratiques des compagnies d'assurances vis-à-vis du sida," in Eric Heilmann, ed., *Sida et libertés: La régulation d'une épidemie dans un état de droit* (n.p., 1991), p. 195.

135. Cornelia Thies, *Die Auswirkungen von AIDS im Privatversicherungsrecht* (Frankfurt, 1991), pp. 4, 22–27, 29, 49.

136. Roth and Gryk, "AIDS and Insurance," pp. 91–94; BT *Drucksache* 10/300, 12 August 1983, No. 66; 11/1548, 17 December 1987, p. 17; Steffen, "France: Social Solidarity," p. 237; Got, *Rapport*, p. 258; Stephan Ruppen, *AIDS: Ein Ratgeber für Rechtsfragen rund um AIDS* (Zurich, 1989), pp. 54–56.

137. Gerald M. Oppenheimer and Robert A. Padgug, "AIDS and the Crisis of Health Insurance," in Frederick G. Reamer, ed., *AIDS and Ethics* (New York, 1991), p. 113; Closen et al., *AIDS*, p. 564.

138. Daniel M. Fox, "Chronic Disease and Disadvantage: The New Politics of HIV Infection," *Journal of Health Politics, Policy, and Law* 15, 2 (summer 1990), pp. 351–52.

139. Got, *Rapport*, p. 259; *Le Monde*, 4 June 1994, p. 24.

140. Arthur S. Leonard, "HIV and United States Workplace Law," in Lawrence Gostin and Lane Porter, eds., *International Law and AIDS* (n.p., 1992), pp. 202–4.

141. Lawrence Bartlett, "Financing Health Care for Persons with AIDS: Balancing Public and Private Responsibilities," in Lawrence O. Gostin, ed., *AIDS and the Health Care System* (New Haven, 1990), p. 215.

142. Lascoumes, "De la sélection des risques à la discrimination," pp. 177–89; Foyer and Khaïat, "Droit et SIDA," pp. 243–45, 253–54; Jean-Luc Fagnart, "Les assurances et le Sida," in Michel Vincineau, ed., *Le Sida: Un défi aux droits* (Brussels, 1991), p. 698; Philippe Pierre, "SIDA: Les implications assurantielles de la pandémie," in Brigitte Feuillet-Le Mintier, ed., *Le SIDA: Aspects juridiques* (Paris, 1995), p. 80; Auvergnon, *Le droit social à l'epreuve du SIDA*, p. 42; Swiss Institute of Comparative Law, *Comparative Study*, pp. 97, 237; Sobel, "Policy Making under Changing Political Situations," pp. 90–91; Steffen, "France: Social Solidarity," pp. 242–44.

143. H. D. C. Roscam Abbing, "AIDS, Human Rights, and Legislation in the Netherlands," in Martin Breum and Aart Hendriks, eds., *AIDS and Human Rights* (Copenhagen, 1988), p. 103; Janherman Veenker, "The Decisive Role of Politics: AIDS Control in the Netherlands," in Theo Sandfort, ed., *The Dutch Response to HIV: Pragmatism and Consensus* (London, 1998), p. 129; Jan K. van Wijngaarden, "The Netherlands: AIDS in a Consensual Society," in David L. Kirp and Ronald Bayer, eds., *AIDS in the Industrialized Democracies* (New Brunswick, 1992), p. 271; Zeegers, "Droit et Sida," p. 330; Swiss Institute of Comparative Law, *Comparative Study*, p. 309; Wayland Kennet, ed., *Parliaments and Screening: A Conference on the Ethical and Social Problems Arising from Testing and Screening for HIV and AIDS* (Paris, 1995), p. 49.

144. Albæk, "AIDS: The Evolution of a Non-Controversial Issue in Denmark," p. 11; Hagstrøm, *AIDS som juridisk problem*, pp. 88–89; Moxnes, "AIDS

and Human Rights," p. 111; Westerhäll and Saldeen, "Réflexions sur le Sida," p. 407; Henriksson and Ytterberg, "Sweden," p. 330.

145. David Hirsch, "SIDA et droit en Australie," in Jacques Foyer and Lucette Khaïat, eds., *Droit et Sida: Comparaison internationale* (Paris, 1994), p. 93; Ruppen, *AIDS*, p. 61; Erwin Deutsch, *Rechtsprobleme von AIDS* (Bergisch Gladbach, 1988), p. 32; Lücke, *Aids*, p. 161; Swiss Institute of Comparative Law, *Comparative Study*, p. 265; Thies, *Die Auswirkungen von AIDS*, pp. 54, 71, 105; BT *Drucksache* 11/2388, Nos. 9–10, 26 May 1988.

146. Nancy J. Haley and Barry S. Reed, "HIV Testing for Life Insurance," in Gerald Schochetman and J. Richard George, eds., *AIDS Testing*, 2d ed. (New York, 1994), p. 255; Brazier and Mulholland, "Droit et Sida," pp. 384–86; Tom Sorell and Heather Draper, "AIDS and Insurance," in Rebecca Bennett and Charles A. Erin, eds., *HIV and AIDS: Testing, Screening, and Confidentiality* (Oxford, 1999), p. 219; House of Commons, *Problems Associated with AIDS*, vol. 1, p. lxii; vol. 2, p. 261; Roth, "AIDS and Insurance," pp. 284–90; Roth and Gryk, "AIDS and Insurance," pp. 91, 95–100, 109–11.

147. Benjamin Schatz, "The AIDS Insurance Crisis: Underwriting or Over-reaching?" *Harvard Law Review* 100, 7 (May 1987), pp. 1786–92; Hermann and Schurgin, *Legal Aspects*, §13:13.

148. Lücke, *Aids*, p. 136; Bartlett, "Financing Health Care," p. 215; Edgar and Sandomire, "Medical Privacy Issues," pp. 215–18; *IDHL* 38, 1 (1987), pp. 42–43; 39, 4 (1988), pp. 833–36; Ford and Quam, "AIDS Quarantine," p. 381; Russel P. Iuculano, "D.C. Act 6–170: The Five-Year Ban on Risk-Based Pricing for AIDS," *AIDS and Public Policy Journal* 2, 1 (1987), pp. 15–17.

149. *Congressional Record* (House), 16 September 1987, 133, pp. 25796–813.

150. Hermann, "AIDS and the Law," p. 291; Mark Scherzer, "Private Insurance," in Scott Burris et al., eds., *AIDS Law Today* (New Haven, 1993), p. 419; Hermann and Schurgin, *Legal Aspects*, §13:14; Tanner and the ALEC National Working Group on State AIDS Policy, *Politics of Health*, pp. 58–59; Haley and Reed, "HIV Testing for Life Insurance," p. 255; Rubenstein et al., *Rights of People*, pp. 31, 131.

151. *IDHL* 44, 2 (1993), p. 231; Deutsche AIDS-Hilfe, Berlin, *Restrictions of Entry and Residence for People with HIV/AIDS: A Global Survey* (Frankfurt, November 1991), pp. 60–61; Swiss Institute of Comparative Law, *Comparative Study*, p. 69; *Le Monde*, 21 January 1988, p. 11; Foyer and Khaïat, "Droit et SIDA," pp. 225, 230; Jaqueline Bouton, "Le secret médical et le sida," in Eric Heilmann, ed., *Sida et libertés: La régulation d'une épidemie dans un état de droit* (n.p., 1991), p. 141; *Le Monde*, 10 February 1988, p. 17.

152. Westerhäll and Saldeen, "Réflexions sur le Sida," p. 412; Rubenstein et al., *Rights of People*, p. 204; Larry O. Gostin, "Public Health Strategies for Confronting AIDS: Legislative and Regulatory Policy in the United States," *JAMA* 261, 11 (17 March 1989), p. 1625; *IDHL* 40, 2 (1989), p. 389.

153. Swiss Institute of Comparative Law, *Comparative Study*, pp. 69–70; Brazier and Mulholland, "Droit et Sida," p. 379.

154. Inge Karin Tiedemann, "Familienrechtliche Probleme im Zusammen-

hang mit AIDS," in Bernd Schünemann and Gerd Pfeiffer, eds., *Die Rechtsprobleme von AIDS* (Baden-Baden, 1988). pp. 338, 347; Gerhard H. Schlund, "Juristische Aspekte beim erworbenen Immun-Defekt-Syndrom (AIDS)," *AIDS-Forschung* 10 (1986), p. 565.

155. Foyer and Khaïat, "Droit et SIDA," pp. 230–31; Swiss Institute of Comparative Law, *Comparative Study,* pp. 69–70; AIDES, *Droit et S.I.D.A,* p. 63; Vèronique Barabe-Bouchard, "La famille et le SIDA," in Brigitte Feuillet-Le Mintier, ed., *Le SIDA: Aspects juridiques* (Paris, 1995), pp. 37–38.

156. Hermann and Schurgin, *Legal Aspects,* §§4:25–26; Robert B. Gainor, "To Have and to Hold: The Tort Liability for the Interspousal Transmission of AIDS," *New England Law Review* 23 (1988–89), p. 895.

6. EVERY MAN HIS OWN QUARANTINE OFFICER: THE VOLUNTARY APPROACH

1. "The Constitutional Rights of AIDS Carriers," *Harvard Law Review* 99 (April 1986), p. 1279; Larry Gostin, "The Future of Communicable Disease Control: Toward a New Concept in Public Health Law," *Milbank Quarterly* 64, suppl. 1 (1986), pp. 80–81; Lawrence O. Gostin, "The Future of Public Health Law," *American Journal of Law and Medicine* 12, 3–4 (1986), pp. 461–90.

2. BT *Drucksache* 11/7200, 31 May 1990, p. 252; David J. Rothman, "Public Policy and Risk Assessment in the AIDS Epidemic," in John Griggs, ed., *AIDS: Public Policy Dimensions* (New York, 1987), p. 66.

3. James F. Childress, "Mandatory HIV Screening and Testing," in Frederick G. Reamer, ed., *AIDS and Ethics* (New York, 1991), p. 63; June E. Osborn, "Public Health and the Politics of AIDS," *Dædalus* 118, 3 (summer 1989), p. 135; Wolfram H. Eberbach, "Seuchenrechtliche Massnahmen gegen AIDS," in Max Busch et al., eds., *HIV/AIDS und Straffälligkeit* (Bonn, 1991), pp. 84–85; House of Commons, 1986–87, Social Services Committee, *Problems Associated with AIDS,* 13 May 1987, vol. 1, p. x.

4. Dale J. Hu et al., "The Emerging Genetic Diversity of HIV: The Importance of Global Surveillance for Diagnostics, Research, and Prevention," *JAMA* 275, 3 (1996), pp. 210–14.

5. Institute of Medicine, *Confronting AIDS: Directions for Public Health, Health Care, and Research* (Washington, DC, 1986), p. 120; Klaus Scherf, *AIDS und Strafrecht* (Baden-Baden, 1992), p. 151; William J. Curran et al., "AIDS: Legal and Policy Implications of the Application of Traditional Disease Control Measures," *Law, Medicine, and Health Care* 15, 1–2 (summer 1987), p. 32; Donald H. J. Hermann, "AIDS and the Law," in Frederick G. Reamer, ed., *AIDS and Ethics* (New York, 1991), p. 294; Larry Gostin, "Traditional Public Health Strategies," in Scott Burris et al., eds., *AIDS Law Today* (New Haven, 1993), pp. 73–74; Larry Gostin, "The Politics of AIDS: Compulsory State Powers, Public Health, and Civil Liberties," *Ohio State Law Journal* 49 (1989), p. 1028; Mark H. Jackson, "The Criminalization of HIV," in Nan D. Hunter and William B. Rubenstein, eds., *AIDS Agenda: Emerging Issues in Civil Rights* (New York, 1992), p. 240.

6. House of Commons, *Problems Associated with AIDS,* vol. 2, p. 10; Peter A. Selwyn, "Tuberculosis and AIDS: Epidemiologic, Clinical, and Social Dimensions," *Journal of Law, Medicine, and Ethics* 21, 3–4 (1993), p. 285; Barbara Breitbach et al., "AIDS-Bekämpfung und Bundes-Seuchengesetz," *Kritische Justiz* 21, 1 (1988), pp. 64–66; Gostin, "Politics of AIDS," p. 1027; Kathleen M. Sullivan and Martha A. Field, "AIDS and the Coercive Power of the State," *Harvard Civil Right–Civil Liberties Law Review* 23 (1988), p. 148.

7. Manfred Bruns, "AIDS, Prostitution und das Strafrecht," *Neue Juristische Wochenschrift* 40, 12 (1987), p. 695; W. H. Eberbach, "Rechtliche Rahmenbedingungen für die Krankheit AIDS in der Bundesrepublik Deutschland 1988," *Das öffentliche Gesundheitswesen* 50 (1988), p. 458; Joseph D. Piorkowski Jr., "Between a Rock and a Hard Place: AIDS and the Conflicting Physician's Duties of Preventing Disease Transmission and Safeguarding Confidentiality," *Georgetown Law Journal* 76 (1987), p. 188; BT *Drucksache* 11/7200, 31 May 1990, p. 175; BT *Verhandlungen* 10/246, 13 November 1986, p. 19094B.

8. Otfried Seewald, "Aids als Herausforderung an den Verfassungsstaat des Grundgesetzes," in Ernst Burkel, ed., *Der AIDS-Komplex: Dimensionen einer Bedrohung* (Frankfurt, 1988), p. 303; *AIDS: Fakten und Konsequenzen: Endbericht der Enquête-Kommission des 11. Deutschen Bundestages "Gefahren von AIDS und wirksame Wege zu ihrer Eindämmung"* (Bonn, 1990), p. 343; *AIDS Nachrichten aus Forschung und Wissenschaft,* 4 (1989), p. 9; Rolf Rosenbrock, "AIDS: Questions and Lessons for Public Health," *AIDS and Public Policy Journal* 8, 1 (1993), p. 11.

9. Martin Sieber, *Die Bedeutung des HIV-Tests für die Aids-Prävention* (Bern, 1995), p. 217; Donna L. Higgins et al., "Evidence for the Effects of HIV Antibody Counseling and Testing on Risk Behaviors," *JAMA* 266, 17 (1991), p. 2424; Hubert Rottleuthner, "Probleme der rechtlichen Regulierung von Aids," and Andreas Salmen, "Aktuelle Erfordernisse der Aidsprävention," in Rolf Rosenbrock and Andreas Salmen, eds., *Aids-Prävention* (Berlin, 1990), pp. 128, 95; Mirko D. Grmek, *History of AIDS* (Princeton, 1990), p. 18; Randy Shilts, *And the Band Played On: Politics, People, and the AIDS Epidemic* (New York, 1988), p. 147; Walt Odets, *In the Shadow of the Epidemic: Being HIV-Negative in the Age of AIDS* (Durham, 1995), pp. 46–47.

10. WHO, *Legislative Responses to AIDS* (Dordrecht, 1989), pp. 256–60; Felix Herzog, "Das Strafrecht im Kampf gegen 'Aids-Desperados,'" in Ernst Burkel, ed., *Der AIDS-Komplex: Dimensionen einer Bedrohung* (Frankfurt, 1988), p. 342; Manfred Steinbach, "Politische Strategien der AIDS-Bekämpfung," in Hans-Ullrich Gallwas et al., eds., *Aids und Recht* (Stuttgart, 1992), p. 64; BT *Drucksache* 10/3749, No. 46; Philip Strong and Virginia Berridge, "No One Knew Anything: Some Issues in British AIDS Policy," in Peter Aggleton et al., eds., *AIDS: Individual, Cultural, and Policy Dimensions* (London, 1990), p. 240.

11. Larry Gostin and William J. Curran, "Legal Control Measures for AIDS: Reporting Requirements, Surveillance, Quarantine, and Regulation of Public

Meeting Places," *American Journal of Public Health* 77, 2 (February 1987), pp. 215–16; William J. Curran, "AIDS and Poverty in the United States of America: A Human Rights Issue," in Martin Breum and Aart Hendriks, eds., *AIDS and Human Rights* (Copenhagen, 1988), p. 153.

12. David L. Kirp and Ronald Bayer, "The Second Decade of AIDS: The End of Exceptionalism?" in Kirp and Bayer, eds., *AIDS in the Industrialized Democracies* (New Brunswick, 1992), p. 365; Patricia Day and Rudolf Klein, "Interpreting the Unexpected: The Case of AIDS Policy Making in Britain," *Journal of Public Policy* 9, 3 (1989), p. 345; Ronald Bayer, "AIDS, Public Health, and Civil Liberties: Consensus and Conflict in Policy," in Frederick G. Reamer, ed., *AIDS and Ethics* (New York, 1991), pp. 26–28; Rolf D. Rosenbrock, "Screening for Human Immunodeficiency Virus," *International Journal of Technology Assessment in Health Care* 7 (1991), p. 267.

13. BT *Drucksache* 11/6485, 15 February 1990; Rolf Rosenbrock, "HIV-Screening," Wissenschaftszentrum Berlin, *Veröffentlichungen der Forschungsgruppe Gesundheitsrisiken und Präventionspolitik*, P90–202 (Berlin, February 1990), p. 9.

14. Peter Roth and Wesley Gryk, "AIDS and Insurance," in Richard Haigh and Dai Harris, eds., *AIDS: A Guide to the Law,* 2d ed. (London, 1995), p. 109; Peter Roth, "AIDS and Insurance: Some Very British Questions," in David FitzSimons et al., eds., *The Economic and Social Impact of AIDS in Europe* (London, 1995), pp. 286–87; BT *Drucksache* 11/2388, Nos. 9–10, 26 May 1988; Benjamin Schatz, "The AIDS Insurance Crisis: Underwriting or Overreaching?" *Harvard Law Review* 100, 7 (May 1987), pp. 1792, 1802; Heather G. Miller et al., eds., *AIDS: The Second Decade* (Washington, DC, 1990), pp. 277–78; Angus Hamilton, "The Criminal Law and HIV Infection," in Richard Haigh and Dai Harris, eds., *AIDS: A Guide to the Law,* 2d ed. (London, 1995), p. 36; Jonathan Glasson, "Public Health and Human Rights: Finding a Balance in HIV Prevention," in David FitzSimons et al., eds., *The Economic and Social Impact of AIDS in Europe* (London, 1995), p. 239.

15. Daniel Defert, "Police sanitaire ou droit commun?" in Emmanuel Hirsch, *Aides: Solidaires* (Paris, 1991), p. 536; Ute Canaris, "Gesundheitspolitische Aspekte im Zusammenhang mit AIDS," in Johannes Korporal and Hubert Malouschek, eds., *Leben mit AIDS—Mit AIDS leben* (Hamburg, 1987), p. 282; Inez de Beaufort, "Individual Responsibility for Health," in Rebecca Bennett and Charles A. Erin, eds., *HIV and AIDS: Testing, Screening, and Confidentiality* (Oxford, 1999), pp. 107–9.

16. Mark H. Jackson, "Health Insurance: The Battle over Limits on Coverage," in Nan D. Hunter and William B. Rubenstein, eds., *AIDS Agenda: Emerging Issues in Civil Rights* (New York, 1992), p. 150.

17. Stephan Ruppen, *AIDS: Ein Ratgeber für Rechtsfragen rund um AIDS* (Zurich, 1989), pp. 54–56; *Aftonbladet* 16 September 2000, p. 15.

18. *Medical Times and Gazette* 11 (1855), pp. 31–35, 84–88.

19. BT *Drucksache* 11/6485, 15 February 1990; Richard D. Mohr, *Gays/Justice: A Study of Ethics, Society, and Law* (New York, 1988), pp. 217–20, 223;

Richard A. Mohr, "AIDS, Gays, and State Coercion," *Bioethics* 1, 1 (1987), pp. 38–40.

20. Rosenbrock, "HIV-Screening," p. 13; Aart Hendriks, "AIDS, AIDS Strategy, and Internationally Recognized Human Rights," in Martin Breum and Aart Hendriks, eds., *AIDS and Human Rights* (Copenhagen, 1988), pp. 19–20; Institute of Medicine, *Confronting AIDS: Update 1988* (Washington, DC, 1988), p. 74; Martin Dannecker, *Homosexuelle Männer und AIDS* (Stuttgart, 1990), p. 228.

21. Gabriel Rotello, *Sexual Ecology: AIDS and the Destiny of Gay Men* (New York, 1997), pp. 106–8; Dieter Meurer, "AIDS und Strafrecht," in Hans-Ullrich Gallwas et al., eds., *Aids und Recht* (Stuttgart, 1992), p. 117; Swiss Institute of Comparative Law, *Comparative Study on Discrimination against Persons with HIV or AIDS* (Strasbourg, 1993), p. 65; Ralph Bolton, "AIDS and Promiscuity: Muddles in the Models of HIV Prevention," *Medical Anthropology* 14 (1992), pp. 177–78; David L. Chambers, "Gay Men, AIDS, and the Code of the Condom," *Harvard Civil Rights–Civil Liberties Law Review* 29 (1994), pp. 353, 366, 377–80.

22. BT *Drucksache* 11/7200, 31 May 1990, p. 368; Lawrence O. Gostin, "The AIDS Litigation Project: A National Review of Court and Human Rights Commission Decisions," *JAMA* 263, 14 (11 April 1990), p. 1966; WHO, *Legislative Responses*, pp. 284–86.

23. David A. Conway, "AIDS and Legal Paternalism," *Social Theory and Practice* 13, 3 (fall 1987), pp. 287–88; Mohr, "AIDS, Gays, and State Coercion," pp. 217–23; Frank Becker and Klaus-Dieter Beisswenger, eds., *Solidarität der Uneinsichtigen: Aktionstag 9. Juli 1988 Frankfurt a.M.* (Berlin, 1988), p. 9.

24. Frédéric Ocqueteau, "La répression pénale dans la lutte contre le sida: Solution ou alibi?" in Eric Heilmann, ed., *Sida et libertés: La régulation d'une épidemie dans un état de droit* (n.p., 1991), pp. 247–49; Rottleuthner, "Probleme der rechtlichen Regulierung," p. 125; Scherf, *AIDS und Strafrecht*, p. 79; Peter Raschke and Claudia Ritter, *Eine Grossstadt lebt mit Aids: Strategien der Prävention und Hilfe am Beispiel Hamburgs* (Berlin, 1991), pp. 212–13.

25. David C. Wyld and David E. Hallock, "Advertising's Response to the AIDS Crisis: The Role of Social Marketing," *AIDS and Public Policy Journal* 4, 4 (1989), p. 201.

26. H. Jäger, ed., *AIDS und HIV-Infektionen* (n.p., n.d.), ix–2.3.4, pp. 1, 5; Andrzej J. Szwarc, ed., *AIDS und Strafrecht* (Berlin, 1996), p. 231; Scherf, *AIDS und Strafrecht*, pp. 85–87, 137; BT *Verhandlungen* 11/110, 24 November 1988, p. 7748B; Rolf Dietrich Herzberg, "Die strafrechtliche Haftung für die Infizierung oder Gefährdung durch HIV," in Andrzej J. Szwarc, ed., *AIDS und Strafrecht* (Berlin, 1996), pp. 82–83; Christoph Knauer, "Die Strafbarkeit des HIV-Infizierten beim Vollziehen sexueller Kontakte mit getroffenen Schutzmassnahmen," *AIDS-Forschung* 9 (1994), pp. 466–68.

27. Markus Müller, *Zwangsmassnahmen als Instrument der Krankheitsbekämpfung: Das Epidemiengesetz und die Persönliche Freiheit* (Basel, 1992), p. 91.

28. *Hansard Parliamentary Debates,* vol. 96 (30 April 1986), col. 918; vol. 113 (27 March 1987), col. 686; Canaris, "Gesundheitspolitische Aspekte," p. 282.

29. Memo by Dr. Ronald Bolton, House of Commons, *Problems Associated with AIDS,* vol. 3, p. 208.

30. Mohr, *Gays/Justice,* pp. 230–38; Patricia Illingworth, *AIDS and the Good Society* (London, 1990), preface, pp. 14–16, 46, 63, 77–79; Larry Kramer, *Reports from the Holocaust:The Making of an AIDS Activist* (New York, 1989), pp. 178–79; Philip M. Kayal, *Bearing Witness: Gay Men's Health Crisis and the Politics of AIDS* (Boulder, 1993), pp. 53–54, 92–95; John Shiers, "One Step to Heaven?" in Bob Cant and Susan Hemmings, eds., *Radical Records:Thirty Years of Lesbian and Gay History, 1957–1987* (London, 1988), pp. 240–41; Marshall Kirk and Hunter Madsen, *After the Ball: How America Will Conquer Its Fear and Hatred of Gays in the '90s* (New York, 1989), pp. xxiv, 356–57; Dan E. Beauchamp, "Morality and the Health of the Body Politic," *Hastings Center Report* 16 (1986), p. 32; RD *Prot,* 1986/87, Bihang, Prop. 149, p. 36.

31. *Hansard,* vol. 108 (23 January 1987), col. 1175. Similar sentiments: Becker and Beisswenger, eds., *Solidarität der Uneinsichtigen,* p. 9; Edward King, *Safety in Numbers: Safer Sex and Gay Men* (London, 1993), p. 246.

32. RD *Prot,* 1986/87, Bihang, Prop. 149, pp. 34–36.

33. Canaris, "Gesundheitspolitische Aspekte," pp. 284–85.

34. Rüdiger Jacob et al., "Problems Associated with Prevention Campaigns," in Dorothee Friedrich and Wolfgang Heckmann, eds., *Aids in Europe: The Behavioural Aspect* (Berlin, 1995), 4:99–107; Jost Reinecke, *AIDS-Prävention und Sexualverhalten: Die Theorie des geplanten Verhaltens im empirischen Test* (Opladen, 1997).

35. Annick Prieur, "Taking Risks Is Rational Behavior," in Behörde für Arbeit, Gesundheit und Soziales der Freien und Hansestadt Hamburg, *Dokumentation des Internationalen Symposiums "HIV/AIDS-Homosexualität/Bisexualität" 6. Oktober 1991 bis 9. Oktober 1991 in Hamburg* (Hamburg, 1991), pp. 177–78; Tim Rhodes, "Risk, Injecting Drug Use, and the Myth of an Objective Social Science," in Joshua Oppenheimer and Helena Reckitt, eds., *Acting on AIDS: Sex, Drugs, and Politics* (London, 1997), p. 64; Gustavo Guizzardi et al., "Rationality and Preventive Measures: The Ambivalence of the Social Discourse on AIDS," in Luc van Campenhoudt et al., eds., *Sexual Interactions and HIV Risk* (London, 1997), pp. 160–62.

36. Peter Davies and Project SIGMA, "On Relapse: Recidivism or Rational Response?" in Peter Aggleton et al., eds., *AIDS: Rights, Risk, and Reason* (London, 1992), pp. 136–37; Peter M. Davies et al., *Sex, Gay Men, and AIDS* (London, 1993), pp. 50–51; Walt Odets, "AIDS Education and Harm Reduction for Gay Men," *AIDS and Public Policy Journal* 9, 1 (1994), p. 10.

37. Szwarc, ed., *AIDS und Strafrecht,* p. 232; Jean-François Fogel and Bertrand Rosenthal, *Fin de siècle à la Havane: Les secrets du pouvoir cubain* (Paris, 1993), p. 359; *Economist,* 15 July 2000, p. 78; Marc Reisinger, "Les avantages d'une prescription détendue de méthadone," in Jean-Marie Guffens, ed.,

Toxicomanie, Hépatites, S.I.D.A. (n.p., 1994), p. 260; Douglas Webb, *HIV and AIDS in Africa* (London, 1997), p. 82.

38. Mary Douglas, *Risk and Blame* (London, 1992), ch. 6; Mary Douglas and Marcel Calvez, "The Self as Risk Taker: A Cultural Theory of Contagion in Relation to AIDS," *Sociological Review* (1990).

39. Michael Bloor, *The Sociology of HIV Transmission* (London, 1995), pp. 85–93; Ronald O. Valdiserri, *Preventing AIDS: The Design of Effective Programs* (New Brunswick, 1989), ch. 3; Michael Pollak, *The Second Plague of Europe: AIDS Prevention and Sexual Transmission among Men in Western Europe* (Binghamton, NY, 1994), p. 63; Graham Hart, "Gay Community Oriented Approaches to Safer Sex," in Tim Rhodes and Richard Hartnoll, eds., *AIDS, Drugs, and Prevention* (London, 1996), p. 88; Allan M. Brandt, "Behavior, Disease, and Health in the Twentieth-Century United States," in Allan M. Brandt and Paul Rozin, eds., *Morality and Health* (New York, 1997), pp. 68–69; Jonathan Mann et al., "Toward a New Health Strategy to Control the HIV/AIDS Pandemic," *Journal of Law, Medicine, and Ethics* 22, 1 (1994), p. 49; Richard G. Parker, "Empowerment, Community Mobilization, and Social Change in the Face of HIV/AIDS," *AIDS* 10, suppl. 3 (1996), pp. S28–29; Samuel R. Friedman et al., "Network and Sociohistorical Approaches to the HIV Epidemic among Drug Injectors," in José Catalán et al., eds., *The Impact of AIDS: Psychological and Social Aspects of HIV Infection* (Amsterdam, 1997), pp. 89–90; Roger Ingham et al., "The Limitations of Rational Decision-Making Models as Applied to Young People's Sexual Behavior," in Peter Aggleton et al., eds., *AIDS: Rights, Risk, and Reason* (London, 1992); Nathalie Bajos and Jacques Marquet, "Research on HIV Sexual Risk: Social Relations-Based Approach in a Cross-Cultural Perspective," *Social Science and Medicine* 50 (2000), pp. 1533–46.

40. Paul Farmer, *Infections and Inequalities: The Modern Plagues* (Berkeley, 1999), p. 86; P. Gillies et al., "Is AIDS a Disease of Poverty?" *AIDS Care* 8, 3 (1996); Richard G. Parker, "Empowerment, Community Mobilization, and Social Change in the Face of HIV/AIDS," *AIDS* 10, suppl. 3 (1996), pp. S28–30; Elizabeth Fee and Nancy Krieger, "Understanding AIDS: Historical Interpretations and the Limits of Biomedical Individualism," *American Journal of Public Health* 83, 10 (October 1993), pp. 1481–83; S. R. Friedman and D. C. Des Jarlais, "HIV among Drug Injectors: The Epidemic and the Response," *AIDS Care* 3, 3 (1991).

41. Michael Pollak and Jean-Paul Moatti, "HIV Risk Perception and Determinants of Sexual Behavior," in Michel Hubert, ed., *Sexual Behaviour and Risks of HIV Infection* (Brussels, 1990), p. 18; Mitchell Cohen and Judy Chwalow, "The Health Belief Model: Always, Sometimes, or Never Useful in Guiding HIV/AIDS Prevention," in Dorothee Friedrich and Wolfgang Heckmann, eds., *Aids in Europe: The Behavioural Aspect* (Berlin, 1995), 4:49–50.

42. J. W. Duyvendak and R. Koopmans, "Resister au Sida: Destin et influence du mouvement homosexuel," in Michael Pollak et al., eds., *Homosexualités et Sida* (n.p., n.d. [1991]), p. 212; Onno de Zwart, Theo Sandfort, and

Marty van Kerkhof, "No Anal Sex Please: We're Dutch: A Dilemma in HIV Prevention Directed at Gay Men," in Sandfort, ed., *The Dutch Response to HIV: Pragmatism and Consensus* (London, 1998), pp. 135–36; King, *Safety in Numbers*, pp. 89–90; Gerjo Kok et al., "Applying Social Psychology to HIV Prevention: Solving a Dilemma in the HIV Prevention Communications on Anal Sex as an Example," in Davidson C. Umeh, ed., *Confronting the AIDS Epidemic: Cross-Cultural Perspectives on HIV/AIDS Education* (Trenton, NJ, 1997), pp. 231–32.

43. Gerry V. Stimson and Martin C. Donoghoe, "Health Promotion and the Facilitation of Individual Change," in Tim Rhodes and Richard Hartnoll, eds., *AIDS, Drugs, and Prevention* (London, 1996), p. 19; Gerry V. Stimson and Rachel Lart, "HIV, Drugs, and Public Health in England: New Words, Old Tunes," *International Journal of the Addictions* 26, 12 (1991), pp. 1272–73.

44. Hendriks, "AIDS, AIDS Strategy," p. 19; Heta Häyry, "Who Should Know about My HIV Positivity and Why?" and Charles A. Erin, "Is There a Right to Remain in Ignorance of HIV Status," in Rebecca Bennett and Charles A. Erin, eds., *HIV and AIDS: Testing, Screening, and Confidentiality* (Oxford, 1999), pp. 242–44, 265–66; H. J. J. Leenen, "Law and AIDS," *AIDS-Forschung* 9 (1986), p. 506; *AIDS: Fakten und Konsequenzen*, p. 329; Klaus Lüderssen, "Die im strafrechtlichen Umgang mit Aids verborgenen Motive: Hypermoral oder Gesinnungsethik?" *Strafverteidiger* 2 (1990), p. 87; Udo Gehring, "Haftpflicht- und Haftpflichtversicherungsrechtliche Fragen bei HIV-Infektionen (AIDS)" (Ph.D. diss., University of Mannheim, 1996), pp. 235–38; Olivier Guillod et al., *Drei Gutachten über rechtliche Fragen im Zusammenhang mit AIDS* (Bern, 1991), pp. 122–23.

45. Cindy Patton, "Save Sex/Save Lives: Evolving Modes of Activism," in Tim Rhodes and Richard Hartnoll, eds., *AIDS, Drugs, and Prevention* (London, 1996), p. 126; Wolf Kirschner, *HIV-Surveillance: Inhaltliche und methodische Probleme bei der Bestimmung der Ausbreitung von HIV-Infektionen* (Berlin, 1993), pp. 64–65.

46. Don C. Des Jarlais et al., "Targeting HIV-Prevention Programs," *New England Journal of Medicine* 331, 21 (1994), pp. 1451–52; David E. Rogers and June E. Osborn, "AIDS Policy: Two Divisive Issues," *JAMA* 270, 4 (1993), p. 494.

47. Day and Klein, "Interpreting the Unexpected," pp. 348–49; Spencer Hagard, "Preventing AIDS through General Public Education: Experience from the United Kingdom," in WHO, *AIDS Prevention and Control* (Geneva, 1988), pp. 41–43; Simon Watney, *Practices of Freedom: Selected Writings on HIV/AIDS* (Durham, NC, 1994), p. 48.

48. Nora Kizer Bell, "Ethical Issues in AIDS Education," in Frederick G. Reamer, ed., *AIDS and Ethics* (New York, 1991), p. 139; Simon Garfield, *The End of Innocence: Britain in the Time of AIDS* (London, 1994), p. 125; Ronald Bayer et al., "Public Health and Private Rights: Health, Social, and Ethical Perspectives," in Robert F. Hummel et al., eds., *AIDS: Impact on Public Policy* (New York, 1986), p. 17; Day and Klein, "Interpreting the Unexpected," p. 349.

49. Swiss Institute of Comparative Law, *Comparative Study*, p. 21; *Public*

Health Reports 103, suppl. 1 (1988), pp. 4, 19; Wyld and Hallock, "Advertising's Response to the AIDS Crisis," p. 199.

50. Cindy Patton, *Last Served? Gendering the HIV Pandemic* (London, 1994), p. 14; Nan D. Hunter, "Censorship and Identity in the Age of AIDS," in Martin P. Levine et al., eds., *In Changing Times: Gay Men and Lesbians Encounter HIV/AIDS* (Chicago, 1997), pp. 45–47; *IDHL* 40, 1 (1989), p. 63; House Committee on Government Operations, *The Politics of AIDS Prevention: Science Takes a Time Out*, 1992, H. Rept. 102–1047, pp. 6–10; Gostin, "AIDS Litigation Project," p. 1961; Larry O. Gostin, "Public Health Strategies for Confronting AIDS: Legislative and Regulatory Policy in the United States," *JAMA* 261, 11 (17 March 1989), p. 1624; Nicholas Freudenberg, "AIDS Prevention in the United States: Lessons from the First Decade," *International Journal of Health Services* 20, 4 (1990), pp. 590–91.

51. Christopher H. Foreman Jr., *Plagues, Products, and Politics: Emergent Public Health Hazards and National Policymaking* (Washington, DC, 1994), p. 80; William DeJong and Jay A. Winsten, "The Strategic Use of the Broadcast Media for AIDS Prevention," in Jaime Sepulveda et al., eds., *AIDS: Prevention through Education* (New York, 1992), pp. 267–69; Karen DeYoung, "Global Politics of AIDS," *Washington Post*, 2 February 1988, pp. 13, 16; BT *Verhandlungen* 11/71, 14 April 1988, p. 4809A-B.

52. June Osborn, "U.S. Response to the AIDS Epidemic: Education Prospects in a Multicultural Society," in Jaime Sepulveda et al., eds., *AIDS: Prevention through Education* (New York, 1992), pp. 343–44; *Public Health Reports* 103, suppl. 1 (1988), p. 20; *Report of the Presidential Commission on the Human Immunodeficiency Virus Epidemic* (Washington, DC, 1988), p. 83; Theodore J. Stein, *The Social Welfare of Women and Children with HIV and AIDS: Legal Protections, Policy, and Programs* (New York, 1998), pp. 125–34; William B. Rubenstein et al., *The Rights of People Who Are HIV Positive* (Carbondale, IL, 1996), p. 292; Peggy Clarke, "Messages Addressed to Women as a Target Audience," in WHO, *AIDS Prevention and Control* (Geneva, 1988), p. 52.

53. Monika Steffen, *The Fight against AIDS: An International Public Policy Comparison between Four European Countries: France, Great Britain, Germany, and Italy* (Grenoble, 1996), p. 58; John Street, "British Government Policy on AIDS: Learning Not to Die of Ignorance," *Parliamentary Affairs* 41 (October 1988), pp. 490–91, 494; Daniel M. Fox, Patricia Day, and Rudolf Klein, "The Power of Professionalism: Policies for AIDS in Britain, Sweden, and the United States," *Dædalus* 118, 2 (spring 1989), p. 97.

54. Hamilton, "The Criminal Law," pp. 31–34; Simon Watney, *Policing Desire: Pornography, AIDS, and the Media* (Minneapolis, 1987), p. 17; Rob Tielman and Hans Hammelburg, "World Survey on the Social and Legal Position of Gays and Lesbians," in Aart Hendriks et al., eds., *The Third Pink Book: A Global View of Lesbian and Gay Liberation and Oppression* (Buffalo, 1993), p. 259; Watney, *Practices of Freedom*, p. 240.

55. RD Prot, 1987/88, Bihang, Prop. 79, pp. 11–13; Kaye Wellings and Becky Field, *Stopping AIDS: AIDS/HIV Education and the Mass Media in Europe*

(London, 1996), pp. 22–24; Benny Henriksson and Hasse Ytterberg, "Sweden: The Power of the Moral(istic) Left," in David L. Kirp and Ronald Bayer, eds., *AIDS in the Industrialized Democracies* (New Brunswick, 1992), p. 331.

56. Harm Hospers and Cor Blom, "HIV Prevention Activities for Gay Men in the Netherlands 1983–93," and Frans van den Boom and Paul Schnabel, "The Impact of AIDS on the Dutch Health Care System," in Theo Sandfort, ed., *The Dutch Response to HIV: Pragmatism and Consensus* (London, 1998), pp. 43–44, 158.

57. Nathalie Bajos et al., "Sexual Behaviour and HIV Epidemiology: Comparative Analysis in France and Britain," *AIDS* 9 (1995), p. 740; Aquilino Morelle, *La défaite de la santé publique* (Paris, 1996), p. 306; Alain Pompidou, "National AIDS Information Programme in France," in WHO, *AIDS Prevention and Control* (Geneva, 1988), pp. 28–31; Pollak, *Second Plague*, p. 38; Murray Pratt, "The Defence of the Straight State: Heteronormativity, AIDS in France, and the Space of the Nation," *French Cultural Studies* 9, 3 (1998), pp. 271–73; Werner Reutter, "Aids, Politik und Demokratie: Ein Vergleich aidspolitischer Massnahmen in Deutschland und Frankreich," Wissenschaftszentrum Berlin für Sozialforschung, *Veröffentlichungsreihe der Forschungsgruppe Gesundheitsrisiken und Präventionspolitik*, P92–205 (Berlin, April 1992), pp. 12–14.

58. Matthias Weikert, "AIDS Prevention: Cooperation of NGOs and GOs," in Dorothee Friedrich and Wolfgang Heckmann, eds., *Aids in Europe: The Behavioural Aspect* (Berlin, 1995), 4:57; Canaris, "Gesundheitspolitische Aspekte," pp. 275, 301; Wolfgang Heckmann and Sabine Reiter, eds., *Community-Oriented Prevention of AIDS and Addiction* (Berlin, 1991; AIDS-Zentrum Hefte 6/1991).

59. Charles Perrow and Mauro F. Guillén, *The AIDS Disaster: The Failure of Organizations in New York and the Nation* (New Haven, 1990), pp. 25–26; Wyld and Hallock, "Advertising's Response to the AIDS Crisis," pp. 201–2.

60. Sandro Cattacin, "Organisatorische Probleme der HIV/AIDS-Politik in föderalen Staaten: Deutschland, Österreich und Schweiz im Vergleich," *Journal für Sozialforschung* 36, 1 (1996), p. 80; Monika Steffen, "AIDS Policies in France," in Virginia Berridge and Philip Strong, eds., *AIDS and Contemporary History* (Cambridge, 1993), p. 252; Monika Steffen, "AIDS and Political Systems," in Dorothee Friedrich and Wolfgang Heckmann, eds., *Aids in Europe: The Behavioural Aspect* (Berlin, 1995), 5:36–37; Steffen, *Fight against AIDS*, pp. 58–59.

61. Mary Catherine Bateson and Richard Goldsby, *Thinking AIDS* (Reading, MA, 1988), p. 122; Wolfgang Heckmann, "AIDS: Soziale Veränderungen und soziale Arbeit," in Max Busch et al., eds., *HIV/AIDS und Straffälligkeit* (Bonn, 1991), p. 4; BT *Drucksache* 11/2495, 16 June 1988, p. 90; BT *Verhandlungen* 11/103, 27 October 1988, p. 7053C.

62. *Harvard Law Review* 110, 5 (1997), pp. 1179–80; Gerlinde Maria Schwarz, *HIV/AIDS Education an den öffentlichen Elementar- und Sekundarschulen der USA: Aufgezeigt am Beispiel von New York City* (Frankfurt, 1997), p. 86.

63. *Hansard*, vol. 144 (13 January 1989), col. 1109; vol. 229 (22 July 1993), col. 618–19; Virginia Berridge, *AIDS in the UK: The Making of Policy, 1981–1994* (Oxford, 1996), p. 265; Glasson, "Public Health and Human Rights," p. 236; Simmy Viinikka, "Children, Young People, and HIV Infection," in Richard Haigh and Dai Harris, eds., *AIDS: A Guide to the Law*, 2d ed. (London, 1995), p. 20.

64. Michael Pollak, *Les homosexuels et le sida: Sociologie d'une épidémie* (Paris, 1988), pp. 206–7; Rolf Rosenbrock, "AIDS: Fragen und Lehren für Public Health," Wissenschaftszentrum Berlin für Sozialforschung, *Veröffentlichungsreihe der Forschungsgruppe Gesundheitsrisiken und Präventionspolitik*, P92–206 (Berlin, April 1992), p. 29; James Kinsella, *Covering the Plague: AIDS and the American Media* (New Brunswick, 1989), ch. 2.

65. Virginia Berridge and Philip Strong, "AIDS in the UK: Contemporary History and the Study of Policy," *Twentieth Century British History* 2, 2 (1991), p. 161; Bayer, "Public Health and Private Rights," p. 21.

66. Pollak, *Les homosexuels et le sida*, pp. 206–7; *RD Prot*, 1988/89:105 (27 April 1989), p. 25.

67. Dwayne C. Turner, *Risky Sex: Gay Men and HIV Prevention* (New York, 1997), pp. 123–27; Marie-Ange Schiltz and Philippe Adam, "Reputedly Effective Risk Reduction Strategies and Gay Men," and Graham Hart and Mary Boulton, "Sexual Behaviour in Gay Men: Towards a Sociology of Risk," in Peter Aggleton et al., eds., *AIDS: Safety, Sexuality, and Risk* (London, 1995), pp. 1, 7, 57; Danièle Peto et al., "Sexual Adaption to HIV Risk," in Michel Hubert, ed., *Sexual Behaviour and Risks of HIV Infection* (Brussels, 1990), pp. 256–57; Turner, *Risky Sex*, pp. 5–16.

68. Wellings and Field, *Stopping AIDS*, pp. 134–35.

69. Ford C. I. Hickson et al., "No Aggregate Change in Homosexual HIV Risk Behaviour among Gay Men Attending the Gay Pride Festivals, United Kingdom, 1993–1995," *AIDS* 10 (1996), p. 773; Peter M. Nardi, "Friends, Lovers, and Families: The Impact of AIDS on Gay and Lesbian Relationships," in Martin P. Levine et al., eds., *In Changing Times: Gay Men and Lesbians Encounter HIV/AIDS* (Chicago, 1997), pp. 77–78.

70. Bloor, *Sociology of HIV Transmission*, p. 127; Dannecker, *Homosexuelle Männer*, pp. 30–31; Joseph A. Kotarba and Norris G. Lang, "Gay Lifestyle Change and AIDS: Preventive Health Care," in Douglas A. Feldman and Thomas M. Johnson, eds., *The Social Dimensions of AIDS* (New York, 1986), p. 138; Michael Bochow, *Die Reaktionen homosexueller Männer auf AIDS in Ost- und Westdeutschland* (Berlin, 1993), pp. 33–34.

71. Rosenbrock, "AIDS: Fragen und Lehren," pp. 9–10; Rolf Rosenbrock, "The Role of Policy in Effective Prevention and Education," in Dorothee Friedrich and Wolfgang Heckmann, eds., *Aids in Europe: The Behavioural Aspect* (Berlin, 1995), 5:22; William A. Rushing, *The AIDS Epidemic: Social Dimensions of an Infectious Disease* (Boulder, 1995), p. 100; Bolton, "AIDS and Promiscuity," pp. 187–88; Peter Scott, "White Noise: How Gay Men's Activism Gets Written Out of AIDS Prevention," in Joshua Oppenheimer and Helena

Reckitt, eds., *Acting on AIDS: Sex, Drugs, and Politics* (London, 1997), p. 311; Marshall H. Becker and Jill G. Joseph, "AIDS and Behavioral Change to Reduce Risk: A Review," *American Journal of Public Health* 78, 4 (1988), p. 407; Jonathan M. Mann, "Human Rights and AIDS," in Mann et al., eds., *Health and Human Rights* (New York, 1999), p. 218.

72. H. Sasse et al., "Pratiques homosexuelles avec partenaires stables et partenaires occasionnels chez les homo/bisexuels en Italie," in Michael Pollak et al., eds., *Homosexualités et Sida* (n.p., n.d. [1991]), p. 73; Pollak and Moatti, "HIV Risk Perception," pp. 26–27; King, *Safety in Numbers*, ch. 1; Martin Dannecker, "Homosexuelle Männer und AIDS," in Wolfgang Heckmann and Meinrad A. Koch, eds., *Sexualverhalten in Zeiten von Aids* (Berlin, 1994), pp. 273–78.

73. Le groupe ACSF, *Les comportements sexuels en France: Rapport au ministre de la Recherche et de l'Espace* (Paris, 1993), p. 212; Susan Kippax et al., *Sustaining Safe Sex: Gay Communities Respond to AIDS* (London, 1993), pp. 80, 82, 84–85.

74. Patrick S. Sullivan et al., "Changes in AIDS Incidence for Men Who Have Sex with Men, United States, 1990–1995," *AIDS* 11 (1997), p. 1644; Pam Rodden et al., "Project Male-Call: Class Differences in Sexual Practice," in Peter Aggleton et al., eds., *AIDS: Foundations for the Future* (London, 1994), pp. 65–66; Nicholas Freudenberg, "AIDS Prevention in the United States: Lessons from the First Decade," *International Journal of Health Services* 20, 4 (1990), p. 592; Heather G. Miller et al., eds., *AIDS: The Second Decade* (Washington, DC, 1990), pp. 40, 82–85; Michael Bochow, "Le safer sex: Une discussion sans fin," in Michael Pollak et al., eds., *Homosexualités et Sida* (n.p., n.d. [1991]), p. 117; Pollak, *Second Plague*, p. 63; Shamil Wanigaratne et al., "Initiating and Maintaining Safer Sex," in José Catalán et al., eds., *The Impact of AIDS: Psychological and Social Aspects of HIV Infection* (Amsterdam, 1997), pp. 27–28; Jeffrey A. Kelly, "HIV Prevention among Gay and Bisexual Men in Small Cities," in Ralph J. DiClemente and John L. Peterson, eds., *Preventing AIDS: Theories and Methods of Behavioral Interventions* (New York, 1994), pp. 299–301.

75. Ralph Bolton, "Mapping Terra Incognita: Sex Research for AIDS Prevention—an Urgent Agenda for the 1990s," in Gilbert Herdt and Shirley Lindenbaum, eds., *The Time of AIDS* (Newbury Park, 1992), pp. 132–36; Hans Bardeleben et al., *Abschied von der sexuellen Revolution: Liebe und Sexualität der "Nach-68er-Generation" in Zeiten von Aids* (Berlin, 1995), pp. 222–26; Gerhard Christiansen and Jürgen Töppich, "Umfragedaten zum Sexualverhalten," in Wolfgang Heckmann and Meinrad A. Koch, eds., *Sexualverhalten in Zeiten von Aids* (Berlin, 1994), p. 26.

76. Giuseppe Ippolito et al., "The Changing Picture of the HIV/AIDS Epidemic," *Annals of the New York Academy of Sciences* 946 (2001), pp. 8–9; Michael Bochow, "Data Deserts and Poverty of Interpretation: Notes on Deficiencies in Prevention-Oriented Research, Taking Gay Men as an Example," in Dorothee Friedrich and Wolfgang Heckmann, eds., *Aids in Europe: The Behavioural Aspect* (Berlin, 1995), 4:249, 256–57; Raschke and Ritter, *Eine Grossstadt*, pp. 95, 98–99; Dannecker, *Homosexuelle Männer*, p. 69, 89, 92–93, 103.

77. Anthony P. M. Coxon, *Between the Sheets: Sexual Diaries and Gay Men's Sex in the Era of AIDS* (London, 1996), pp. 5, 171–72; Graham Hart et al., " 'Relapse' to Unsafe Sexual Behavior among Gay Men: A Critique of Recent Behavioural HIV/AIDS Research," *Sociology of Health and Illness* 14, 2 (1992), pp. 226–27.

78. Robert B. Hays and John L. Peterson, "HIV Prevention for Gay and Bisexual Men in Metropolitan Cities," in Ralph J. DiClemente and Peterson, eds., *Preventing AIDS: Theories and Methods of Behavioral Interventions* (New York, 1994), p. 268.

79. Bernd Schünemann, "Die Rechtsprobleme der AIDS-Eindämmung," in Schünemann and Gerd Pfeiffer, eds., *Die Rechtsprobleme von AIDS* (Baden-Baden, 1988), p. 415; Willy H. Eirmbter et al., *AIDS und die gesellschaftliche Folgen* (Frankfurt, 1993), p. 52; Lenore Manderson et al., "Condom Use in Heterosexual Sex," in José Catalán et al., eds., *The Impact of AIDS: Psychological and Social Aspects of HIV Infection* (Amsterdam, 1997), p. 10.

80. Paula A. Treichler, "How to Use a Condom: Lessons from the AIDS Epidemic," in Joshua Oppenheimer and Helena Reckitt, eds., *Acting on AIDS: Sex, Drugs, and Politics* (London, 1997), pp. 53–54; Steven D. Pinkerton and Paul R. Abramson, "The Joys of Diversification: Vaccines, Condoms, and AIDS Prevention," *AIDS and Public Policy Journal* 10, 3 (1995), p. 152; *Economist*, 2 March 2002, p. 99.

81. Susan J. Palmer, "AIDS as Metaphor," *Society* 26 (1989), p. 48; Robin Gorna, *Vamps, Virgins, and Victims: How Can Women Fight AIDS?* (London, 1996), pp. 338–39, 350–51, 354, 357, 365, 369; Tessa Boffin, "Fairy Tales, 'Facts' and Gossip: Lesbians and AIDS," in Boffin and Sunil Gupta, eds., *Ecstatic Antibodies: Resisting the AIDS Mythology* (London, 1990), pp. 163–64.

82. Fee and Krieger, "Understanding AIDS," p. 1479; Nicolas Mauriac, *Le mal entendu: Le sida et les médias* (Paris, 1990), pp. 98–101.

83. Quoted in Kayal, *Bearing Witness*, p. 80. On O'Connor: Peter Lewis Allen, *The Wages of Sin: Sex and Disease, Past and Present* (Chicago, 2000), pp. 142–43. Conservative Jews took a similar position: Inon I. Schenker and Galia Sabar-Friedman, "The Jewish Religion and the HIV/AIDS Challenge," in Inon I. Schenker et al., eds., *AIDS Education: Interventions in Multi-Cultural Societies* (New York, 1996), p. 252.

84. Rotello, *Sexual Ecology*, pp. 10–13.

85. *Le Monde*, 5 July 1986, p. 12; *IDHL* 39, 2 (1988), p. 363; Pascal Vennesson, "Une gestion sans incidences politiques: L'action du service de santé des armées," in Pierre Favre, ed., *Sida et politique: Les premiers affrontements (1981–1987)* (Paris, 1992), p. 98; Lucette Khaïat, "Nouveau virus et vieux démons: Le droit face au sida, une approache comparative," in Eric Heilmann, ed., *Sida et libertés: La régulation d'une épidemie dans un état de droit* (n.p., 1991), p. 79.

86. *Le Monde*, 11 January 1989, p. 17; Virginie Linhart, "Le silence de l'église," in Pierre Favre, ed., *Sida et politique: Les premiers affrontements (1981–1987)* (Paris, 1992), pp. 132–33; Frédéric Martel, *Le rose et le noir: Les ho-*

mosexuels en France depuis 1968 (Paris, 1996), p. 289. Historical background: Martine Sevegrand, *Les enfants du bon dieu: Les catholiques français et la procréation au XXe siècle* (Paris, 1995). On U.S. Catholics: David Sadofsky, *The Question of Privacy in Public Policy* (Westport, CT, 1993), p. 89.

87. J.-F. Malherbe and S. Zorrilla, *Le citoyen, le medecin et le sida: L'exigence de vérité* (Louvain-la-Neuve, 1988), pp. 63–64.

88. Peter Gould, *The Slow Plague: A Geography of the AIDS Pandemic* (Cambridge, MA, 1993), ch. 5.

89. Paul W. Ewald, *Evolution of Infectious Diseases* (Oxford, 1994), p. 198.

90. Françoise Dubois-Arber and Brenda Spencer, "Condom Use," in Michel Hubert, ed., *Sexual Behaviour and Risks of HIV Infection* (Brussels, 1990), p. 266; B. D. Bytchenko, "A Search for Effective Strategies against AIDS: Points for Discussion," in M. A. Koch and F. Deinhardt, eds., *AIDS Diagnosis and Control: Current Situation* (Munich, 1988), p. 59; Saulius Chaplinskas, "The Impact of HIV/AIDS in Lithuania," in David FitzSimons et al., eds., *The Economic and Social Impact of AIDS in Europe* (London, 1995), p. 159; Pollak, *Second Plague*, p. 8; Klaus Schuller and Heino Stöver, "AIDS und Drogenkonsum," in Johannes Korporal and Hubert Malouschek, eds., *Leben mit AIDS—Mit AIDS leben* (Hamburg, 1987), p. 229.

91. *Le Monde*, 20 November 1986, p. 25a; Claude Got, *Rapport sur le SIDA* (Paris, 1989), pp. 109, 224.

92. Pollak, *Les homosexuels et le sida*, p. 74.

93. D. C. Jayasuriya, *AIDS: Public Health and Legal Dimensions* (Dordrecht, 1988), p. 53; Reutter, "Aids, Politik und Demokratie," p. 11; Got, *Rapport*, p. 104.

94. William H. Masters, Virginia E. Johnson, and Robert C. Kolodny, *Crisis: Heterosexual Behavior in the Age of AIDS* (New York, 1988), p. 118; Patton, *Last Served?* pp. 116–18; Diane K. Lewis, "African-American Women at Risk: Notes on the Sociocultural Context of HIV Infection," in Beth E. Schneider and Nancy E. Stoller, eds., *Women Resisting AIDS: Feminist Strategies of Empowerment* (Philadelphia, 1995), p. 64; Rafael M. Díaz, *Latino Gay Men and HIV: Culture, Sexuality, and Risk Behavior* (New York, 1998), p. 33.

95. *Le Monde*, 5 April 1995, pp. 1, 11; Dominique Hausser et al., "Effectiveness of the AIDS Prevention Campaigns in Switzerland," in Alan F. Fleming et al., *The Global Impact of AIDS* (New York, 1988), p. 225; D. Hausser et al., "Assessing AIDS Prevention in Switzerland," in F. Paccaud et al., eds., *Assessing AIDS Prevention* (Basel, 1992), pp. 117–18; Raschke and Ritter, *Eine Grossstadt*, pp. 207–8; Bundeszentrale für gesundheitliche Aufklärung, *Aids im öffentlichen Bewusstsein der Bundesrepublik 1996* (Cologne, 1997), pp. 58–59.

96. *Hansard*, vol. 106 (2 December 1986), col. 612; Malcolm Potts and Roger V. Short, "Condoms for the Prevention of HIV Transmission: Cultural Dimensions," *AIDS* 3, suppl. (1989), p. S262.

97. Jürgen Kölzsch, "HIV-/Aids-Beratungs- und Betreuungsmodell an der Charité-Hautklinik Berlin," in Doris Schaeffer et al., eds., *Aids-Krankenversorgung* (Berlin, 1992), p. 189; Zhores A. Medvedev, "Evolution of AIDS Policy

in the Soviet Union," *British Medical Journal* 300 (7 April 1990), p. 933; Juan Vicente Aliaga, "A Land of Silence: Political, Cultural, and Artistic Responses to AIDS in Spain," in Joshua Oppenheimer and Helena Reckitt, eds., *Acting on AIDS: Sex, Drugs, and Politics* (London, 1997), p. 395.

98. Heather G. Miller et al., eds., *AIDS: The Second Decade* (Washington, DC, 1990), pp. 277–78; Hamilton, "The Criminal Law," p. 36; Glasson, "Public Health and Human Rights," p. 239; Schwarz, *HIV/AIDS Education*, pp. 74–76.

99. *RD Prot*, 1986/87:110 (24 April 1987), pp. 46–47.

100. *Le Monde*, 29 November 1986, p. 11a; 21 October 1992, p. 2; *IDHL* 38, 2 (1987), p. 249; Martel, *Le rose et le noir*, p. 289; Pollak, *Les homosexuels et le sida*, p. 74; Sevegrand, *Les enfants du bon dieu*, p. 286; *Journal Officiel, Lois et Decrets*, 28 January 1987, No. 23, pp. 991–96.

101. House of Commons, *Problems Associated with AIDS*, vol. 1, p. xxxi; Denis Parisot, "Café Branché: A Metaphor against AIDS," in Dorothee Friedrich and Wolfgang Heckmann, eds., *Aids in Europe: The Behavioural Aspect* (Berlin, 1995), 3:19; Roger Staub, "The Swiss Hot Rubber Campaign: Self-Proclaimed Gays Take Responsibility for Informing their Community," in WHO, *AIDS Prevention through Health Promotion: Facing Sensitive Issues* (Geneva, 1991), p. 47.

102. *Le Monde*, 3 December 1986, p. 36; House Committee on Government Operations, *The Politics of AIDS Prevention*, pp. 11–12.

103. *AIDS-Forschung* 10, 10 (October 1995), p. 512; John Bongaarts et al., "The Relationship between Male Circumcision and HIV Infection in African Populations," *AIDS* 3 (1989), p. 373; Marc Urassa et al., "Male Circumcision and Susceptibility to HIV Infection among Men in Tanzania," *AIDS* 11 (1997), p. 73; World Bank, *Confronting AIDS: Public Priorities in a Global Epidemic* (Oxford, 1997), pp. 64–65; Janneke H. H. M. Van de Wijgert and Nancy S. Padian, "Heterosexual Transmission of HIV," in Lorraine Sherr, ed., *AIDS and the Heterosexual Population* (Chur, 1993), p. 10; *Los Angeles Times*, 11 July 2000, p. A18; *New Scientist* 167, 2246 (8 July 2000), pp. 18–19.

104. Maurice Tournier et al., *SIDA'venture: SIDA, Ethique, Discriminations* (Paris, 1989), pp. 10–11.

105. Michael Smithurst, "AIDS: Risks and Discrimination," in Brenda Almond, ed., *AIDS: A Moral Issue* (London, 1990), p. 100; Baldwin, *Contagion and the State*, p. 409; Nancy Tomes, *The Gospel of Germs: Men, Women, and the Microbe in American Life* (Cambridge, MA, 1998), pp. 132–34; Bernard Paillard, *Notes on the Plague Years: AIDS in Marseilles* (New York, 1998), p. 213.

106. Georges Vigarello, *Le sain et le malsain* (Paris, 1993), p. 292.

107. *RD Prot*, 1986/87, Bihang, Socialutskottets betänkande 19, p. 25; Rhodes, "Risk, Injecting Drug Use," pp. 67–68; Mark Blumberg, *AIDS: The Impact on the Criminal Justice System* (Columbus, 1990), p. 152; William B. Johnston and Kevin R. Hopkins, *The Catastrophe Ahead: AIDS and the Case for a New Public Policy* (New York, 1990), pp. 94–95; Neil McKeganey, "Le contexte social du comportement à risques des utilisateurs de seringues," in Nathalie

Bajos et al., *Le sida en Europe: Nouveaux enjeux pour les sciences sociales* (Paris, 1998), pp. 82–83.

108. M. Daniel Fernando, *AIDS and Intravenous Drug Use* (Westport, CT, 1993), p. 60; Robert Heimer et al., "Three Years of Needle Exchange in New Haven: What Have We Learned?" *AIDS and Public Policy Journal* 9, 2 (1993), p. 59; Elaine O'Keefe, "Altering Public Policy on Needle Exchange: The Connecticut Experience," *AIDS and Public Policy Journal* 6, 4 (1991), p. 160.

109. Jonathan Mann et al., "Toward a New Health Strategy to Control the HIV/AIDS Pandemic," *Journal of Law, Medicine, and Ethics* 22, 1 (1994), p. 43; Fox, Day, and Klein, "Power of Professionalism," p. 98; Institute of Medicine, *Confronting AIDS*, p. 105; *Report of the Presidential Commission*, p. 94; *Public Health Reports*, 103, suppl. 1 (1988), pp. 7–8; *RD Prot*, 1986/87, Bihang, Socialutskottets betänkande 19, p. 25; 1987/88, Bihang, Prop. 79, p. 16; *Hansard*, vol. 107 (18 December 1986), col. 701; vol. 144 (13 January 1989), col. 1102, 1115, 1125, 1151; June Crawford et al., "Not Gay, Not Bisexual, but Polymorphously Sexually Active: Male Bisexuality and AIDS in Australia," in Peter Aggleton, ed., *Bisexualities and AIDS: International Perspectives* (London, 1996), p. 57; Michael Bartos, "Community vs. Population: The Case of Men Who Have Sex with Men," in Peter Aggleton et al., eds., *AIDS: Foundations for the Future* (London, 1994), p. 94; Jan Zita Grover, "AIDS: Keywords," in Douglas Crimp, ed., *AIDS: Cultural Analysis, Cultural Activism* (Cambridge, 1988), p. 21; Masters, Johnson, and Kolodny, *Crisis*, p. 4.

110. Phillip Brian Harper, "Eloquence and Epitaph: Black Nationalism and the Homophobic Impulse in Responses to the Death of Max Robinson," in Timothy F. Murphy and Suzanne Poirier, eds., *Writing AIDS: Gay Literature, Language, and Analysis* (New York, 1993), p. 132; Lewis, "African-American Women at Risk," p. 65; Cathy Jean Cohen, "Power, Resistance, and the Construction of Crisis: Marginalized Communities Respond to AIDS" (Ph.D. diss., University of Michigan, 1993), p. 335.

111. Don C. Des Jarlais and Samuel R. Friedman, "HIV Infection among Intravenous Drug Users: Epidemiology and Risk Reduction," *AIDS* 1 (1987), p. 67.

112. Becker and Joseph, "AIDS and Behavioral Change to Reduce Risk: A Review," p. 407.

113. Stimson and Donoghoe, "Health Promotion," pp. 10, 14; Andy D. Peters et al., "Edinburgh Drug Users: Are They Injecting and Sharing Less?" *AIDS* 8 (1994), p. 527; Rushing, *AIDS Epidemic*, pp. 101–2; Don C. Des Jarlais and Samuel R. Friedman, "The Epidemic of HIV Infection among Injecting Drug Users in New York City," in John Strang and Gerry V. Stimson, eds., *AIDS and Drug Misuse: The Challenge for Policy and Practice in the 1990s* (London, 1990), p. 90.

114. Kyung-Hee Choi and Laurie A. Wermuth, "Unsafe Sex and Behavior Change," in James L. Sorensen et al., eds., *Preventing AIDS in Drug Users and their Sexual Partners* (New York, 1991), pp. 54–56; Neil McKeganey et al., "The Social Context of Injectors' Risk Behaviour," in Gerry V. Stimson et al., eds.,

Drug Injecting and HIV Infection: Global Dimensions and Local Responses (London, 1998), p. 22.

115. Stimson and Donoghoe, "Health Promotion," pp. 17–18; Raschke and Ritter, *Eine Grossstadt*, p. 76.

116. Des Jarlais and Friedman, "HIV Infection among Intravenous Drug Users," p. 69; John K. Watters, "Americans and Syringe Exchange: Roots of Resistance," in Tim Rhodes and Richard Hartnoll, eds., *AIDS, Drugs, and Prevention* (London, 1996), p. 23; Garfield, *End of Innocence*, p. 99; Enrico Tempesta and Massimo di Giannantonio, "The Italian Epidemic: A Case Study," in John Strang and Gerry V. Stimson, eds., *AIDS and Drug Misuse: The Challenge for Policy and Practice in the 1990s* (London, 1990), p. 112.

117. *Congressional Record* (Senate), 16 May 1990, p. 6289; *RD Prot*, 1986/87, Bihang, Socialutskottets betänkande 19, p. 25.

118. House of Commons, *Problems Associated with AIDS*, vol. 3, pp. 180–81; Samuel Walker, *The Rights Revolution: Rights and Community in Modern America* (New York, 1998), pp. 149–50.

119. John Street and Albert Weale, "Britain: Policy-Making in a Hermetically Sealed System," in David L. Kirp and Ronald Bayer, eds., *AIDS in the Industrialized Democracies* (New Brunswick, 1992), p. 208.

120. Richard Hartnoll and Dagmar Hedrich, "AIDS Prevention and Drug Policy," in Tim Rhodes and Hartnoll, eds., *AIDS, Drugs, and Prevention* (London, 1996), p. 47; Guenter Frankenberg, "Germany: The Uneasy Triumph of Pragmatism," David L. Kirp and Ronald Bayer, eds., *AIDS in the Industrialized Democracies* (New Brunswick, 1992), p. 119; H.-J. Albrecht, "Drug Policy in the Federal Republic of Germany," in Albrecht and Anton van Kalmthout, eds., *Drug Policies in Western Europe* (Freiburg, 1989), p. 183; Raschke and Ritter, *Eine Grossstadt*, p. 142; Ingo Ilja Michels, " 'Harm Reduction' and the Political Concept of the 'War on Drugs' in Germany," in AIDS-Forum D.A.H., *Aspects of AIDS and AIDS-Hilfe in Germany* (Berlin, 1993), pp. 51–53; BT *Drucksache* 11/2495, 16 June 1988, pp. 12, 106–7.

121. "Entschliessung der Konferenz der für das Gesundheitswesen zuständigen Minister und Senatoren der Länder (GMK) vom 27. 3. 1987," in Günter Frankenberg, *AIDS-Bekämpfung im Rechtsstaat* (Baden-Baden, 1988), p. 177; Bundesrat, *Drucksache*, 396/87, 22 September 1987.

122. Klaus Geppert, "AIDS und Strafvollzug," in Andrzej J. Szwarc, ed., *AIDS und Strafrecht* (Berlin, 1996), p. 253; BT Drucksache 11/6551, 1 March 1990; Karl-Heinz Reuband, *Drogenkonsum und Drogenpolitik: Deutschland und die Niederlande im Vergleich* (Opladen, 1992), pp. 83–84; *Bundesgesetzblatt*, 1992, 1:1593, §29.

123. Mildred Blaxter, *AIDS: Worldwide Policies and Problems* (London, 1991), p. 23; Martin C. Donoghoe et al., *Syringe-Exchange in England* (London, 1992); Street and Weale, "Britain," pp. 207–9; Fox, Day, and Klein, "Power of Professionalism," p. 98; *Hansard*, vol. 93 (6 March 1986), col. 564; vol. 144 (13 January 1989), col. 1107; vol. 107 (18 December 1986), col. 701.

124. Rachel Anne Lart, "HIV and English Drugs Policy" (Ph.D., University of London, 1996), ch. 3; Richard Davenport-Hines, *The Pursuit of Oblivion: A Global History of Narcotics, 1500–2000* (London, 2001), p. 381.

125. Garfield, *End of Innocence*, pp. 97–99, 102; Berridge, *AIDS in the UK*, p. 287; Chris Bennett and Ewan Ferlie, *Managing Crisis and Change in Health Care: The Organizational Response to HIV/AIDS* (Buckingham, 1994), p. 24; Street, "British Government Policy on AIDS," p. 497; Alison M. Richardson and Philip A. Gaskell, "HIV Infection and AIDS in Lothian," in Maryan Pye et al., eds., *Responding to the AIDS Challenge: A Comparative Study of Local AIDS Programmes in the United Kingdom* (Harlow, 1989), p. 83.

126. *Le Monde*, 29 November 1986, p. 11a; Geneviève Pinet, "AIDS, Legislative Measures, and Ethical Issues," in M. A. Koch and F. Deinhardt, eds., *AIDS Diagnosis and Control: Current Situation* (Munich, 1988), pp. 49–50; Monika Steffen, "France: Social Solidarity and Scientific Expertise," in David L. Kirp and Ronald Bayer, eds., *AIDS in the Industrialized Democracies* (New Brunswick, 1992), pp. 236–37; WHO, *Legislative Responses*, p. 75.

127. *Le Monde*, 22 October 1994; Steffen, *Fight against AIDS*, p. 109; Jacques Foyer and Lucette Khaïat "Droit et SIDA: La situation française," in Foyer and Khaïat, *Droit et Sida: Comparaison internationale* (Paris, 1994), p. 222; Monika Steffen, "Les modèles nationaux d'adaptation aux défis d'une épidémie," *Revue française de sociologie* 41, 1 (2000), p. 19; Ph. Duneton, "Toxicomanie, quelle réponse sanitaire à l'heure du S.I.D.A.?" in Jean-Marie Guffens, ed., *Toxicomanie, Hépatites, S.I.D.A.* (n.p., 1994), p. 121.

128. Claude Évin and Bruno Durieux, *La lutte contre le sida en France* (Paris, 1992), p. 48; Steffen, *Fight against AIDS*, p. 103; Magguy Coulouarn, "The French Experience," in Wolfgang Heckmann and Sabine Reiter, eds., *Community-Oriented Prevention of AIDS and Addiction* (Berlin, 1991; AIDS-Zentrum Hefte 6/1991), p. 102; France Lert, "Drug Use, AIDS, and Social Exclusion in France," in Jean-Paul Moatti et al., eds., *AIDS in Europe: New Challenges for the Social Sciences* (London, 2000), p. 195.

129. *RD Prot*, 1985/86:33 (21 November 1985), p. 20; 1986/87, Bihang, Socialutskottets betänkande 19, p. 25; 1988/89:105 (27 April 1989), p. 20, 30; 1985/86, Bihang, Socialutskottets betänkande 15, pp. 20–21; 1986/87, Bihang, Socialutskottets betänkande 19, pp. 2, 23, 25; 1987/88, Bihang, Prop. 79, pp. 38–39; 1988/89, Bihang, Socialutskottets betänkande 21, pp. 1, 5, 7, 11–12, 44–45; 1988/89:105 (27 April 1989), pp. 7–8, 11.

130. *RD Prot*, 1985/86:33 (21 November 1985), p. 10; Michael G. Koch, *AIDS: Vom Molekül zur Pandemie* (Heidelberg, 1987), p. 153; Gerry V. Stimson et al., "Distributing Sterile Needles and Syringes to People Who Inject Drugs: The Syringe-Exchange Experiment," in John Strang and Stimson, eds., *AIDS and Drug Misuse: The Challenge for Policy and Practice in the 1990s* (London, 1990), p. 222.

131. Fox, Day, and Klein, "Power of Professionalism," p. 103; Henriksson and Ytterberg, "Sweden," p. 327.

132. *RD Prot*, 1986/87, Bihang, Socialutskottets betänkande 19, p. 24.

133. *RD Prot*, 1986/87:110 (24 April 1987), pp. 39–40, 47; 1986/87:109 (23 April 1987), p. 140.

134. Annika Snare, "The Legal Treatment of AIDS in Denmark," in Martin Breum and Aart Hendriks, eds., *AIDS and Human Rights* (Copenhagen, 1988), p. 39; J. Jepsen, "Drug Policies in Denmark," in Hans-Jörg Albrecht and Anton van Kalmthout, eds., *Drug Policies in Western Europe* (Freiburg, 1989), pp. 107–8; Birgit Westphal Christensen et al., *AIDS: Prævention og kontrol i Norden* (Stockholm, 1988), p. 203.

135. A. M. van Kalmthout, "Characteristics of Drug Policy in the Netherlands," in Hans-Jörg Albrecht and van Kalmthout, eds., *Drug Policies in Western Europe* (Freiburg, 1989), pp. 261–71; Jan K. van Wijngaarden, "The Netherlands: AIDS in a Consensual Society," in David L. Kirp and Ronald Bayer, eds., *AIDS in the Industrialized Democracies* (New Brunswick, 1992), pp. 261–65; Erik van Ameijden and Anneke van den Hoek, "AIDS among Injecting Drug Users in the Netherlands," in Theo Sandfort, ed., *The Dutch Response to HIV: Pragmatism and Consensus* (London, 1998).

136. *New York Times*, 6 May 2000, p. B2; Bytchenko, "A Search for Effective Strategies," p. 58; Rubenstein et al., *Rights of People*, pp. 338–39; Chris B. Pascal, "Selected Issues in AIDS and Drug Abuse: Prevention, Treatment, and Criminal Justice," in Lawrence Gostin and Lane Porter, eds., *International Law and AIDS* (n.p., 1992), pp. 231–34.

137. Stein, *Social Welfare of Women and Children*, p. 135; Stimson and Donoghoe, "Health Promotion," p. 13; Heather G. Miller et al., eds., *AIDS: The Second Decade* (Washington, DC, 1990), pp. 124–26; Scott Burris, "Education to Reduce the Spread of HIV," in Burris et al., eds., *AIDS Law Today* (New Haven, 1993), pp. 103–5.

138. Elaine O'Keefe, "Altering Public Policy on Needle Exchange: The Connecticut Experience," *AIDS and Public Policy Journal* 6, 4 (1991); Watters, "Americans and Syringe Exchange," pp. 29, 34–35; *IDHL* 41, 4 (1990), pp. 607–9; 42, 2 (1991), pp. 245–54; *Congressional Record* (Senate), 16 May 1990, pp. 6290–91; Tim Rhodes and Richard Hartnoll, "Reaching the Hard to Reach: Models of HIV Outreach Health Education," in Peter Aggleton et al., eds., *AIDS: Responses, Interventions, and Care* (London, 1991), p. 238; Gerald M. Oppenheimer, "To Build a Bridge: The Use of Foreign Models by Domestic Critics of U.S. Drug Policy," in Ronald Bayer and Gerald M. Oppenheimer, eds., *Confronting Drug Policy: Illicit Drugs in a Free Society* (Cambridge, 1993), pp. 215–20.

139. Fee and Krieger, "Understanding AIDS," p. 1479; Institute of Medicine, *Confronting AIDS: Update 1988*, p. 86; Warwick Anderson, "The New York Needle Trial: The Politics of Public Health in the Age of AIDS," in Virginia Berridge and Philip Strong, eds., *AIDS and Contemporary History* (Cambridge, 1993), pp. 157–58, 164–69; Cohen, "Power, Resistance, and the Construction of Crisis," ch. 6; Fernando, *AIDS and Intravenous Drug Use*, p. 138; Watters, "Americans and Syringe Exchange," pp. 30–32; Elinor Burkett, *The Gravest*

Show on Earth: America in the Age of AIDS (Boston, 1995), pp. 183–85; Mark Smith, "AIDS and Minority Health," in Caroline Hannaway et al., eds., *AIDS and the Public Debate* (Amsterdam, 1995), p. 104.

140. Garfield, *End of Innocence*, p. 96; Fernando, *AIDS and Intravenous Drug Use*, p. 43; Stimson and Donoghoe, "Health Promotion," p. 14; Blumberg, *AIDS*, p. 170; *Hansard*, vol. 93 (6 March 1986), col. 564; Memo from the Home Office, House of Commons, *Problems Associated with AIDS*, vol. 3, p. 79; Hamilton, "The Criminal Law," p. 36; BT *Drucksache 11/2495*, 16 June 1988, pp. 106–7.

141. Richard Hartnoll, "The International Context," in Susanne MacGregor, ed., *Drugs and British Society: Responses to a Social Problem in the Eighties* (London, 1989), pp. 36–42.

142. Sebastian Scheerer, *Die Genese der Betäubungsmittelgesetze in der Bundesrepublik Deutschland und in den Niederlanden* (Göttingen, 1982), p. 70; Hartnoll and Hedrich, "AIDS Prevention," p. 44; Hans-Jörg Albrecht, "Les politiques de la drogue en Allemagne," in Alain Ehrenberg, ed., *Vivre avec les drogues: Régulations, politiques, marchés, usages* (Paris, 1996), p. 47; BT *Drucksache 11/6163*, 22 December 1989; BT *Verhandlungen 11/216*, 20 June 1990, pp. 17099C ff.

143. Massimo Campedelli, "Entre répression, indifférence et réduction des risques," in Alain Ehrenberg, ed., *Vivre avec les drogues: Régulations, politiques, marchés, usages* (Paris, 1996), p. 73; A. Manna and E. Barone Ricciardelli, "The Limitations and Formalities of Criminal Law Provisions Concerning Narcotics: Considerations on Legislation in Italy," in Hans-Jörg Albrecht and Anton van Kalmthout, eds., *Drug Policies in Western Europe* (Freiburg, 1989), pp. 195–98; Adolf Ceretti and Isabella Merzagora, "AIDS in Prisons in Italy," in Philip A. Thomas and Martin Moerings, eds., *AIDS in Prison* (Aldershot, U.K., 1994), p. 85.

144. *RD Prot*, 1987/88, Bihang, Prop. 79, pp. 17–18; A. Solarz, "Drug Policy in Sweden," in Hans-Jörg Albrecht and Anton van Kalmthout, eds., *Drug Policies in Western Europe* (Freiburg, 1989), pp. 346–48; Jepsen, "Drug Policies," pp. 107–8, 114; Albrecht, "Drug Policy," pp. 176–77; Ragnar Hauge, "Drug Control Policies," in Ole-Jørgen Skog and Ragnar Waahlberg, eds., *Alcohol and Drugs: The Norwegian Experience* (Oslo, 1988), p. 157; Richard Hartnoll, *Multi-City Study: Drug Misuse Trends in Thirteen European Cities* (Strasbourg, 1994), p. 32; Börje Olsson, ed., *Narkotikasituationen i Norden: Utvecklingen 1987–1991* (Copenhagen, 1993), pp. 85, 122.

145. Morelle, *La défaite de la santé publique*, pp. 145, 149; Alain Ehrenberg, "Comment vivre avec les drogues?" in Ehrenberg, ed., *Vivre avec les drogues: Régulations, politiques, marchés, usages* (Paris, 1996), p. 6; J. Bernat de Celis, "France's Policy Concerning Illegal Drug Users," in Hans-Jörg Albrecht and Anton van Kalmthout, eds., *Drug Policies in Western Europe* (Freiburg, 1989), pp. 143–45; Robert Power, "Drug-Using Trends and HIV Risk Behaviour," in John Strang and Gerry V. Stimson, eds., *AIDS and Drug Misuse: The Challenge for Policy and Practice in the 1990s* (London, 1990), p. 71.

146. Virginia Berridge, *Opium and the People: Opiate Use and Drug Con-

trol Policy in Nineteenth and Early Twentieth Century England, rev. ed. (London, 1999), pp. 279–80, 286; Virginia Berridge, "Historical Issues," in Susanne MacGregor, ed., Drugs and British Society: Responses to a Social Problem in the Eighties (London, 1989), pp. 29–30; Govert Frank van de Wijngaart, Competing Perspectives on Drug Use: The Dutch Experience (Amsterdam, 1991), pp. 123–25; van Kalmthout, "Characteristics of Drug Policy," pp. 261–71; van Wijngaarden, "The Netherlands," pp. 261–65; van Ameijden and van den Hoek, "AIDS among Injecting Drug Users."

147. A. Rutherford and P. Green, "Illegal Drugs and British Criminal Justice Policy," in Hans-Jörg Albrecht and Anton van Kalmthout, eds., Drug Policies in Western Europe (Freiburg, 1989), pp. 384–85; James B. Bakalar and Lester Grinspoon, Drug Control in a Free Society (Cambridge, 1984), p. 94; Gerry V. Stimson and Edna Oppenheimer, Heroin Addiction: Treatment and Control in Britain (London, 1982), pp. 60–61; Virginia Berridge, "AIDS and British Drug Policy: Continuity or Change?" in Berridge and Philip Strong, eds., AIDS and Contemporary History (Cambridge, 1993), p. 136; Ehrenberg, "Comment vivre avec les drogues?" p. 16.

148. Virginia Berridge, "AIDS, Drugs, and History," British Journal of Addiction 87, 3 (1992), p. 367; Virginia Berridge, "AIDS and British Drug Policy: History Repeats Itself . . . ?" in David K. Whynes and Philip T. Bean, eds., Policing and Prescribing: The British System of Drug Control (Houndmills, U.K., 1991), pp. 176, 180–88; Gerry Stimson et al., "The Future of Syringe Exchange in the Public Health Prevention of HIV Infection," in Peter Aggleton et al., eds., AIDS: Responses, Interventions, and Care (London, 1991), pp. 225, 230; Rutherford and Green, "Illegal Drugs," pp. 383–84; Stimson and Lart, "HIV, Drugs, and Public Health in England," pp. 1264–65; Susanne MacGregor, "Choices for Policy and Practice," in MacGregor, ed., Drugs and British Society: Responses to a Social Problem in the Eighties (London, 1989), p. 194; Robert Power et al., "Drug Prevention and HIV Policy," AIDS 4, suppl. 1 (1990), p. S264.

149. David F. Musto, The American Disease: Origins of Narcotic Control, exp. ed. (New York, 1987), chs. 5, 10; Watters, "Americans and Syringe Exchange," pp. 27–28; Robert Power et al., "Drug Prevention and HIV Policy," AIDS 4, suppl. 1 (1990), p. S263; Fernando, AIDS and Intravenous Drug Use, p. 75.

150. Ehrenberg, "Comment vivre avec les drogues?" pp. 7–8; Lert, "Drug Use, AIDS, and Social Exclusion in France," pp. 190–91; Morelle, La défaite de la santé publique, pp. 151–53.

151. Raschke and Ritter, Eine Grossstadt, p. 134; Steffen, Fight against AIDS, p. 99; RD Prot, 1988/89:105 (27 April 1989), pp. 16, 19, 35.

152. RD Prot, 1986/87:110 (24 April 1987), p. 47; Berridge, "AIDS and British Drug Policy: History Repeats Itself . . . ?" p. 176; Berridge, "AIDS, Drugs, and History," p. 367; Stimson and Lart, "HIV, Drugs, and Public Health in England," p. 1265.

153. Steffen, Fight against AIDS, p. 129; Jeff Stryker, "IV Drug Use and AIDS: Public Policy and Dirty Needles," Journal of Health Politics, Policy, and Law 14, 4 (1989), p. 732.

154. Morelle, *La défaite de la santé publique*, pp. 145–51; Coulouarn, "The French Experience," p. 102.

155. Annie Serfaty, "L'infection par le VIH liée à l'usage de drogues en France," *Sida, toxicomanie: Une lecture documentaire* (November 1993), p. 73; Anne Coppel, "Peut-on soigner les toxicomanes? Les enseignements de l'histoire," in Jean-Marie Guffens, ed., *Toxicomanie, Hépatites, S.I.D.A.* (n.p., 1994), pp. 44–45; *Sida et toxicomanie: Répondre: Actes du colloque international organisé par FIRST* (Paris, 1989), p. 20; Steffen, "France: Social Solidarity," p. 221; Jean de Savigny, *Le Sida et les fragilités françaises: Nos réactions face à l'épidémie* (Paris, 1995), pp. 80–86, 94–97.

156. *Sida et toxicomanie: Répondre*, pp. 179–80; Duneton, "Toxicomanie," p. 122; Davenport-Hines, *Pursuit of Oblivion*, p. 292; *Le Monde*, 23 September 1993, p. 13.

157. De Celis, "France's Policy," pp. 153–54; Anne Coppel, "Les intervenants en toxicomanie, le sida et la réduction des risques en France," in Alain Ehrenberg, ed., *Vivre avec les drogues: Régulations, politiques, marchés, usages* (Paris, 1996), pp. 75–77, 100–101.

158. *Le Monde*, 23 September 1993, p. 13.

159. *Journal Officiel, Débats*, Assemblée Nationale, 31 May 1994, p. 2407; Lert, "Drug Use, AIDS, and Social Exclusion in France," p. 195; François-Régis Cerruti, *Medilex: Guide juridique médical* (Levallois-Perret, 1996), pp. 231–32.

160. Coppel, "Les intervenants en toxicomanie," pp. 77, 91–92.

161. Steffen, *Fight against AIDS*, pp. 106–8.

162. F. M. Böcker, "HIV and Methadone Treatment: The German Experience," in N. Loimer et al., eds., *Drug Addiction and AIDS* (Vienna, 1991), p. 216; Hartnoll and Hedrich, "AIDS Prevention," p. 52; Canaris, "Gesundheitspolitische Aspekte," pp. 284–85; BT *Drucksache* 11/2495, 16 June 1988, pp. 104–5.

163. Carmen Stürzel, "Aids und Obdachlosigkeit: New York und Berlin—ein Metropolenvergleich," Wissenschaftszentrum Berlin für Sozialforschung, *Veröffentlichungsreihe der Forschungsgruppe Gesundheitsrisiken und Präventionspolitik*, P94–203 (Berlin, May 1994), p. 13; Norbert Kathke and Stefan Schweitzer, "Ersatzdrogenvergabe in München: Ein Erfahrungsbericht der Städtischen Gesundheitsbehörde," *AIDS-Forschung* 10 (1992), p. 524.

164. BT *Drucksache* 11/2495, 16 June 1988, pp. 14, 101–8; BT *Verhandlungen* 11/103, 27 October 1988, p. 7054B; Geppert, "AIDS und Strafvollzug," pp. 258–59; "Zu den rechtspolitischen Konsequenzen der Methadon-Entscheidung des BGH," *AIDS-Forschung* 7 (1992), p. 345.

165. BT *Drucksache* 11/608, No. 106–07, 10 July 1987; Albrecht, "Drug Policy," p. 187; S. Scheerer, "Killing the Ill? Heroin and AIDS in West Germany," in Hans-Jörg Albrecht and Anton van Kalmthout, eds., *Drug Policies in Western Europe* (Freiburg, 1989), pp. 170–71; Raschke and Ritter, *Eine Grossstadt*, p. 135; BT *Drucksache* 10/5307, 11 April 1986, p. 3; 11/5856, 16 July 1986, p. 24; 11/2495, 16 June 1988, pp. 103–4.

166. Wolfgang Heckmann, "Die Reorganisation der Drogenhilfe angesichts

der Aids-Krise," in Doris Schaeffer et al., eds., *Aids-Krankenversorgung* (Berlin, 1992), pp. 67–68; Raschke and Ritter, *Eine Grossstadt*, p. 135.

167. *RD Prot*, 1987/88, Bihang, Prop. 79, pp. 39–40; 1987/88, Bihang, Socialutskottets betänkande 10, p. 21; 1988/89, Bihang, Socialutskottets betänkande 21, pp. 34–35; Christensen et al., *AIDS*, pp. 204–5; *RD Prot*, 1985/86, Bihang, Socialutskottets betänkande 15, pp. 20–21; Solarz, "Drug Policy in Sweden," p. 349.

168. *RD Prot*, 1987/88, Bihang, Prop. 79, pp. 16, 38; 1988/89:105 (27 April 1989), pp. 23, 25; 1986/87, Bihang, Prop. 2, p. 26.

169. *SFS* 1981:1243; *RD Prot*, 1986/87:109 (23 April 1987), pp. 143–44; 1986/87:110 (24 April 1987), p. 43; 1985/86, Bihang, Prop. 171, pp. 12, 17; 1985/86:33 (21 November 1985), p. 17; 1985/86:157 (30 May 1986), p. 11.

170. *RD Prot*, 1986/87, Bihang, Prop. 2, pp. 26–28; *SFS* 1988:870; 1987/88, Bihang, Prop. 147, pp. 1–3.

171. *RD Prot*, 1987/88, Bihang, Socialutskottets betänkande 25, pp. 5–6; 1987/88:136 (8 June 1988), pp. 10–12, 19, 32.

172. BT *Verhandlungen* 12/12, 28 February 1991, p. 584C; Albrecht, "Les politiques de la drogue," p. 60; Berridge, "AIDS and British Drug Policy: History Repeats Itself . . . ?" p. 190.

173. Watters, "Americans and Syringe Exchange," pp. 24–26; N. Christie, "Reflections on Drugs," in Hans-Jörg Albrecht and Anton van Kalmthout, eds., *Drug Policies in Western Europe* (Freiburg, 1989), p. 43.

174. Berridge, "AIDS, Drugs, and History," p. 366.

175. Patricia van der Smissen and Jean-Marc Picard, "Dépénaliser la consommation et le commerce des stupéfiants? L'opinion de juristes," in Michel Vincineau, ed., *Le Sida: Un défi aux droits* (Brussels, 1991), p. 178; *Public Health Reports*, 103, suppl. 1 (1988), pp. 66–67; *Report of the Presidential Commission*, p. 95; Gerry V. Stimson, "Revising Policy and Practice: New Ideas about the Drugs Problem," in John Strang and Stimson, eds., *AIDS and Drug Misuse: The Challenge for Policy and Practice in the 1990s* (London, 1990), p. 126; Lewis, "African-American Women at Risk," pp. 61–62.

176. Fernando, *AIDS and Intravenous Drug Use*, p. 120.

7. THE POLYMORPHOUS POLITICS OF PREVENTION

1. *Hansard Parliamentary Debates*, vol. 229 (22 July 1993), col. 617; Chris Bennett and Ewan Ferlie, *Managing Crisis and Change in Health Care: The Organizational Response to HIV/AIDS* (Buckingham, 1994), pp. 25–29; Patricia Day and Rudolf Klein, "Interpreting the Unexpected: The Case of AIDS Policy Making in Britain," *Journal of Public Policy* 9, 3 (1989), pp. 348–49.

2. Jonathan Glasson, "Public Health and Human Rights: Finding a Balance in HIV Prevention," in David FitzSimons et al., eds., *The Economic and Social Impact of AIDS in Europe* (London, 1995), p. 235; David Goss and Derek Adam-Smith, *Organizing AIDS: Workplace and Organizational Responses to the HIV/AIDS Epidemic* (London, 1995), p. 150; Richard Haigh and Dai Harris,

eds., *AIDS: A Guide to the Law*, 2d ed. (London, 1995), p. 3; Geneviève Pinet, "AIDS, Legislative Measures, and Ethical Issues," in M. A. Koch and F. Deinhardt, eds., *AIDS Diagnosis and Control: Current Situation* (Munich, 1988), p. 49; John Street and Albert Weale, "Britain: Policy-Making in a Hermetically Sealed System," in David L. Kirp and Ronald Bayer, eds., *AIDS in the Industrialized Democracies* (New Brunswick, 1992), pp. 191–92; Marlene C. McGuirl and Robert N. Gee, "AIDS: An Overview of the British, Australian, and American Responses," *Hofstra Law Review* 14, 107 (1985), pp. 110, 113.

3. Virginia Berridge, *AIDS in the UK: The Making of Policy, 1981–1994* (Oxford, 1996), pp. 245–49; Michel Setbon, *Pouvoirs contre SIDA: De la transfusion sanguine au dépistage: Decisions et pratiques en France, Grande-Bretagne et Suède* (Paris, 1993), p. 385; Daniel M. Fox, Patricia Day, and Rudolf Klein, "The Power of Professionalism: Policies for AIDS in Britain, Sweden, and the United States," *Dædalus* 118, 2 (spring 1989), p. 98.

4. Lesley A. Hall, " 'The Cinderella of Medicine': Sexually-Transmitted Diseases in Britain in the Nineteenth and Twentieth Centuries," *Genitourinary Medicine* 69 (1993), p. 318.

5. *RD Prot*, 1986/87, Bihang, Prop. 149, p. 8; 1988/89:105 (27 April 1989), pp. 13–14, 24–25.

6. *RD Prot*, 1988/89, Bihang, Prop. 5, p. 26.

7. Werner Reutter, "Aids, Politik und Demokratie: Ein Vergleich aidspolitischer Massnahmen in Deutschland und Frankreich," Wissenschaftszentrum Berlin für Sozialforschung, *Veröffentlichungsreihe der Forschungsgruppe Gesundheitsrisiken und Präventionspolitik*, P92–205 (Berlin, April 1992), p. 11; Setbon, *Pouvoirs contre SIDA*, pp. 384–85; René Bernex, *SIDA: Nous sommes tous concernés* (Paris, 1985), pp. 149–50; Gérard Bach-Ignasse, "Le Sida et la vie politique française," in Michael Pollak et al., eds., *Homosexualités et Sida* (n.p., n.d. [1991]), pp. 97–98.

8. Monika Steffen, "AIDS Policies in France," in Virginia Berridge and Philip Strong, eds., *AIDS and Contemporary History* (Cambridge, 1993), p. 243; Monika Steffen, *The Fight against AIDS: An International Public Policy Comparison between Four European Countries: France, Great Britain, Germany, and Italy* (Grenoble, 1996), p. 12; Matthew Ramsey, "Public Health in France," in Dorothy Porter, ed., *The History of Public Health and the Modern State* (Amsterdam, 1994), pp. 92–93.

9. *Report of the Presidential Commission on the Human Immunodeficiency Virus Epidemic* (Washington, DC, 1988).

10. *IDHL* 38, 3 (1987), pp. 504–7.

11. Scott Burris and Lawrence O. Gostin, "The Impact of HIV/AIDS on the Development of Public Health Law," in Ronald O. Valdiserri, ed., *Dawning Answers: How the HIV/AIDS Epidemic Has Helped to Strengthen Public Health* (Oxford, 2003), p. 100.

12. Setbon, *Pouvoirs contre SIDA*, pp. 172–73.

13. Bernd Schünemann, "Die Rechtsprobleme der AIDS-Eindämmung," in Schünemann and Gerd Pfeiffer, eds., *Die Rechtsprobleme von AIDS* (Baden-

Baden, 1988), p. 417; Michael G. Koch, "Stellungnahme zur AIDS-Problematik: Antworten auf Fragen der Presse," *AIDS-Forschung* 3, 10 (October 1988), p. 543; Klaus Scherf, *AIDS und Strafrecht* (Baden-Baden, 1992), pp. 148–49; Smittskyddskommittén, *Om smittskydd,* SOU 1985:37, pp. 106, 155; *RD Prot,* 1985/86, Bihang, Prop. 13, p. 16; "Socialminister Gertrud Sigurdsens inledningsanförande," in Benny Henriksson, ed., *Aids: Föreställningar om en verklighet* (Stockholm, 1987), p. 107.

14. Gunnar Broberg and Mattias Tydén, *Oönskade i folkhemmet: Rashygien och sterilisering i Sverige* (Stockholm, 1991); Maija Runcis, *Steriliseringar i folkhemmet* (Stockholm, 1998); Maciej Zaremba, *De rena och de andra: Om tvångssteriliseringar, rashygien och arvsynd* (n.p., 1999); Gunnar Broberg and Nils Roll-Hansen, eds., *Eugenics and the Welfare State* (East Lansing, MI, 1996); Stefan Kuhl, *The Nazi Connection: Eugenics, American Racism, and German National Socialism* (Oxford, 1994).

15. Michael F. Marmor, "The Ophthalmic Trials of G. H. A. Hansen," *Survey of Ophthalmology* 47, 3 (2002), pp. 282–84.

16. Wendy E. Parmet, "Legal Rights and Communicable Disease: AIDS, the Police Power, and Individual Liberty," *Journal of Health Politics, Policy, and Law* 14, 4 (1989), pp. 746–48.

17. Tonny Dina Maria Zeegers Paget, *AIDS and Public Health Measures: A Global Survey of the Activities of Legislatures, 1983–1993* (Groningen, 1996), p. 16; Vera Boltho-Massarelli and Michael O'Boyle, "Droits de l'homme et santé publique, une nouvelle alliance," in Eric Heilmann, ed., *Sida et libertés: La régulation d'une épidemie dans un état de droit* (n.p., 1991), p. 40.

18. Edward P. Richards, "The Jurisprudence of Prevention: The Right of Societal Self-Defense against Dangerous Individuals," *Hastings Constitutional Law Quarterly* 16, 329 (1989), pp. 336–37.

19. James B. Bakalar and Lester Grinspoon, *Drug Control in a Free Society* (Cambridge, 1984), p. 69.

20. S. Fluss and J. Lau Hansen, "La réponse du législateur face au Vih/Sida: Aperçu international," in Jacques Foyer and Lucette Khaïat, *Droit et Sida: Comparaison internationale* (Paris, 1994), p. 470; Michael Pollak, "Introduction à la discussion: Systèmes de lutte contre les MST et sciences sociales," in Nadine Job-Spira et al., eds., *Santé publique et maladies à transmission sexuelle* (Montrouge, 1990), pp. 107–8; Daniel Defert, "Police sanitaire ou droit commun?" in Emmanuel Hirsch, *Aides: Solidaires* (Paris, 1991), p. 539; Françoise Héritier-Augé, preface to Eric Heilmann, ed., *Sida et libertés: La régulation d'une épidemie dans un état de droit* (n.p., 1991), p. 12; Koch, "Stellungnahme zur AIDS-Problematik," p. 545; Berridge, *AIDS in the UK,* p. 55; Jonathan M. Mann, "AIDS: Discrimination and Public Health," in WHO, *Legislative Responses to AIDS* (Dordrecht, 1989), p. 292; Lawrence O. Gostin and Zita Lazzarini, *Human Rights and Public Health in the AIDS Pandemic* (New York, 1997), pp. xv, 2, 51–52; Sev S. Fluss, "National AIDS Legislation: An Overview of Some Global Developments," in Lawrence Gostin and Lane Porter, eds., *International Law*

and AIDS (n.p., 1992), pp. 22–23, 259 ff; "Conclusions and Recommendations," in Koch and Deinhardt, eds., *AIDS Diagnosis and Control*, p. 178.

21. Dorothy Porter, *Health, Civilization, and the State: A History of Public Health from Ancient to Modern Times* (London, 1999), ch. 3.

22. George Rosen, "Political Order and Human Health in Jeffersonian Thought," *Bulletin of the History of Medicine* 26, 1 (1952); George Rosen, *From Medical Police to Social Medicine* (New York, 1974), pp. 246–58.

23. Dora B. Weiner, *The Citizen-Patient in Revolutionary and Imperial Paris* (Baltimore, 1993).

24. From the now massive literature: Colin Jones and Roy Porter, eds., *Reassessing Foucault: Power, Medicine, and the Body* (London, 1994); Graham Burchell et al., eds., *The Foucault Effect: Studies in Governmentality* (Chicago, 1991); Johan Goudsblom, "Zivilisation, Ansteckungsangst und Hygiene: Betrachtungen über ein Aspekt des europäischen Zivilisationsprozesses," in Peter Gleichmann et al., eds., *Materialen zu Norbert Elias' Zivilisationstheorie* (Frankfurt, 1977); Nikolas Rose, *Governing the Soul: The Shaping of the Private Self* (London, 1990); Peter N. Stearns, *Battleground of Desire: The Struggle for Self-Control in Modern America* (New York, 1999).

25. Patrick Nützi, *Rechtsfragen verhaltenslenkender staatlicher Information: Strukturen-Zulässigkeit-Haftung, illustriert an den Beispielen AIDS und Listeriose* (Bern, 1995), ch. 1.

26. Pollak, "Introduction à la discussion," pp. 107–8; Jean-Baptiste Brunet, "Évolution de la législation française sur les maladies sexuellement transmissibles," in Nadine Job-Spira et al., eds., *Santé publique et maladies à transmission sexuelle* (Montrouge, 1990), pp. 113–16.

27. Bryan S. Turner, *The Body and Society: Explorations in Social Theory*, 2d ed. (London, 1996), p. 210; Stephen Davies, *The Historical Origins of Health Fascism* (London, 1991); Robert N. Proctor, *The Nazi War on Cancer* (Princeton, 1999), p. 12.

28. Deborah Jones Merritt, "The Constitutional Balance between Health and Liberty," *Hastings Center Report* 16, 6 (December 1986), suppl., pp. 7–8.

29. William J. Curran et al., "AIDS: Legal and Policy Implications of the Application of Traditional Disease Control Measures," *Law, Medicine, and Health Care* 15, 1–2 (summer 1987), pp. 32–33; Wendy E. Parmet, "AIDS and Quarantine: The Revival of an Archaic Doctrine," *Hofstra Law Review* 14, 1 (fall 1985), pp. 54–55, 89; Thomas B. Stoddard and Walter Rieman, "AIDS and the Rights of the Individual," in Dorothy Nelkin et al., eds., *A Disease of Society: Cultural and Institutional Responses to AIDS* (Cambridge, 1991), p. 243.

30. Broberg and Tydén, *Oönskade i folkhemmet*, p. 189.

31. Nancy Ford and Michael D. Quam, "AIDS Quarantine: The Legal and Practical Implications," *Journal of Legal Medicine* 8, 3 (1987), pp. 367, 396; Richards, "Jurisprudence of Prevention," pp. 340–42.

32. Stoddard and Rieman, "AIDS and the Rights of the Individual," p. 241; Ford and Quam, "AIDS Quarantine," pp. 389–90.

33. William Curran et al., *AIDS: Legal and Regulatory Policy* (Frederick, MD, 1988), pp. 103–6; Michael Mills et al., "The Acquired Immunodeficiency Syndrome: Infection Control and Public Health Law," *New England Journal of Medicine* 314, 14 (3 April 1986), p. 934.

34. *RD Prot*, 1986/87, Bihang, Prop. 2, pp. 22–23, 26; Larry Gostin, "The Future of Communicable Disease Control: Toward a New Concept in Public Health Law," *Milbank Quarterly* 64, suppl. 1 (1986), pp. 80–81; Lawrence O. Gostin, "The Future of Public Health Law," *American Journal of Law and Medicine* 12, 3–4 (1986), pp. 461–90; Hugh Davis Graham, "The Political Culture of Rights: Postwar Germany and the United States in Comparative Perspective," in Manfred Berg and Martin H. Geyer, eds., *Two Cultures of Rights: The Quest for Inclusion and Participation in Modern America and Germany* (Cambridge, 2002); Roland Czada and Heidi Friedrich-Czada, "Aids als politisches Konfliktfeld und Verwaltungsproblem," in Rolf Rosenbrock and Andreas Salmen, eds., *Aids-Prävention* (Berlin, 1990), p. 272; Jean-Paul Jean, "Les problèmes juridiques soulevés par le développement des MST et leur prévention," in Nadine Job-Spira et al., eds., *Santé publique et maladies à transmission sexuelle* (Montrouge, 1990), p. 122; Brunet, "Évolution de la législation française," pp. 113–16; Boltho-Massarelli and O'Boyle, "Droits de l'homme," p. 41; Larry Gostin, "The Politics of AIDS: Compulsory State Powers, Public Health, and Civil Liberties," *Ohio State Law Journal* 49 (1989), p. 1030.

35. Monroe E. Price, *Shattered Mirrors: Our Search for Identity and Community in the AIDS Era* (Cambridge, MA, 1989), p. 9.

36. Markus Müller, *Zwangsmassnahmen als Instrument der Krankheitsbekämpfung: Das Epidemiengesetz und die Persönliche Freiheit* (Basel, 1992), p. 89; Swiss Institute of Comparative Law, *Comparative Study on Discrimination against Persons with HIV or AIDS* (Strasbourg, 1993), pp. 257, 264; Otfried Seewald, "Aids als Herausforderung an den Verfassungsstaat des Grundgesetzes," in Ernst Burkel, ed., *Der AIDS-Komplex: Dimensionen einer Bedrohung* (Frankfurt, 1988), pp. 318–19.

37. Ronald Elsberry, "AIDS Quarantine in England and the United States," *Hastings International and Comparative Law Review* 10 (1986), pp. 133–34; Curran, *AIDS*, pp. 259–62; Jochen Hofmann, "Verfassungs- und verwaltungsrechtliche Probleme der Virus-Erkrankung Aids unter besonderer Berücksichtigung des bayerischen Massnahmenkatalogs," *Neue Juristische Wochenschrift* 41 (1988), p. 1491.

38. Mark H. Jackson, "The Criminalization of HIV," in Nan D. Hunter and William B. Rubenstein, eds., *AIDS Agenda: Emerging Issues in Civil Rights* (New York, 1992), pp. 240–41; Larry Gostin, "Traditional Public Health Strategies," in Scott Burris et al., eds., *AIDS Law Today* (New Haven, 1993), p. 63–65; Terry Morehead Dworkin and Elies Steyger, "AIDS Victims in the European Community and the United States: Are They Protected from Unjustified Discrimination?" *Texas International Law Journal* 24 (1989), pp. 311–12; "The Constitutional Rights of AIDS Carriers," *Harvard Law Review* 99 (April 1986), pp. 1276–85; William J. Curran et al., "AIDS: Legal and Policy Implications of

the Application of Traditional Disease Control Measures," *Law, Medicine, and Health Care* 15, 1–2 (1987), p. 32; Parmet, "AIDS and Quarantine," pp. 65–79; Curran, *AIDS*, pp. 252–58.

39. John David Skrentny, *The Ironies of Affirmative Action: Politics, Culture, and Justice in America* (Chicago, 1996), ch. 1.

40. Samuel Walker, *The Rights Revolution: Rights and Community in Modern America* (New York, 1998), ch. 1.

41. Mona Ozouf, *Women's Words: Essay on French Singularity* (Chicago, 1997); Frédéric Martel, *Le rose et le noir: Les homosexuels en France depuis 1968* (Paris, 1996); Birte Siim, "Gender and Citizenship in France: Feminist Perspectives," in Denis Bouget and Bruno Palier, eds., *Comparing Social Welfare Systems in Nordic Europe and France* (Paris, n.d.), pp. 202–4; Birte Siim, *Gender and Citizenship: Politics and Agency in France, Britain, and Denmark* (Cambridge, 2000); Pierre Rosanvallon, *Le sacre du citoyen* (Paris, 1992).

42. House of Commons, 1986–87, Social Services Committee, *Problems Associated with AIDS*, 13 May 1987, vol. 2, p. 298; Michael Pollak, *Les homosexuels et le sida: Sociologie d'une épidémie* (Paris, 1988), p. 157; Paul Sieghart, *AIDS and Human Rights: A UK Perspective* (London, 1989), p. 54.

43. Andrei S. Markovitz and Philip S. Gorski, *The German Left: Red, Green, and Beyond* (Cambridge, 1988), p. 18; Sander L. Gilman, "Plague in Germany, 1939/1989: Cultural Images of Race, Space, and Disease," in Andrew Porter et al., eds., *Nationalisms and Sexualities* (New York, 1992), p. 185.

44. Willy H. Eirmbter et al., *AIDS und die gesellschaftliche Folgen* (Frankfurt, 1993), pp. 34, 38; Frank Becker and Klaus-Dieter Beisswenger, eds., *Solidarität der Uneinsichtigen: Aktionstag 9. Juli 1988 Frankfurt a.M.* (Berlin, 1988), pp. 5–9; Patrick Wachsmann, "Le sida ou la gestion de la peur par l'état de droit," in Eric Heilmann, ed., *Sida et libertés: La régulation d'une épidemie dans un état de droit* (n.p., 1991), p. 103; Ute Canaris, "Gesundheitspolitische Aspekte im Zusammenhang mit AIDS," in Johannes Korporal and Hubert Malouschek, eds., *Leben mit AIDS—Mit AIDS leben* (Hamburg, 1987), p. 299; BT *Verhandlungen* 11/71, 14 April 88, p. 4800C; Günter Frankenberg, *AIDS-Bekämpfung im Rechtsstaat* (Baden-Baden, 1988), pp. 14, 26; BT *Drucksache* 11/2495, 16 June 1988, p. 122; Uta Gerhardt, "Zur Effektivität der konkurrierenden Programme der AIDS-Kontrolle," in Bernd Schünemann and Gerd Pfeiffer, eds., *Die Rechtsprobleme von AIDS* (Baden-Baden, 1988), p. 78.

45. Günter Grau, *AIDS: Krankheit oder Katastrophe?* (Berlin, 1990), pp. 188–89. A garbled version of this story is in Michael Kirby, "AIDS: Return to Sachsenhausen?" in Alan F. Fleming et al., *The Global Impact of AIDS* (New York, 1988), pp. 318–19.

46. Karl Otto Hondrich, "Risikosteuerung durch Nichtwissen," in Ernst Burkel, ed., *Der AIDS-Komplex: Dimensionen einer Bedrohung* (Frankfurt, 1988), p. 136. Similar fears: Rita Süssmuth, *AIDS: Wege aus der Angst* (Hamburg, 1987), p. 95; Wolfgang Haug, "Das historische Syphilis-Paradigma und die Gefahr eines analogen AIDS-Paradigmas der Moral," in *AIDS: Fakten und Konsequenzen*, pp. 78 ff; BT *Drucksache* 11/7200, 31 May 1990, pp. 39–45.

47. BT *Verhandlungen*, 1 March 1950, p. 1461A-B; 23 April 1952, pp. 8859D. 8862A, 8863A-64A; 12 June 1953, pp. 13419D-20D; 3 May 1961, pp. 8978C-79C.

48. Art. 11, Abs. 2; Art. 13 Abs. 3. Andreas Costard, *Öffentlich-rechtliche Probleme beim Auftreten einer neuen übertragbaren Krankheit am Beispiel AIDS* (Berlin, 1989), pp. 29–39; Hofmann, "Verfassungs- und verwaltungsrechtliche Probleme," p. 1488; Seewald, "Aids als Herausforderung," pp. 305–16.

49. BT *Drucksache* 11/7200, 31 May 1990, pp. 176–77.

50. RD *Prot*, 1988/89, Bihang, Prop. 5, pp. 27–28.

51. Sydney M. Laird, *Venereal Disease in Britain* (Harmondsworth, 1943), p. 45; Thomas Parran, *Shadow on the Land: Syphilis* (New York, 1937), p. 105; Félix Regnault, *L'évolution de la prostitution* (Paris, n.d. [1906?]), pp. 262–68. And later too: Charles F. Clark, *AIDS and the Arrows of Pestilence* (Golden, CO, 1994), pp. 79–80.

8. TO DIE LAUGHING:
GAYS AND OTHER INTEREST GROUPS

1. Paul Farmer, *Infections and Inequalities: The Modern Plagues* (Berkeley, 1999), ch. 2.

2. William Muraskin, "The Silent Epidemic: The Social, Ethical, and Medical Problems Surrounding the Fight against Hepatitis B," *Journal of Social History* 22, 2 (1988), pp. 281–83.

3. World Bank, *Confronting AIDS: Public Priorities in a Global Epidemic* (Oxford 1997), p. 273.

4. Peter Baldwin, *Contagion and the State in Europe, 1830–1930* (Cambridge, 1999), chs. 4–5.

5. Mariana Valverde, *Diseases of the Will: Alcohol and the Dilemmas of Freedom* (Cambridge, 1998), p. 137.

6. Jonathan M. Mann and Daniel J. M. Tarantola, eds., *AIDS in the World II* (New York, 1996), p. 347.

7. Edward King, *Safety in Numbers: Safer Sex and Gay Men* (London, 1993), p. 250; Volker Koch, *Zu einer sozialen Ätiologie von AIDS: Der soziologische Beitrag zur Krankheitserklärung* (Bremen, 1989), p. 106.

8. Virginia Berridge and Philip Strong, eds., *AIDS and Contemporary History* (Cambridge, 1993), pp. 49–50; Elizabeth W. Etheridge, *Sentinel for Health: A History of the Centers for Disease Control* (Berkeley, 1992), chs. 18, 24; Virginia Berridge and Philip Strong, "AIDS in the UK: Contemporary History and the Study of Policy," *Twentieth Century British History* 2, 2 (1991), p. 158.

9. Joseph B. McCormick and Susan Fisher-Hoch, *Level 4: Virus Hunters of the CDC* (Atlanta, 1996); Richard Preston, *Hot Zone* (New York, 1994); Laurie Garrett, *The Coming Plague: Newly Emerging Diseases in a World Out of Balance* (New York, 1995); Frank Ryan, *Virus X: Tracking the New Killer Plagues*

(New York, 1998); C. J. Peters and Mark Olshaker, *Virus Hunter: Thirty Years of Battling Hot Viruses around the World* (New York, 1998).

10. James Harvey Young, "AIDS and Deceptive Therapies," in Young, *American Health Quackery* (Princeton, 1992); James Harvey Young, "AIDS and the FDA," in Caroline Hannaway et al., eds., *AIDS and the Public Debate* (Amsterdam, 1995), pp. 51–53; Bernard Paillard, *Notes on the Plague Years: AIDS in Marseilles* (New York, 1998), ch. 6; Virginia Berridge, *AIDS in the UK: The Making of Policy, 1981–1994* (Oxford, 1996), pp. 270–71; Jean de Savigny, *Le Sida et les fragilités françaises: Nos réactions face à l'épidémie* (Paris, 1995), pp. 235–36; Boris Velimirovic, "NATC: A Delusive Approach," *AIDS-Forschung* 5 (1993), pp. 257–64; *Los Angeles Times*, 30 May 2000, p. A20; K. S. Kermani, "Stress, Emotions, Autogenic Training, and AIDS: A Holistic Approach to the Management of HIV-Infected Individuals," *Holistic Medicine* 2 (1987); Wolfgang Wiesner, ed., *Texte zur Behandlung von AIDS im Rahmen der traditionellen Chinesischen Medizin* (Petershausen, 1994).

11. *AIDS: Fakten und Konsequenzen: Endbericht der Enquête-Kommission des 11. Deutschen Bundestages "Gefahren von AIDS und wirksame Wege zu ihrer Eindämmung"* (Bonn, 1990), pp. 32, 166, 353; BT *Verhandlungen* 11/8, 2 April 1987, pp. 452B-C; BT *Drucksache* 11/7200, 31 May 1990, pp. 14, 85, 189–90; Walter Bachmann, "Seuchenrechtliche Aspekte der HIV-Infektion," *AIDS-Forschung* 2, 2 (1987), p. 102.

12. BT *Drucksache* 11/7200, 31 May 1990, p. 185; "Die rechtliche Beurteilung von Eingriffsmassnahmen und ihre Gewichtung im Rahmen der Gesamtstrategie der AIDS-Bekämpfung," *AIDS-Forschung* 5 (1989), p. 265.

13. In Portland, Maine, a mother whose one child, treated with AZT, nonetheless died, rejected letting the other one take a three-drug cocktail. The state Supreme Court ruled that her refusal did not amount to child abuse or neglect, but left the door open if the child's condition worsened or new medical treatments developed. *Los Angeles Times*, 20 November 1998, p. A24; 27 October 1998, p. A5.

14. Steven Epstein, *Impure Science: AIDS, Activism, and the Politics of Knowledge* (Berkeley, 1996); Ian Young, *The AIDS Dissidents: An Annotated Bibliography* (Metuchen, NJ, 1993).

15. Robert M. Wachter, *The Fragile Coalition: Scientists, Activists, and AIDS* (New York, 1991), pp. 78–79.

16. Martin A. Levin and Mary Bryna Sanger, *After the Cure: Managing AIDS and Other Public Health Crises* (Lawrence, 2000), p. ix; Mark Schoofs, "An AIDS Vaccine," in Dangerous Bedfellows, eds., *Policing Public Sex: Queer Politics and the Future of AIDS Activism* (Boston, 1996), pp. 177–78.

17. Barry D. Adam, "Mobilizing around AIDS," in Martin P. Levine et al., eds., *In Changing Times: Gay Men and Lesbians Encounter HIV/AIDS* (Chicago, 1997), p. 25; Hong Sik Cho, "L'association des hémophiles: De la réserve à la lutte," in Pierre Favre, ed., *Sida et politique: Les premiers affrontements (1981–1987)* (Paris, 1992), pp. 100–101.

18. Ronald Bayer and Eric Feldman, "Understanding the Blood Feuds," in Feldman and Bayer, eds., *Blood Feuds: AIDS, Blood, and the Politics of Medical Disaster* (New York, 1999), p. 11.

19. Jamie L. Feldman, *Plague Doctors: Responding to the AIDS Epidemic in France and America* (Westport, CT, 1995), p. 149; Dennis Altman, *Power and Community: Organizational and Cultural Responses to AIDS* (London, 1994), p. 78; Peter Raschke and Claudia Ritter, *Eine Grossstadt lebt mit Aids: Strategien der Prävention und Hilfe am Beispiel Hamburgs* (Berlin, 1991), pp. 180–81; Nancy E. Stoller, "From Feminism to Polymorphous Activism: Lesbians in AIDS Organizations," in Martin P. Levine et al., eds., *In Changing Times: Gay Men and Lesbians Encounter HIV/AIDS* (Chicago, 1997), pp. 183–84; Janherman Veenker, "The Decisive Role of Politics: AIDS Control in the Netherlands," in Theo Sandfort, ed., *The Dutch Response to HIV: Pragmatism and Consensus* (London, 1998), p. 124; Amber Hollibaugh, "Lesbian Denial and Lesbian Leadership in the AIDS Epidemic," in Beth E. Schneider and Nancy E. Stoller, eds., *Women Resisting AIDS: Feminist Strategies of Empowerment* (Philadelphia, 1995), pp. 219, 225; David Wilson, "Preventing Transmission of HIV in Heterosexual Prostitution," in Lorraine Sherr, ed., *AIDS and the Heterosexual Population* (Chur, 1993), p. 74; Chetan Bhatt and Robert Lee, "Official Knowledges: The Free Market, Identity Formation, Sexuality, and Race in the HIV/AIDS Sector," in Joshua Oppenheimer and Helena Reckitt, eds., *Acting on AIDS: Sex, Drugs, and Politics* (London, 1997), pp. 206–8, 227–28; Mehboob Dada, "Race and the AIDS Agenda," in Tessa Boffin and Sunil Gupta, eds., *Ecstatic Antibodies: Resisting the AIDS Mythology* (London, 1990), pp. 92–93; James Monroe Smith, *AIDS and Society* (Upper Saddle River, NJ, 1996), pp. 278–81; Le groupe ACSF, *Les comportements sexuels en France: Rapport au ministre de la Recherche et de l'Espace* (Paris, 1993), p. 212.

20. Judy Bury, "Women and HIV/AIDS: Medical Issues," in Lesley Doyal et al., eds., *AIDS: Setting a Feminist Agenda* (London, 1994), p. 32; Sheila Henderson, "Living with the Virus: Perspectives from HIV-Positive Women in London," in Nicholas Dorn et al., eds., *AIDS: Women, Drugs, and Social Care* (London, 1992), p. 116; Tamsin Wilton, *EnGendering AIDS: Deconstructing Sex, Text, and Epidemic* (London, 1997), pp. 24–29; Cynthia A. Gomez, "Lesbians at Risk for HIV: The Unresolved Debate," in Gregory M. Herek and Beverly Greene, eds., *AIDS, Identity, and Community: The HIV Epidemic and Lesbians and Gay Men* (Thousand Oaks, 1995); Amber Hollibaugh, "Seducing Women into 'A Lifestyle of Vaginal Fisting': Lesbian Sex Gets Virtually Dangerous," in Dangerous Bedfellows, eds., *Policing Public Sex: Queer Politics and the Future of AIDS Activism* (Boston, 1996), pp. 328–29; *Women's Health* 2, 1–2 (1996); Elinor Burkett, *The Gravest Show on Earth: America in the Age of AIDS* (Boston, 1995), p. 212; Altman, *Power and Community*, pp. 47–48; Frédéric Martel, *Le rose et le noir: Les homosexuels en France depuis 1968* (Paris, 1996), pp. 376–77; Simon Garfield, *The End of Innocence: Britain in the Time of AIDS* (London, 1994), p. 89; Robin Gorna, *Vamps, Virgins, and Victims: How Can Women Fight AIDS?* (London, 1996), pp. 348–51; Joyce Hunter and Priscilla

Alexander, "Women Who Sleep with Women," in Lynellyn D. Long and E. Maxine Ankrah, eds., *Women's Experiences with HIV/AIDS* (New York, 1996), p. 44; *Hansard Parliamentary Debates*, vol. 73 (21 February 1985), col. 585.

21. Ronald Bayer, "Politics, Social Sciences, and HIV Prevention in the United States," in Dorothee Friedrich and Wolfgang Heckmann, eds., *Aids in Europe: The Behavioural Aspect* (Berlin, 1995), 1:46–47; Burkett, *Gravest Show on Earth*, pp. 148–50; Dudley Clendinen and Adam Nagourney, *Out for Good: The Struggle to Build a Gay Rights Movement in America* (New York, 1999), pp. 494–99; Cathy Jean Cohen, "Power, Resistance, and the Construction of Crisis: Marginalized Communities Respond to AIDS" (Ph.D. diss., University of Michigan, 1993), p. 255.

22. Barry D. Adam, *The Rise of a Gay and Lesbian Movement* (Boston, 1987), pp. 93–97; Clendinen and Nagourney, *Out for Good*, ch. 6; Diana Fuss, *Essentially Speaking: Feminism, Nature, and Difference* (New York, 1989), p. 47; Cindy Patton, "Save Sex/Save Lives: Evolving Modes of Activism," in Tim Rhodes and Richard Hartnoll, eds., *AIDS, Drugs, and Prevention* (London, 1996), pp. 127–28; Gabriel Rotello, *Sexual Ecology: AIDS and the Destiny of Gay Men* (New York, 1997), pp. 203, 209; Stoller, "From Feminism to Polymorphous Activism," pp. 176–77, 180; Nancy E. Stoller, "Lesbian Involvement in the AIDS Epidemic: Changing Roles and Generational Differences," in Beth E. Schneider and Stoller, eds., *Women Resisting AIDS: Feminist Strategies of Empowerment* (Philadelphia, 1995), pp. 273–75; Cindy Patton, *Fatal Advice: How Safe-Sex Education Went Wrong* (Durham, 1996), p. 4; Robin Gorna, "Dangerous Vessels: Feminism and the AIDS Crisis," in Joshua Oppenheimer and Helena Reckitt, eds., *Acting on AIDS: Sex, Drugs, and Politics* (London, 1997), p. 150; Gorna, *Vamps, Virgins, and Victims*, pp. 262, 274.

23. Lynne Segal, "Lessons from the Past: Feminism, Sexual Politics, and the Challenge of AIDS," and Simon Watney, "Taking Liberties," in Erica Carter and Simon Watney, eds., *Taking Liberties* (London, 1989), pp. 31, 135–39; Janet Holland et al., "Pressure, Resistance, Empowerment: Young Women and the Negotiation of Safer Sex," in Peter Aggleton et al., eds., *AIDS: Rights, Risk, and Reason* (London, 1992), p. 144; Henderson, "Living with the Virus," p. 16; Gorna, *Vamps, Virgins, and Victims*, pp. 46, 295, 310–11.

24. Mann and Tarantola, *AIDS in the World II*, p. 254.

25. Kajo Pieper, "On the History of the AIDS-Hilfe," in AIDS-Forum D.A.H., *Aspects of AIDS and AIDS-Hilfe in Germany* (Berlin, 1993), pp. 15–16.

26. Walt Odets, "Why We Do Not Do Primary Prevention for Gay Men," in Joshua Oppenheimer and Helena Reckitt, eds., *Acting on AIDS: Sex, Drugs, and Politics* (London, 1997), pp. 136–37; Marita Sturken, *Tangled Memories: The Vietnam War, the AIDS Epidemic, and the Politics of Remembering* (Berkeley, 1997), p. 166; Alvin Novick, "Conflict within the HIV/AIDS Advocate/Activist Communities," *AIDS and Public Policy Journal* 8, 4 (1993), p. 156.

27. Simon LeVay and Elisabeth Nonas, *City of Friends: A Portrait of the Gay and Lesbian Community in America* (Cambridge, MA, 1995), p. 259; Michael Bartos, "Governing AIDS," *Australian Left Review* 148 (March 1993),

pp. 55–56; Virginia Berridge, " 'Unambiguous Voluntarism?' AIDS and the Voluntary Sector in the United Kingdom, 1981–1992," in Caroline Hannaway et al., eds., *AIDS and the Public Debate* (Amsterdam, 1995), p. 156.

28. Michael P. Brown, *RePlacing Citizenship: AIDS Activism and Radical Democracy* (New York, 1997), pp. xv, 81–82; Paula A. Treichler, "How to Have Theory in an Epidemic: The Evolution of AIDS Treatment Activism," Constance Penley and Andrew Ross, eds., *Technoculture* (Minneapolis, 1991), pp. 79–93.

29. *Hansard*, vol. 121 (26 October 1987), col. 187; Jacques Foyer and Lucette Khaïat "Droit et SIDA: La situation française," in Foyer and Khaïat, *Droit et Sida: Comparaison internationale* (Paris, 1994), p. 216; Alain Sobel, "Policy Making under Changing Political Situations: The French National AIDS Council and AIDS Control Policies," in Dorothee Friedrich and Wolfgang Heckmann, eds., *Aids in Europe: The Behavioural Aspect* (Berlin, 1995), 4:89.

30. Leon Gordenker et al., *International Cooperation in Response to AIDS* (London, 1995), pp. 103–6; Chris Bennett and Ewan Ferlie, *Managing Crisis and Change in Health Care: The Organizational Response to HIV/AIDS* (Buckingham, 1994), pp. 35–36; Albert R. Jonsen and Jeff Stryker, eds., *The Social Impact of AIDS in the United States* (Washington, DC, 1993), p. 173; Rolf Rosenbrock, "The Role of Policy in Effective Prevention and Education," in Dorothee Friedrich and Wolfgang Heckmann, eds., *Aids in Europe: The Behavioural Aspect* (Berlin, 1995), 5:23; Peter Söderholm, *Global Governance of AIDS: Partnerships with Civil Society* (Lund, 1997).

31. Theodore J. Stein, *The Social Welfare of Women and Children with HIV and AIDS: Legal Protections, Policy, and Programs* (New York, 1998), p. 54; Jonathan Mann et al., "Toward a New Health Strategy to Control the HIV/AIDS Pandemic," *Journal of Law, Medicine, and Ethics* 22, 1 (1994), p. 45; Philip M. Kayal, *Bearing Witness: Gay Men's Health Crisis and the Politics of AIDS* (Boulder, 1993), p. 62; Charles Perrow and Mauro F. Guillén, *The AIDS Disaster: The Failure of Organizations in New York and the Nation* (New Haven, 1990), pp. 107–12.

32. Altman, *Power and Community*, pp. 100–101; Monika Steffen, "AIDS Policies in France," in Virginia Berridge and Philip Strong, eds., *AIDS and Contemporary History* (Cambridge, 1993), p. 257; Berridge and Strong, "AIDS in the UK," p. 167.

33. Michael Pollak, "Organizing the Fight against AIDS," in Michael Pollak, ed. *AIDS: A Problem for Sociological Research* (London, 1992), pp. 41–42; Michael Pollak, "Les visages multiples de la mobilisation contre le Sida," in Michael Pollak et al., eds., *Homosexualités et Sida* (n.p. n.d. [1991]), pp. 22–24; Jeffrey Weeks et al., "An Anatomy of the HIV/AIDS Voluntary Sector in Britain," in Peter Aggleton et al., eds., *AIDS: Foundations for the Future* (London, 1994), p. 14; Emmanuel Hirsch, *Le SIDA: Rumeurs et faits* (Paris, 1987), p. 119; *Le Monde*, 29 November 1986, p. 11a; Richard Dunne, "New York City: Gay Men's Health Crisis," in John Griggs, ed., *AIDS: Public Policy Dimensions* (New York, 1987), p. 155–56; Perrow and Guillén, *AIDS Disaster*, p. 117.

34. Weeks et al., "An Anatomy of the HIV/AIDS Voluntary Sector," p. 2; Guenter Frankenberg, "Germany: The Uneasy Triumph of Pragmatism," in David L. Kirp and Ronald Bayer, eds., *AIDS in the Industrialized Democracies* (New Brunswick, 1992), p. 120; Ute Canaris, "Gesundheitspolitische Aspekte im Zusammenhang mit AIDS," in Johannes Korporal and Hubert Malouschek, eds., *Leben mit AIDS—Mit AIDS leben* (Hamburg, 1987), p. 294; Bennett and Ferlie, *Managing Crisis and Change*, p. 22; Matthias Weikert, "AIDS Prevention: Cooperation of NGOs and GOs," in Dorothee Friedrich and Wolfgang Heckmann, eds., *Aids in Europe: The Behavioural Aspect* (Berlin, 1995), 4:58–59; Raschke and Ritter, *Eine Grossstadt*, p. 89.

35. Susan M. Allen et al., "The Organizational Transformation of Advocacy: Growth and Development of AIDS Community-Based Organizations," *AIDS and Public Policy Journal* 10, 1 (1995), pp. 50–51.

36. Canaris, "Gesundheitspolitische Aspekte," pp. 294–95; Werner Reutter, "Aids, Politik und Demokratie: Ein Vergleich aids-politischer Massnahmen in Deutschland und Frankreich," Wissenschaftszentrum Berlin für Sozialforschung, *Veröffentlichungsreihe der Forschungsgruppe Gesundheitsrisiken und Präventionspolitik*, P92–205 (Berlin, April 1992), p. 30; Tim Rhodes, "Outreach, Community Change, and Community Empowerment: Contradictions for Public Health and Health Promotion," in Peter Aggleton et al., eds., *AIDS: Foundations for the Future* (London, 1994), pp. 49, 58–60.

37. Altman, *Power and Community*, pp. 10–11; Brown, *RePlacing Citizenship*, ch. 4; Cindy Patton, *Inventing AIDS* (New York, 1990), p. 22; Mark Smith, "AIDS and Minority Health," in Caroline Hannaway et al., eds., *AIDS and the Public Debate* (Amsterdam, 1995), p. 101.

38. Weeks et al., "An Anatomy of the HIV/AIDS Voluntary Sector," p. 2.

39. Raschke and Ritter, *Eine Grossstadt*, pp. 88–89.

40. Pollak, "Organizing the Fight," pp. 45–46; Garfield, *End of Innocence*, p. 130; Erik Albæk, "AIDS: The Evolution of a Non-Controversial Issue in Denmark" (paper presented at the American Political Science Association, 1990), pp. 14, 29.

41. Robert A. Padgug and Gerald M. Oppenheimer, "Riding the Tiger: AIDS and the Gay Community," in Elizabeth Fee and Daniel M. Fox, eds., *AIDS: The Making of a Chronic Disease* (Berkeley, 1992), pp. 256, 268, 271–72.

42. Michael Pollak, *The Second Plague of Europe: AIDS Prevention and Sexual Transmission among Men in Western Europe* (Binghamton, NY, 1994), p. 19; Pollak, "Les visages multiples," pp. 22–23; Martel, *Le rose et le noir*, ch. 14; *AIDS-Nachrichten aus Forschung und Wissenschaft* 1 (1991), p. 1; Berridge, *AIDS in the UK*, pp. 272–74; Maxine Wolfe, "The AIDS Coalition to Unleash Power (ACT UP): A Direct Model of Community Research for AIDS Prevention," in Johannes P. Van Vugt, edz., *AIDS Prevention and Services: Community Based Research* (Westport, 1994); Andreas Salmen, ed., *ACT UP: Feuer unterm Arsch: Die AIDS-Aktionsgruppen in Deutschland und den USA* (Berlin, 1991). Though local political styles varied, and in some places—Vancouver, for ex-

ample—ACT UP's tactics rubbed instincts the wrong way: Brown, *RePlacing Citizenship*, pp. 74–77.

43. Albæk, "AIDS: Evolution of a Non-Controversial Issue," p. 29; Patton, "Save Sex/Save Lives," p. 118; Altman, *Power and Community*, p. 72; Gordenker et al., *International Cooperation*, pp. 103–6.

44. Jan Willem Duyvendak, *The Power of Politics: New Social Movements in France* (Boulder, 1995), p. 49; Roland Czada and Heidi Friedrich-Czada, "Aids als politisches Konfliktfeld und Verwaltungsproblem," in Rolf Rosenbrock and Andreas Salmen, eds., *Aids-Prävention* (Berlin, 1990), pp. 261–64.

45. Bayer, "Politics, Social Sciences, and HIV Prevention," 1:46–47; Burkett, *Gravest Show on Earth*, p. 147; Lois M. Takahashi, *Homelessness, AIDS, and Stigmatization: The NIMBY Syndrome in the United States at the End of the Twentieth Century* (Oxford, 1998), pp. 173–74; Ronald O. Valdiserri, ed., *Dawning Answers: How the HIV/AIDS Epidemic Has Helped to Strengthen Public Health* (Oxford, 2003), ch. 3.

46. Jan K. van Wijngaarden, "The Netherlands: AIDS in a Consensual Society," in David L. Kirp and Ronald Bayer, eds., *AIDS in the Industrialized Democracies* (New Brunswick, 1992), p. 256; Theo Sandfort, ed., *The Dutch Response to HIV: Pragmatism and Consensus* (London, 1998), passim; Canaris, "Gesundheitspolitische Aspekte," p. 269; BT *Verhandlungen* 11/8, 2 April 1987, p. 430B; Ian Schäfer, "Die Deutsche AIDS-Hilfe: Ihre Aktivitäten, Präventionsstrategien und Kooperationsansätze," in Josef Faltermeier and Ionka Senger, eds., *AIDS und soziale Arbeit* (Frankfurt, 1988), pp. 65–67.

47. Gary W. Dowsett, *Practicing Desire: Homosexual Sex in the Era of AIDS* (Stanford, 1996), pp. 65–68; Susan Kippax et al., *Sustaining Safe Sex: Gay Communities Respond to AIDS* (London, 1993), pp. 9, 13; Barbara A. Misztal, "AIDS in Australia: Diffusion of Power and Making of Policy," in Misztal and David Moss, eds., *Action on AIDS: National Policies in Comparative Perspective* (New York, 1990), p. 197; Deborah Lupton, *Moral Threats and Dangerous Desires: AIDS in the News Media* (London, 1994), p. 117.

48. Peter M. Davies et al., *Sex, Gay Men, and AIDS* (London, 1993), p. 17; Daniel M. Fox, Patricia Day, and Rudolf Klein, "The Power of Professionalism: Policies for AIDS in Britain, Sweden, and the United States," *Dædalus* 118, 2 (spring 1989), p. 96; John Street, "British Government Policy on AIDS: Learning Not to Die of Ignorance," *Parliamentary Affairs* 41 (October 1988), pp. 504–5; John Street and Albert Weale, "Britain: Policy-Making in a Hermetically Sealed System," in David L. Kirp and Ronald Bayer, eds., *AIDS in the Industrialized Democracies* (New Brunswick, 1992), p. 193.

49. Birgit Westphal Christensen et al., *AIDS: Prævention og kontrol i Norden* (Stockholm, 1988), pp. 53–54, 222; RD *Prot*, 1985/86, Bihang, Prop. 13, p. 9; Reutter, "Aids, Politik und Demokratie," pp. 29–30.

50. An attempt at a tabulation of attitudes and legal instruments: Rob Tielman and Hans Hammelburg, "World Survey on the Social and Legal Position of Gays and Lesbians," in Aart Hendriks et al., eds., *The Third Pink Book: A Global View of Lesbian and Gay Liberation and Oppression* (Buffalo, 1993).

51. Michael Dreyer, "Minorities, Civil Rights, and Political Culture: Homosexuality in Germany and the United States," in Manfred Berg and Martin H. Geyer, eds., *Two Cultures of Rights: The Quest for Inclusion and Participation in Modern America and Germany* (Cambridge, 2002), pp. 254–57; Adam, *Rise of a Gay and Lesbian Movement*, ch. 2.

52. David Moss, "AIDS in Italy: Emergency in Slow Motion," in Barbara A. Misztal and Moss, eds., *Action on AIDS: National Policies in Comparative Perspective* (New York, 1990), p. 150.

53. Olli Stålström and Outi Lithén, "AIDS in Finland," in Martin Breum and Aart Hendriks, eds., *AIDS and Human Rights* (Copenhagen, 1988), p. 46.

54. David Rayside, *On the Fringe: Gays and Lesbians in Politics* (Ithaca, 1998), pp. 26–27, 38–39; Leslie J. Moran, *The Homosexual(ity) of Law* (London, 1996), p. 206; David Feldman, *Civil Liberties and Human Rights in England and Wales* (Oxford, 1993), pp. 512–15; Philip A. Thomas, "AIDS in Prisons in England and Wales," in Thomas and Martin Moerings, eds., *AIDS in Prison* (Aldershot, U.K., 1994), p. 48; Paul Skidmore, "Sexuality and the UK Armed Forces: Judicial Review of the Ban on Homosexuality," in Terrell Carver and Véronique Mottier, eds., *Politics of Sexuality: Identity, Gender, Citizenship* (London, 1998); *Economist*, 5 February 2000, p. 52.

55. Richard A. Posner, *Sex and Reason* (Cambridge, MA, 1992), pp. 60–66; Adam, *Rise of a Gay and Lesbian Movement*, pp. 43–44; Rayside, *On the Fringe*, ch. 7.

56. Posner, *Sex and Reason*, p. 24, ch. 6. Though for a corrective on the ancient Greeks, see James Davidson, *Courtesans and Fishcakes: The Consuming Passions of Classical Athens* (London, 1997), pp. 167–82.

57. Peter Aggleton, "Priorities for Social and Behavioural Research on AIDS," in Dorothee Friedrich and Wolfgang Heckmann, eds., *Aids in Europe: The Behavioural Aspect* (Berlin, 1995), 1:57–58; Sophie Day, "Anthropological perspectives on sexually transmitted diseases," in Nadine Job-Spira et al., eds., *Santé publique et maladies à transmission sexuelle* (Montrouge, 1990), pp. 92–93; Richard G. Parker, *Bodies, Pleasures, and Passions: Sexual Culture in Contemporary Brazil* (Boston, 1991), pp. 43–54; Ana Luisa Liguori et al., "Bisexuality and HIV/AIDS in Mexico," in Peter Aggleton, ed., *Bisexualities and AIDS: International Perspectives* (London, 1996), p. 79; Richard Parker, "AIDS in Brazil," in Herbert Daniel and Richard Parker, eds., *Sexuality, Politics, and AIDS in Brazil: In Another World?* (London, 1993), pp. 15–16; John L. Peterson, "AIDS-Related Risks and Same-Sex Behaviors among African American Men," in Martin P. Levine et al., eds., *In Changing Times: Gay Men and Lesbians Encounter HIV/AIDS* (Chicago, 1997), pp. 287–88; John L. Peterson, "Black Men and Their Same-Sex Desires and Behaviors," in Gilbert Herdt, ed., *Gay Culture in America* (Boston, 1992), pp. 149–50; John L. Peterson, "AIDS-Related Risks and Same-Sex Behaviors among African American Men," in Gregory M. Herek and Beverly Greene, eds., *AIDS, Identity, and Community: The HIV Epidemic and Lesbians and Gay Men* (Thousand Oaks, 1995), pp. 85–90; *Los Angeles Times*, 14 January 2000, p. A13. Doubts about the hermetic quality of such clas-

sifications: Stephen O. Murray, "Machismo, Male Homosexuality, and Latino Culture," in Murray, *Latin American Male Homosexualities* (Albuquerque, 1995), pp. 50–55.

58. Joseph Carrier, *De Los Otros: Intimacy and Homosexuality among Mexican Men* (New York, 1995), pp. 3–6, 17; E. Antonio de Moya and Rafael Garcia, "Three Decades of Male Sex Work in Santo Domingo," in Peter Aggleton, ed., *Men Who Sell Sex: International Perspectives on Male Prostitution and HIV/AIDS* (Philadelphia, 1999), pp. 127–29. But see, in contradiction to this dichotomy: Anja Bestmann, "Mexikanische Mannsbilder: Eine geschlechterbezogene Analyse mexikanischer Hiv/Aids-Forschungen," in Bestmann et al., eds., *Aids—weltweit und dichtdran* (Saarbrücken, 1997).

59. Michael Warner, *The Trouble with Normal: Sex, Politics, and the Ethics of Queer Life* (New York, 1999), p. 38; George Stambolian, *Male Fantasies/Gay Realities* (New York, 1984), p. 155; Hans A. M. von Druten et al., "Homosexual Role Behavior and the Spread of HIV," in Dorothee Friedrich and Wolfgang Heckmann, eds., *Aids in Europe: The Behavioural Aspect* (Berlin, 1995), 4:259; Mirko D. Grmek, *History of AIDS* (Princeton, 1990), pp. 168–69; Anthony P. M. Coxon et al., "Sex Role Separation in Sexual Diaries of Homosexual Men," *AIDS* 7 (1993), p. 881; Rotello, *Sexual Ecology*, pp. 77–78; Joseph M. Carrier and J. Raul Magana, "Use of Ethnosexual Data on Men of Mexican Origin for HIV/AIDS Prevention Programs," in Gilbert Herdt and Shirley Lindenbaum, eds., *The Time of AIDS* (Newbury Park, 1992), pp. 252–56; Joseph Carrier, "Miguel: Sexual Life History of a Gay Mexican American," in Gilbert Herdt, ed., *Gay Culture in America* (Boston, 1992), pp. 205–6; Daniel Mendelsohn, *The Elusive Embrace: Desire and the Riddle of Identity* (New York, 1999), pp. 73–74.

60. Richard G. Parker, "Responding to AIDS in Brazil," in Barbara A. Misztal and David Moss, eds., *Action on AIDS: National Policies in Comparative Perspective* (New York, 1990), p. 59; Paul Farmer, *AIDS and Accusation: Haiti and the Geography of Blame* (Berkeley, 1992), p. 135; Diane K. Lewis, "African-American Women at Risk: Notes on the Sociocultural Context of HIV Infection," in Beth E. Schneider and Nancy E. Stoller, eds., *Women Resisting AIDS: Feminist Strategies of Empowerment* (Philadelphia, 1995), pp. 64–65; Rafael M. Díaz, *Latino Gay Men and HIV: Culture, Sexuality, and Risk Behavior* (New York, 1998), p. 7; Paillard, *Notes on the Plague Years*, p. 228.

61. Ernest Quimby, "Anthropological Witnessing for African Americans: Power, Responsibility, and Choice in the Age of AIDS," in Gilbert Herdt and Shirley Lindenbaum, eds., *The Time of AIDS* (Newbury Park, 1992), p. 165; Michael Pollak, *Les homosexuels et le sida: Sociologie d'une épidémie* (Paris, 1988), p. 45.

62. Jacobo Schifter and Peter Aggleton, "*Cacherismo* in a San José Brothel: Aspects of Male Sex Work in Costa Rica," in Peter Aggleton, ed., *Men Who Sell Sex: International Perspectives on Male Prostitution and HIV/AIDS* (Philadelphia, 1999), p. 151.

63. David Arnold, *Colonizing the Body: State Medicine and Epidemic Disease in Nineteenth-Century India* (Berkeley, 1993), pp. 183–85. Or the black-

ness of Africans: Samuel V. Duh, *Blacks and Aids: Causes and Origins* (Newbury Park, 1991), ch. 6.

64. Frank Rühmann, *AIDS: Eine Krankheit und ihre Folgen*, 2d ed. (Frankfurt, 1985), p. 119; Michael G. Koch, "Stellungnahme zur AIDS-Problematik: Antworten auf Fragen der Presse," *AIDS-Forschung* 3, 11 (November 1988), p. 604.

65. *Congressional Record* (House), 13 December 1982, 128, p. 30377; C. Everett Koop, "The Early Days of AIDS As I Remember Them," in Caroline Hannaway et al., eds., *AIDS and the Public Debate* (Amsterdam, 1995), p. 10.

66. Douglas Crimp, "Accommodating Magic," in Marjorie Garber et al., eds., *Media Spectacles* (New York, 1993), pp. 258–59; Evelynn Hammonds, "Race, Sex, AIDS: The Construction of 'Other,'" *Radical America* 20 (1986), p. 29.

67. Gayle S. Rubin, "Elegy for the Valley of the Kings: AIDS and the Leather Community in San Francisco, 1981–1996," in Martin P. Levine et al., eds., *In Changing Times: Gay Men and Lesbians Encounter HIV/AIDS* (Chicago, 1997), pp. 103, 111; LeVay and Nonas, *City of Friends*, pp. 61–63.

68. Rotello, *Sexual Ecology*, p. 9, 40–42, 51, 86; Ilan H. Meyer and Laura Dean, "Patterns of Sexual Behavior and Risk Taking among Young New York City Gay Men," *AIDS Education and Prevention* 7, suppl. 13–23 (1995), pp. 17, 19, 21–22; World Bank, *Confronting AIDS*, pp. 68, 139–56.

69. Jean-Florian Mettetal quoted in Daniel Defert, "Discours social, consensus et épidemie," in Emmanuel Hirsch, ed., *Aides: Solidaires* (Paris, 1991), pp. 352–53, 665; Daniel Defert "L'enjeu des gais," *Gai Pied Hebdo* 446 (29 November 1990), pp. 61–62; John Ballard, "The Constitution of AIDS in Australia: Taking 'Governance at a Distance' Seriously," in Mitchell Dean and Barry Hindess, eds., *Governing Australia: Studies in Contemporary Rationalities of Government* (Cambridge, 1998), p. 127.

70. Elaine Showalter, *Sexual Anarchy: Gender and Culture at the Fin de Siècle* (New York, 1990), p. 200; Richard D. Mohr, *Gays/Justice: A Study of Ethics, Society, and Law* (New York, 1988), p. 252 and passim; Stein, *Social Welfare*, p. 12; Dan E. Beauchamp, *The Health of the Republic: Epidemics, Medicine, and Moralism as Challenges to Democracy* (Philadelphia, 1988), p. 208.

71. Kathleen M. Sullivan and Martha A. Field, "AIDS and the Coercive Power of the State," *Harvard Civil Rights–Civil Liberties Law Review* 23 (1988), p. 150; *Hansard*, vol. 112 (10 March 1987), col. 139–40; vol. 114 (7 April 1987), col. 152; House of Commons, 1986–87, Social Services Committee, *Problems Associated with AIDS*, 13 May 1987, vol. 3, p. 35; Garfield, *End of Innocence*, p. 113.

72. Rühmann, *AIDS*, p. 86; Larry Kramer, *Reports from the Holocaust: The Making of an AIDS Activist* (New York, 1989), p. 233.

73. Antony A. Vass, *AIDS: A Plague in Us* (St. Ives, 1986), p. 58.

74. Simon Watney, *Practices of Freedom: Selected Writings on HIV/AIDS* (Durham, NC, 1994), pp. 48–49; Norman Naimark, *The Russians in Germany: A History of the Soviet Zone of Occupation, 1945–1949* (Cambridge, MA, 1995), p. 97; Dennis Altman, *Global Sex* (Chicago, 2001), p. 98; Marco Pulver,

Tribut der Seuche oder: Seuchenmythen als Quelle sozialer Kalibrierung: Eine Rekonstruktion des AIDS-Diskurses vor dem Hintergrund von Studien zur Historizität des Seuchendispositivs (Frankfurt, 1999), pp. 520–21.

75. Martin Dannecker, *Homosexuelle Männer und AIDS* (Stuttgart, 1990), p. 40; Martin Dannecker, "Homosexuelle Männer und AIDS," in Wolfgang Heckmann and Meinrad A. Koch, eds., *Sexualverhalten in Zeiten von Aids* (Berlin, 1994), p. 273; Anthony P. M. Coxon, *Between the Sheets: Sexual Diaries and Gay Men's Sex in the Era of AIDS* (London, 1996), pp. 65, 69; Davies et al., *Sex, Gay Men, and AIDS*, p. 107; A. P. M. Coxon, "The Effect of Age and Relationship on Gay Men's Sexual Behavior," *Project SIGMA Working Paper* 13 (June 1990), pp. 14–15; Michael Bochow, *Die Reaktionen homosexueller Männer auf AIDS in Ost- und Westdeutschland* (Berlin, 1993), pp. 31–32.

76. Bernd Schünemann, "AIDS und Strafrecht," in Andrzej J. Szwarc, ed., *AIDS und Strafrecht* (Berlin, 1996), pp. 41, 126; Weikert, "AIDS Prevention," p. 58; Larry O. Gostin, "Public Health Strategies for Confronting AIDS: Legislative and Regulatory Policy in the United States," *JAMA* 261, 11 (17 March 1989), p. 1621; Paula A. Treichler, "AIDS, Homophobia, and Biomedical Discourse: An Epidemic of Signification," in Douglas Crimp, ed., *AIDS: Cultural Analysis, Cultural Activism* (Cambridge, 1988), p. 51; *Hansard*, 11 March 1994, col. 546.

77. Schünemann, "AIDS und Strafrecht," p. 37; Johannes Frhr. v. Gayl, *Das Parlamentarische Institut der Enquête-Kommission am Beispiel der Enquête-Kommission "AIDS" des Deutschen Bundestages* (Frankfurt, 1993), p. 80; Wolfgang Steinke et al., "Die seuchenpolitische Reaktion auf die HIV/AIDS-Epidemie in der Schweiz," *AIDS-Forschung* 1 (1994), pp. 7–8, 15.

78. House of Commons, *Problems Associated with AIDS*, vol. 3, pp. 141–47.

79. Jean-Jacques Amy and Walter Foulon, "Sida et grossesse," in Michel Vincineau, ed., *Le Sida: Un défi aux droits* (Brussels, 1991), p. 397; *Congressional Record* (House), 30 June 1987, p. 18379; (House) 13 June 1990, p. 3522; (House) 11 March 1993, p. 1208; Bernd Schünemann, "Die Rechtsprobleme der AIDS-Eindämmung," in Schünemann and Gerd Pfeiffer, eds., *Die Rechtsprobleme von AIDS* (Baden-Baden, 1988), p. 390.

80. *Congressional Record* (Senate), 25 January 1989, p. 396; (House) 13 June 1990, p. 3547; (Senate) s 14 January 1991, pp. 878–79.

81. Samuel R. Friedman et al., "AIDS and Self-Organization among Intravenous Drug Users," *International Journal of the Addictions* 22, 3 (1987), pp. 201–19; Jeff Stryker, "IV Drug Use and AIDS: Public Policy and Dirty Needles," *Journal of Health Politics, Policy, and Law* 14, 4 (1989), p. 731.

82. Wachter, *Fragile Coalition*, p. 65; Tomas J. Philipson and Richard A. Posner, *Private Choices and Public Health: The AIDS Epidemic in an Economic Perspective* (Cambridge, MA, 1993), p. 204; Michel Setbon, *Pouvoirs contre SIDA: De la transfusion sanguine au dépistage: Decisions et pratiques en France, Grande-Bretagne et Suède* (Paris, 1993), p. 242; Showalter, *Sexual Anarchy*, p. 192; B. Velimirovic, "AIDS as a Social Phenomenon," in M. A. Koch and F. Deinhardt, eds., *AIDS Diagnosis and Control: Current Situation* (Munich, 1988), p. 43.

83. Treichler, "AIDS, Homophobia, and Biomedical Discourse," p. 51.

84. Epstein, *Impure Science*, pp. 31–38, chs. 5–6; Arthur D. Kahn, *AIDS: The Winter War* (Philadelphia, 1993), chs. 3, 5, 7; Altman, *Power and Community*, p. 72.

85. George A. Gellert et al., "Manging the Non-Compliant HIV-Infected Individual: Experiences from a Local Health Department," *AIDS and Public Policy Journal* 8, 1 (1993), p. 24.

86. Burkett, *Gravest Show on Earth*, p. 304; Martel, *Le rose et le noir*, p. 245.

87. Kramer, *Reports from the Holocaust*, pp. 158, 173, 263–65; Kayal, *Bearing Witness*, p. 40; Epstein, *Impure Science*, pp. 221–22; Lewis, "African-American Women at Risk," p. 67; Gena Corea, *The Invisible Epidemic: The Story of Women and AIDS* (New York, 1992), p. 230; Wilton, *EnGendering AIDS*, p. 119; Ronald Bayer, "Blood and AIDS in America," in Eric Feldman and Bayer, eds., *Blood Feuds: AIDS, Blood, and the Politics of Medical Disaster* (New York, 1999), p. 38.

88. Dennis Altman, "Legitimation through Disaster: AIDS and the Gay Movement," in Elizabeth Fee and Daniel M. Fox, eds., *AIDS: The Burdens of History* (Berkeley, 1988), p. 301 and passim; Jeffrey Weeks, "AIDS and the Regulation of Sexuality," in Virginia Berridge and Philip Strong, eds., *AIDS and Contemporary History* (Cambridge, 1993), p. 31; Rolf Rosenbrock, "AIDS: Fragen und Lehren für Public Health," Wissenschaftszentrum Berlin für Sozialforschung, *Veröffentlichungsreihe der Forschungsgruppe Gesundheitsrisiken und Präventionspolitik*, P92–206 (Berlin, April 1992), pp. 30–31.

89. John-Manuel Andriote, *Victory Deferred: How AIDS Changed Gay Life in America* (Chicago, 1999), p. xi.

90. Horst Stipp and Dennis Kerr, "Determinants of Public Opinion about AIDS," *Public Opinion Quarterly* 53 (1989), p. 102; Dreyer, "Minorities, Civil Rights, and Political Culture," p. 271.

91. Swiss Institute of Comparative Law, *Comparative Study on Discrimination against Persons with HIV or AIDS* (Strasbourg, 1993), pp. 171, 177.

92. Peter M. Nardi, "Friends, Lovers, and Families: The Impact of AIDS on Gay and Lesbian Relationships," in Martin P. Levine et al., eds., *In Changing Times: Gay Men and Lesbians Encounter HIV/AIDS* (Chicago, 1997), pp. 70–71; Andrew Sullivan, *Virtually Normal: An Argument about Homosexuality* (New York, 1995), pp. 179–87; William B. Rubenstein, ed., *Lesbians, Gay Men, and the Law* (New York, 1993), pp. 398–405; Helmut Blazek, *Rosa Zeiten für rosa Liebe: Geschichte der Homosexualität* (Frankfurt, 1996), pp. 266–67, 296–98; Bruce Bawter, *A Place at the Table: The Gay Individual in American Society* (New York, 1993).

93. Bent Hansen and Henning Jørgensen, "The Danish Partnership Law," in Aart Hendriks et al., eds., *The Third Pink Book: A Global View of Lesbian and Gay Liberation and Oppression* (Buffalo, 1993); Albæk, "AIDS: Evolution of a Non-Controversial Issue," p. 5; *Los Angeles Times*, 14 October 1999, p. A6.

94. Rayside, *On the Fringe*, ch. 2, pp. 310–11; Clendinen and Nagourney, *Out for Good*, pp. 531–39; Rubenstein, *Lesbians, Gay Men, and the Law*, p. xvii;

Jonathan Glasson, "Public Health and Human Rights: Finding a Balance in HIV Prevention," in David FitzSimons et al., eds., *The Economic and Social Impact of AIDS in Europe* (London, 1995), p. 237.

95. Nancy Goldstein, introduction to Nancy Goldstein and Jennifer L. Manlowe, eds., *The Gender Politics of HIV/AIDS in Women* (New York, 1997), pp. 2–3; Ken Plummer, "Organizing AIDS," in Peter Aggleton and Hilary Homans, eds., *Social Aspects of Aids* (London, 1988), p. 25.

96. Edwin Hackney, "Low-Incidence Community Response to AIDS," in Richard Ulack and William F. Skinner, eds., *AIDS and the Social Sciences* (Lexington, KT, 1991), pp. 69–70, 79; Beth E. Schneider, "Owning an Epidemic: The Impact of AIDS on Small-City Lesbian and Gay Communities," in Martin P. Levine et al., eds., *In Changing Times: Gay Men and Lesbians Encounter HIV/AIDS* (Chicago, 1997), pp. 146–47, 153–54; "J. Stephan McDaniel et al., "Delivering Culturally Sensitive AIDS Education in Rural Communities," in Davidson C. Umeh, ed., *Confronting the AIDS Epidemic: Cross-Cultural Perspectives on HIV/AIDS Education* (Trenton, NJ, 1997), p. 171; Jeffrey A. Kelly, "HIV Prevention among Gay and Bisexual Men in Small Cities," in Ralph J. DiClemente and John L. Peterson, eds., *Preventing AIDS: Theories and Methods of Behavioral Interventions* (New York, 1994), p. 302; King, *Safety in Numbers*, p. 42.

97. Sandra Panem, *AIDS Bureaucracy* (Cambridge, MA, 1988), p. 16; Richard Dunne, "New York City: Gay Men's Health Crisis," in John Griggs, ed., *AIDS: Public Policy Dimensions* (New York, 1987), p. 164; Perrow and Guillén, *AIDS Disaster*, pp. 107–12; Aran Ron and David E. Rogers, "AIDS in the United States: Patient Care and Politics," *Dædalus* 118, 2 (spring 1989), p. 50; Dennis Altman, *AIDS and the New Puritanism* (London, 1986), pp. 127 ff.

98. Gilbert Herdt, ed., *Gay Culture in America* (Boston, 1992); Simon Watney, *Policing Desire: Pornography, AIDS, and the Media* (Minneapolis, 1987), p. 128; Erik Albæk, "Denmark: AIDS and the Political 'Pink Triangle,'" in David L. Kirp and Ronald Bayer, eds., *AIDS in the Industrialized Democracies* (New Brunswick, 1992), pp. 285, 289; Frans van den Boom and Paul Schnabel, "The Impact of AIDS on the Dutch Health Care System," in Theo Sandfort, ed., *The Dutch Response to HIV: Pragmatism and Consensus* (London, 1998), p. 166; J. W. Duyvendak and R. Koopmans, "Resister au Sida: Destin et influence du mouvement homosexuel," in Michael Pollak et al., eds., *Homosexualités et Sida* (n.p. n.d. [1991]), p. 217; Dreyer, "Minorities, Civil Rights, and Political Culture," p. 271.

99. Pollak, *Second Plague*, pp. 11–16; Pollak, "Organizing the Fight against AIDS," pp. 38–44; Altman, *AIDS and the New Puritanism*, p. 108; Dominique Brenky and Olivia Zémor, *La route du SIDA* (Paris, 1985), p. 72; Nathalie Bajos et al., "Sexual Behaviour and HIV Epidemiology: Comparative Analysis in France and Britain," *AIDS* 9 (1995), p. 741.

100. Roger Charbonney and Philippe Esnault, "Ecce homos . . . " in Jean Martin, ed., *Faire face au SIDA* (Lausanne, 1988), pp. 146–47; Rühmann, *AIDS*, pp. 119, 134; Altman, *AIDS and the New Puritanism*, pp. 91, 108; Setbon, *Pouvoirs contre SIDA*, p. 231; Altman, *Power and Community*, p. 20.

101. Kayal, *Bearing Witness;* Perrow and Guillén, *AIDS Disaster,* pp. 107–12; Gerd Paul and Loretta Walz, eds., *Eine Stadt Lebt mit AIDS: Hilfe und Selbsthilfe in San Francisco* (Berlin, 1986), p. 72.

102. Ira Cohen and Ann Elder, "Major Cities and Disease Crises: A Comparative Perspective," *Social Science History* 13, 1 (1989), pp. 45–46.

103. Doris Schaeffer et al., eds., *Aids-Krankenversorgung* (Berlin, 1992), pp. 270, 291; Hans Halter, "Die dunklen Flügel der Seuche," in Hans Halter, ed., *Todesseuche AIDS* (Reinbek, 1985), p. 151; Carmen Stürzel, "Aids und Obdachlosigkeit: New York und Berlin—ein Metropolenvergleich," Wissenschaftszentrum Berlin für Sozialforschung, *Veröffentlichungsreihe der Forschungsgruppe Gesundheitsrisiken und Präventionspolitik,* P94–203 (Berlin, May 1994), p. 28; Loretta Walz, "AIDS und Prävention: Das Beispiel San Francisco," in Johannes Korporal and Hubert Malouschek, eds., *Leben mit AIDS—Mit AIDS leben* (Hamburg, 1987), pp. 187–89; Paul and Walz, *Eine Stadt;* Andrew Bebbington and Pat Warren, *AIDS: The Local Authority Response* (Canterbury, December 1988), p. 1.

104. Pollak, *Second Plague,* p. 38; Lisa Power and Tim Barnett, "Gathering Strength and Gaining Power: How Lesbians and Gay Men Began to Change their Fortunes in Britain in the Nineties," in Aart Hendriks et al., eds., *The Third Pink Book: A Global View of Lesbian and Gay Liberation and Oppression* (Buffalo, 1993); *Economist,* 5 February 2000, p. 52; Martin J. Walker, *Dirty Medicine: Science, Big Business, and the Assault on Health Care,* rev. ed. (London, 1994), p. 181.

105. Bajos et al., "Sexual Behaviour and HIV Epidemiology," pp. 740–41; Martel, *Le rose et le noir,* p. 265; Duyvendak and Koopmans, "Resister au Sida," pp. 202–4; Jan Willem Duyvendak, "From Revolution to Involution: The Disappearance of the Gay Movement in France," in Gert Hekma et al., eds., *Gay Men and the Sexual History of the Political Left* (New York, 1995); Pollak, *Les homosexuels et le sida,* p. 132; Frank Arnal, "The Gay Press and Movement in France," in Aart Hendriks et al., eds., *The Third Pink Book: A Global View of Lesbian and Gay Liberation and Oppression* (Buffalo, 1993), pp. 41–42; Hanspeter Kriesi et al., *New Social Movements in Western Europe: A Comparative Analysis* (Minneapolis, 1995), pp. 170–71.

106. Martel, *Le rose et le noir,* pp. 226–29; Fabienne Dulac, "Du refus de la maladie a une prise en charge exigeante," in Pierre Favre, ed., *Sida et politique: Les premiers affrontements (1981–1987)* (Paris, 1992), pp. 62–63.

107. Emmanuel Hirsch, *Aides: Solidaires* (Paris, 1991), pp. 30, 83, 87, 123–24; Pollak, "Organizing the Fight," p. 42; Pollak, *Second Plague,* p. 15; Monika Steffen, *The Fight against AIDS: An International Public Policy Comparison between Four European Countries: France, Great Britain, Germany, and Italy* (Grenoble, 1996), p. 24; Reutter, "Aids, Politik und Demokratie," p. 8; Dulac, "Du refus de la maladie a une prise en charge exigeante," p. 71; Martel, *Le rose et le noir,* pp. 260–61.

108. David Vital, *The Origins of Zionism* (Oxford, 1975), p. 25; Adrian Favell, *Philosophies of Integration: Immigration and the Idea of Citizenship in France and Britain* (Houndmills, 1998), p. 61.

109. Watney, *Practices of Freedom*, p. 235; Martel, *Le rose et le noir*, passim; David Caron, "Liberté, Égalité, Séropositivité: AIDS, the French Republic, and the Question of Community," *French Cultural Studies* 9, 3 (1998), pp. 284–85.

110. Frances FitzGerald, *Cities on a Hill: A Journey through Contemporary American Cultures* (New York, 1986), p. 58.

111. Judith Butler, *Bodies That Matter: On the Discursive Limits of "Sex"* (London, 1993); David Plummer and Doug Porter, "The Use and Misuse of Epidemiological Categories," in Godfrey Linge and Doug Porter, eds., *No Place for Borders: The HIV/AIDS Epidemic and Development in Asia and the Pacific* (New York, 1997), pp. 42–43.

112. Lisa Duggan and Nan D. Hunter, *Sex Wars: Sexual Dissent and Political Culture* (New York, 1995), pp. 159–65. This is the problem that Joan Scott touched on in analyzing the tensions between postmodern and feminist historiography. If there is no coherent individual with an identity based in gender, or anything else, then there cannot be women's history. Joan Wallach Scott, "Gender: A Useful Category of Social Analysis," in Scott, *Gender and the Politics of History*, rev. ed. (New York, 1999). Similarly it is the logical conundrum that lies at the heart of multiculturalist ideologies: presupposing the very ethnic and national identities among the individuals who, when aggregated, are supposed to break down the inherited identity of the nation. Anthony Giddens, *The Third Way: The Renewal of Social Democracy* (Cambridge, 1998), p. 133. For related issues, see Diana Fuss, "The 'Risk' of Essence," in Fuss, *Essentially Speaking: Feminism, Nature, and Difference* (New York, 1989).

113. Duyvendak, *Power of Politics*, pp. 39–40; Alan R. H. Baker, *Fraternity among the French Peasantry: Sociability and Voluntary Associations in the Loire Valley, 1815–1914* (Cambridge, 1999).

114. Jean Cavailhes et al., *Rapport gai: Enquête sur les modes de vie homosexuels en France* (Paris, 1984), pp. 92–95; Christophe Martet, *Les combattants du sida* (Paris, 1993), p. 46; Jacques Girard, *Le mouvement homosexuel en France, 1945–1980* (Paris, 1981), pp. 187–88.

115. Duyvendak, *Power of Politics*, pp. 3–5, 166; Duyvendak and Koopmans, "Resister au Sida," pp. 202–4; Gert Hekma et al., "Leftist Sexual Politics and Homosexuality: A Historical Overview," in Hekma et al., eds., *Gay Men and the Sexual History of the Political Left* (New York, 1995), pp. 3–16.

116. Paul Smith, *Feminism in the Third Republic: Women's Political and Civil Rights in France, 1918–1945* (Oxford, 1996), pp. 5, 43–62; Christine Bard, *Les Filles de Marianne: Histoire des féminismes, 1914–1940* (Paris, 1995), p. 358; Harry Oosterhuis, "The 'Jews' of the Antifascist Left: Homosexuality and Socialist Resistance to Nazism," and Randall Halle, "Between Marxism and Psychoanalysis: Antifascism and Antihomosexuality in the Frankfurt School," in Gert Hekma et al., eds., *Gay Men and the Sexual History of the Political Left* (New York, 1995).

117. Martel, *Le rose et le noir*, pp. 150–57; Cavailhes, *Rapport gai*, pp. 10, 17, 130–31; Arnal, *Résister ou disparaître?* pp. 56–59.

118. Duyvendak, *Power of Politics*, pp. 188–93; Jan Willem Duyvendak,

"From Revolution to Involution: The Disappearance of the Gay Movement in France," *Journal of Homosexuality* 29 (1995), pp. 376–77.

119. As analyzed in a series of excellent articles in *French Cultural Studies* 9, 3 (1998).

120. Pollak, *Second Plague*, pp. 38–39; Steffen, "AIDS Policies in France," p. 250; Moss, "AIDS in Italy," pp. 150–51, 163; Altman, *Power and Community*, p. 21; Carrier and Magana, "Use of Ethnosexual Data," p. 256.

121. Robert A. Nye, *Masculinity and Male Codes of Honor in Modern France* (New York, 1993), ch. 6.

122. Pierre Favre, "La gestion administrative du Sida," in Favre, ed., *Sida et politique: Les premiers affrontements (1981–1987)* (Paris, 1992), p. 91; Monika Steffen, "AIDS and Political Systems," in Dorothee Friedrich and Wolfgang Heckmann, eds., *Aids in Europe: The Behavioural Aspect* (Berlin, 1995), 5:36; Steffen, "AIDS Policies in France," p. 259.

123. Pollak, *Second Plague*, p. 9.

124. Michael Bochow, "Reactions of the Gay Community to AIDS in East and West Berlin," in AIDS-Forum D.A.H., *Aspects of AIDS and AIDS-Hilfe in Germany* (Berlin, 1993), p. 23.

125. Ronald Bayer, "AIDS, Public Health, and Civil Liberties: Consensus and Conflict in Policy," in Frederick G. Reamer, ed., *AIDS and Ethics* (New York, 1991), pp. 26–28; Ronald Bayer and David L. Kirp, "The United States: At the Center of the Storm," in Kirp and Bayer, eds., *AIDS in the Industrialized Democracies* (New Brunswick, 1992), p. 14.

126. Patton, *Inventing AIDS*, p. 22; Kayal, *Bearing Witness*, pp. xv, 5, 7, 26–27, 34, 62, 72.

127. Albæk, "AIDS: Evolution of a Non-Controversial Issue," p. 8.

128. Kaye Wellings, "HIV/AIDS Prevention: The European Approach," in Dorothee Friedrich and Wolfgang Heckmann, eds., *Aids in Europe: The Behavioural Aspect* (Berlin, 1995), 1:52; Street and Weale, "Britain," p. 189; Coxon, *Between the Sheets*, p. 128; John Shiers, "One Step to Heaven?" in Bob Cant and Susan Hemmings, eds., *Radical Records: Thirty Years of Lesbian and Gay History, 1957–1987* (London, 1988), p. 235.

129. Bochow, "Reactions of the Gay Community," p. 29; Michael Pollak, "AIDS Policy in France," in Barbara A. Misztal and David Moss, eds., *Action on AIDS: National Policies in Comparative Perspective* (New York, 1990), p. 84; Monika Steffen, "France: Social Solidarity and Scientific Expertise," in David L. Kirp and Ronald Bayer, eds., *AIDS in the Industrialized Democracies* (New Brunswick, 1992), p. 236.

130. However, early in the new millennium, the Parisians reintroduced bathhouses and back rooms, both hetero- and homosexual, while the rest of the world was still suffering from post-AIDS sex shock. Guy Trebay, "Le Relapse: Libertinism Makes a Comeback in French Clubs," *New York Times*, 28 April 2002, sec. 9, p. 1.

131. James Miller, *The Passion of Michel Foucault* (New York, 1993), pp. 259–62.

132. Frank Becker and Klaus-Dieter Beisswenger, eds., *Solidarität der Uneinsichtigen: Aktionstag 9. Juli 1988 Frankfurt a.M.* (Berlin, 1988), p. 17.

133. Rayside, *On the Fringe*, pp. 276–77.

134. Janine Mossuz-Lavau, *Les lois de l'amour: Les politiques de la sexualité en France de 1950 à nos jours* (Paris, 1991), pp. 249–51; Girard, *Le mouvement homosexuel*, pp. 89, 95–98, 127–31.

135. John Nguyet Erni, *Unstable Frontiers: Technomedicine and the Cultural Politics of "Curing" AIDS* (Minneapolis, 1994), pp. 12–13; Jonsen and Stryker, *Social Impact of AIDS*, pp. 82–83, 90–94; Lynn Payer, *Medicine and Culture: Varieties of Treatment in the United States, England, West Germany, and France* (New York, 1988), p. 110; Lucette Khaïat, "Nouveau virus et vieux démons: Le droit face au sida, une approache comparative," in Eric Heilmann, ed., *Sida et libertés: La régulation d'une épidemie dans un état de droit* (n.p., 1991), p. 68; Nicolas Dodier and Janine Barbot, "Le temps des tensions épistémiques: Le développement des essais thérapeutiques dans le cadre du sida," *Revue française de sociologie* 41, 1 (2000), pp. 83–89.

136. Lawrence O. Gostin, "The AIDS Litigation Project: A National Review of Court and Human Rights Commission Decisions," *JAMA* 263, 15 (18 April 1990), p. 2090; George J. Annas, "Faith (Healing), Hope, and Charity at the FDA: The Politics of AIDS Drug Trials," in Lawrence O. Gostin, ed., *AIDS and the Health Care System* (New Haven, 1990), pp. 183–86, 190; Epstein, *Impure Science*, passim; Christine Grady, *The Search for an AIDS Vaccine: Ethical Issues in the Development and Testing of a Preventive HIV Vaccine* (Bloomington, 1995), pp. 47–59; Jonathan Kwitny, *Acceptable Risks* (New York, 1992); Peter S. Arno and Karyn L. Feiden, *Against the Odds: The Story of AIDS Drug Development, Politics, and Profits* (New York, 1992), ch. 6.

137. *Report of the Presidential Commission on the Human Immunodeficiency Virus Epidemic* (Washington, DC, 1988), pp. 37, 47–54; Norman Daniels, *Seeking Fair Treatment: From the AIDS Epidemic to National Health Care Reform* (New York, 1995), ch. 5; Young, "AIDS and the FDA," pp. 54–60; Jeffrey Levi, "Unproven AIDS Therapies: The Food and Drug Administration and ddI," in Kathi E. Hanna, ed., *Biomedical Politics* (Washington, DC, 1991), pp. 14–18.

138. Altman, *Power and Community*, p. 73; Burkett, *Gravest Show on Earth*, p. 272; Arno and Feiden, *Against the Odds*, pp. 33, 99; Stuart Marshall, "Picturing Deviancy," in Boffin and Gupta, *Ecstatic Antibodies*, pp. 33–34; BT *Drucksache* 11/2495, 16 June 1988, p. 5; *Report of the Presidential Commission*, p. xviii.

139. Lars Trägårdh, *Patientmakt i Sverige, USA och Holland: Individuella kontra sociala rättigheter* (Stockholm, 1999); Berridge, *AIDS in the UK*, pp. 184–87; Lawrence O. Gostin, "Hospitals, Health Care Professionals, and Persons with AIDS," in Lawrence O. Gostin, ed., *AIDS and the Health Care System* (New Haven, 1990), pp. 8–9.

140. Mary Douglas and Marcel Calvez, "The Self as Risk Taker: A Cultural Theory of Contagion in Relation to AIDS," *Sociological Review* (1990), p. 463.

141. *Congressional Record* (Senate), 14 January 1991, pp. 878–79; (Senate) 21 January 1993, pp. 145–46.

142. Aran Ron and David E. Rogers, "AIDS in the United States: Patient Care and Politics," *Dædalus* 118, 2 (spring 1989), p. 47; Wachter, *Fragile Coalition*, p. 82; Bayer and Kirp, "The United States," p. 44; Victoria A. Harden and Dennis Rodrigues, "Context for a New Disease: Aspects of Biomedical Research Policy in the United States before AIDS," in Virginia Berridge and Philip Strong, eds., *AIDS and Contemporary History* (Cambridge, 1993), p. 192; Nadine Job-Spira, "Une approche commune pour la lutte contre les MST et le SIDA," in Job-Spira et al., eds., *Santé publique et maladies à transmission sexuelle* (Montrouge, 1990), pp. 3–5; Burkett, *Gravest Show on Earth*, pp. 155–58; William Winkenwerder et al., "Federal Spending for Illness Caused by the Human Immunodeficiency Virus," *New England Journal of Medicine* 320, 24 (1989), p. 1602; *Congressional Record* (Senate), 12 October 1990, pp. 15070–73.

143. Evridiki Hatziandreu et al., "AIDS and Biomedical Research Funding: Comparative Analysis," *Reviews of Infectious Diseases* 10, 1 (January-February 1988), pp. 159–67; Alan N. Schechter, "Basic Research Related to AIDS," in Victoria A. Harden and Guenter B. Risse, eds., *AIDS and the Historian* (n.p. 1991), pp. 45–50; World Bank, *Confronting AIDS*, p. 245.

144. Mossuz-Lavau, *Les lois de l'amour*, p. 272; Koch, *Zu einer sozialen Ätiologie von AIDS*, p. 42.

145. Howard M. Leichter, *Free to Be Foolish: Politics and Health Promotion in the United States and Great Britain* (Princeton, 1991), p. 221; Berridge, *AIDS in the UK*, p. 19.

146. Johann Valentin Müller, *Praktisches Handbuch der medicinischen Galanteriekrankheiten* (Marburg, Germany, 1788), p. 21; Wilhelm Rudeck, *Syphilis und Gonorrhoe vor Gericht: Die sexuellen Krankheiten in ihrer juristischen Tragweite nach der Rechtsprechung Deutschlands, Österreichs und der Schweiz*, 2d ed. (Berlin, 1902), pp. 28–34.

147. Patton, *Fatal Advice*, p. 107.

148. John Rechy, *The Sexual Outlaw* (New York, 1977), p. 31.

149. Guy Hocquenghem, *Homosexual Desire* (Durham, NC, 1993), ch. 4; Mendelsohn, *Elusive Embrace*, pp. 73–74; Davies et al., *Sex, Gay Men, and AIDS*, pp. 127–29; Mario Mieli, *Homosexuality and Liberation: Elements of a Gay Critique* (London, 1980), pp. 148–49.

150. Michael Pollak and Marie-Ange Schiltz, "Les homosexuels français face au sida: Modifications des pratiques sexuelles et émergence de nouvelles valeurs," *Anthropologie et sociétés* 15, 2–3 (1991), p. 56; Walt Odets, *In the Shadow of the Epidemic: Being HIV-Negative in the Age of AIDS* (Durham, NC, 1995), p. 130; Bochow, "Reactions of the Gay Community," pp. 41–42.

151. John Lauritsen, *The AIDS War: Propaganda, Profiteering, and Genocide from the Medical-Industrial Complex* (New York, 1993), pp. 188–90; Kramer, *Reports from the Holocaust*, pp. 27–28, 46; James Kinsella, *Covering the Plague: AIDS and the American Media* (New Brunswick, NJ, 1989), pp.

34–36, 174–81; Ralph Bolton, "AIDS and Promiscuity: Muddles in the Models of HIV Prevention," *Medical Anthropology* 14 (1992), pp. 153–54.

152. "The Constitutional Rights of AIDS Carriers," *Harvard Law Review* 99 (April 1986), p. 1285; Judith A. Rabin, "The AIDS Epidemic and Gay Bathhouses: A Constitutional Analysis," *Journal of Health Politics, Policy, and Law* 10, 4 (winter 1986), pp. 733–36; Bayer and Kirp, "The United States," p. 20; D. C. Jayasuriya, *AIDS: Public Health and Legal Dimensions* (Dordrecht, 1988), p. 81; WHO, *Legislative Responses to AIDS* (Dordrecht, 1989), p. 228; *IDHL* 37, 3 (1986), p. 544; *RD Prot*, 1986/87, Bihang, Prop. 149, p. 40; FitzGerald, *Cities on a Hill*, pp. 97–101.

153. Ronald Bayer, "AIDS, Power, and Reason," *Milbank Quarterly* 64, suppl. 1 (1986), p. 172; Allan Bérubé, "The History of Gay Bathhouses," in Dangerous Bedfellows, eds., *Policing Public Sex: Queer Politics and the Future of AIDS Activism* (Boston, 1996). On the other hand, in Rita Mae Brown's account of crashing a bath in New York, she describes the regulars' behavior as a distillation of traditional male hypergenitalized sex. Rita Mae Brown, "Queen for a Day: A Stranger in Paradise," in Karla Jay and Allen Young, eds., *Lavender Culture* (New York, 1978).

154. L. A. Gosse, *Rapport sur l'épidémie de choléra en Prusse, en Russie et en Pologne* (Geneva, 1833), pp. 329–33.

155. Bayer, "AIDS, Public Health, and Civil Liberties," pp. 30–31; James W. Dearing and Everett M. Rogers, "AIDS and the Media Agenda," in Timothy Edgar et al., eds., *AIDS: A Communication Perspective* (Hillsdale, NJ, 1992), p. 179; Benjamin Heim Shepard, *White Nights and Ascending Shadows: An Oral History of the San Francisco AIDS Epidemic* (London, 1997), pp. 219–20.

156. Burkett, *Gravest Show on Earth*, p. 6; Clendinen and Nagourney, *Out for Good*, pp. 479–83, 499–503; Peter Jobst, "La creation litteraire et le Sida," in Michael Pollak et al., eds., *Homosexualités et Sida* (n.p. n.d. [1991]), p. 191; Michael Callen and Richard Berkowitz, "We Know Who We Are: Two Gay Men Declare War on Promiscuity," *New York Native* 8 November 1982. Similar was the approach taken in Marshall Kirk and Hunter Madsen, *After the Ball: How America Will Conquer Its Fear and Hatred of Gays in the '90s* (New York, 1989).

157. Halter, "Die dunklen Flügel," p. 149; Kuno Kruse, "AIDS in den Medien," in Johannes Korporal and Hubert Malouschek, eds., *Leben mit AIDS — Mit AIDS leben* (Hamburg, 1987), p. 311; Blazek, *Rosa Zeiten für rosa Liebe*, pp. 288–89; Pulver, *Tribut der Seuche*, pp. 406–10; Bochow, "Reactions of the Gay Community," pp. 29–30; Martel, *Le rose et le noir*, pp. 233, 237, 242, 339.

158. Dannecker, *Homosexuelle Männer und AIDS*, pp. 30–31; Raschke and Ritter, *Eine Grossstadt*, p. 89; *RD Prot*, 1986/87, Bihang, Prop. 149, pp. 34–36; Rotello, *Sexual Ecology*, pp. 6–8 and passim.

159. Rühmann, *AIDS*, pp. 123–27, 141; Becker and Beisswenger, *Solidarität der Uneinsichtigen*, pp. 10, 25; Andreas Salmen, "Aktuelle Erfordernisse der Aidsprävention," in Rolf Rosenbrock and Salmen, eds., *Aids-Prävention* (Berlin,

1990),p. 95; Dangerous Bedfellows, eds., *Policing Public Sex: Queer Politics and the Future of AIDS Activism* (Boston, 1996), pt. 1.

160. Rubin, "Elegy for the Valley of the Kings," p. 117; FitzGerald, *Cities on a Hill*, pp. 97–111; Ronald Bayer, *Private Acts, Social Consequences: AIDS and the Politics of Public Health* (New York, 1989), ch. 2.

161. SFS 1987:375; Staatssekretärsausschuss "AIDS" der Bayerischen Staatsregierung, *Konzept der Bayerischen Staatsregierung zur Bekämpfung der Immunschwächekrankheit AIDS* (Munich, n.d.), p. 15; Wellings, "HIV/AIDS Prevention," p. 52; RD Prot, 1986/87, Bihang, Prop. 149, pp. 5–15, 37; 1986/87, Bihang, Socialutskottets betänkande 38. Surprisingly similar regulations (bright lighting, no cubicles) had been used against Italian ice-cream shops, those dens of iniquity, in Scotland early in the twentieth century. Roger Davidson, *Dangerous Liaisons: A Social History of Venereal Disease in Twentieth-Century Scotland* (Amsterdam, 2000), p. 31.

162. Martel, *Le rose et le noir*, p. 234.

163. King, *Safety in Numbers*, p. 40; Epstein, *Impure Science*, p. 97; Rotello, *Sexual Ecology*, p. 109; Odets, "Why We Do Not Do Primary Prevention," pp. 136–37; BT *Verhandlungen* 11/71, 14 April 1988, p. 4803C.

164. Duyvendak and Koopmans, "Resister au Sida," p. 212; Onno de Zwart, Theo Sandfort, and Marty van Kerkhof, "No Anal Sex Please: We're Dutch: A Dilemma in HIV Prevention Directed at Gay Men," in Sandfort, ed., *The Dutch Response to HIV: Pragmatism and Consensus* (London, 1998), pp. 135–36; King, *Safety in Numbers*, pp. 89–90; Patton, *Fatal Advice*, p. 106.

165. Rayside, *On the Fringe*, pp. 5–6; Mendelsohn, *Elusive Embrace*, pp. 30–35.

166. Jonsen and Stryker, *Social Impact*, p. 223; Duggan and Hunter, *Sex Wars*, pp. 101–6.

167. Warner, *Trouble with Normal*, chs. 2, 3.

168. Patton, *Inventing AIDS*, pp. 8, 14, 21–22; Michael Bartos, "Community vs. Population: The Case of Men Who Have Sex with Men," in Peter Aggleton et al., eds., *AIDS: Foundations for the Future* (London, 1994), pp. 86, 94; Adam, "Mobilizing around AIDS," p. 25; King, *Safety in Numbers*, pp. 203–5.

169. Ronald Bayer, "The Dependent Center: The First Decade of the AIDS Epidemic in New York City," in David Rosner, ed., *Hives of Sickness: Public Health and Epidemics in New York City* (New Brunswick, 1995), p. 134.

170. Rotello, *Sexual Ecology*, pp. 89, 202–3.

171. Miller, *Passion of Michel Foucault*.

172. Garfield, *End of Innocence*, p. 111; Luc Montagnier, *Vaincre le SIDA: Entretiens avec Pierre Bourget* (Paris, 1986), p. 145; Berridge, *AIDS in the UK*, p. 189; Street, "British Government Policy on AIDS," p. 503; Hirsch, *Le SIDA: Rumeurs et faits*, p. 42.

173. Patricia Day and Rudolf Klein, "Interpreting the Unexpected: The Case of AIDS Policy Making in Britain," *Journal of Public Policy* 9, 3 (1989), pp. 347, 350; RD Prot, 1985/86, Bihang, Socialutskottets betänkande 15, p. 17; 1988/89:105 (27

April 1989), pp. 13–14; 1986/87, Bihang, Socialutskottets betänkande 19, p. 27; 1987/88, Bihang, Prop. 79, p. 29; Peter Baldwin, "Beveridge in the Longue Durée," in John Hills et al., eds., *Beveridge and Social Security: An International Retrospective* (Oxford, 1994), p. 43.

174. Schäfer, "Die Deutsche AIDS-Hilfe," p. 71; Peter Scott, "White Noise: How Gay Men's Activism Gets Written Out of AIDS Prevention," in Joshua Oppenheimer and Helena Reckitt, eds., *Acting on AIDS: Sex, Drugs, and Politics* (London, 1997), pp. 313–15; King, *Safety in Numbers*, ch. 5; Rotello, *Sexual Ecology*, ch. 7, pp. 165–66, 176; Bayer, "Politics, Social Sciences, and HIV Prevention," 1:43–44.

175. Glasson, "Public Health and Human Rights," p. 238; Simon Watney, "The Spectacle of AIDS," in Douglas Crimp, ed., *AIDS: Cultural Analysis, Cultural Activism* (Cambridge, 1988), p. 72; Garfield, *End of Innocence*, pp. 130–31, 226.

176. S. A. Månsson, "Psycho-Social Aspects of HIV Testing: The Swedish Case," *AIDS Care* 2, 1 (1990), p. 8; Benny Henriksson, *Social Democracy or Societal Control? A Critical Analysis of Swedish AIDS Policy* (Stockholm, 1988), p. 17; Don C. Des Jarlais et al., "Targeting HIV-Prevention Programs," *New England Journal of Medicine* 331, 21 (1994), p. 1451.

177. One of the themes of Peter Baldwin, *The Politics of Social Solidarity: Class Bases of the European Welfare State, 1875–1975* (Cambridge, 1990).

178. Michael Fumento, *The Myth of Heterosexual AIDS* (New York, 1990), p. 211; Canaris, "Gesundheitspolitische Aspekte," p. 293; Richard A. Mohr, "AIDS, Gays, and State Coercion," *Bioethics* 1, 1 (1987), pp. 35–38.

179. Berridge, *AIDS in the UK*, pp. 237–40; Pollak, *Les homosexuels et le sida*, pp. 162–64; Reutter, "Aids, Politik und Demokratie," p. 12.

180. House of Commons, *Problems Associated with AIDS*, vol. 3, pp. 141–47; Rotello, *Sexual Ecology*, p. 115.

181. *Los Angeles Times*, 14 January 2000, p. A13; Smith, "AIDS and Minority Health," p. 102.

182. Peterson, "Black Men and Their Same-Sex Desires," p. 150; Gregory M. Herek and Eric K. Glunt, "AIDS-Related Attitudes in the United States: A Preliminary Conceptualization," *Journal of Sex Research* 28, 1 (1991), p. 111; Harlon L. Dalton, "AIDS in Blackface," *Dædalus* 118, 3 (summer 1989), p. 211; Barbara G. Sosnowitz, "AIDS Prevention, Minority Women, and Gender Assertiveness," in Beth E. Schneider and Nancy E. Stoller, eds., *Women Resisting AIDS: Feminist Strategies of Empowerment* (Philadelphia, 1995), pp. 140–41; Benjamin P. Bowser, "HIV Prevention and African Americans: A Difference of Class," in Johannes P. Van Vugt, ed., *AIDS Prevention and Services: Community Based Research* (Westport, 1994), pp. 94–95.

183. *Congressional Record* (Senate), 1 August 1986, 132, pp. 18692–96; Quimby, "Anthropological Witnessing," p. 170; Daniel M. Fox, "Chronic Disease and Disadvantage: The New Politics of HIV Infection," *Journal of Health Politics, Policy, and Law* 15, 2 (summer 1990), p. 348.

184. Harlon L. Dalton, "AIDS in Blackface," *Dædalus* 118, 3 (summer 1989),

pp. 209–11; Cohen, "Power, Resistance, and the Construction of Crisis," pp. 430–35; Fox, "Chronic Disease and Disadvantage," p. 348.

185. Philipson and Posner, *Private Choices and Public Health*, p. 204.

186. France Lert, "Drug Use, AIDS, and Social Exclusion in France," in Jean-Paul Moatti et al., eds., *AIDS in Europe: New Challenges for the Social Sciences* (London, 2000), p. 197; Benny Jose et al., "Collective Organisation of Injecting Drug Users and the Struggle against AIDS," in Tim Rhodes and Richard Hartnoll, eds., *AIDS, Drugs, and Prevention* (London, 1996), p. 221; Czada and Friedrich-Czada, "Aids als politisches Konfliktfeld," p. 261; Pollak, "Organizing the Fight," p. 36; Samuel R. Friedman et al., "Organizing Drug Users against AIDS," in Joan Huber and Beth E. Schneider, eds., *The Social Context of AIDS* (Newbury Park, CA, 1992), p. 116; Curtis Price, "AIDS, Organization of Drug Users, and Public Policy," *AIDS and Public Policy Journal* 7, 3 (1992), pp. 143; Samuel R. Friedman and Cathy Casriel, "Drug Users' Organisations and AIDS Policy," *AIDS and Public Policy Journal* 3, 2 (1987), pp. 31–35; Werner Hermann, "JES: History, Demands, and Future," in AIDS-Forum D.A.H., *Aspects of AIDS and AIDS-Hilfe in Germany* (Berlin, 1993), pp. 65–74.

187. Etheridge, *Sentinel for Health*, p. 332; Danièle Carricaburu, "L'Association Française des Hémophiles face au danger de contamination par le virus du sida: Stratégie de normalisation de la maladie et définition collective du risque," *Sciences sociales et santé* 11, 3–4 (1993), pp. 64–65; Stephan Dressler, "Blood 'Scandal' and AIDS in Germany," in Eric Feldman and Ronald Bayer, eds., *Blood Feuds: AIDS, Blood, and the Politics of Medical Disaster* (New York, 1999), p. 196; Hans Halter, " 'Das Unrecht, das einem einzelnen widerfährt, ist eine Bedrohung für alle': Zur Situation der HIV-infizierten Hämophilen in Frankreich und Deutschland," *AIDS-Forschung* 2 (1993), pp. 63–64.

188. Anne-Marie Casteret, *L'affaire du sang* (Paris, 1992), p. 209; Pollak, "Organizing the Fight," p. 36; Altman, *Power and Community*, p. 21; David Kirp, "The Politics of Blood: Hemophilia Activism in the AIDS Crisis," in Eric Feldman and Ronald Bayer, eds., *Blood Feuds: AIDS, Blood, and the Politics of Medical Disaster* (New York, 1999), pp. 302–5.

189. Becker and Beisswenger, *Solidarität der Uneinsichtigen*, pp. 40–41.

190. Virginia van der Vliet, *The Politics of AIDS* (London, 1996), pp. 102–3; J. N. Hays, *The Burdens of Disease: Epidemics and Human Response in Western History* (New Brunswick, 1998), p. 302.

191. Jacques du Guerny and Elisabeth Sjöberg, "Interrelationship between Gender Relations and the HIV/AIDS Epidemic," in Jonathan M. Mann et al., eds., *Health and Human Rights* (New York, 1999), pp. 202–5; Priscilla R. Ulin et al., "Bargaining for Life: Women and the AIDS Epidemic in Haiti," in Lynellyn D. Long and E. Maxine Ankrah, eds., *Women's Experiences with HIV/AIDS* (New York, 1996), pp. 98–102.

192. *RD Prot*, 1986/87:109 (23 April 1987), p. 143; Nan D. Hunter, "Complications of Gender: Women and HIV Disease," in Nan D. Hunter and William B. Rubenstein, eds., *AIDS Agenda: Emerging Issues in Civil Rights* (New York, 1992), p. 7; Mann and Tarantola, *AIDS in the World II*, pp. 196–200.

193. Burkett, *Gravest Show on Earth,* p. 208; *Congressional Record* (Senate), 15 May 1990, p. 6224.

194. Stein, *Social Welfare,* pp. ix, 7, 42; Bury, "Women and HIV/AIDS: Medical Issues," pp. 35–37; Goldstein and Manlowe, *Gender Politics;* Burkett, *Gravest Show on Earth,* pp. 192–93; Arno and Feiden, *Against the Odds,* pp. 200–202; Christopher H. Foreman Jr., *Plagues, Products, and Politics: Emergent Public Health Hazards and National Policymaking* (Washington, DC, 1994), pp. 49–50. Generally: Cindy Patton, *Last Served? Gendering the HIV Pandemic* (London, 1994).

195. Wilton, *EnGendering AIDS,* pp. 92, 102.

9. VOX POPULI SUPREMA LEX EST: EXPERTISE, AUTHORITY, AND DEMOCRACY

1. Stanislav Andreski, *Syphilis, Puritanism, and Witch Hunts* (London, 1989); Alan Mayne, " 'The Dreadful Scourge': Responses to Smallpox in Sydney and Melbourne, 1881–82," in Roy Macleod and Milton Lewis, eds., *Disease, Medicine, and Empire* (London, 1988), p. 226; Nayan Shah, *Contagious Divides: Epidemics and Race in San Francisco's Chinatown* (Berkeley, 2001); František Graus, *Pest- Geissler- Judenmorde: Das 14. Jahrhundert als Krisenzeit* (Göttingen, 1987).

2. Richard Goldstein, "AIDS and the Social Contract," in Erica Carter and Simon Watney, eds., *Taking Liberties* (London, 1989), p. 84; James W. Jones, "Discourses on and of AIDS in West Germany, 1986–90," in John C. Fout, ed., *Forbidden History* (Chicago, 1992), pp. 364–65.

3. BT *Verhandlungen* 10/114, 17 January 1985, p. 8505C; 10/187, 16 January 1986, p. 14234A; William A. Rushing, *The AIDS Epidemic: Social Dimensions of an Infectious Disease* (Boulder, 1995), pp. 156–58; Michael L. Closen et al., *AIDS: Cases and Materials* (Houston, 1989), p. 183; Ian Young, *The AIDS Dissidents: An Annotated Bibliography* (Metuchen, NJ, 1993), p. 56; Michael Fumento, *The Myth of Heterosexual AIDS* (New York, 1990), p. 108; Jacob Segal and Lilli Segal, *AIDS: Die Spur führt ins Pentagon* (Essen, 1990); Leonard G. Horowitz, *Emerging Viruses: AIDS and Ebola: Nature, Accident, or Intentional?* (Rockport, MA, 1997).

4. Closen, *AIDS,* p. 77; Fumento, *Myth of Heterosexual AIDS,* p. 200; Randy Shilts, *And the Band Played On: Politics, People, and the AIDS Epidemic* (New York, 1988), p. 309; Günter Grau, *AIDS: Krankheit oder Katastrophe?* (Berlin, 1990), p. 101.

5. Vagn Greve and Annika Snare, *AIDS: Nogle retspolitiske spørgsmål,* 5th ed. (Copenhagen, 1987), p. 7; House of Commons, 1986–87, Social Services Committee, *Problems Associated with AIDS,* 13 May 1987, vol. 3, pp. 180–81; Albert R. Jonsen and Jeff Stryker, eds., *The Social Impact of AIDS in the United States* (Washington, DC, 1993), p. 131; Johannes Gründel, "AIDS—eine ethische Herausforderung an die Christen," in Bistum Essen, ed., *AIDS—eine medizinische und eine moralische Herausforderung* (Nettetal, n.d.), pp. 39–40, 66;

Charles Perrow and Mauro F. Guillén, *The AIDS Disaster: The Failure of Organizations in New York and the Nation* (New Haven, 1990), pp. 98–101; Barbara Venrath, *AIDS, die soziale Definition einer Krankheit* (Oldenburg, 1994), pp. 167–68; Patricia L. Jakobi, "Medical Science, Christian Fundamentalism, and the Etiology of AIDS," *AIDS and Public Policy Journal* 5, 2 (1990).

6. Jean-François Revel, "AIDS and Political Manipulation," in Charles Mérieux, ed., *SIDA: Épidémies et sociétés* (n.p., 1987), p. 36; Renée Sabatier, *Blaming Others: Prejudice, Race, and Worldwide AIDS* (London, 1988), pp. 110–14; Mukesh Kapila and Maryan J. Pye, "The European Response to AIDS," in Jaime Sepulveda et al., eds., *AIDS: Prevention through Education* (New York, 1992), p. 215; Mary Haour-Knipe, "Prévention du sida ou discrimination? Les migrants et les minorités ethniques," in Nathalie Bajos et al., *Le sida en Europe: Nouveaux enjeux pour les sciences sociales* (Paris, 1998), pp. 164–65.

7. Sander L. Gilman, "AIDS and Syphilis: The Iconography of Disease," in Douglas Crimp, ed., *AIDS: Cultural Analysis, Cultural Activism* (Cambridge, 1988), pp. 100–101; Elaine Showalter, *Sexual Anarchy: Gender and Culture at the Fin de Siècle* (New York, 1990), p. 190; Michael Pollak, *Les homosexuels et le sida: Sociologie d'une épidémie* (Paris, 1988), p. 145; Sander Gilman, *Disease and Representation: Images of Illness from Madness to AIDS* (Ithaca, 1988), pp. 262–66; Virginia Berridge, *AIDS in the UK: The Making of Policy, 1981–1994* (Oxford, 1996), p. 116.

8. Jonathan Mann, "Facteurs epidemiologiques et impact social," in Charles Mérieux, ed., *SIDA: Épidémies et sociétés* (n.p., 1987), p. 45; Sunil Gupta, "No Solutions," in Tessa Boffin and Sunil Gupta, eds., *Ecstatic Antibodies: Resisting the AIDS Mythology* (London, 1990), p. 103; Katharine Park, "Kimberly Bergalis, AIDS, and the Plague Metaphor," in Marjorie Garber et al., eds., *Media Spectacles* (New York, 1993), p. 244.

9. Henning Machein, "Mythen sterben langsam: Aids in Mali," in Anja Bestmann et al., eds., *Aids—weltweit und dichtdran* (Saarbrücken, 1997), pp. 185–86; Sarah N. Qureshi, "Global Ostracism of HIV-Positive Aliens: International Restrictions Barring HIV-Positive Aliens," *Maryland Journal of International Law and Trade* 19 (1995), p. 116; Dana Lear, "AIDS in the African Press," in David Buchanan and George Cernada, eds., *Progress in Preventing AIDS? Dogma, Dissent, and Innovation* (Amityville, NY, 1998), p. 222.

10. Vera Boltho-Massarelli and Michael O'Boyle, "Droits de l'homme et santé publique, une nouvelle alliance," in Eric Heilmann, ed., *Sida et libertés: La régulation d'une épidemie dans un état de droit* (n.p., 1991), p. 58; *Congressional Record* (Senate), 10 July 1991, p. 9476.

11. Institute of Medicine, *Confronting AIDS: Directions for Public Health, Health Care, and Research* (Washington, DC, 1986), p. 127; Nicholas Freudenberg, "AIDS Prevention in the United States: Lessons from the First Decade," *International Journal of Health Services* 20, 4 (1990), p. 591; Arnold J. Rosoff, "The AIDS Crisis: Constitutional Turning Point?," *Law, Medicine, and Health Care* 15, 1–2 (summer 1987), p. 83; Ronald Bayer and David L. Kirp, "The United States: At the Center of the Storm," in Kirp and Bayer, eds., *AIDS in the*

Industrialized Democracies (New Brunswick, 1992), pp. 25–26; Nancy Ford and Michael D. Quam, "AIDS Quarantine: The Legal and Practical Implications," *Journal of Legal Medicine* 8, 3 (1987), p. 392.

12. Willy H. Eirmbter et al., *AIDS und die gesellschaftliche Folgen* (Frankfurt, 1993), pp. 107–9; Guenter Frankenberg, "Germany: The Uneasy Triumph of Pragmatism," Ronald Bayer and David L. Kirp, eds., *AIDS in the Industrialized Democracies* (New Brunswick, 1992), p. 112; Swiss Institute of Comparative Law, *Comparative Study on Discrimination against Persons with HIV or AIDS* (Strasbourg, 1993), p. 16; BT *Verhandlungen* 11/8, 2 April 1987, p. 428D.

13. Berridge, *AIDS in the UK*, pp. 84, 134; Memo by Dr. Ronald Bolton, House of Commons, *Problems Associated with AIDS*, vol. 3, pp. 206–11; *Hansard Parliamentary Debates*, vol. 144 (13 January 1989), col. 1158.

14. *Le Monde*, 2 June 1987, p. 9; Michel Setbon, *Pouvoirs contre SIDA: De la transfusion sanguine au dépistage: Decisions et pratiques en France, Grande-Bretagne et Suède* (Paris, 1993), p. 181; J. P. Moatti et al., "Social Perception of AIDS in the General Public: A French Study," *Health Policy* 9 (1988), p. 5.

15. Greve and Snare, *AIDS*, p. 18; Erik Albæk, "Denmark: AIDS and the Political 'Pink Triangle,'" in Ronald Bayer and David L. Kirp, eds., *AIDS in the Industrialized Democracies* (New Brunswick, 1992), p. 300; *RD Prot*, 1986/87:109 (23 April 1987), p. 140; 1986/87, Bihang, Prop. 2, p. 23; 1985/86, Bihang, Socialutskottets betänkande 15, pp. 3, 16–17.

16. *RD Prot*, 1988/89, Bihang, Prop. 5, pp. 26, 51, 54; 1986/87, Bihang, Prop. 2, p. 23.

17. Claude-B. Blouin et al., *Sida Story* (Paris, 1986), pp. 50–51; Gérard Bach-Ignasse, "Le Sida et la vie politique française," in Michael Pollak et al., eds., *Homosexualités et Sida* (n.p., n.d. [1991]), p. 96; Claudine Herzlich and Janine Pierret, "Une maladie dans l'espace public: Le sida dans six quotidiens français," *Annales, ESC*, 43, 5 (1988), p. 1123; Michel Danti-Juan, "Quelques reflexions en droit penal français sur les problemes posés par le sida," *Revue de droit penal et de criminologie* 68 (1988), p. 631; Ute Canaris, "Gesundheitspolitische Aspekte im Zusammenhang mit AIDS," in Johannes Korporal and Hubert Malouschek, eds., *Leben mit AIDS—Mit AIDS leben* (Hamburg, 1987), p. 295; Jean-Paul Moatti, "Les nouveaux enjeux pour les sciences socio-comportementales face à l'épidémie de sida," in Nathalie Bajos et al., *Le sida en Europe: Nouveaux enjeux pour les sciences sociales* (Paris, 1998), p. 59.

18. Dominique Brenky and Olivia Zémor, *La route du SIDA* (Paris, 1985), p. 170; Michael Kirby, "AIDS and the Law," *Dædalus* 118, 3 (summer 1989), p. 113; Joseph Wayne Smith, *AIDS, Philosophy, and Beyond: Philosophical Dilemmas of a Modern Pandemic* (Aldershot, U.K., 1991), pp. 119–22.

19. Aran Ron and David E. Rogers, "AIDS in the United States: Patient Care and Politics," *Dædalus* 118, 2 (spring 1989), p. 45; Greve and Snare, *AIDS*, p. 75; Luc Montagnier, *Vaincre le SIDA: Entretiens avec Pierre Bourget* (Paris, 1986), p. 148; Lill Scherdin, "AIDS in Prisons in Norway," in Philip A. Thomas and Martin Moerings, eds., *AIDS in Prison* (Aldershot, U.K., 1994), p. 11; Wolf-Rüdiger Schenke, "Die Bekämpfung von AIDS als verfassungsrechtliches und

polizeirechtliches Problem," in Bernd Schünemann and Gerd Pfeiffer, eds., *Die Rechtsprobleme von AIDS* (Baden-Baden, 1988), p. 142; Kuno Kruse, "AIDS in den Medien," in Johannes Korporal and Hubert Malouschek, eds., *Leben mit AIDS—Mit AIDS leben* (Hamburg, 1987), p. 313; René Martin, *Eine Krankheit zum Tode: Aids in der deutschsprachigen Literatur* (St. Ingbert, 1995), pp. 304–5; Benny Henriksson, "Aids—föreställningar om en verklighet," in Henriksson, ed., *Aids: Föreställningar om en verklighet* (Stockholm, 1987), p. 64; Simon Watney, *Practices of Freedom: Selected Writings on HIV/AIDS* (Durham, NC, 1994), p. 191; Fritz Erik Hoevels, *Zwischen Monogamie-Propaganda und grünem Licht für Virus-Überträger: Tabuthema AIDS-Stop* (Freiburg, 1986), p. 23; Johann Singhartinger, *AIDS als Anlass—Kontrolle als Konzept: Entwicklungen am Beispiel Strafvollzug* (Munich, 1987), p. 73.

20. Roger Ingham, "AIDS: Knowledge, Awareness, and Attitudes," in John Cleland and Benoît Ferry, eds., *Sexual Behavior and AIDS in the Developing World* (London, 1995), p. 69; Douglas Webb, *HIV and AIDS in Africa* (London, 1997), pp. 167–68; Jakobi, "Medical Science, Christian Fundamentalism, and the Etiology of AIDS," p. 90; Grau, *AIDS*, p. 10; C. Everett Koop, *Koop: The Memoirs of America's Family Doctor* (New York, 1991), p. 208.

21. Rita Süssmuth, *AIDS: Wege aus der Angst* (Hamburg, 1987), p. 27; Olli Stålström and Outi Lithén, "AIDS in Finland," in Martin Breum and Aart Hendriks, eds., *AIDS and Human Rights* (Copenhagen, 1988), pp. 46–47; Closen, *AIDS*, p. 182; Martti Grönfors and Olli Stålström, "Power, Prestige, Profit: AIDS and the Oppression of Homosexual People," *Acta Sociologica* 30, 1 (1987), p. 58.

22. Wolfgang Steinke et al., "Die seuchenpolitische Reaktion auf die HIV/AIDS-Epidemie in der Schweiz," *AIDS-Forschung* 1 (1994), p. 15.

23. Carl F. Stychin, *Law's Desire: Sexuality and the Limits of Justice* (London, 1995), ch. 2; Jonathan Glasson, "Public Health and Human Rights: Finding a Balance in HIV Prevention," in David FitzSimons et al., eds., *The Economic and Social Impact of AIDS in Europe* (London, 1995), p. 238; Noel Annan, *Our Age: Portrait of a Generation* (London, 1990), p. 152; Peter M. Davies et al., *Sex, Gay Men, and AIDS* (London, 1993), pp. 31–32; *Hansard* (15 December 1987), col. 1000–01, 1009–10, 1022.

24. Arnaud Mercier, "Les médias comme espace scénique," in Pierre Favre, ed., *Sida et politique: Les premiers affrontements (1981–1987)* (Paris, 1992), p. 116; Susan Sontag, *AIDS and Its Metaphors* (New York, 1988), p. 62; Jean-Marie Guffens and Caroline Guffens, "Guerre et folie, Guerre et SIDA," in Jean-Marie Guffens, ed., *Toxicomanie, Hépatites, S.I.D.A.* (n.p., 1994), p. 24. Though anti-Semitism did also leave a trace in attacks by blacks in the United States on the medical establishment, another alleged bastion of Jewish hegemony. Fumento, *Myth of Heterosexual AIDS*, p. 138. Even among people with AIDS, with one group accusing another of delaying distribution of AL721, one of many failed therapies on which the sick staked hopes, anti-Semitic canards were put to use. Arthur D. Kahn, *AIDS, The Winter War* (Philadelphia, 1993), p. 91.

25. Maurice Tournier et al., *SIDA'venture: SIDA, Ethique, Discriminations*

(Paris, 1989), pp. 9–11, 18. The National Front's term for AIDS patients, *sidaique* was taken to echo that for Jews, *hébraique*.

26. *Le Monde*, 16 April 1987; 3 December 1986, p. 36; François Bachelot and Pierre Lorane, *Une société au risque du sida* (Paris, 1988), pp. 22, 52–53, 265–87; Pollak, *Les homosexuels*, pp. 167–68; Michael Pollak, "AIDS Policy in France: Biomedical Leadership and Preventive Impotence," in Barbara A. Misztal and David Moss, eds., *Action on AIDS: National Policies in Comparative Perspective* (New York, 1990), p. 95; Patrick Wachsmann, "Le Sida ou la gestion de la peur par l'état de droit," in Daniel Borrillo and Anne Masseran, eds., *Sida et droits de l'homme: L'épidémie dans un Etat de droit* (Strasbourg, 1991), pp. 15–16; Michel Hastings, "La rhétorique hygiéniste de Jean-Marie Le Pen," *Revue politique et parlementaire* 90, 933 (1988), pp. 55–58; Frédéric Martel, *Le rose et le noir: Les homosexuels en France depuis 1968* (Paris, 1996), p. 285. Similar opinions could also be heard from renegade Gaullists. *Le Monde*, 23 December 1991, p. 8.

27. Nicolas Mauriac, *Le mal entendu: Le sida et les médias* (Paris, 1990), pp. 141–43; Bernard Seytre, *Sida: Les secrets d'une polémique* (Paris, 1993), pp. 24–25; Bernard Paillard, *Notes on the Plague Years: AIDS in Marseilles* (New York, 1998), p. 23. Lyndon LaRouche was probably the closest one came to this in the English-speaking world.

28. Vagn Greve and Annika Snare, "Retssystemet v. Aids?" *Retfærd* 9, 34 (1986), p. 15; J. N. Hays, *The Burdens of Disease: Epidemics and Human Response in Western History* (New Brunswick, 1998), p. 297; *Hansard*, vol. 90 (29 January 1986), col. 793.

29. *Hansard*, vol. 122 (10 November 1987), col. 107; James D. Slack, *AIDS and the Public Work Force: Local Government Preparedness in Managing the Epidemic* (Tuscaloosa, 1991), p. 3; Marco Pulver, *Tribut der Seuche oder: Seuchenmythen als Quelle sozialer Kalibrierung: Eine Rekonstruktion des AIDS-Diskurses vor dem Hintergrund von Studien zur Historizität des Seuchendispositivs* (Frankfurt, 1999), p. 459; C. Manuel et al., "The Ethical Approach to AIDS: A Bibliographical Review," *Journal of Medical Ethics* 16 (1990), p. 14.

30. BT *Drucksache* 11/274, 14 May 1987, p. 2; Frank Rühmann, *AIDS: Eine Krankheit und ihre Folgen*, 2d ed. (Frankfurt, 1985), pp. 77–80, 93; Canaris, "Gesundheitspolitische Aspekte," p. 278; Kruse, "AIDS in den Medien," p. 310; Edward Albert, "Illness and Deviance: The Response of the Press to AIDS," in Douglas A. Feldman and Thomas M. Johnson, eds., *The Social Dimensions of AIDS* (New York, 1986), pp. 168–76;

31. Seymour Martin Lipset, *Political Man: The Social Bases of Politics*, exp. ed. (Baltimore, 1981), pp. 127–152; Richard Hamilton, *Who Voted for Hitler?* (Princeton, 1982), chs. 1–3, 14; Thomas Childers, *The Nazi Voter: The Social Foundations of Fascism in Germany, 1919–1933* (Chapel Hill, 1983), pp. 262–69; Peter Baldwin, "Social Interpretations of Nazism: Renewing a Tradition," *Journal of Contemporary History* 25, 1 (January 1990).

32. Michael Pollak and Jean-Paul Moatti, "HIV Risk Perception and Deter-

minants of Sexual Behavior," in Michel Hubert, ed., *Sexual Behaviour and Risks of HIV Infection* (Brussels, 1990), pp. 32–34; Michael Pollak, "Attitudes, Beliefs, and Opinions," in Pollak, ed. *AIDS: A Problem for Sociological Research* (London, 1992), p. 29; Michael Pollak et al., "Systèmes de réaction au SIDA et action préventive," *Sciences sociales et santé* 7, 1 (1989), pp. 116–21; Elizabeth Ioannidi and Michael Haeder, "Attitudes towards People with HIV/AIDS," in Michel Hubert et al., eds., *Sexual Behaviour and HIV/AIDS in Europe* (London, 1998), p. 373; Eirmbter, *AIDS*, pp. 34, 38; Rüdiger Jacob, *Krankheitsbilder und Deutungsmuster: Wissen über Krankheit und dessen Bedeutung für die Praxis* (Opladen, 1995), pp. 165–69; Rüdiger Jacob et al., *Aids-Vorstellungen in Deutschland: Stabilität und Wandel* (Berlin, 1997), pp. 68, 141; Canaris, "Gesundheitspolitische Aspekte," p. 296; Gregory M. Herek and Eric K. Glunt, "AIDS-Related Attitudes in the United States: A Preliminary Conceptualization," *Journal of Sex Research* 28, 1 (1991), pp. 111–13; Robert Allard, "Beliefs about AIDS as Determinants of Preventive Practices and of Support for Coercive Measures," *American Journal of Public Health* 79, 4 (1989), p. 450; Beth A. Le Poire et al., "Who Wants to Quarantine Persons with AIDS? Patterns of Support for California's Proposition 64," *Social Science Quarterly* 71, 2 (1990); Claes Herlitz and Bengt Brorsson, "AIDS in the Minds of Swedish People: 1986–1989," *AIDS* 4 (1990), p. 1014.

33. Achim Hättich et al., "Predictors of Discrimination against AIDS Patients and Cancer Patients: A Multivariate Comparison," in Dorothee Friedrich and Wolfgang Heckmann, eds., *Aids in Europe: The Behavioural Aspect* (Berlin, 1995), 5:235–41.

34. Barry D. Adam, "Sociology and People Living with AIDS," in Joan Huber and Beth E. Schneider, eds., *The Social Context of AIDS* (Newbury Park, CA, 1992), p. 12; Ronald Bayer, "Politics, Social Sciences, and HIV Prevention in the United States," in Dorothee Friedrich and Wolfgang Heckmann, eds., *Aids in Europe: The Behavioural Aspect* (Berlin, 1995), 1:46–47; Roland Czada and Heidi Friedrich-Czada, "Aids als politisches Konfliktfeld und Verwaltungsproblem," in Rolf Rosenbrock and Andreas Salmen, eds., *Aids-Prävention* (Berlin, 1990), p. 257.

35. Dorothy Nelkin and Stephen Hilgartner, "Disputed Dimensions of Risk: A Public School Controversy over AIDS," *Milbank Quarterly* 64, suppl. 1 (1986), pp. 118 ff; Virginia Berridge and Philip Strong, "AIDS in the UK: Contemporary History and the Study of Policy," *Twentieth Century British History* 2, 2 (1991), p. 152.

36. Norbert Schmacke, "Aids und Seuchengesetze," in Cornelius Prittwitz, ed., *Aids, Recht und Gesundheitspolitik* (Berlin, 1990), p. 17; Barbara A. Misztal, "AIDS in Australia: Diffusion of Power and Making of Policy," in Misztal and David Moss, eds., *Action on AIDS: National Policies in Comparative Perspective* (New York, 1990), p. 205.

37. House of Commons, *Problems Associated with AIDS*, vol. 3, pp. 23–25; Patricia Day and Rudolf Klein, "Interpreting the Unexpected: The Case of AIDS Policy Making in Britain," *Journal of Public Policy* 9, 3 (1989), p. 346.

38. Sheila M. Rothman, *Living in the Shadow of Death: Tuberculosis and the Social Experience of Illness in American History* (New York, 1994), p. 189; John Duffy, *A History of Public Health in New York City, 1625–1866* (New York, 1968), pp. 102–3.

39. In Britain, home tests were forbidden by the 1988 Health and Medicines Act, 1988 c 49, sect. 23.

40. "Entschliessung der 63. Konferenz der für das Gesundheitswesen zuständigen Minister und Senatoren der Länder vom 22. bis 23. November 1990 in Berlin," *AIDS-Forschung* 6, 1 (January 1991), p. 28.

41. House of Commons, *Problems Associated with AIDS*, vol. 2, pp. 64–77; Berridge, *AIDS in the UK*, p. 138; "Stellungnahme der Deutschen Gesellschaft für Innere Medizin zu AIDS," *AIDS-Forschung* 7 (1989), p. 379.

42. Michael Kirby, "The Ten Paradoxes of AIDS: Summing Up the Conference," in Alan F. Fleming et al., *The Global Impact of AIDS* (New York, 1988), p. 397; Day and Klein, "Interpreting the Unexpected," pp. 351–52.

43. *Le Monde*, 1 July 1987, p. 15e.

44. Sev S. Fluss, "National AIDS Legislation: An Overview of Some Global Developments," in Lawrence Gostin and Lane Porter, eds., *International Law and AIDS* (n.p., 1992), pp. 4–6.

45. Sandro Cattacin, "Organisatorische Probleme der HIV/AIDS-Politik in föderalen Staaten: Deutschland, Österreich und Schweiz im Vergleich," *Journal für Sozialforschung* 36, 1 (1996), p. 74.

46. Day and Klein, "Interpreting the Unexpected," pp. 347, 349–52; Daniel M. Fox, Patricia Day, and Rudolf Klein, "The Power of Professionalism: Policies for AIDS in Britain, Sweden, and the United States," *Dædalus* 118, 2 (spring 1989), passim; Neil Small, "The Changing Context of Health Care in the UK: Implications for HIV/AIDS," in Peter Aggleton et al., eds., *AIDS: Foundations for the Future* (London, 1994), p. 24; Berridge, *AIDS in the UK*, pp. 55, 150–51.

47. John Street and Albert Weale, "Britain: Policy-Making in a Hermetically Sealed System," in Ronald Bayer and David L. Kirp, eds., *AIDS in the Industrialized Democracies* (New Brunswick, 1992), p. 215; John Street, "A Fall in Interest? British AIDS Policy, 1986–1990," in Virginia Berridge and Philip Strong, eds., *AIDS and Contemporary History* (Cambridge, 1993), pp. 234–35; Berridge, *AIDS in the UK*, pp. 84, 134; Chris Bennett and Ewan Ferlie, *Managing Crisis and Change in Health Care: The Organizational Response to HIV/AIDS* (Buckingham, 1994), pp. 60–70.

48. *Le Monde*, 30 June 1987, p. 18d; 16 April 1987.

49. *Le Monde*, 11 December 1987, p. 10e; Pierre Mathiot, "Le sida dans la stratégie et la rhétorique du Front national," in Pierre Favre, ed., *Sida et politique: Les premiers affrontements (1981–1987)* (Paris, 1992), p. 199; Monika Steffen, "AIDS Policies in France," in Virginia Berridge and Philip Strong, eds., *AIDS and Contemporary History* (Cambridge, 1993), p. 253; Jean de Savigny, *Le Sida et les fragilités françaises: Nos réactions face à l'épidémie* (Paris, 1995), pp. 217–18; Martel, *Le rose et le noir*, p. 285.

50. Monika Steffen, "France: Social Solidarity and Scientific Expertise," in

Ronald Bayer and David L. Kirp, eds., *AIDS in the Industrialized Democracies* (New Brunswick, 1992), p. 221; *Le Monde*, 17 December 1988, p. 1.

51. Monika Steffen, *The Fight against AIDS: An International Public Policy Comparison between Four European Countries: France, Great Britain, Germany, and Italy* (Grenoble, 1996), pp. 42, 47; Setbon, *Pouvoirs contre SIDA*, p. 186; Monika Steffen, "AIDS and Political Systems," in Dorothee Friedrich and Wolfgang Heckmann, eds., *Aids in Europe: The Behavioural Aspect* (Berlin, 1995), 5:31–34.

52. Werner Reutter, "Aids, Politik und Demokratie: Ein Vergleich aids-politischer Massnahmen in Deutschland und Frankreich," Wissenschaftszentrum Berlin für Sozialforschung, *Veröffentlichungsreihe der Forschungsgruppe Gesundheitsrisiken und Präventionspolitik*, P92–205 (Berlin, April 1992), pp. 28, 31; Wolfgang Haug, "Das historische Syphilis-Paradigma und die Gefahr eines analogen AIDS-Paradigmas der Moral," in *AIDS: Fakten und Konsequenzen: Endbericht der Enquête-Kommission des 11. Deutschen Bundestages "Gefahren von AIDS und wirksame Wege zu ihrer Eindämmung"* (Bonn, 1990), p. 88.

53. BT *Verhandlungen* 11/8, 2 April 1987, p. 429A; Canaris, "Gesundheits-politische Aspekte," p. 299.

54. Larry Gostin, "The Politics of AIDS: Compulsory State Powers, Public Health, and Civil Liberties," *Ohio State Law Journal* 49 (1989), p. 1019.

55. Timothy F. Murphy, *Ethics in an Epidemic: AIDS, Morality, and Culture* (Berkeley, 1994), p. 131; *AIDS-Nachrichten aus Forschung und Wissenschaft*, 3 (1991), pp. 1–2; *Congressional Record* (House), 24 April 1991, p. 2476; Michael L. Closen and Mark E. Wojcik, "Living with HIV and without Discrimination," in Lawrence Gostin and Lane Porter, eds., *International Law and AIDS* (n.p., 1992), pp. 157–59; Robert M. Wachter, *The Fragile Coalition: Scientists, Activists, and AIDS* (New York, 1991), pp. 113–15, 124–25, 134.

56. *Congressional Record* (House), 11 March 1993, pp. 1206–8; (Senate) 17 February 1993, pp. 1709–10.

57. David L. Kirp et al., *Learning by Heart: AIDS and Schoolchildren in America's Communities* (New Brunswick, 1989), p. 23; Nelkin and Hilgartner, "Disputed Dimensions of Risk," pp. 118 ff.

58. Simmy Viinikka, "Children, Young People, and HIV Infection," in Richard Haigh and Dai Harris, eds., *AIDS: A Guide to the Law*, 2d ed. (London, 1995), p. 19; Simon Garfield, *The End of Innocence: Britain in the Time of AIDS* (London, 1994), p. 71; AIDES, *Droit et S.I.D.A.: Guide juridique*, 3d ed. (Paris, 1996), p. 224.

59. Daniel T. Rodgers, *Atlantic Crossings: Social Politics in a Progressive Age* (Cambridge, MA, 1998), ch. 4; Susan Wade Peabody, *Historical Study of Legislation Regarding Public Health in the States of New York and Massachusetts* (Chicago, 1909), p. 34.

60. Lois M. Takahashi, *Homelessness, AIDS, and Stigmatization: The NIMBY Syndrome in the United States at the End of the Twentieth Century* (Oxford, 1998), pp. 49–51 and passim; Jane Balin, *A Neighborhood Divided: Community Resistance to an AIDS Care Facility* (Ithaca, 1999).

61. Though, of course, there were examples of objections raised by neighbors in European cities: to hospices for AIDS patients in Rome: *Sida et toxicomanie: Répondre: Actes du colloque international organisé par FIRST* (Paris, 1989), p. 67. In Glasgow to needle exchanges: Martin C. Donoghoe et al., *Syringe-Exchange in England* (London, 1992), p. 7. And in Switzerland to drug treatment centers: Dominique Malatesta et al., "Between Public Health and Public Order: Harm Reduction Facilities and Neighbourhood Problems," in Jean-Paul Moatti et al., eds., *AIDS in Europe: New Challenges for the Social Sciences* (London, 2000), pp. 178–87.

62. C. Everett Koop, "The Early Days of AIDS As I Remember Them," in Caroline Hannaway et al., eds., *AIDS and the Public Debate* (Amsterdam, 1995); Charles Backstrom and Leonard Robins, "State AIDS Policy Making: Perspectives of Legislative Health Committee Chairs," *AIDS and Public Policy Journal* 10, 4 (1995–96), p. 247.

63. J. Rogers Hollingsworth, *A Political Economy of Medicine: Great Britain and the United States* (Baltimore, 1986); Walter W. Powell and Paul J. Dimaggio, eds., *The New Institutionalism in Organizational Analysis* (Chicago, 1991); Malcolm Rutherford, *Institutions in Economics: The Old and New Institutionalism* (Cambridge, 1984); B. Guy Peters, *Institutional Theory in Political Science: The "New Institutionalism"* (London, 1999).

64. Czada and Friedrich-Czada, "Aids als politisches Konfliktfeld," pp. 259–61.

65. *Hansard*, vol. 127 (9 February 1988), col. 135; vol. 133 (20 May 1988), col. 612.

66. Marlene C. McGuirl and Robert N. Gee, "AIDS: An Overview of the British, Australian, and American Responses," *Hofstra Law Review* 14, 107 (1985), p. 135.

67. Czada and Friedrich-Czada, "Aids als politisches Konfliktfeld," pp. 259–60.

68. Martin Dinges, "Pest und Staat: Von der Institutionengeschichte zur sozialen Konstruktion," in Martin Dinges and Thomas Schlich, eds., *Neue Wege in der Seuchengeschichte* (Stuttgart, 1995), p. 83; Peter Baldwin, *Contagion and the State in Europe, 1830–1930* (Cambridge, 1999), ch. 2.

69. Hans-Volker Happel and Werner Schneider, "L'expérience allemande et la Charte de Francfort," in Jean-Marie Guffens, ed., *Toxicomanie, Hépatites, S.I.D.A.* (n.p., 1994), pp. 267–68; Massimo Campedelli, "Entre répression, indifférence et réduction des risques," and Anne Coppel, "Les intervenants en toxicomanie, le sida et la réduction des risques en France," in Alain Ehrenberg, ed., *Vivre avec les drogues: Régulations, politiques, marchés, usages* (Paris, 1996), pp. 73, 76; Steffen, *Fight against AIDS*, pp. 106–8.

70. Virginia Berridge, "AIDS and British Drug Policy: Continuity or Change?" in Berridge and Philip Strong, eds., *AIDS and Contemporary History* (Cambridge, 1993), p. 146; Donoghoe et al., *Syringe-Exchange in England*, pp. 7–8; Gerry Stimson et al., "The Future of Syringe Exchange in the Public Health Prevention of HIV Infection," in Peter Aggleton et al., eds., *AIDS: Responses, Interventions and Care* (London, 1991), pp. 225, 230.

71. Richard Pates, "The Initiatives Used in South Glamorgan to Combat the Spread of HIV amongst Drug Users in the County," in Wolfgang Heckmann and Sabine Reiter, eds., *Community-Oriented Prevention of AIDS and Addiction* (Berlin, 1991; AIDS-Zentrum Hefte 6/1991), p. 54; Berridge, *AIDS in the UK*, p. 287.

72. Eric Heilmann, "La protection des données nominatives consacrées au VIH," in Heilmann, ed., *Sida et libertés: La régulation d'une épidemie dans un état de droit* (n.p., 1991), p. 146.

73. Jeffrey Levi, "Unproven AIDS Therapies: The Food and Drug Administration and ddI," in Kathi E. Hanna, ed., *Biomedical Politics* (Washington, DC, 1991), pp. 35–36.

74. William B. Rubenstein et al., *The Rights of People Who Are HIV Positive* (Carbondale, IL, 1996), p. 204.

75. BT *Drucksache* 11/274, 14 May 1987, p. 2; BT *Verhandlungen* 11/71, 14 April 1988, p. 4801A; Martin Grieser, "Immundefektsyndrom und Seuchenrecht," in Johannes Korporal and Hubert Malouschek, eds., *Leben mit AIDS— Mit AIDS leben* (Hamburg, 1987), p. 245.

76. J. Lallement, "Les assurances face à l'épidémie," in J. M. Dupuy et al., eds., *SIDA 2001: AIDS 2001* (Paris, 1989), p. 186; Pierre Lascoumes, "De la sélection des risques à la discrimination: Les pratiques des compagnies d'assurances vis-à-vis du sida," in Eric Heilmann, ed., *Sida et libertés: La régulation d'une épidemie dans un état de droit* (n.p., 1991), p. 173; *Congressional Record* (House), 16 September 1987, 133, pp. 25796–25813.

77. Richard Freeman, "The Politics of AIDS in Britain and Germany," in Peter Aggleton et al., eds., *AIDS: Rights, Risk, and Reason* (London, 1992), p. 57.

78. Reutter, "Aids, Politik und Demokratie " pp. 29–30; *Congressional Record* (Senate), 15 May 1990, p. 6229; Bayer, "Politics, Social Sciences and HIV Prevention," pp. 46–47.

79. Christopher H. Foreman Jr., *Plagues, Products, and Politics: Emergent Public Health Hazards and National Policymaking* (Washington, DC, 1994), pp. 15–16; Edward P. Richards III, "HIV Testing, Screening, and Confidentiality: An American Perspective," in Rebecca Bennett and Charles A. Erin, eds., *HIV and AIDS: Testing, Screening, and Confidentiality* (Oxford, 1999), p. 77; Martin A. Levin and Mary Bryna Sanger, *After the Cure: Managing AIDS and Other Public Health Crises* (Lawrence, 2000), pp. 11–12; Marlene C. McGuirl and Robert N. Gee, "AIDS: An Overview of the British, Australian, and American Responses," *Hofstra Law Review* 14, 107 (1985), p. 124.

80. Sandra Panem, *The AIDS Bureaucracy* (Cambridge, MA, 1988), pp. 39–47; Ronald Elsberry, "AIDS Quarantine in England and the United States," *Hastings International and Comparative Law Review* 10 (1986), pp. 130–31.

81. David E. Rogers, "Federal Spending on AIDS: How Much Is Enough?" *New England Journal of Medicine* 320, 24 (1989), p. 1624; *Congressional Record* (House), 3 August 1990, p. 6915.

82. A. E. Benjamin and Philip R. Lee, "Public Policy, Federalism, and AIDS,"

Death Studies 12, 5–6 (1988), pp. 577, 580 ff; Czada and Friedrich-Czada, "Aids als politisches Konfliktfeld," pp. 257–58.

83. Donna I. Dennis, "HIV Screening and Discrimination: The Federal Example," in Scott Burris et al., eds., *AIDS Law Today* (New Haven, 1993), p. 187.

84. Robert D. Leigh, *Federal Health Administration in the United States* (New York, 1927), p. 80; John Duffy, *The Sanitarians: A History of American Public Health* (Urbana, 1990), pp. 242–43; Margaret Humphreys, *Yellow Fever and the South* (New Brunswick, 1992).

85. Bundesrat, *Verhandlungen* 580, 25 September 1987, p. 306C.

86. BT *Verhandlungen* 10/254, 5 December 1986, p. 19825D; BT *Drucksache* 11/213, 4 May 1987; 11/341, 22 May 1987.

87. BT *Drucksache* 12/2344, 25 March 1992, p. 28; BT *Verhandlungen* 12/147, 12 March 1993, p. 12631B; 12/23, 25 April 1991, p. 1605; Reutter, "Aids, Politik und Demokratie," p. 21.

88. RD *Prot*, 1988/89, Bihang, Prop. 5, pp. 24–26.

89. Jean-Baptiste Brunet, "Évolution de la législation française sur les maladies sexuellement transmissibles," in Nadine Job-Spira et al., eds., *Santé publique et maladies à transmission sexuelle* (Montrouge, 1990), p. 118; Louis Lebrun, "Les institutions médicales et le sida: Le cadre juridique français," in Eric Heilmann, ed., *Sida et libertés: La régulation d'une épidemie dans un état de droit* (n.p., 1991), pp. 117–18; Louis Lebrun, "Les institutions medicales et le Sida: Le cadre juridique français," in Daniel Borrillo and Anne Masseran, eds., *Sida et droits de l'homme: L'épidémie dans un Etat de droit* (Strasbourg, 1991), p. 78.

90. *Le Monde*, 30 June 1987, p. 18d; Setbon, *Pouvoirs contre SIDA*, pp. 173–75, 192; Claude Got, *Rapport sur le SIDA* (Paris, 1989), p. 42; Steffen, "AIDS Policies in France," p. 253.

91. Gertrud Lenzer, "Aids in Amerika," in Ernst Burkel, ed., *Der AIDS-Komplex: Dimensionen einer Bedrohung* (Frankfurt, 1988), pp. 198–203; Michael Pollak, "Organizing the Fight against AIDS," in Pollak, ed. *AIDS: A Problem for Sociological Research* (London, 1992), pp. 50–51; David Moss, "AIDS in Italy: Emergency in Slow Motion," in Barbara A. Misztal and Moss, eds., *Action on AIDS: National Policies in Comparative Perspective* (New York, 1990), p. 137; Fluss, "National AIDS Legislation," p. 6.

92. Walter Satzinger and Eva Bujok, "Zwischen Seuchenprävention und Sozialfürsorge: Bemerkungen über Aids-Beratung unter bayerischen Bedingungen," in Rolf Rosenbrock and Andreas Salmen, eds., *Aids-Prävention* (Berlin, 1990), p. 68; Reutter, "Aids, Politik und Demokratie," p. 26; Bundesrat, *Verhandlungen* 580, 25 September 1987, p. 303B; Virginie Linhart, "L'intervention tardive et dispersée des partis et des syndicats," in Pierre Favre, ed., *Sida et politique: Les premiers affrontements (1981–1987)* (Paris, 1992), p. 140.

93. *Report of the Presidential Commission on the Human Immunodeficiency Virus Epidemic* (Washington, DC, 1988), p. 77.

94. Bernd Schünemann, "Die Rechtsprobleme der AIDS-Eindämmung," in

Schünemann and Gerd Pfeiffer, eds., *Die Rechtsprobleme von AIDS* (Baden-Baden, 1988), p. 435.

95. Elsberry, "AIDS Quarantine," p. 128; Alistair Orr, "Legal AIDS: Implications of AIDS and HIV for British and American Law," *Journal of Medical Ethics* 15 (1989), p. 62.

96. Leigh, *Federal Health Administration*, pp. 26–27; Deborah Jones Merritt, "The Constitutional Balance between Health and Liberty," *Hastings Center Report* 16, 6 (December 1986), suppl., pp. 8–9; Scott Burris, "Public Health, 'AIDS Exceptionalism' and the Law," *John Marshall Law Review* 27 (1994), p. 271.

97. Rolf Rosenbrock, "AIDS: Fragen und Lehren für Public Health," Wissenschaftszentrum Berlin für Sozialforschung, *Veröffentlichungsreihe der Forschungsgruppe Gesundheitsrisiken und Präventionspolitik,* P92–206 (Berlin, April 1992), p. 34.

98. James C. Mohr, *Doctors and the Law: Medical Jurisprudence in Nineteenth-Century America* (New York, 1993), pp. 112–13; Marilynn M. Rosenthal, *Dealing with Medical Malpractice: The British and Swedish Experience* (Durham, NC, 1988).

99. Rodgers, *Atlantic Crossings,* pp. 245–50; Lawrence M. Friedman, *The Republic of Choice: Law, Authority, and Culture* (Cambridge, MA, 1990), p. 191; David A. Moss, *When All Else Fails: Government as the Ultimate Risk Manager* (Cambridge, MA, 2002), ch. 8.

100. Peter W. Huber, *Liability: The Legal Revolution and Its Consequences* (New York, 1988), chs. 1, 9.

101. Dieter Geisen, *International Medical Malpractice Law: A Comparative Law Study of Civil Liability Arising from Medical Care* (Dordrecht, 1988), p. 542; David M. Studdert and Troyen A. Brennan, "No Fault Compensation for Medical Injuries: The Prospect for Error Prevention," *JAMA* 286, 2 (2001), p. 220; R. Ian McEwin, "No-Fault Compensation Systems," in Gerrit de Geest and Boudewijn Bouckaert, eds., *Encyclopedia of Law and Economics,* vol. 3 (Cheltenham, U.K., 2000).

102. Georges Vigarello, *Le sain et le malsain* (Paris, 1993), p. 318.

103. Bill W. Dufwa, "Compensation for Personal Injury in Sweden," in Bernhard A. Koch and Helmut Koziol, eds., *Compensation for Personal Injury in Comparative Perspective* (Vienna, 2003); Lotta Westerhäll and Ake Saldeen, "Réflexions sur le Sida et le droit suédois," in Jacques Foyer and Lucette Khaïat, *Droit et Sida: Comparaison internationale* (Paris, 1994), pp. 406–9. Analogously, auto insurance in the well-developed welfare states of northern Europe played only a residual and complementary role to the primary one assumed by social insurance. Henri Margeat, "L'expérience française en matière de réparation," *Revue générale de droit* 18 (1987), p. 235.

104. "Bundesgerichtshof, Urteil vom 30.4.1991," *AIDS-Forschung* 6, 8 (August 1991), pp. 422–23.

105. *RD Prot* 1992/93, Lagutskottets betänkande 46, pp. 6, 8–10, 14.

106. "Bericht des Bundesministers für Gesundheit an den Ausschuss für Gesundheit des Deutschen Bundestages zur HIV-Infektionsgefährdung durch Blutprodukte vom 30. November 1992," *AIDS-Forschung* 12 (1993), p. 668.

107. Jonathan M. Mann and Daniel J. M. Tarantola, eds., *AIDS in the World II* (New York, 1996), p. 288; Ronald Bayer, "Blood and AIDS in America," in Eric A. Feldman and Bayer, eds., *Blood Feuds: AIDS, Blood, and the Politics of Medical Disaster* (New York, 1999), p. 47; Xavière Perron, "L'indemnisation des malades atteints du SIDA: Le cas des hémophiles et des transfusés approché de droit comparé," in Brigitte Feuillet-Le Mintier, ed., *Le SIDA: Aspects juridiques* (Paris, 1995).

108. BT *Drucksache* 11/2495, 16 June 1988, p. 5; *Report of the Presidential Commission*, p. xviii; Mann and Tarantola, *AIDS in the World II*, p. 190.

109. Andrew Grubb and David S. Pearl, *Blood Testing, AIDS and DNA Profiling: Law and Policy* (Bristol, 1990), pp. 140–41.

110. Dieter Giesen, "Compensation and Consent: A Brief Comparative Examination of Liability for HIV-Infected Blood," in Rebecca Bennett and Charles A. Erin, eds., *HIV and AIDS: Testing, Screening, and Confidentiality* (Oxford, 1999), pp. 94–100, 105; Dieter Giesen and Jens Poll, "Zur Haftung für infizierte Blutkonserven im amerikanischen und deutschen Recht," *Recht der Internationalen Wirtschaft* 39, 4 (1993), pp. 270–71; "Hanseatisches Oberlandesgericht: Urteil vom 30. März 1990," *AIDS-Forschung* 10 (1990), p. 547.

111. Anne Marie Moulin, "Reversible History: Blood Transfusion and the Spread of AIDS in France," in Caroline Hannaway et al., eds., *AIDS and the Public Debate* (Amsterdam, 1995), pp. 179, 183–84.

112. Michael G. Koch, "Stellungnahme zur AIDS-Problematik: Antworten auf Fragen der Presse," *AIDS-Forschung* 3, 10 (October 1988), p. 541; Schünemann, "Die Rechtsprobleme der AIDS-Eindämmung," p. 395.

113. Staatssekretärsausschuss "AIDS" der Bayerischen Staatsregierung, *Konzept der Bayerischen Staatsregierung zur Bekämpfung der Immunschwächekrankheit AIDS* (Munich, n.d.), p. 15.

114. Richard Titmuss, *The Gift Relationship: From Human Blood to Social Policy* (London, 1970).

115. *Hansard*, vol. 74 (25 February 1985), col. 65–66.

116. Martha A. Field and Kathleen M. Sullivan, "AIDS and the Criminal Law," *Law, Medicine, and Health Care* 15, 1–2 (summer 1987), p. 46; Sherry Glied, "The Circulation of the Blood: AIDS, Blood, and the Economics of Information," in Eric A. Feldman and Ronald Bayer, eds., *Blood Feuds: AIDS, Blood, and the Politics of Medical Disaster* (New York, 1999), p. 330; D. Reviron et al., "Prevention of HIV Infection by Transfusion: Comparative Analysis of Systems Adopted in Developed Countries," *AIDS and Public Policy Journal* 6, 1 (1991), p. 26; *Congressional Record* (Senate), 16 May 1990, pp. 6294–95.

117. Rubenstein et al., *Rights of People*, pp. 35–36; James W. Buehler, "HIV and AIDS Surveillance: Public Health Lessons Learned," in Ronald O. Valdiserri, ed., *Dawning Answers: How the HIV/AIDS Epidemic Has Helped to Strengthen Public Health* (New York, 2003), pp. 42–44.

118. *RD Prot,* 1985/86, Bihang, Prop. 171, p. 18; Erik Albæk, "AIDS: The Evolution of a Non-Controversial Issue in Denmark" (paper presented at the American Political Science Association), 1990, p. 28; *Hansard,* vol. 144 (13 January 1989), col. 1110.

119. Elinor Burkett, *The Gravest Show on Earth: America in the Age of AIDS* (Boston, 1995), pp. 141–43; Philip R. Lee and Peter S. Arno, "AIDS and Health Policy," in John Griggs, ed., *AIDS: Public Policy Dimensions* (New York, 1987), pp. 8–14; *Congressional Record* (House), 14 June 1993, p. 3491; (House) 18 June 1993, p. 3820; (Senate) 18 February 1993, p. 1766; (Senate) 16 May 1990, p. 6307; Jacob Levenson, *The Secret Epidemic: The Story of AIDS and Black America* (New York, 2004), pp. 135–40.

120. Glimpses into this netherworld of AIDS patients in public hospitals is provided in Victor Ayala, *Falling through the Cracks: AIDS and the Urban Poor* (Bayside, NY, 1996).

121. *Report of the Presidential Commission,* p. 17, ch. 10; National Commission on AIDS, *American Living with AIDS* (Washington, DC, 1991), ch. 4.

122. Theodore J. Stein, *The Social Welfare of Women and Children with HIV and AIDS: Legal Protections, Policy, and Programs* (New York, 1998), pp. 55–58.

123. Raymond A. Smith, *Encyclopedia of AIDS* (Chicago, 1998), pp. 58–60; Rosenbrock, "AIDS: Fragen und Lehren," pp. 21–22; Robin Gorna, *Vamps, Virgins, and Victims: How Can Women Fight AIDS?* (London, 1996), p. 116; R. A. Ancelle Park, "European AIDS Definition," *Lancet* 339 (1992), p. 671; G. J. P. van Griensven et al., "Expansion of AIDS Case Definition," *Lancet* 338 (1991), p. 1012; Joan H. Fujimura and Danny Y. Chou, "Dissent in Science: Styles of Scientific Practice and the Controversy over the Cause of AIDS," *Social Science and Medicine* 38, 8 (1994), p. 1031.

124. Daniel Shacknai, "Wealth = Health: The Public Financing of AIDS Care," in Nan D. Hunter and William B. Rubenstein, eds., *AIDS Agenda: Emerging Issues in Civil Rights* (New York, 1992), p. 181; Rubenstein et al., *Rights of People,* pp. 143, 175–76.

125. Stein, *Social Welfare,* p. 49; Dennis Altman, "The Politics of AIDS," in John Griggs, ed., *AIDS: Public Policy Dimensions* (New York, 1987), p. 26; William Winkenwerder et al., "Federal Spending for Illness Caused by the Human Immunodeficiency Virus," *New England Journal of Medicine* 320, 24 (1989), p. 1600; Robert J. Buchanan et al., "Medicaid Coverage of AIDS-Related Care: Attitudes of State Legislators Serving on Health-Related Committees," *AIDS and Public Policy Journal* 6, 3 (1991), p. 135.

126. Anthony H. Pascal et al., *The Effects of the AIDS Epidemic on Traditional Medicaid Populations,* Rand R-4148-HCFA (Santa Monica, 1992); Gerald M. Oppenheimer and Robert A. Padgug, "AIDS and the Crisis of Health Insurance," in Frederick G. Reamer, ed., *AIDS and Ethics* (New York, 1991), pp. 106, 114; Lawrence C. Shulman and Joanne E. Mantell, "The AIDS Crisis: A United States Health Care Perspective," *Social Science and Medicine* 26, 10 (1988), p. 981.

127. Mark H. Jackson, "Health Insurance: The Battle over Limits on Cover-

age," in Nan D. Hunter and William B. Rubenstein, eds., *AIDS Agenda: Emerging Issues in Civil Rights* (New York, 1992), pp. 148–63; John F. Dudley, "The Medical Costs of AIDS: Abandoning the HIV-Infected Employee," *Duquesne Law Review* 30 (1992), pp. 920–21; Ronald Turner, "ERISA and Employer Capping of Medical Benefits for Treatment of AIDS and Related Illnesses," *AIDS and Public Policy Journal* 7, 2 (1992), p. 90.

128. Mark Blumberg, *AIDS: The Impact on the Criminal Justice System* (Columbus, 1990), p. 205; Fitzhugh Mullan, *Plagues and Politics: The Story of the United States Public Health Service* (New York, 1989), p. 96; National Commission on AIDS, *Report: HIV Disease in Correctional Facilities* (Washington, DC, 1991), p. 10; John Kleinig, "The Ethical Challenge of AIDS to Traditional Liberal Values," *AIDS and Public Policy Journal* 5, 1 (1990), p. 43.

129. Pierre Darbeda, "Les prisons face au Sida: Vers des normes européennes," *Revue de science criminelle et de droit pénal comparé*, 4 (1990), p. 826; AIDES, *Droit et S.I.D.A.: Guide juridique*, p. 160.

130. Peter Roth, "AIDS and Insurance: Some Very British Questions," in David FitzSimons et al., eds., *The Economic and Social Impact of AIDS in Europe* (London, 1995), p. 283.

131. Cornelia Thies, *Die Auswirkungen von AIDS im Privatversicherungsrecht* (Frankfurt, 1991), p. 81.

132. Swiss Institute, *Comparative Study*, p. 395; Wesley Gryk, "AIDS and Immigration," in Richard Haigh and Dai Harris, eds., *AIDS: A Guide to the Law*, 2d ed. (London, 1995), pp. 82–83; *Hansard*, vol. 146 (10 February 1989), col. 820.

133. Claude Évin and Bruno Durieux, *La lutte contre le sida en France* (Paris, 1992), p. 77; Manuel Carballo and Harald Siem, "Migration, Migration Policy, and AIDS," in Mary Haour-Knipe and Richard Rector, eds., *Crossing Borders: Migration, Ethnicity, and AIDS* (London, 1996), p. 34; Philippe Auvergnon, ed., *Le droit social à l'epreuve du SIDA* (n.p., n.d.), p. 112.

134. *Congressional Record* (House), 3 March 1993, p. 973; (House) 11 March 1993, p. 1208; (House) 17 June 1993, p. 3706; Nancy E. Allin, "The AIDS Pandemic: International Travel and Immigration Restrictions and the World Health Organization's Response," *Virginia Journal of International Law* 28 (1988), p. 1055; Murphy, *Ethics in an Epidemic*, p. 131.

135. *Congressional Record* (House), 16 June 1993, p. 3695. Similarly: *Congressional Record* (Senate), 17 February 1993, p. 1709.

136. Gunnar Broberg and Mattias Tydén, "Eugenics in Sweden: Efficient Care," in Broberg and Nils Roll-Hansen, eds., *Eugenics and the Welfare State: Sterilization Policy in Denmark, Sweden, Norway, and Finland* (East Lansing, MI, 1996), pp. 104–5.

137. Gregor Heemann, *AIDS und Arbeitsrecht: Rechtliche Fragen bei der Begründung und Beendigung von Arbeitsverhältnissen in der Bundesrepublik Deutschland und in England* (Baden-Baden, 1992), p. 101; Hans-Ulrich Gallwas, "AIDS und Recht aus verfassungsrechtlicher Sicht," in Gallwas et al., eds., *Aids und Recht* (Stuttgart, 1992), p. 31; Wolfgang Loschelder, "Die Bekämpfung von AIDS als gesundheitsrechtliches Problem," in Bernd Schünemann and Gerd

Pfeiffer, eds., *Die Rechtsprobleme von AIDS* (Baden-Baden, 1988), p. 168; Manfred Seume, "Der HIV-Antikörpertest bei Einstellungsuntersuchungen von Beamtenbewerbern," *AIDS-Forschung* 12 (1987), pp. 703–7.

138. Annika Snare, "The Legal Treatment of AIDS in Denmark," in Martin Breum and Aart Hendriks, eds., *AIDS and Human Rights* (Copenhagen, 1988), p. 41.

139. Winfried Mummenhoff, "Arbeitsrechtliche Problemkreise bei HIV-Infektionen," in Hans-Ulrich Gallwas et al., eds., *Aids und Recht* (Stuttgart, 1992), pp. 162–65; Maren Sedelies, *Arbeitsrechtliche Probleme im Umgang mit der Immunschwächekrankheit Aids* (Aachen, 1992), pp. 129–31.

140. *Congressional Record* (House), 13 August 1986, p. 21428.

141. *Congressional Record* (Senate), 11 July 1990, pp. 9529–30.

142. Richards, "HIV Testing, Screening, and Confidentiality," p. 79.

143. *RD Prot*, 1988/89, Bihang, Prop. 112; *SFS* 1989:225; 1961 Bundesseuchengesetz, §49.

144. BT *Drucksache* 11/7200, 31 May 1990, p. 181; Andreas Costard, *Öffentlich-rechtliche Probleme beim Auftreten einer neuen übertragbaren Krankheit am Beispiel AIDS* (Berlin, 1989), pp. 110–11; Wolf-Rüdiger Schenke, "AIDS aus verwaltungsrechtlicher Perspektive," in Hans-Ulrich Gallwas et al., eds., *Aids und Recht* (Stuttgart, 1992), pp. 51–53; Manfred Bruns in Vereinigung Berliner Strafverteidiger, *AIDS im Strafvollzug: Strafe wegen AIDS?* (Berlin, n.d. [1987]), p. 33.

145. BT *Drucksache* 11/4043, 21 February 1989; Berridge, *AIDS in the UK*, p. 116; BT *Drucksache* 11/503, No. 37–38, 19 June 1987; 11/5856, 16 July 1986, p. 24; 11/7200, 31 May 1990, p. 239.

146. Alain Ehrenberg, "Comment vivre avec les drogues?" in Ehrenberg, ed., *Vivre avec les drogues: Régulations, politiques, marchés, usages* (Paris, 1996), pp. 6–7.

147. Nan D. Hunter, "Complications of Gender: Women and HIV Disease," in Hunter and William B. Rubenstein, eds., *AIDS Agenda: Emerging Issues in Civil Rights* (New York, 1992), p. 25–26.

148. Rubenstein et al., *Rights of People*, pp. 42–43; Dieter Meurer, "AIDS und strafrechtliche Probleme der Schweigepflicht," in Andrzej J. Szwarc, ed., *AIDS und Strafrecht* (Berlin, 1996), p. 141.

149. *IDHL* 39, 3 (1988), p. 631.

150. Swiss Institute, *Comparative Study*, p. 46.

151. Jörg Lücke, *Aids im amerikanischen und deutschen Recht* (Berlin, 1989), pp. 145–47; John Borneman, "AIDS in the Two Berlins," in Douglas Crimp, ed., *AIDS: Cultural Analysis, Cultural Activism* (Cambridge, 1988), p. 225; Kelvin Widdows, "AIDS and the Workplace: Some Approaches at the National Level," *International Journal of Comparative Labour Law and Industrial Relations* 4, 3 (1988), p. 150.

152. Lücke, *Aids*, pp. 153–54.

153. Anne-Sophie Rieben Schizas, "Employment, the Law, and HIV: An Overview of European Legislation," in David FitzSimons et al., eds., *The Economic and Social Impact of AIDS in Europe* (London, 1995), p. 305.

154. Virginia Berridge, "'Unambiguous Voluntarism?' AIDS and the Voluntary Sector in the United Kingdom, 1981–1992," in Caroline Hannaway et al., eds., *AIDS and the Public Debate* (Amsterdam, 1995), p. 153; Peter Raschke and Claudia Ritter, *Eine Grossstadt lebt mit Aids: Strategien der Prävention und Hilfe am Beispiel Hamburgs* (Berlin, 1991), pp. 33–34, 82.

10. CLIO INTERVENES: THE EFFECT OF THE PAST ON PUBLIC HEALTH

1. Unless otherwise noted, the historical details in this chapter rest on Peter Baldwin, *Contagion and the State in Europe, 1830–1930* (Cambridge, 1999).

2. Michel Setbon, *Pouvoirs contre SIDA: De la transfusion sanguine au dépistage: Decisions et pratiques en France, Grande-Bretagne et Suède* (Paris, 1993), p. 316.

3. Anthony S. Wohl, *Endangered Lives: Public Health in Victorian Britain* (Cambridge, 1983), p. 164; Dorothy Porter, *Health, Civilization, and the State: A History of Public Health from Ancient to Modern Times* (London, 1999), ch. 7.

4. Christopher Hamlin, *Public Health and Social Justice in the Age of Chadwick: Britain, 1800–1854* (Cambridge, 1998).

5. Monika Steffen, "Les modèles nationaux d'adaptation aux défis d'une épidémie," *Revue française de sociologie* 41, 1 (2000), p. 25.

6. Virginia Berridge, "AIDS and Contemporary History," in Berridge and Philip Strong, eds., *AIDS and Contemporary History* (Cambridge, 1993), pp. 2–3; Virginia Berridge, "AIDS: History and Contemporary History," in Gilbert Herdt and Shirley Lindenbaum, eds., *The Time of AIDS* (Newbury Park, 1992), pp. 57–58; Paul Sieghart, *AIDS and Human Rights: A UK Perspective* (London, 1989), p. 21; Virginia Berridge, "AIDS, Drugs, and History," *British Journal of Addiction* 87, 3 (1992), p. 364.

7. Robert F. Hummel et al., eds., *AIDS: Impact on Public Policy* (New York, 1986), p. 92; Rolf Jansen-Rosseck, ed., "Integrating AIDS and STD Programmes: Documentation of a Symposium," *AIDS-Themen und Konzepte* 9 (1994), p. 22.

8. House of Commons, 1986–87, Social Services Committee, *Problems Associated with AIDS*, 13 May 1987, vol. 1, pp. lviii, lix; vol. 2, p. 73; vol. 3, p. 45; *Hansard Parliamentary Debates*, vol. 113 (27 March 1987), col. 678.

9. *Hansard*, vol. 73 (20 February 1985), col. 499; Ronald Elsberry, "AIDS Quarantine in England and the United States," *Hastings International and Comparative Law Review* 10 (1986), p. 141.

10. Roy Porter, "Plague and Panic," *New Society* (12 December 1986), p. 13; Roy Porter, "History Says No to the Policeman's Response to AIDS," *British Medical Journal* 293, 6562 (1986) p. 1589.

11. Laurence Brockliss and Colin Jones, *The Medical World of Early Modern France* (Oxford, 1997), pp. 352–53; Ann F. La Berge, *Mission and Method: The Early Nineteenth-Century French Public Health Movement* (Cambridge,

1992); Lion Murard and Patrick Zylberman, *L'hygiène dans la république: La santé publique en France, ou l'utopie contrariée (1870–1918)* (Paris, 1996).

12. Aquilino Morelle, *La défaite de la santé publique* (Paris, 1996), pp. 209–11, 221–31 320–21, 330–31; Claude Évin and Bruno Durieux, *La lutte contre le sida en France* (Paris, 1992), p. 36.

13. William Coleman, *Death Is a Social Disease: Public Health and Political Economy in Early Industrial France* (Madison, 1982), pp. 207, 277.

14. Monika Steffen, *The Fight against AIDS: An International Public Policy Comparison between Four European Countries: France, Great Britain, Germany, and Italy* (Grenoble, 1996), pp. 158–61.

15. Ronald Bayer et al., "Public Health and Private Rights: Health, Social, and Ethical Perspectives," in Robert F. Hummel et al., eds., *AIDS: Impact on Public Policy* (New York, 1986), p. 16.

16. William J. Novak, *The People's Welfare: Law and Regulation in Nineteenth-Century America* (Chapel Hill, 1996), ch. 6 and passim; William R. Brock, *Investigation and Responsibility: Public Responsibility in the United States, 1865–1900* (Cambridge, 1984); Daniel T. Rodgers, *Atlantic Crossings: Social Politics in a Progressive Age* (Cambridge, MA, 1998), pp. 80–81.

17. Sheila M. Rothman, *Living in the Shadow of Death: Tuberculosis and the Social Experience of Illness in American History* (New York, 1994), p. 188.

18. Evelynn Maxine Hammonds, *Childhood's Deadly Scourge: The Campaign to Control Diphtheria in New York City, 1880–1930* (Baltimore, 1999), p. 15.

19. Margaret Humphreys, *Yellow Fever and the South* (New Brunswick, 1992), p. 33; Paul Starr, *The Social Transformation of American Medicine* (New York, 1982), pp. 189–94.

20. John Andrew Mendelsohn, "Cultures of Bacteriology: Formation and Transformation of a Science in France and Germany, 1870–1914" (Ph.D. diss., Princeton University, 1996); Elizabeth Fee and Dorothy Parker, "Public Health, Preventive Medicine, and Professionalization: Britain and the United States in the Nineteenth Century," in Elizabeth Fee and Roy M. Acheson, eds., *A History of Education in Public Health* (Oxford, 1991), pp. 33–34.

21. Alan M. Kraut, *Silent Travelers: Germs, Genes, and the "Immigrant Menace"* (New York, 1994), pp. 23–30.

22. John Duffy, *A History of Public Health in New York City, 1625–1866* (New York, 1968), p. 440; Arno Karlen, *Plague's Progress: A Social History of Man and Disease* (London, 1995), p. 108.

23. Barbara Gutmann Rosenkrantz, *Public Health and the State: Changing Views in Massachusetts, 1842–1936* (Cambridge, MA, 1972), p. 1.

24. John Duffy, *The Sanitarians: A History of American Public Health* (Urbana, 1990), p. 23.

25. Duffy, *History of Public Health*, pp. 125–26.

26. Humphreys, *Yellow Fever*, pp. 8–11, ch. 1; Richard Harrison Shryock, *The Development of Modern Medicine* (New York, 1947), p. 240.

27. Michael L. Closen et al., *AIDS: Cases and Materials* (Houston, 1989), pp. 893–94; Faith G. Pendleton, "The United States Exclusion of HIV-Positive Aliens: Realities and Illusions," *Suffolk Transnational Law Review* 18 (1995), p. 288.

28. Robert D. Leigh, *Federal Health Administration in the United States* (New York, 1927), pp. 33–35, chs. 2, 3.

29. Duffy, *Sanitarians*, pp. 165–68.

30. Harry F. Dowling, *Fighting Infection: Conquests of the Twentieth Century* (Cambridge, MA, 1977), pp. 97–103.

31. Alan M. Kraut, "Plagues and Prejudice: Nativism's Construction of Disease in Nineteenth- and Twentieth-Century New York City," in David Rosner, ed., *Hives of Sickness: Public Health and Epidemics in New York City* (New Brunswick, 1995), p. 66; Rupert E. D. Whitaker and Richard K. Edwards, "An Ethical Analysis of the US Immigration Policy of Screening Foreigners for the Human Immunodeficiency Virus," *AIDS and Public Policy Journal* 5, 4 (1990), p. 147.

32. David McBride, *From TB to AIDS: Epidemics among Urban Blacks since 1900* (Albany, 1991), pp. 59, 86, 111; Nayan Shah, *Contagious Divides: Epidemics and Race in San Francisco's Chinatown* (Berkeley, 2001).

33. Rosenkrantz, *Public Health and the State*, pp. 19–20, 30; Duffy, *History of Public Health*, pp. 192–93; Suellen Hoy, *Chasing Dirt: The American Pursuit of Cleanliness* (New York, 1995), chs. 4, 5.

34. Fitzhugh Mullan, *Plagues and Politics: The Story of the United States Public Health Service* (New York, 1989), pp. 40, 48; Ralph Chester Williams, *The United States Public Health Service, 1798–1950* (Washington, DC, 1951), pp. 88, 102; Juan P. Osuna, "The Exclusion from the United States of Aliens Infected with the AIDS Virus," *Houston Journal of International Law* 16, 1 (1993), pp. 5–6; Duffy, *Sanitarians*, p. 194.

35. Amy L. Fairchild, *Science at the Borders: Immigrant Medical Inspection and the Shaping of the Modern Industrial Labor Force* (Baltimore, 2003), p. 3.

36. Kraut, *Silent Travelers*, p. 51; Baldwin, *Contagion and the State*, ch. 3.

37. *Protocoles et procès-verbaux de la conférence sanitaire internationale de Rome inaugurée le 20 Mai 1885* (Rome, 1885), p. 116.

38. *Conférence sanitaire internationale de Paris, 7 Février–3 Avril 1894* (Paris, 1894), p. 100, 283–84; *Journal Officiel*, 1911, Chambre, Doc., Annexe 1218, p. 1062; *Proceedings of the International Sanitary Conference Provided for by Joint Resolution of the Senate and House of Representatives in the Early Part of 1881* (Washington, DC, 1881) pp. 76–77; Paul Weindling, *International Health Organisations and Movements, 1918–1939* (Cambridge, 1995), p. 5.

39. Leigh, *Federal Health Administration*, pp. 291–93.

40. Shah, *Contagious Divides*, ch. 5.

41. Howard Markel, *Quarantine: East European Jewish Immigrants and the New York City Epidemics of 1892* (Baltimore, 1997), pp. 5–6, 95–100, ch. 5–6.

42. Rosenkrantz, *Public Health and the State*, pp. 31–32; Hammonds, *Childhood's Deadly Scourge*, p. 41.

43. Hoy, *Chasing Dirt*, pp. 24–27.

44. Rosenkrantz, *Public Health and the State*, pp. 30–31.

45. Peter N. Stearns, *Battleground of Desire: The Struggle for Self-Control in Modern America* (New York, 1999), pp. 58–66, 259; Hoy, *Chasing Dirt*, ch. 4.

46. *Conférence sanitaire internationale de Paris, 7 Février–3 Avril 1894* (Paris, 1894), pp. 97–100; Public Record Office, FO 83/1330, Paris Sanitary Conference, No. 9, Phipps, 1 March 1894.

47. *Conférence sanitaire internationale de Paris, 7 Février–3 Avril 1894*, pp. 280, 482.

48. Lawrence C. Kleinman, "To End an Epidemic: Lessons from the History of Diphtheria," *New England Journal of Medicine* 326, 11 (1991), pp. 774–75; Hammonds, *Childhood's Deadly Scourge*, pp. 79–80, 151 and passim.

49. Duffy, *Sanitarians*, p. 195.

50. Jean Humbert, *Du role de l'administration en matière de prophylaxie des maladies épidémiques* (Paris, 1911), pp. 183–84.

51. Rothman, *Living in the Shadow*, p. 181.

52. On Koch's autocratic leanings: H. Oidtmann, "Beschwerdeschrift gegen den Geh.-Rath Dr. Koch, den Verfechter der Impfschutzlehre—aus dem Jahre 1889" *Der Impfgegner* 8, 1 (January 1890); Richard J. Evans, *Death in Hamburg: Society and Politics in the Cholera Years, 1830–1910* (Oxford, 1987), pp. 265–69, 313 ff; Mendelsohn, "Cultures of Bacteriology"; Daniel M. Fox, "From TB to AIDS: Value Conflicts in Reporting Disease," *Hastings Center Report* 16, 6 (December 1986), suppl., p. 12.

53. Sheila M. Rothman, "Seek and Hide: Public Health Departments and Persons with Tuberculosis, 1890–1940," *Journal of Law, Medicine, and Ethics* 21, 3–4 (1993), p. 292.

54. John M. Eyler, *Sir Arthur Newsholme and State Medicine, 1885–1935* (Cambridge, 1997), p. 150.

55. Jeffrey P. Baker, "Immunization and the American Way: Four Childhood Vaccines," *American Journal of Public Health* 90, 2 (2000), pp. 200–201.

56. Duffy, *Sanitarians*, p. 28; Duffy, *History of Public Health*, p. 340; James C. Mohr, *Doctors and the Law: Medical Jurisprudence in Nineteenth-Century America* (New York, 1993), p. 110.

57. Judith Walzer Leavitt, *The Healthiest City: Milwaukee and the Politics of Health Reform* (Princeton, 1982), pp. 89–90.

58. Leigh, *Federal Health Administration*, p. 308.

59. Ibid., p. 143; Dowling, *Fighting Infection*, pp. 97–103.

60. Brock, *Investigation and Responsibility*, p. 144; Humphreys, *Yellow Fever*, pp. 121–22, 138; Jo Ann Carrigan, "Yellow Fever: Scourge of the South," in Todd L. Savitt and James Harvey Young, eds., *Disease and Distinctiveness in the American South* (Knoxville, 1988), p. 68.

61. Williams, *United States Public Health Service*, p. 82–86.

62. Leigh, *Federal Health Administration*, pp. 320–21.

63. Christopher H. Foreman Jr., *Plagues, Products, and Politics: Emergent Public Health Hazards and National Policymaking* (Washington, DC, 1994), p. 61.

64. Elizabeth W. Etheridge, *Sentinel for Health: A History of the Centers for Disease Control* (Berkeley, 1992), pp. 121, 157–58, 178–79, 184–86.

65. *Los Angeles Times*, 5 May 2000, p. A15.

66. *New York Times*, 28 April 2003; 7 May 2003.

67. Barron H. Lerner, *Contagion and Confinement: Controlling Tuberculosis along the Skid Road* (Baltimore, 1998).

68. During the 1980s, some four hundred were incarcerated for this reason. Sixty million dollars were spent in New York building 140 isolation units on Rikers Island. Foreman, *Plagues, Products, and Politics*, p. 63; Martin A. Levin and Mary Bryna Sanger, *After the Cure: Managing AIDS and Other Public Health Crises* (Lawrence, 2000), p. 111; Kraut, *Silent Travelers*, pp. 262–63.

69. Zachary Gussow, *Leprosy, Racism, and Public Health: Social Policy in Chronic Disease Control* (Boulder, 1989), p. 22.

70. Timothy F. Murphy, *Ethics in an Epidemic: AIDS, Morality, and Culture* (Berkeley, 1994), p. 129.

71. *Congressional Record* (House), 11 March 1993, pp. 1204, 1208.

72. Ibid., p. 1208; (House) 14 June 1993, p. 3491; (House) 16 June 1993, p. 3599; (House) 17 June 1993, p. 3704.

73. Baldwin, *Contagion and the State*, ch. 2.

74. Evans, *Death in Hamburg*.

75. Rolf Rosenbrock, "AIDS: Fragen und Lehren für Public Health," Wissenschaftszentrum Berlin für Sozialforschung, *Veröffentlichungsreihe der Forschungsgruppe Gesundheitsrisiken und Präventionspolitik*, P92–206 (Berlin, April 1992), pp. 33–34; Rolf Rosenbrock, "Aids-Prävention und die Aufgaben der Sozialwissenschaften," in Rosenbrock and Andreas Salmen, eds., *Aids-Prävention* (Berlin, 1990), pp. 16–17; Wolf Kirschner, *HIV-Surveillance: Inhaltliche und methodische Probleme bei der Bestimmung der Ausbreitung von HIV-Infektionen* (Berlin, 1993), p. 45, 53–60.

76. Gunnar Broberg and Mattias Tydén, *Oönskade i folkhemmet: Rashygien och sterilisering i Sverige* (Stockholm, 1991); Maija Runcis, *Steriliseringar i folkhemmet* (Stockholm, 1998); Maciej Zaremba, *De rena och de andra: Om tvångssteriliseringar, rashygien och arvsynd* (n.p., 1999); Gunnar Broberg and Nils Roll-Hansen, eds., *Eugenics and the Welfare State* (East Lansing, MI, 1996); Stefan Kuhl, *The Nazi Connection: Eugenics, American Racism, and German National Socialism* (Oxford, 1994).

77. James M. Glass, *"Life Unworthy of Life": Racial Phobia and Mass Murder in Hitler's Germany* (New York, 1997), pp. 79–83; Paul Weindling, *Epidemics and Genocide in Eastern Europe, 1890–1945* (Oxford, 2000).

78. Wolfgang Schumacher and Egon Meyn, *Bundes-Seuchengesetz*, 4th ed. (Cologne, 1992), p. 3.

79. Yvonne Hirdman, "Utopia in the Home," *International Journal of Political Economy* 22, 2 (1992), pp. 1–99.

80. Neil Gilbert, *Transformation of the Welfare State: The Silent Surrender of Public Responsibility* (New York, 2002), p. 147.

81. Patrick Zylberman, "Les damnés de la démocratie puritaine: Stérilisations en Scandinavie, 1929–1977," *Le Mouvement Social* 187 (1999), pp. 99–125.

82. Madeleine Leijonhufvud, *HIV-smitta: Straff- och skadeståndsansvar* (Stockholm, 1993), p. 49; Benny Henriksson and Hasse Ytterberg, "Sweden: The Power of the Moral(istic) Left," in David L. Kirp and Ronald Bayer, eds., *AIDS in the Industrialized Democracies* (New Brunswick, 1992), p. 335; Michael Pollak, *The Second Plague of Europe: AIDS Prevention and Sexual Transmission among Men in Western Europe* (Binghamton, NY, 1994), pp. 77–78; Benny Henriksson, *Social Democracy or Societal Control? A Critical Analysis of Swedish AIDS Policy* (Stockholm, 1988), pp. 54–55.

83. BT *Drucksache* 11/2495, 16 June 1988, p. 122; Michael G. Koch, "Stellungnahme zur AIDS-Problematik: Antworten auf Fragen der Presse," *AIDS-Forschung* 3, 10 (October 1988), p. 545; Peter Gauweiler, "Zur Notwendigkeit eines geschlossenen Gesamtkonzepts staatlicher Massnahmen zur Bekämpfung der Weltseuche AIDS," in Bernd Schünemann and Gerd Pfeiffer, eds., *Die Rechtsprobleme von AIDS* (Baden-Baden, 1988), pp. 50–51; Edmund Stoiber, "Kontinuität bayerischer AIDS-Politik," *AIDS-Forschung* 11 (1989), p. 571.

84. BT *Verhandlungen* 11/71, 14 April 1988, p. 4809D; Bernd Schünemann, "AIDS und Strafrecht," in Andrzej J. Szwarc, ed., *AIDS und Strafrecht* (Berlin, 1996), p. 45; Peter Gauweiler, *Was tun gegen AIDS?* (Percha am Starnberger See, 1989), p. 155.

85. Bundesrat, *Verhandlungen* 580, 25 September 1987, pp. 295D, 296D–97A; 11/185, 14 December 1989, pp. 14354D, 14355D.

11. LIBERTY, AUTHORITY, AND
THE STATE IN THE AIDS ERA

1. Jamie L. Feldman, *Plague Doctors: Responding to the AIDS Epidemic in France and America* (Westport, CT, 1995), pp. 101–6; Lynn Payer, *Medicine and Culture: Varieties of Treatment in the United States, England, West Germany, and France* (New York, 1988), pp. 61–62.

2. Françoise F. Hamers et al., "The HIV Epidemic Associated with Injecting Drug Use in Europe: Geographic and Time Trends," *AIDS* 11 (1997), p. 1371; Nathalie Bajos et al., "Sexual Behaviour and HIV Epidemiology: Comparative Analysis in France and Britain," *AIDS* 9 (1995), p. 742; David Moss, "AIDS in Italy: Emergency in Slow Motion," in Barbara A. Misztal and Moss, eds., *Action on AIDS: National Policies in Comparative Perspective* (New York, 1990), p. 137.

3. Ronald Bayer, "Politics, Social Sciences, and HIV Prevention in the

United States," in Dorothee Friedrich and Wolfgang Heckmann, eds., *Aids in Europe: The Behavioural Aspect* (Berlin, 1995), 1:44–45.

4. Nan D. Hunter and William B. Rubenstein, eds., *AIDS Agenda: Emerging Issues in Civil Rights* (New York, 1992), p. 3.

5. S. Fluss and J. Lau Hansen, "La réponse du législateur face au Vih/Sida: Aperçu international," in Jacques Foyer and Lucette Khaïat, *Droit et Sida: Comparaison internationale* (Paris, 1994), pp. 444, 456; André Glucksmann, *La fêlure du monde: Éthique et sida* (n.p., 1994), p. 51; Michel Setbon, *Pouvoirs contre SIDA: De la transfusion sanguine au dépistage: Decisions et pratiques en France, Grande-Bretagne et Suède* (Paris, 1993), pp. 293–94.

6. S. Eric Lamboi and Francisco S. Sy, "The Impact of AIDS on State Public Health Legislation in the United States: A Critical Review," *AIDS Education and Prevention* 1, 4 (1989), p. 337; Albert R. Jonsen and Jeff Stryker, eds., *The Social Impact of AIDS in the United States* (Washington, DC, 1993), p. 33, ch. 2; Roland Czada and Heidi Friedrich-Czada, "Aids als politisches Konfliktfeld und Verwaltungsproblem," in Rolf Rosenbrock and Andreas Salmen, eds., *Aids-Prävention* (Berlin, 1990), pp. 259–61; Edward P. Richards III, "HIV Testing, Screening, and Confidentiality: An American Perspective," in Rebecca Bennett and Charles A. Erin, eds., *HIV and AIDS: Testing, Screening, and Confidentiality* (Oxford, 1999), p. 77; Michael Kirby, "AIDS and the Law," in *Dædalus* 118, 3 (summer 1989), p. 110. An exception to this claim: David C. Colby and David G. Baker, "State Policy Responses to the AIDS Epidemic," *Publius* 18, 3 (summer 1988), p. 121.

7. Margaret Duckett and Andrew J. Orkin, "AIDS-Related Migration and Travel Policies and Restrictions: A Global Survey," *AIDS* 3, suppl. 1 (1989), p. S251; Lawrence Gostin et al., "Screening and Restrictions on International Travellers for Public Health Purposes: An Evaluation of United States Travel and Immigration Policy," in Gostin and Lane Porter, eds., *International Law and AIDS* (n.p., 1992), p. 135; James F. Childress, "Mandatory HIV Screening and Testing," in Frederick G. Reamer, ed., *AIDS and Ethics* (New York, 1991), p. 68; Larry O. Gostin et al., "Screening Immigrants and International Travelers for the Human Immunodeficiency Virus," *New England Journal of Medicine*, 322, 24 (14 June 1990), p. 1743.

8. Jean-Pierre Cabestan, "SIDA et droit en Chine populaire," in Jacques Foyer and Lucette Khaïat, *Droit et Sida: Comparaison internationale* (Paris, 1994), p. 105; Susan Scholle Connor, "AIDS and International Ethical and Legal Standards: Role of the World Health Organization," in Lawrence Gostin and Lane Porter, eds., *International Law and AIDS* (n.p., 1992), p. 42.

9. Jean-Baptiste Brunet, "Évolution de la législation française sur les maladies sexuellement transmissibles," in Nadine Job-Spira et al., eds., *Santé publique et maladies à transmission sexuelle* (Montrouge, 1990), pp. 113–16; Jonathan Mann, "Global AIDS: Revolution, Paradigm, and Solidarity," *AIDS* 4, suppl. 1 (1990), p. S249; Lawrence O. Gostin, *Public Health Law: Power, Duty, Restraint* (Berkeley, 2000), pp. 107–9.

10. Sundhedsbestyrelsen, *AIDS: Sygdommen AIDS og retningslinier til forebyggelse af HIV-infektion* (n.p., [Copenhagen], 1988), p. 18.

11. John Harris and Søren Holm, "If Only AIDS Were Different!" *Hastings Center Report* 23, 6 (1993), pp. 6–7.

12. J. P. Moatti et al., "Social Perception of AIDS in the General Public: A French Study," *Health Policy* 9 (1988), p. 7; Knud S. Larsen et al., "Acquired Immune Deficiency Syndrome: International Attitudinal Comparisons," *Journal of Social Psychology* 131, 2 (1991), pp. 289–91; Michael G. Koch, "Stellungnahme zur AIDS-Problematik: Antworten auf Fragen der Presse," *AIDS-Forschung* 3, 10 (October 1988), p. 545; *Le Monde*, 3 December 1986, p. 36; Aquilino Morelle, *La défaite de la santé publique* (Paris, 1996), pp. 272 ff.

13. Bayer, "Politics, Social Sciences, and HIV Prevention," pp. 38–40; David L. Kirp and Ronald Bayer, "The Second Decade of AIDS: The End of Exceptionalism?" in Kirp and Bayer, eds., *AIDS in the Industrialized Democracies* (New Brunswick, 1992), p. 365.

14. Dennis Altman, *AIDS and the New Puritanism* (London, 1986), p. 26; John Street, "A Fall in Interest? British AIDS Policy, 1986–1990," in Virginia Berridge and Philip Strong, eds., *AIDS and Contemporary History* (Cambridge, 1993), pp. 234–35.

15. Czada and Friedrich-Czada, "Aids als politisches Konfliktfeld," p. 258.

16. Howard M. Leichter, *Free to Be Foolish: Politics and Health Promotion in the United States and Great Britain* (Princeton, 1991), p. 243; Elinor Burkett, *The Gravest Show on Earth: America in the Age of AIDS* (Boston, 1995), p. 293.

17. Curiously, it was precisely the Hollywood connection from his earlier days that helped bring AIDS to Reagan's attention: the peril of being a conservative from a liberal milieu. C. Everett Koop, "The Early Days of AIDS As I Remember Them," in Caroline Hannaway et al., eds., *AIDS and the Public Debate* (Amsterdam, 1995), p. 10.

18. Robert M. Wachter, *The Fragile Coalition: Scientists, Activists, and AIDS* (New York, 1991), p. 104; Philip M. Kayal, *Bearing Witness: Gay Men's Health Crisis and the Politics of AIDS* (Boulder, 1993), p. 44; Simon Garfield, *The End of Innocence: Britain in the Time of AIDS* (London, 1994), p. 114; Frédéric Martel, *Le rose et le noir: Les homosexuels en France depuis 1968* (Paris, 1996), pp. 333–34.

19. Nicolas Mauriac, *Le mal entendu: Le sida et les médias* (Paris, 1990), pp. 138–41; Michael Bochow, "Reactions of the Gay Community to AIDS in East and West Berlin," in AIDS-Forum D.A.H., *Aspects of AIDS and AIDS-Hilfe in Germany* (Berlin, 1993), p. 27.

20. Claudine Herzlich and Janine Pierret, "Une maladie dans l'espace public: Le sida dans six quotidiens français," *Annales, ESC* 43, 5 (1988), p. 1123.

21. Frank Arnal, *Résister ou disparaître? Les homosexuels face au sida* (Paris, 1993), pp. 123–24.

22. *BT Verhandlungen* 11/71, 14 April 1988, p. 4810C; Virginie Linhart, "Le silence de l'église," in Pierre Favre, ed., *Sida et politique: Les premiers affronte-*

ments (1981–1987) (Paris, 1992), p. 128; Deborah Lupton, Moral Threats and Dangerous Desires: AIDS in the News Media (London, 1994), pp. 74–75; Gabriel Rotello, Sexual Ecology: AIDS and the Destiny of Gay Men (New York, 1997), pp. 10–13.

23. Stephanie C. Kane, AIDS Alibis: Sex, Drugs, and Crime in the Americas (Philadelphia, 1998), p. 33; Nancy Krieger, introduction to Krieger and Glen Margo, eds., AIDS: The Politics of Survival (Amityville, NY, 1994), p. ix.

24. Peter H. Duesberg, Infectious AIDS: Have We Been Misled? (Berkeley, 1995), p. 336; Frank Rühmann, AIDS: Eine Krankheit und ihre Folgen, 2d ed. (Frankfurt, 1985), pp. 31–32.

25. Joan Shenton, Positively False: Exposing the Myths around HIV and AIDS (London, 1998), pp. xxvi, xxxii, 21.

26. Duesberg, Infectious AIDS, pp. 333, 515.

27. Neville Hodgkinson, AIDS, the Failure of Contemporary Science: How a Virus That Never Was Deceived the World (London, 1996), p. 5; Gordon T. Stewart, "The Epidemiology and Transmission of AIDS: A Hypothesis Linking Behavioural and Biological Determinants to Time, Person and Place," in Peter Duesberg, ed., AIDS: Virus- or Drug Induced? (Dordrecht, 1996), pp. 179–80; Congressional Record (Senate), 14 May 1990, p. 6128.

28. Peter S. Arno and Karyn L. Feiden, Against the Odds: The Story of AIDS Drug Development, Politics, and Profits (New York, 1992), p. 33.

29. Peter Pulzer, The Rise of Political Anti-Semitism in Germany and Austria, rev. ed. (Cambridge, 1988); Dan Diner, America in the Eyes of the Germans: An Essay on Anti-Americanism (Princeton, 1996).

30. Elizabeth Fee and Nancy Krieger, "Thinking and Rethinking AIDS: Implications for Health Policy," International Journal of Health Sciences 23, 2 (1993), p. 326; Rotello, Sexual Ecology, pp. 10–13.

31. Gerald M. Oppenheimer, "In the Eye of the Storm: The Epidemiological Construction of AIDS," in Elizabeth Fee and Daniel M. Fox, eds., AIDS: The Burdens of History (Berkeley, 1988), pp. 267–72, 279.

32. Nancy Goldstein and Jennifer L. Manlowe, eds., The Gender Politics of HIV/AIDS in Women (New York, 1997), pp. 29–30, 68; Sylvia Noble Tesh, Hidden Arguments: Political Ideology and Disease Prevention Policy (New Brunswick, 1988), pp. 33, 40; Steven Epstein, Impure Science: AIDS, Activism, and the Politics of Knowledge (Berkeley, 1996), pp. 95–96, 158.

33. Michael Pollak, The Second Plague of Europe: AIDS Prevention and Sexual Transmission among Men in Western Europe (Binghamton, NY, 1994), pp. 77–78; Karl Otto Hondrich, "Risikosteuerung durch Nichtwissen," in Ernst Burkel, ed., Der AIDS-Komplex: Dimensionen einer Bedrohung (Frankfurt, 1988), p. 136.

34. RD Prot, 1988/89, Bihang, Prop. 5, p. 53.

35. Martel, Le rose et le noir; Edmund White, "AIDS Awareness and Gay Culture in France," in Joshua Oppenheimer and Helena Reckitt, eds., Acting on AIDS: Sex, Drugs, and Politics (London, 1997), pp. 339–45; David Caron, "Lib-

erté, Égalité, Séropositivité: AIDS, the French Republic, and the Question of Community," *French Cultural Studies* 9, 3 (1998), pp. 282–83.

36. Jaqueline Bouton, "Le secret médical et le sida," in Eric Heilmann, ed., *Sida et libertés: La régulation d'une épidemie dans un état de droit* (n.p., 1991), pp. 139–40; Françoise Barré-Sinoussi et al., *Le SIDA en questions* (Paris, 1987), p. 59.

37. Fabienne Dulac, "Du refus de la maladie a une prise en charge exigeante," in Pierre Favre, ed., *Sida et politique: Les premiers affrontements (1981–1987)* (Paris, 1992), pp. 63–64; Dennis Altman, *Power and Community: Organizational and Cultural Responses to AIDS* (London, 1994), pp. 22–23.

38. Guenter Frankenberg, "Germany: The Uneasy Triumph of Pragmatism," and John Street and Albert Weale, "Britain: Policy-Making in a Hermetically Sealed System," in David L. Kirp and Ronald Bayer, eds., *AIDS in the Industrialized Democracies* (New Brunswick, 1992), pp. 120, 197.

39. *IDHL* 38, 4 (1987), pp. 769–71; 41, 3 (1990), pp. 431–32; 42, 1 (1991), pp. 20–21, 21–25; 44, 2 (1993), pp. 223–28; 46, 3 (1995); Nadine Marie, "Le Sida dans l'ex-URSS," in Jacques Foyer and Lucette Khaïat, *Droit et Sida: Comparaison internationale* (Paris, 1994), pp. 434–38; Christopher Williams, *AIDS in Post-Communist Russia and Its Successor States* (Aldershot, U.K., 1995), p. 59, 73–74, 160–61.

40. *IDHL* 37, 1 (1986), pp. 21–23; 38, 4 (1987), pp. 768–69; 39, 4 (1988), pp. 830–32; 41, 2 (1990), pp. 246–47; 46, 4 (1995); WHO, *Legislative Responses to AIDS* (Dordrecht, 1989), pp. 92–95; D. C. Jayasuriya, *AIDS: Public Health and Legal Dimensions* (Dordrecht, 1988), p. 28; Swiss Institute of Comparative Law, *Comparative Study on Discrimination against Persons with HIV or AIDS* (Strasbourg, 1993), p. 18.

41. Roger Davidson, *Dangerous Liaisons: A Social History of Venereal Disease in Twentieth-Century Scotland* (Amsterdam, 2000), pp. 321–22.

42. Peter Baldwin, *Contagion and the State in Europe* (Cambridge, 1999), pp. 88, 131–32, ch. 3.

43. Wolf-Dieter Narr, "Aids: Prävention, Aufklärung, Demokratie—Steinige Wege, Fluchtwege und Abwege," in Rolf Rosenbrock and Andreas Salmen, eds., *Aids-Prävention* (Berlin, 1990), p. 244.

44. Hondrich, "Risikosteuerung," p. 136.

45. *IDHL* 34, 2 (1983), pp. 252–55.

46. Niels Sönnichsen, "Überlegungen und Erfahrungen zur Verhütung und Bekämpfung des Syndroms des erworbenen Immundefektes (AIDS) in der DDR," *AIDS-Forschung* 2, 10 (October 1987), p. 552; *AIDS-Forschung* 3, 2 (February 1988), p. 107.

47. *IDHL* 40, 3 (1989), p. 585; Ehrhart Neubert, "A Critical Analysis of the Social Consequences of AIDS in the German Democratic Republic," in Martin Breum and Aart Hendriks, eds., *AIDS and Human Rights* (Copenhagen, 1988), pp. 61–62.

48. "Protokoll zwischen dem Bayerischen Staatsministerium für Wis-

senschaft und Kunst und dem Ministerium für Gesundheitswesen der Deutschen Demokratischen Republik über die Zusammenarbeit auf dem Gebiet der AIDS-Forschung," *AIDS-Forschung* 1 (1990), pp. 51–52; Peter Gauweiler, *Was tun gegen AIDS?* (Percha am Starnberger See, 1989), pp. 119, 132. Michael G. Koch, who was advisor to Peter Gauweiler during the implementation phase of the Bavarian measures, had trained in the DDR and was to spend his later career in Sweden (where he called himself Michael von Koch!). The Bavarians also admired the Cuban example of traditional public health techniques: Gert G. Frösner, "AIDS-Bekämpfung: Die unterschiedliche Seuchenbekämpfung in verschiedenen Ländern," *AIDS-Forschung* 11 (1989), pp. 598–99.

49. Ronald Bayer et al., "The American, British, and Dutch Responses to Unlinked Anonymous HIV Seroprevalence Studies: An International Comparison," *AIDS* 4 (1990), pp. 285–86.

50. Mary Catherine Bateson and Richard Goldsby, *Thinking AIDS* (Reading, MA, 1988), p. 122.

51. Signild Vallgårda, *Folkesundhed som Politik: Danmark og Sverige fra 1930 til i Dag* (Århus, 2003), ch. 10; Vagn Greve and Annika Snare, "Retssystemet v. Aids?" *Retfærd* 9, 34 (1986), pp. 7–11; Sundhedsbestyrelsen, *AIDS: Sygdommen AIDS og retningslinier til forebyggelse af HIV-infektion*, p. 18; Vagn Greve and Annika Snare, *AIDS: Nogle retspolitiske spørgsmål*, 5th ed. (Copenhagen, 1987), p. 19.

52. *BT Drucksache* 10/5430, No. 54, 2 May 1986.

53. Department of Health and Human Services, Public Health Service, *AIDS: A Public Health Challenge* (Washington, DC, October 1987), 1:3–38; Allyn K. Nakashima et al., "Effect of HIV Reporting by Name on Use of HIV Testing in Publicly Funded Counselling and Testing Programs," *JAMA* 280, 16 (1998), pp. 1421–26; Brian C. Castrucci et al., "The Elimination of Anonymous HIV Testing: A Case Study in North Carolina," *Journal of Public Health Management Practice* 8, 6 (2002), pp. 30–37. Similar results in Canada: Gayatri C. Jayaraman et al., "Mandatory Reporting of HIV Infection and Opt-Out Prenatal Screening for HIV Infection: Effect on Testing Rates," *Canadian Medical Association Journal* 168, 6 (2003).

54. Lutz Horn, "Die Behandlung von AIDS in ausgewählten Mitgliedstaaten des Europarates—ein rechtsvergleichender Überblick," in Hans-Ullrich Gallwas et al., eds., *Aids und Recht* (Stuttgart, 1992), p. 212. Though for the opposite view, see Arthur Kreuzer, "Sozialwissenschaftlich-kriminologische Vorbehalte gegenüber der strafrechtsdogmatisch-kriminalpolitischen Aids-Diskussion," in Cornelius Prittwitz, ed., *Aids, Recht und Gesundheitspolitik* (Berlin, 1990), p. 118.

55. Albert Palmberg, *A Treatise on Public Health* (London, 1895), p. iii; Henri Monod, *La santé publique* (Paris, 1904), p. 3; Morelle, *La défaite de la santé publique*, pp. 308–9.

56. Monika Steffen, "AIDS and Political Systems," 5:36; Jean-Marie Auby, "SIDA: Problématique de droit de la santé," in Philippe Auvergnon, ed., *Le droit social à l'epreuve du SIDA* (n.p., n.d.), p. 21.

57. Richards, "HIV Testing, Screening, and Confidentiality," pp. 88–90.

58. Baldwin, *Contagion and the State*, pp. 350, 520, 539; Franz v. Liszt, "Der strafrechtliche Schutz gegen Gesundheitsgefährdung durch Geschlechtskranke," *Zeitschrift für die Bekämpfung der Geschlechtskrankheiten* 1, 1 (1903), pp. 21–22.

59. Koch, "Stellungnahme zur AIDS-Problematik," p. 545.

60. Reichstag, *Stenographische Berichte der Verhandlungen* 1892/93, 21 April 1893, pp. 1959D–1960A, 1964D–1965D.

61. *RD Prot*, 1988/89:44 (13 December 1988), p. 12.

62. Such were the battles fought out surrounding a court case in Hamburg in 1989: Madeleine Leijonhufvud, *HIV-smitta: Straff- och skadeståndsansvar* (Stockholm, 1993), pp. 48–49; Klaus Scherf, *AIDS und Strafrecht* (Baden-Baden, 1992), pp. 63–66.

63. Michael Bess, *The Light-Green Society: Ecology and Technological Modernity in France, 1960–2000* (Chicago, 2003), passim.

64. Gérard Bach-Ignasse, "Le Sida et la vie politique française," in Michael Pollak et al., eds., *Homosexualités et Sida* (n.p., n.d. [1991]), p. 101.

65. *BT Verhandlungen* 11/4, 18 March 1987, p. 118D.

66. *Le Monde*, 11 January 1989, p. 17.

67. Of the sort painfully laid bare in Morelle, *La défaite de la santé publique*.

68. Martel, *Le rose et le noir*; Monika Steffen, "Les modèles nationaux d'adaptation aux défis d'une épidémie," *Revue française de sociologie*, 41, 1 (2000), p. 24; Michael Pollak and Marie-Ange Schiltz, "Les homosexuels français face au sida: Modifications des pratiques sexuelles et émergence de nouvelles valeurs," *Anthropologie et sociétés* 15, 2–3 (1991), p. 54.

69. Stephen P. Strickland, *Politics, Science, and Dread Disease: A Short History of United States Research Policy* (Cambridge, MA, 1972), p. 213.

70. David Kirp, "The Politics of Blood: Hemophilia Activism in the AIDS Crisis," in Eric A. Feldman and Ronald Bayer, eds., *Blood Feuds: AIDS, Blood, and the Politics of Medical Disaster* (New York, 1999), p. 312.

71. Although, of course, there are debates over whether multiculturalism in fact throws up real differences or merely masks a fundamental assimilation beneath a veneer of difference. Stanley Fish, *The Trouble with Principle* (Cambridge, MA, 1999), ch. 4; John A. Hall and Charles Lindholm, *Is America Breaking Apart?* (Princeton, 1999).

72. Matti Hayry and Heta Hayry, "AIDS and a Small North European Country: A Study in Applied Ethics," *International Journal of Applied Philosophy* 3, 3 (1987), p. 59.

73. Peter Baldwin, "The Return of the Coercive State? Behavioral Control in Multicultural Society," in John A. Hall et al., eds., *The Nation-State under Challenge: Autonomy and Capacity in a Changing World* (Princeton, 2003); Elizabeth Fee, "Public Health and the State: The United States," in Dorothy Porter, ed., *The History of Public Health and the Modern State* (Amsterdam, 1994), p. 260; Alfred Yankauer, "Sexually Transmitted Diseases: A Neglected Public Health Priority," *American Journal of Public Health* 84, 12 (1994), p. 1896.

74. "Stellungnahme der Deutschen Gesellschaft für Innere Medizin zu AIDS," *AIDS-Forschung* 7 (1989), p. 379.

75. *International Herald Tribune,* 30 May 2003, p. 9.

76. John R. Lott, *More Guns, Less Crime: Understanding Crime and Gun-Control Laws* (Chicago, 1998).

77. Norman Fowler, *Ministers Decide: A Personal Memoir of the Thatcher Years* (London, 1991), p. 253.

78. Rita Süssmuth, AIDS: Wege aus der Angst (Hamburg, 1987), p. 93; Staatssekretärsausschuss "AIDS" der Bayerischen Staatsregierung, *Konzept der Bayerischen Staatsregierung zur Bekämpfung der Immunschwächekrankheit AIDS* (Munich, n.d.), p. 1.

79. Lawrence M. Friedman, *The Republic of Choice: Law, Authority, and Culture* (Cambridge, MA, 1990), p. 2.

80. Nikolas Rose, *Governing the Soul: The Shaping of the Private Self,* 2d ed. (London, 1999); Nikolas Rose, *Powers of Freedom: Reframing Political Thought* (Cambridge, 1999); Peter N. Stearns, *Battleground of Desire: The Struggle for Self-Control in Modern America* (New York, 1999); Mariana Valverde, *Diseases of the Will: Alcohol and the Dilemmas of Freedom* (Cambridge, 1998), p. 17; Helmut Willke, *Ironie des Staates: Grundlinien einer Staatstheorie polyzentrischer Gesellschaft* (Frankfurt, 1992).

81. Alfons Labisch, " 'Hygiene ist Moral—Moral ist Hygiene': Soziale Disziplinierung durch Ärzte und Medizin," in Christoph Sachsse and Florian Tennstedt, eds., *Soziale Sicherheit und soziale Disziplinierung* (Frankfurt, 1986), p. 280.

82. Markus Müller, *Zwangsmassnahmen als Instrument der Krankheitsbekämpfung: Das Epidemiengesetz und die Persönliche Freiheit* (Basel, 1992), pp. 63–64; Michael Ramah and Claire M. Cassidy, "Social Marketing and Prevention of AIDS," in Jaime Sepulveda et al., eds., *AIDS: Prevention through Education* (New York, 1992); David C. Wyld and David E. Hallock, "Advertising's Response to the AIDS Crisis: The Role of Social Marketing," *AIDS and Public Policy Journal* 4, 4 (1989).

83. Kenneth F. Kiple, ed. *The Cambridge World History of Human Disease* (Cambridge, 1993), p. 205; Rüdiger Jacob, *Krankheitsbilder und Deutungsmuster: Wissen über Krankheit und dessen Bedeutung für die Praxis* (Opladen, 1995), pp. 37–38; Nora Kizer Bell, "Ethical Issues in AIDS Education," in Frederick G. Reamer, ed., *AIDS and Ethics* (New York, 1991), p. 137; Arnold J. Rosoff, "The AIDS Crisis: Constitutional Turning Point?" *Law, Medicine, and Health Care* 15, 1–2 (summer 1987), p. 81.

84. Ronald Bayer, *Private Acts, Social Consequences: AIDS and the Politics of Public Health* (New York, 1989), p. 11.

85. Joachim Israel, "Sykdom og sosial kontroll," in Turid Eikvam and Arne Grønningsæter, eds., *AIDS og samfunnet* (n.p., 1987), p. 21. Similarly: Felix Herzog, "Das Strafrecht im Kampf gegen 'Aids-Desperados,'" in Ernst Burkel, ed., *Der AIDS-Komplex: Dimensionen einer Bedrohung* (Frankfurt, 1988), p. 342; Roy Porter, "History Says No to the Policeman's Response to AIDS,"

British Medical Journal 293, 6562 (1986), p. 1590; *BT Verhandlungen* 12/12, 28 February 1991, p. 593B-C; F. Grémy and A. Bouckaert, "Santé publique et sida: Contribution du sida à la critique de la raison médicale," *Ethique* 12, 2 (1994), pp. 16, 20–21.

86. Koch, "Stellungnahme zur AIDS-Problematik," pp. 541–42.

87. *RD Prot*, 1985/86:109 (4 April 1986), p. 9.

88. Aart Hendriks, *AIDS and Mobility: The Impact of International Mobility on the Spread of HIV and the Need and Possibility for AIDS/HIV Prevention Programmes* (Copenhagen, 1991), p. 18.

89. Hannah Arendt, *The Origins of Totalitarianism* (New York, 1968), pt. 2, pp. 55–66.

90. Klaus Scherf, *AIDS und Strafrecht* (Baden-Baden, 1992), p. 83.

91. Ute Canaris, "Gesundheitspolitische Aspekte im Zusammenhang mit AIDS," in Johannes Korporal and Hubert Malouschek, eds., *Leben mit AIDS — Mit AIDS leben* (Hamburg, 1987), p. 282; M. A. Schiltz and Th. G. M. Sandfort, "HIV-Positive People, Risk, and Sexual Behaviour," *Social Science and Medicine* 50 (2000), p. 573.

92. Johan Goudsblom, "Zivilisation, Ansteckungsangst und Hygiene: Betrachtungen über ein Aspekt des europäischen Zivilisationsprozesses," in Peter Gleichmann et al., eds., *Materialen zu Norbert Elias' Zivilisationstheorie* (Frankfurt, 1977), pp. 216–18.

93. Carl Wilhelm Streubel, *Wie hat der Staat der Prostitution gegenüber sich zu verhalten?* (Leipzig, 1862), pp. 50–51.

94. Georges Vigarello, *Le sain et le malsain* (Paris, 1993), pp. 57–58.

95. Johan Goudsblom, "Public Health and the Civilizing Process," *Milbank Quarterly* 64, 2 (1986), p. 175.

96. Louis Fiaux, *Le délit pénal de contamination intersexuelle* (Paris, 1907), p. 16.

97. Lassar, "Quelle part revient, en dehors de la prostitution, aux autres modes de dissémination de la syphilis et des maladies vénériennes?" in Dubois-Havenith, ed., *Conférence internationale pour la prophylaxie de la syphilis et des maladies vénériennes: Rapports préliminaires* (Brussels, 1899), vol. 1, pt. 1, p. 10; Allan M. Brandt, "AIDS: From Social History to Social Policy," *Law, Medicine, and Health Care* 14, 5–6 (December 1986), p. 232.

98. Friedrich Weinbrenner, *Wie schützt man sich vor Ansteckung?* (Bonn, 1908), pp. 7–9.

99. Michael Pollak, "Introduction à la discussion: Systèmes de lutte contre les MST et sciences sociales," in Nadine Job-Spira et al., eds., *Santé publique et maladies à transmission sexuelle* (Montrouge, 1990), p. 110.

100. Goudsblom, "Public Health and the Civilizing Process," pp. 185–86.

101. Vigarello, *Le sain et le malsain*, pp. 291–98.

102. "Entschliessung der Sondersitzung der Konferenz der für das Gesundheitswesen zuständigen Minister und Senatoren der Länder (GMK) vom 27.3.1987 in Bonn," in Bundesministerium für Jugend, Familie, Frauen und Gesundheit, *Aidsbekämpfung in der Bundesrepublik Deutschland* (n.p., n.d.), p.

87, and in Günter Frankenberg, *AIDS-Bekämpfung im Rechtsstaat* (Baden-Baden, 1988), p. 176; *BT Verhandlungen* 11/43, 26 November 1987, p. 2965B; 11/71, 14 April 1988, p. 4806D; *BT Drucksache* 11/2495, 16 June 1988, p. 9. Similarly: Herzog, "Das Strafrecht im Kampf gegen 'Aids-Desperados,'" p. 342; Jonathan Mann, "Global AIDS: Epidemiology, Impact, Projections, Global Strategy," in World Health Organization, *AIDS Prevention and Control* (Geneva, 1988), p. 9; *BT Verhandlungen* 12/12, 28 February 1991, p. 592B-C.

103. *BT Drucksache* 11/1364, 26 November 1987.

104. Sundhedsbestyrelsen, *AIDS: Sygdommen AIDS og retningslinier til forebyggelse af HIV-infektion*, p. 18.

105. Theo Sandfort, "Pragmatism and Consensus: The Dutch Response to HIV," in Sandfort, ed., *The Dutch Response to HIV: Pragmatism and Consensus* (London, 1998), p. 7; Jan K. van Wijngaarden, "The Netherlands: AIDS in a Consensual Society," in David L. Kirp and Ronald Bayer, eds., *AIDS in the Industrialized Democracies* (New Brunswick, 1992), p. 264.

106. Frédéric Ocqueteau, "La répression pénale dans la lutte contre le sida: Solution ou alibi?" in Eric Heilmann, ed., *Sida et libertés: La régulation d'une épidemie dans un état de droit* (n.p., 1991), p. 249; Hubert Rottleuthner, "Probleme der rechtlichen Regulierung von Aids," in Rolf Rosenbrock and Andreas Salmen, eds., *Aids-Prävention* (Berlin, 1990), p. 125; *BT Drucksache* 11/2495, 16 June 1988, p. 79.

107. Porter, "History Says No," p. 1590; Jean de Savigny, *Le Sida et les fragilités françaises: Nos réactions face à l'épidémie* (Paris, 1995), pp. 307–8; Rotello, *Sexual Ecology*, p. 10.

108. *BT Verhandlungen* 11/4, 18 March 1987, p. 118D.

109. John Hardie, *AIDS, Dentistry, and the Illusion of Infection Control: Questioning the HIV Hypothesis* (Lewiston, NY, 1995), p. v; Bernard Paillard, *Notes on the Plague Years: AIDS in Marseilles* (New York, 1998), ch. 5.

110. *Report of the Presidential Commission on the Human Immunodeficiency Virus Epidemic* (Washington, DC, 1988), pp. 30–32; Justizminister des Landes Nordrhein-Westfalen, *Im Gespräch: AIDS im Strafvollzug: Protokoll des Symposiums am 2. Oktober 1985 in Düsseldorf* (Düsseldorf, n.d.), p. 35.

111. *BT Verhandlungen* 11/103, 27 October 1988, p. 7057B-C; Peter Gould, *The Slow Plague: A Geography of the AIDS Pandemic* (Cambridge, MA, 1993), p. 25; Michael Fumento, *The Myth of Heterosexual AIDS* (New York, 1990), p. 164; Jean-François Rouge, "L'economie du sida," *L'Expansion* (24 January–6 February 1991), pp. 47–48.

112. Elizabeth Fee and Nancy Krieger, "Understanding AIDS: Historical Interpretations and the Limits of Biomedical Individualism," *American Journal of Public Health* 83, 10 (October 1993), p. 1479.

113. Wolfram H. Eberbach, "Aktuelle Rechtsprobleme der HIV-Infektion," *AIDS-Forschung* 6 (1988), pp. 308–9. Echoes of this: "Die rechtliche Beurteilung von Eingriffsmassnahmen und ihre Gewichtung im Rahmen der Gesamtstrategie der AIDS-Bekämpfung," *AIDS-Forschung* 5 (1989), p. 267.

114. Staatssekretärsausschuss "AIDS" der Bayerischen Staatsregierung, *Konzept der Bayerischen Staatsregierung;* Bayerisches Staatsministerium des Innern, *Strategie gegen AIDS* (Munich [1989]); Bundesrat, *Verhandlungen* 580, 25 September 1987, p. 296D; "Entschliessung der Sondersitzung der Konferenz der für das Gesundheitswesen zuständigen Minister und Senatoren der Länder (GMK) vom 27.3.1987 in Bonn," in Bundesministerium für Jugend, *Familie, Frauen und Gesundheit, Aidsbekämpfung in der Bundesrepublik Deutschland* (n.p., n.d.), p. 87; *BT Verhandlungen* 11/103, 27 October 1988, p. 7050B-C; House of Commons, 1986–87, Social Services Committee, *Problems Associated with AIDS,* 13 May 1987, vol. 1, p. xxx; Dominique Hausser et al., "Effectiveness of the AIDS Prevention Campaigns in Switzerland," in Alan F. Fleming et al., *The Global Impact of AIDS* (New York, 1988), p. 220; WHO, *AIDS Diagnosis and Control: Current Situation* (Copenhagen, 1987), p. 5; Lawrence Gostin and Lane Porter, eds., *International Law and AIDS* (n.p., 1992), p. 263; *Report of the Presidential Commission,* pp. 83–85; Lupton, *Moral Threats,* pp. 53, 62; Kaye Wellings and Becky Field, *Stopping AIDS: AIDS/HIV Education and the Mass Media in Europe* (London, 1996), pp. 31–32.

115. *BT Verhandlungen* 12/12, 28 February 1991, p. 587B.

116. Ronald Bayer and David L. Kirp, "The United States: At the Center of the Storm," in Kirp and Bayer, eds., *AIDS in the Industrialized Democracies* (New Brunswick, 1992), p. 35; Simmy Viinikka, "Children, Young People, and HIV Infection," in Richard Haigh and Dai Harris, eds., *AIDS: A Guide to the Law,* 2d ed. (London, 1995), p. 20; Swiss Institute, *Comparative Study,* p. 18; Barbara A. Misztal, "AIDS in Poland: The Fear of Unmasking Intolerance," in Misztal and David Moss, eds., *Action on AIDS: National Policies in Comparative Perspective* (New York, 1990), p. 169.

117. *IDHL* 37, 1 (1986), p. 26; Lotta Westerhäll and Ake Saldeen, "Réflexions sur le Sida et le droit suédois," in Jacques Foyer and Lucette Khaïat, *Droit et Sida: Comparaison internationale* (Paris, 1994), p. 394; *RD Prot,* 1988/89, Bihang, Prop. 5, p. 3; Timothy Harding and Marinette Ummel, "Consensus on Non-Discrimination in HIV Policy," *Lancet* 341, 8836 (1993), pp. 24–25.

118. Vincent Sterner, "Rättsläget kring AIDS i Sverige," *Retfærd* 11, 1 (1988), p. 35; *RD Prot,* 1988/89, Bihang, Prop. 5, p. 89; 1988/89:105 (27 April 1989), p. 26.

119. Sigfried Borelli et al., eds., *Geschichte der Deutschen Gesellschaft zur Bekämpfung der Geschlechtskrankheiten* (Berlin, 1992), p. 79.

120. Fee and Krieger, "Understanding AIDS," pp. 1482–83; Tim Rhodes, "Individual and Community Action in HIV Prevention," in Rhodes and Richard Hartnoll, eds., *AIDS, Drugs, and Prevention* (London, 1996), pp. 1–2.

121. *BT Verhandlungen* 11/8, 2 April 1987, pp. 430C-431A.

122. Narr, "Aids: Prävention, Aufklärung, Demokratie," p. 245.

123. *RD Prot,* 1988/89, Bihang, Prop. 5, p. 205.

124. Lynne Segal, "Lessons from the Past: Feminism, Sexual Politics, and the Challenge of AIDS," in Erica Carter and Simon Watney, eds., *Taking Liberties*

(London, 1989), pp. 135–39; Walt Odets, "AIDS Education and Harm Reduction for Gay Men," *AIDS and Public Policy Journal* 9, 1 (1994), pp. 5–6.

125. Pollak and Schiltz, "Les homosexuels français face au sida," p. 56; Michael Pollak, *Les homosexuels et le sida: Sociologie d'une épidémie* (Paris, 1988), pp. 81–82.

126. Greve and Snare, *AIDS,* p. 52; Noel Annan, *Our Age: Portrait of a Generation* (London, 1990), p. 153.

127. J. W. Duyvendak and R. Koopmans, "Resister au Sida: Destin et influence du mouvement homosexuel," in Michael Pollak et al., eds., *Homosexualités et Sida* (n.p., n.d. [1991]), p. 212; van Wijngaarden, "The Netherlands," p. 260; Birgit Westphal Christensen et al., *AIDS: Prævention og kontrol i Norden* (Stockholm, 1988), p. 82.

128. Richard D. Mohr, *Gays/Justice: A Study of Ethics, Society, and Law* (New York, 1988), p. 252; Andreas Salmen, "Aktuelle Erfordernisse der Aidsprävention," in Rolf Rosenbrock and Salmen, eds., *Aids-Prävention* (Berlin, 1990), p. 95; Frank Becker and Klaus-Dieter Beisswenger, eds., *Solidarität der Uneinsichtigen: Aktionstag 9. Juli 1988 Frankfurt a.M.* (Berlin, 1988), pp. 10, 25.

129. Cindy Patton, "Save Sex/Save Lives: Evolving Modes of Activism," in Tim Rhodes and Richard Hartnoll, eds., *AIDS, Drugs, and Prevention* (London, 1996), pp. 125–28; Cindy Patton, *Fatal Advice: How Safe-Sex Education Went Wrong* (Durham, NC, 1996), passim; Graham Hart et al., " 'Relapse' to Unsafe Sexual Behavior among Gay Men: A Critique of Recent Behavioural HIV/AIDS Research," *Sociology of Health and Illness* 14, 2 (1992), pp. 226–27.

130. Mitchell Cohen, "The Place of Time in Understanding Risky Behaviour Related to HIV Infection," in Dorothee Friedrich and Wolfgang Heckmann, eds., *Aids in Europe: The Behavioural Aspect* (Berlin, 1995), 4:27–28; Jared Diamond, *Why Is Sex Fun?* (New York, 1997), p. 65; Priscilla Alexander, "Sex Workers Fight against AIDS: An International Perspective," in Beth E. Schneider and Nancy E. Stoller, eds., *Women Resisting AIDS: Feminist Strategies of Empowerment* (Philadelphia, 1995), p. 106; Brooke Grundfest Schoepf, "AIDS, Sex, and Condoms: African Healers and the Reinvention of Tradition in Zaire," *Medical Anthropology* 14 (1992), p. 231; Gilbert H. Herdt, "Semen Depletion and the Sense of Maleness," in Stephen O. Murray, ed., *Oceanic Homosexualities* (New York, 1992), pp. 37–41.

131. Rafael Miguel Diaz, "Latino Gay Men and Psycho-Cultural Barriers to AIDS Prevention," in Martin P. Levine et al., eds., *In Changing Times: Gay Men and Lesbians Encounter HIV/AIDS* (Chicago, 1997), pp. 228–31.

132. Meredeth Turshen, "Is AIDS Primarily a Sexually Transmitted Disease?" in Nadine Job-Spira et al., eds., *Santé publique et maladies à transmission sexuelle* (Montrouge, 1990), p. 347; Henning Machein, "Mythen sterben langsam: Aids in Mali," in Anja Bestmann et al., eds., *Aids—weltweit und dichtdran* (Saarbrücken, 1997), pp. 188–89; Beth E. Schneider and Valerie Jenness, "Social Control, Civil Liberties, and Women's Sexuality," in Schneider and

Nancy E. Stoller, eds., *Women Resisting AIDS: Feminist Strategies of Empowerment* (Philadelphia, 1995), pp. 80–81.

133. *BT Drucksache* 11/7200, 31 May 1990, p. 340; House of Commons, *Problems Associated with AIDS*, vol. 1, pp. xxvii–viii.

134. Michael T. Isbell, "AIDS and Public Health: The Enduring Relevance of a Communitarian Approach to Disease Prevention," *AIDS and Public Policy Journal* 8, 4 (1993), pp. 160, 168.

135. Ronald Bayer, "AIDS Prevention and Cultural Sensitivity: Are They Compatible?" *American Journal of Public Health* 84, 6 (1994), pp. 895–97.

136. James Miller, *The Passion of Michel Foucault* (New York, 1993), ch. 8.

137. Marco Pulver, *Tribut der Seuche oder: Seuchenmythen als Quelle sozialer Kalibrierung: Eine Rekonstruktion des AIDS-Diskurses vor dem Hintergrund von Studien zur Historizität des Seuchendispositivs* (Frankfurt, 1999), pp. 438–40; Michael Bartos, "Community vs. Population: The Case of Men Who Have Sex with Men," in Peter Aggleton et al., eds., *AIDS: Foundations for the Future* (London, 1994), pp. 82–85.

138. Wolf Kirschner, *HIV-Surveillance: Inhaltliche und methodische Probleme bei der Bestimmung der Ausbreitung von HIV-Infektionen* (Berlin, 1993), pp. 10, 64–65, 70.

139. John Rechy, *The Sexual Outlaw* (New York, 1977), p. 31.

140. François Bachelot and Pierre Lorane, *Une société au risque du sida* (Paris, 1988), pp. 22, 52–53, 265–87; Staatssekretärsausschuss "AIDS" der Bayerischen Staatsregierung, *Konzept der Bayerischen Staatsregierung*, p. 15; Bayer and Kirp, "The United States," p. 21; Dudley Clendinen and Adam Nagourney, *Out for Good: The Struggle to Build a Gay Rights Movement in America* (New York, 1999), p. 502; Randy Shilts, *And the Band Played On: Politics, People, and the AIDS Epidemic* (New York, 1988), p. 443.

141. David Rayside, *On the Fringe: Gays and Lesbians in Politics* (Ithaca, 1998), pp. 304–5 and passim; Barry D. Adam, *The Rise of a Gay and Lesbian Movement* (Boston, 1987), ch. 6; Clendinen and Nagourney, *Out for Good*, pt. 3.

142. Peter Duesberg, *Inventing the AIDS Virus* (Washington, DC, 1996), pp. 369–70.

143. Baldwin, *Contagion and the State*, ch. 1.

144. For similar themes, see Baldwin, "Return of the Coercive State?"

145. Zachary Gussow, *Leprosy, Racism, and Public Health: Social Policy in Chronic Disease Control* (Boulder, 1989), pp. 19–20, ch. 4.

146. Mary Douglas and Marcel Calvez, "The Self as Risk Taker: A Cultural Theory of Contagion in Relation to AIDS," *Sociological Review* (1990), p. 462.

147. Félix Regnault, *L'Évolution de la prostitution* (Paris, n.d. [1906?]), pp. 250–57.

148. J. Courmont, "La lutte contre les maladies infectieuses en Suède et en Norvège," *Annales d'hygiène publique et de médecine légale* 4, 12 (1909), pp. 239–43; Yves-Marie Bercé, *Le chaudron et la lancette: Croyances populaires et médecine préventive* (Paris, 1984), p. 302.

149. Barron H. Lerner, *Contagion and Confinement: Controlling Tuberculosis along the Skid Road* (Baltimore, 1998).

150. Renée Dubos and Jean Dubos, *The White Plague: Tuberculosis, Man, and Society* (Boston, 1952), p. 172.

151. Virginia Berridge, *AIDS in the UK: The Making of Policy, 1981–1994* (Oxford, 1996), pp. 278–79; Lois M. Takahashi, *Homelessness, AIDS, and Stigmatization: The NIMBY Syndrome in the United States at the End of the Twentieth Century* (Oxford, 1998), pp. 18–19; Altman, *Power and Community*, pp. 3–4; Jonathan M. Mann and Daniel J. M. Tarantola, eds., *AIDS in the World II* (New York, 1996), p. 63.

152. Jonsen and Stryker, *Social Impact of AIDS*, p. 9; Monroe E. Price, *Shattered Mirrors: Our Search for Identity and Community in the AIDS Era* (Cambridge, MA, 1989), pp. 64–65; David McBride, *From TB to AIDS: Epidemics among Urban Blacks since 1900* (Albany, 1991), ch. 6; Sarah Santana et al., "Human Immunodeficiency Virus in Cuba: The Public Health Response of a Third World Country," in Nancy Krieger and Glen Margo, eds., *AIDS: The Politics of Survival* (Amityville, NY, 1994), p. 169.

153. Gregory M. Herek and Eric K. Glunt, "AIDS-Related Attitudes in the United States: A Preliminary Conceptualization," *Journal of Sex Research* 28, 1 (1991), pp. 107, 111.

154. Benjamin P. Bowser, "HIV Prevention and African Americans: A Difference of Class," in Johannes P. Van Vugt, ed., *AIDS Prevention and Services: Community Based Research* (Westport, 1994), pp. 96–100.

155. Michael Bloor, *The Sociology of HIV Transmission* (London, 1995), p. 60; *Los Angeles Times*, 14 January 2000, p. A13.

156. Ronald Bayer, "Perinatal Transmission of HIV Infection: The Ethics of Prevention," in Lawrence O. Gostin, ed., *AIDS and the Health Care System* (New Haven, 1990), pp. 64–65, 69–70.

157. Nonetheless, mandatory universal testing gained favor again, as for AIDS, once penicillin was thought to reduce mortality in infants. Katherine L. Acuff and Ruth R. Faden, "A History of Prenatal and Newborn Screening Programs: Lessons for the Future," in Ruth R. Faden et al., eds., *AIDS, Women, and the Next Generation* (New York, 1991), pp. 67–71.

158. Bayer, "Politics, Social Sciences, and HIV Prevention," pp. 46–47; Ken Rigby et al., "The Theory of Reasoned Action as Applied to AIDS Prevention for Australian Ethnic Groups," in Deborah J. Terry et al., eds., *The Theory of Reasoned Action: Its Application to Aids-Preventive Behaviour* (Oxford, 1993); Rinske van Duifhuizen, "HIV/AIDS Prevention Programmes for Migrants and Ethnic Minorities in Europe," in Mary Haour-Knipe and Richard Rector, eds., *Crossing Borders: Migration, Ethnicity, and AIDS* (London, 1996), p. 121.

159. Loes Singels, "AIDS Prevention for Migrants in the Netherlands," in Theo Sandfort, ed., *The Dutch Response to HIV: Pragmatism and Consensus* (London, 1998), pp. 110–11; de Savigny, *Le Sida et les fragilités françaises*, pp. 108–16; Caren Weilandt et al., "HIV-Prevention for Migrants: Integration of HIV-Prevention into Social Work among Migrant Populations," in Inon I.

Schenker et al., eds., *AIDS Education: Interventions in Multi-Cultural Societies* (New York, 1996), pp. 141–47.

160. *Public Health Reports,* 103, suppl. 1 (1988), p. 20; Charles Perrow and Mauro F. Guillén, *The AIDS Disaster: The Failure of Organizations in New York and the Nation* (New Haven, 1990), p. 25.

161. Claudia L. Windal, "Cultural and Societal Impediments to HIV/AIDS Education in the American Indian Community: Mitakuye Oyasin," in Davidson C. Umeh, ed., *Confronting the AIDS Epidemic: Cross-Cultural Perspectives on HIV/AIDS Education* (Trenton, NJ, 1997), p. 7; Gregory M. Herek, "AIDS and Stigma," *American Behavioral Scientist* 42, 7 (1999), p. 1109.

162. For an approach to the now enormous literature on this subject, see Adrian Favell, *Philosophies of Integration: Immigration and the Idea of Citizenship in France and Britain* (Houndmills, 1998).

163. RD Prot, 1985/86, Bihang, Prop. 13, p. 11; 1986/87, Bihang, Prop. 149, p. 8.

164. RD Prot, 1985/86:33 (21 November 1985), pp. 7, 17; 1985/86:157 (30 May 1986), p. 11.

165. RD Prot, 1986/87, Bihang, Prop. 2, pp. 21, 26–28; 1986/87:50 (16 December 1986), p. 4; 1988/89, Bihang, Prop. 5, p. 90; 1988/89:105 (27 April 1989), pp. 19, 31; Vallgårda, *Folkesundhed som Politik,* pp. 250–51.

166. RD Prot, 1988/89, Bihang, Prop. 5, pp. 263–64, 273; 1986/87:50 (16 December 1986), p. 7.

167. BT Drucksache 11/1548, 17 December 1987, pp. 3, 5; 11/680, 7 August 1987; BT Verhandlungen 11/43, 26 November 1987, p. 2965B; BT Drucksache 11/54, No. 36, 13 March 1987; BT Verhandlungen 11/5, 19 March 87, pp. 230D–31A; "Entschliessung der 63. Konferenz der für das Gesundheitswesen zuständigen Minister und Senatoren der Länder vom 22. bis 23. November 1990 in Berlin," *AIDS-Forschung* 6, 1 (January 1991), pp. 28–29; Bundesrat, *Verhandlungen* 580, 25 September 1987, pp. 307A, 295C–96D.

168. Davidson, *Dangerous Liaisons,* p. 321; *Congressional Record* (House), 3 August 1990, p. 6917; (Senate) 11 July 1990, p. 9542.

169. Baldwin, *Contagion and the State.*

170. Feldman, *Plague Doctors,* p. 37; Meinrad A. Koch, "Surveys on AIDS in Europe (What Do They Tell Us?)," in Koch and F. Deinhardt, eds., *AIDS Diagnosis and Control: Current Situation* (Munich, 1988), p. 72; François Bachelot and Pierre Lorane, *Une société au risque du sida* (Paris, 1988), p. 98.

171. Michel Hubert, "AIDS in Belgium: Africa in Microcosm," Barbara A. Misztal and David Moss, eds., *Action on AIDS: National Policies in Comparative Perspective* (New York, 1990), p. 101; M. Pollak, "Assessing AIDS Prevention among Male Homo- and Bisexuals," in F. Paccaud et al., eds., *Assessing AIDS Prevention* (Basel, 1992), p. 153; J. B. Brunet et al., "La surveillance du SIDA en Europe," *Revue d'epidemiologie et de santé publique* 34 (1986), pp. 127–28, 132; Georges Verhaegen, "Allocution de bienvenue," in Michel Vincineau, ed., *Le Sida: Un défi aux droits* (Brussels, 1991), p. 12.

172. *Hansard Parliamentary Debates,* vol. 108 (22 January 1987), col. 732; vol. 120 (21 October 1987), col. 742.

173. B. D. Bytchenko, "A Search for Effective Strategies against AIDS: Points for Discussion," in M. A. Koch and F. Deinhardt, eds., *AIDS Diagnosis and Control: Current Situation* (Munich, 1988), p. 55; Hendriks, *AIDS and Mobility*, p. 20.

174. Christine Ann McGarrigle and Owen Noel Gill, "UK HIV Testing Practice: By How Much Might the Infection Diagnosis Rate Increase through Normalisation?" in Jean-Paul Moatti et al., eds., *AIDS in Europe: New Challenges for the Social Sciences* (London, 2000), pp. 225–26; Anthony Browne, "How the Government Endangers British Lives," *Spectator* 25 January 2003, p. 13; Ministère des affaires sociales et de l'intégration, *La lutte contre le sida en France* (Paris, 1991), p. 8; Mission SIDA du Profeseur Luc Montagnier, *Le Sida et la société française: Décembre 1993* (Paris, 1994), p. 112.

175. Anders Foldspang and Else Smith, *Overvågning af HIV og AIDS i Danmark* (Copenhagen, 1992), pp. 18, 45, 47; Beatrice Irene Tschumi Sangvik, *Dänemark, Norwegen, Schweden und die Schweiz in Auseinandersetzung mit HIV und Aids* (Zürich, 1994), p. 106; Renée Danziger, "HIV Testing and HIV Prevention in Sweden," *British Medical Journal* 7127 (24 January 1994), pp. 293–96; Mary Haour-Knipe, "Prévention du sida ou discrimination? Les migrants et les minorités ethniques," in Nathalie Bajos et al., *Le sida en Europe: Nouveaux enjeux pour les sciences sociales* (Paris, 1998), pp. 164–65.

176. *Economist*, 14 August 1999, p. 18.

177. *RD Prot*, 1985/86, Bihang, Prop. 13, pp. 10–11; 1985/86:33 (21 November 1985), p. 20; 1988/89:105 (27 April 1989), p. 25.

178. *Aftonbladet* 16 September 2000.

179. De Savigny, *Le Sida et les fragilités françaises*, p. 17; Ministère des affaires sociales et de l'intégration, *La lutte contre le sida en France*, p. 7; Monika Steffen, "France: Social Solidarity and Scientific Expertise," in David L. Kirp and Ronald Bayer, eds., *AIDS in the Industrialized Democracies* (New Brunswick, 1992), p. 229.

180. Altman, *Power and Community*, pp. 3–4; Mann and Tarantola, *AIDS in the World II*, p. 63; Julia M. Dayton and Michael H. Merson, "Global Dimensions of the AIDS Epidemic: Implications for Prevention and Care," *Infectious Disease Clinics of North America* 14, 4 (2000), p. 796.

181. Peter Gould, *The Slow Plague: A Geography of the AIDS Pandemic* (Cambridge, MA, 1993), ch. 13; S. A. Månsson, "Psycho-Social Aspects of HIV Testing: The Swedish Case," *AIDS Care* 2, 1 (1990), pp. 8–10; Benny Henriksson, "Swedish AIDS Policy from a Human Rights Perspective," in Martin Breum and Aart Hendriks, eds., *AIDS and Human Rights* (Copenhagen, 1988), p. 126; Olivier Guillod et al., *Drei Gutachten über rechtliche Fragen im Zusammenhang mit AIDS* (Bern, 1991), pp. 156–57.

182. Sandra Panem, *The AIDS Bureaucracy* (Cambridge, MA, 1988), pp. 16–17; Ira Cohen and Ann Elder, "Major Cities and Disease Crises: A Comparative Perspective," *Social Science History* 13, 1 (1989), pp. 45–46.

183. *RD Prot*, 1986/87:110 (24 April 1987), pp. 41–42.

184. Peter Piot et al., "The Global Impact of HIV/AIDS," *Nature* 410 (2001),

pp. 971–72; Dayton and Merson, "Global Dimensions of the AIDS Epidemic: Implications for Prevention and Care," pp. 791–99.

185. De Savigny, *Le Sida et les fragilités françaises,* p. 315.

186. Ronald O. Valdiserri, ed., *Dawning Answers: How the HIV/AIDS Epidemic Has Helped to Strengthen Public Health* (Oxford, 2003).

187. John A. Harrington, "The Instrumental Uses of Autonomy: A Review of AIDS Law and Policy in Europe," *Social Science and Medicine* 55, 8 (2002), pp. 1425–34.

188. *New York Times,* 28 April 2003; 7 May 2003; *International Herald Tribune,* 3–4 May 2003, p. 6; 7 May 2003; *Economist,* 3 May 2003, p. 65.

189. Raffaele d'Amelio et al., "A Global Review of Legislation on HIV/AIDS: The Issue of HIV Testing," *Journal of Acquired Immune Deficiency Syndromes* 28, 2 (2001), pp. 174–76.

190. *East African Standard,* 6 August 2003, p. 13.

191. *Financial Times,* 3 August 2003, p. 24.

192. Catherine Campbell, *"Letting Them Die": Why HIV/AIDS Intervention Programmes Fail* (Oxford, 2003), pp. 25–28.

193. David Patterson and Leslie London, "International Law, Human Rights, and HIV/AIDS," *Bulletin of the World Health Organization* 80, 12 (2002), pp. 965–66.

194. Tony Barnett and Alan Whiteside, *AIDS in the Twenty-First Century: Disease and Globalization* (Houndmills, 2002), pp. 73–74.

195. Michael Hardt and Antonio Negri, *Empire* (Cambridge, MA, 2000), p. 136.

196. Abram de Swaan, *In Care of the State: Health Care, Education, and Welfare in Europe and the USA in the Modern Era* (New York, 1988).

197. Peter Baldwin, *The Politics of Social Solidarity: Class Bases of the European Welfare State, 1875–1975* (Cambridge, 1990), p. 299.

Index

Child abuse, 77
Chile, 79
China, 8, 35, 37, 78, 202, 232, 247, 284, 287, 289
Chinatown, San Francisco, 234
Chirac, Jacques, administration of, 144
Cholera, 2, 3, 4, 18, 19, 24, 26, 28, 41, 46, 48, 87, 129, 193, 202, 212, 228, 233, 234, 235, 240, 244, 253, 281, 281, 284, 289
Christian, Marc, 97
Christian Democratic Union, Germany, 56, 68, 136, 210, 248
Christian Social Union, Bavaria, 57, 248, 253
Christians, fundamentalist, 175
Chronic disease, 16, 18, 26, 87, 128, 160, 286
Churchill, Winston, 7
CIA, 202
Circumcision, 141, 205
Civil law, 97
Civil rights, 32, 156ff, 208, 230, 231, 246, 252, 255, 262, 288, 289
Civil Rights Act (U.S., 1964), 102, 105
Civil rights movement, 188
Civil Rights Restoration Act (U.S., 1987), 105
Civil servants, 37, 39, 57, 64, 106–08, 217, 223, 273
Clark, Hilton B., 145
Clausewitz, Carl von, 19
Clermont-Tonnerre, Count Stanislas de, 184
Climate change, 17, 18
Clinical ecology, 18
Clinton, Bill, administration of, 135, 175, 223
COBRA, 120, 221
Cold war, 8
Collard, Cyril, 127
Colonies, 282f
Colorado, 51, 69, 255
Comité d'urgence antirépression homosexuelle, 184, 185
Communicable Disease Surveillance Centre, UK, 68, 166

Communism, 156, 252
Communists, in Sweden, 63, 151, 153, 256, 280
Condom code, 129–30, 267
Condoms, 16, 17, 23, 33, 34, 54, 58, 59, 71, 93, 194, 200, 249, 254, 260, 267, 270, 288; change in attitude to, 139–40; as evidence of prostitution, 128, 141; increasing use of, 137; instead of discouraging anal sex, 133, 269; in prisons, 114; promotion of, 135
Conference of State and Territorial Epidemiologists, U.S., 215
Confidentiality, 37, 43, 52, 61, 65, 69, 72–77, 113–14, 127, 207, 215, 225, 251, 280
Congress, U.S., 106, 155, 240
Conservative Family Campaign, UK, 33
Conservatives, and AIDS, 51, 73, 136, 190, 198, 202, 204, 226, 247, 248, 255, 273
Constitution, U.S., 161, 214, 217, 231
Consular officials, 234
Consumption, 9
Contact tracing, 32, 37, 45, 48, 51, 52, 54, 69–71, 200
Contagion and the State in Europe, 1830–1930, 3
Contagious disease laws, 41–42; in Denmark, 53; in East Germany (1982), 254; in Germany (1900), 44, 45, 163, 241, 253, 254; in Germany (1961), 42, 45, 51, 55–56, 115, 163, 224, 241, 253; in Sweden (1968), 45, 53, 55, 60, 61, 91, 154, 164, 251; in UK, 47, 229
Contraception, 33, 139, 140, 161, 186, 260
Contributory negligence, 93, 256, 264
Copenhagen, 203, 283, 285
Corpses, 59
Costa Rica, 79, 100
Council of Europe, 114, 157
Courts: and AIDS regulations, 217f; and antidiscrimination, 101; and HIV transmission, 90–91

Compositor:	Binghamton Valley Composition
Text:	10/13 Aldus
Display:	Aldus
Printer and binder:	Thomson-Shore, Inc.